MW00606882

Practical Viewing of the Optic Disc

Practical Viewing of the Optic Disc

KATHLEEN B. DIGRE, M.D.
Professor of Neurology and Ophthalmology, University of Utah School of Medicine, Salt Lake City; Neuro-Ophthalmologist, Moran Eye Center, University of Utah Health Sciences Center, Salt Lake City

JAMES J. CORBETT, M.D.
McCarty Professor, Chairman of Neurology, Professor of Ophthalmology, University of Mississippi School of Medicine, University of Mississippi Medical Center, Jackson

Artist: Michael Schenk
University of Mississippi, Jackson

Computer Graphic Artist: Jean Henderson
University of Mississippi, Jackson

Photographers: Doug Blanchard, Elizabeth Snodgrass, and Paula Morris
Moran Eye Center, University of Utah Health Sciences Center, Salt Lake City

CD Design: Nancy Lombardo, MLS
and the University of Utah Eccles Health Sciences Library, Salt Lake City, with HTML support from Yusup Alimov, Derek Cowan, Jeremy Smith, and Valeri Craigle, University of Utah, Salt Lake City

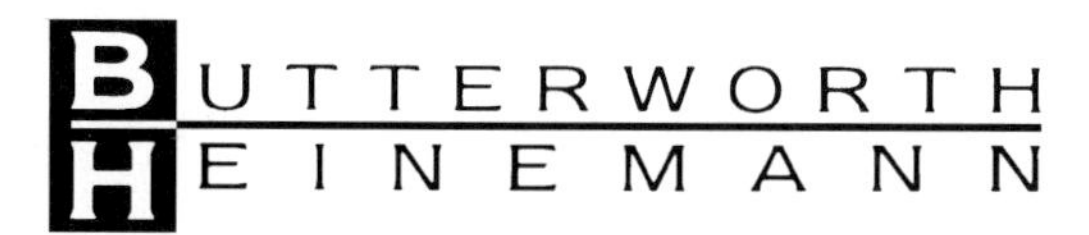

An Imprint of Elsevier Science
Amsterdam Boston London Oxford New York Paris
San Diego San Francisco Singapore Sydney Tokyo

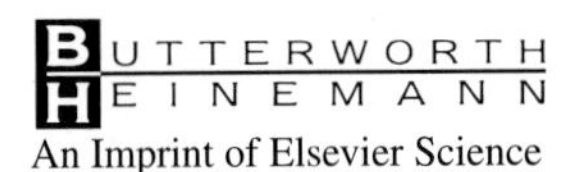

An Imprint of Elsevier Science

200 Wheeler Road
Burlington, MA 01803

Practical Viewing of the Optic Disc
ISBN 0-7506-7289-7

Notice

Neurology and ophthalmology are ever-changing fields. Standard safety precautions must be followed, but as new research and clinical experience broaden our knowledge, changes in treatment and drug therapy may become necessary or appropriate. Readers are advised to check the most current product information provided by the manufacturer of each drug to be administered to verify the recommended dose, the method and duration of administration, and contraindications. It is the responsibility of the treating physician, relying on experience and knowledge of the patient, to determine dosages and the best treatment for each individual patient. Neither the Publisher nor the author assume any liability for any injury and/or damage to persons or property arising from this publication.

The Publisher

Library of Congress Cataloging-in-Publication Data

Digre, Kathleen B.
Practical viewing of the optic disc / Kathleen B. Digre, James J. Corbett ; artist, Michael Schenk ; computer graphic artist, Jean Henderson ; photographers, Doug Blanchard ... [et al.].
p. ; cm.
Includes bibliographical references and index.
ISBN 0-7506-7289-7
1. Optic disc—Examination. 2. Ophthalmoscopes. 3. Optic disc—Abnormalities—Diagnosis. I. Corbett, James J. (James John), 1940- II. Title.
[DNLM: 1. Optic Disk—physiopathology. 2. Optic Nerve Diseases—diagnosis. 3. Physical Examination. WW 280 D575v 2002]
RE728.O67 D544 2003
617.7'1545—dc21

2002023238

SSC/MVY

Printed in the United States of America

9 8 7 6 5 4 3 2 1

This book is dedicated to our parents,
Clifford and Bernice Digre and Maxwell and Rose Corbett
Who made us practical.
Our children,
Johanna, Gita, and Jennifer, Jillian, John
Who taught us what essentials were.
Our spouses,
Michael Varner and Joyce Corbett
Who keep us viewing the big picture.

Contents

Preface

Viewing the optic disc provides the physician a close-up look into the health of an individual. The technique and its instrument, the ophthalmoscope, were developed 150 years ago, and, yet, the facility most physicians have with the instrument is marginal. Although all physicians are at least acquainted with the ophthalmoscope in medical school, many leave the use of the instrument to ophthalmologists or optometrists due to lack of training in viewing. Even many neurologists, who have great facility with examination of the cranial nerves, sometimes refrain from the close examination of the second cranial nerve—the only site in the body where the brain can be observed "head-on."

We wrote this book to help all of us physicians learn to better use this valuable tool for the diagnosis of neurologic and systemic conditions. When we started this book, it was our hope that it would spur physicians to once again pick up the ophthalmoscope and view the disc with more confidence. We hope that it allows the ophthalmoscopist to view the fundus of the eye with a purpose and with an expectation of what one may see.

We also hope that this book will help teachers better instruct students about the fundus and the disc.

Some of the videos on the CD are mini-tutorials designed to help the practitioner master the techniques of the examination. Other videos give live demonstrations of the dynamic fundus.

We see the book as a guide for the viewer in understanding what the possible abnormalities are once a certain disc or retinal variation is identified. The CD and the book are to be viewed and studied together. The CD is designed to visually assist the individual to recognize abnormalities that may be encountered. The book complements the CD with further information about some of the conditions and when further evaluation is required. Finally, the information contained in the CD and the book is meant to excite all who use it into being better observers of a structure that lies in our viewing path—the back of the human eye.

K. B. D.
J. J. C.

Acknowledgments

We wish to thank the following people who have been generous with their time and commitment to our project:

Dr. David Luehr, M.D., family physician, Cloquet, Minnesota, who helped review the scope of information presented.

Nancy Lombardo, librarian at The Spencer Eccles Health Sciences Library, University of Utah, who oversaw the CD development. Yusup Alimov, Derek Cowan, Jeremy Smith, Valeri Craigle, and Wayne Peay, who helped with portions of the CD development

Elizabeth Wako and Colleen Parker, medical students at the University of Utah who helped with the video production and initial CD development.

Our reviewers, Dr. William T. Shults and Dr. Shirley Wray, and sub-reviewers, Dr. F. Jane Durcan and Dr. Michael Brodsky.

Our colleague and mentor, Dr. William F. Hoyt, who supplied many of the lovely photographs of the nerve fiber layer.

Jon Lingren, PA-C, who modeled for many of the photographs. Elaine Thompson, Alexander Ingold, Johanna Varner, Anne Chisolm, and Bernice and Clifford Digre, who modeled for some photographs and videos.

Our colleagues who provided photographs, including Dr. Paul Zimmerman, Dr. F. Jane Durcan, Dr. Marie Acierno, Dr. William T. Shults, Dr. C. J. Chen, Dr. Michael Brodsky, Dr. Judith Warner, Dr. William Fletcher, Paula Morris, Dr. Daniel Jacobson,

Dr. Takahashi, Dr. George Cioffi, Dr. Michael van Buskirk, Dr. Madison Slusher, Dr. Sohan Hayreh, Lee Allen, Dr. Nick Mammalis, Dr. Robert Hoffman, Dr. Norman Schatz, Dr. Martin Lubow, Dr. Christopher Blodi, Dr. Roger Harrie, Dr. Bradley Katz, Dr. Shelly Cross, Dr. Robert Saul, Dr. Lanning Kline, Dr. Donnel Creel, and Dr. Hussein Wafapoor.

We also wish to thank the National Library of Medicine and the Mayo Historical Unit Foundation, Rochester, Minnesota, for the contribution of historical material, and the Welch-Allyn Company for supplying photographs and historical information.

Our publisher, Susan Pioli, for her advice and enthusiasm; editor Lucinda Ewing and CD editor Robert Browne for all their hard work.

And finally, we owe a special thanks to Dr. H. Stanley Thompson, our mentor, colleague, and friend.

1 Getting Ready—Preparing to View the Optic Disc

I could not too strongly recommend you to seek in the application of Helmholtz's mirror the invaluable assistance which it is capable of yielding in such circumstances. Cases abound in this hospital, and, in a very short time, you will be able, with a little practice, to put yourselves abreast of the fundamental facts.

Jean-Martin Charcot[1]

For the efficient use of the ophthalmoscope in medical practice, the student must be familiar, first, with the use of the instrument . . .

William Gowers[2]

The ability to view the back of the eye—the fundus and disc—is a relatively recent discovery in medicine. We have known that we could view the disc for only approximately 150 years. We have had the tool of ophthalmoscopy—the direct ophthalmoscope—in a useable, portable, and ubiquitous form for less than 100 years. How this instrument came to be is a great story.

History of Ophthalmoscopy

Humans have observed for years that the eyes of certain animals reflect light. For example, a wolf's eye appears to glow. It took a while to realize that the light was not emanating from the animal, but was a light reflection from the choroidal tapetum lucidum (a membrane between the choroid and retina in certain animals that reflects any light). Animals that have this reflex include the cat, dog, sheep, rabbit, goat, and wolf.[3]

Observing the optic nerve of a cat after submerging the cat's head in water, Jean Méry of France in 1703 viewed the optic disc not only through a dilated pupil, but improved optics of seeing by using the refractive power of water.[4] Bénédict Prevost in France in 1810 concluded after performing multiple experiments on his house cats in the dark and in the light under multiple conditions—fright, sleeping, and excitement—that the eyes do not shine, but instead reflect light.

Then Johannes E. Purkinje, a Czech, while in Breslau, Germany in 1823, examined the insides of a human and a dog eye using a candle as a light source and a concave spherical lens.[5,6] Although Purkinje tried to popularize the technique, few heeded his findings. He wrote the following, later quoted by Rucker:

Thus, from now on practically no membrane or liquid content of the eye will escape the properly reflected eye, and if practitioners, spurning the painstaking inquiry of physiologists, will not disdain or fear this method, they will find it useful in ocular diagnosis.[5]

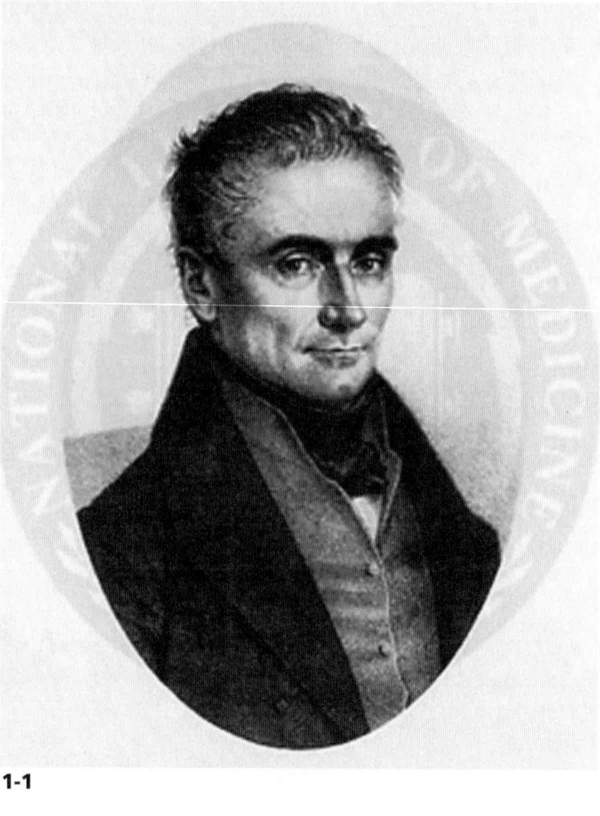

1-1

Figure 1-1. Johannes Evangelista Purkinje (1787–1869) was a professor of physiology and pathology in Breslau, Germany, and later in Prague. Although he is chiefly known for the cells in the cerebellum that bear his name (Purkinje cells), his doctoral dissertation was on the subjective aspects of vision, including entoptic phenomena.[6,7] (Photograph courtesy of the National Library of Medicine.)

Further observations were made by William Cumming in London, who reported in 1846 that he viewed the red reflex in normal and albino human beings.[5] The stage was set to view the retina by early work such as that of von Brücke (1847), who independently viewed the retina of a patient while looking through a tube by light of a candle.[8] Helmholtz later credited von Brücke's observations as leading him to his discovery.

At approximately the same time, Charles Babbage (1847), an English mathematician and "engineer" who invented the precursor to modern computers, reported to a friend that he was able to view the optic fundus with an instrument. Dr. Babbage's instrument used a parabolic mirror as a reflecting light source, with a hole in the center. Through this hole, he was able to view the disc. Babbage never formally reported his results, however, and, as did Purkinje, lost his place as "discoverer" of the ophthalmoscope to Helmholtz.[5]

Credit therefore goes to Helmholtz for developing the first apparatus for viewing the human fundus, as reported on December 17, 1850. While a 29-year-old professor at Königsberg University, he developed an "Augenspiegel," or "eye mirror." This ophthalmoscope was composed of a light source, a concave lens, and three glass plates. The glass plates reflected light to illuminate the inside of the patient's eye, thereby permitting the examiner to view the retina and optic disc through a concave lens held at the correct focal distance. This was the first direct ophthalmoscope.

Helmholtz wrote the following to his father:

It was so obvious, requiring, moreover no knowledge beyond the optics I learned at the Gymnasium, that it seems almost ludicrous that I and others should have been so slow as not to see it. It is, namely, combination of glasses, by means of which it is possible to illuminate the dark background of the eye, through the pupil, without employing any dazzling light, and to obtain a view of all the elements of the retina at

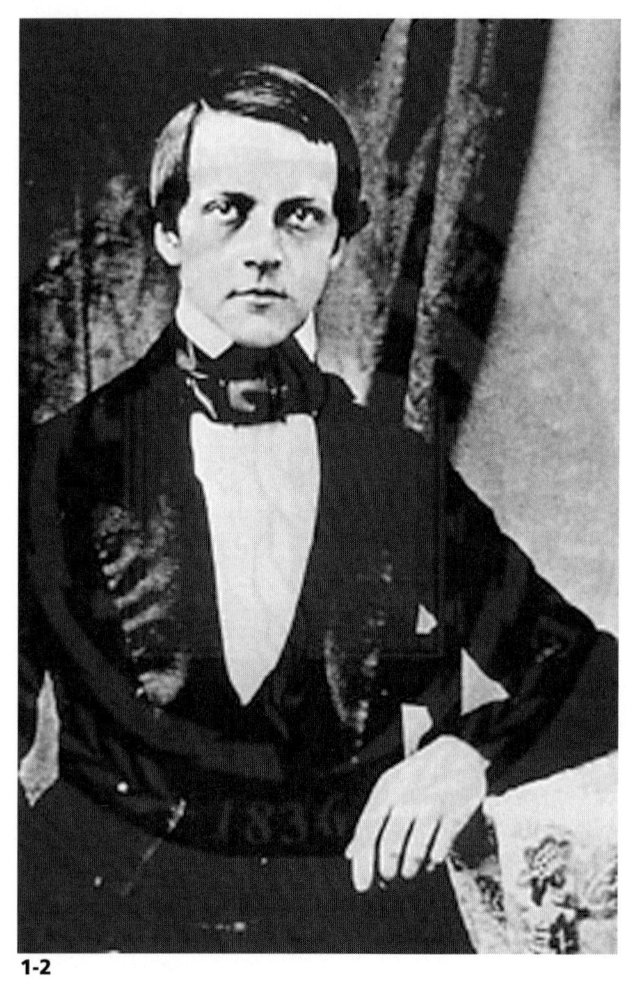

1-2

once, more exactly than one can see the external parts of the eye without magnification . . . The blood-vessels are displayed in the neatest way, with the branching arteries and veins, the entrance of the optic nerve into the eye . . . My discovery makes the minute investigation of the internal structures of the eye a possibility.[5]

To secure his right as "inventor," Helmholtz presented the ophthalmoscope to the Physical Society of Berlin in 1850 and published his monograph in 1851.

Figure 1-2. Hermann Ludwig Ferdinand von Helmholtz was born in 1821 in Germany (Potsdam). His father was a professor of philosophy. Although Helmholtz graduated from medical school in Berlin in 1843, he devoted most of his time and attention to the study of physiology at the University of Königsberg. While still quite young, he reported the invention of the ophthalmoscope on December 6, 1850. He was a great scientist as well and published a definitive text on optics, titled *Handbook of Physiological Optics*. He also is known for the description of the physical law of conservation of energy. He died in 1894.[9] (Photograph courtesy of the National Library of Medicine.)

In the monograph, Helmholtz not only described the optics and the instrument itself, but also what he believed to be the importance of his findings[10]:

After one learns to recognize the characteristics of the retina in the normal eye, I have no doubt that it will be possible to diagnose all the pathologic conditions of the retina by visual observation . . . Engorgement of the vessels or varicosities of the vessels can easily be perceived. Exudates in the substance of the retina, or between the retina and pigment layer, can be recognized by their light appearance against the dark background . . . In short, I believe I do not exaggerate when I anticipate that all those changes in the vitreous body and the retina previously noted in cadavers will be recognized in the living eye. This fact appears to offer the greatest impetus to development of the pathologic study of these structures. . . .

Figure 1-3. A. **The title page from Helmholtz's 1851 monograph.** B. **His labeled Figure 1 (*bottom right corner*) shows the position of the examiner (G), examinee (D), and external light; in his case, the flame (A). The light reflects off of the glass plate reflector (C) slightly turned toward (H) (C and F are the makings of the ophthalmoscope) the examinee's eye (D) when the observer peers through the lens (F). Helmholtz also had a description of the optics. In Figure 2, he depicts the ophthalmoscope and a horizontal cross-section through the mirrors (glass plate reflectors) (h to h) that are fastened by a brass plate (g to g) onto the circular plate (a). There are openings (f) through which screws could pass to hold various removable and interchangeable concave lenses (n to n), shown in Figure 3. The apparatus is then fastened to the handle (m). (Photographs courtesy of the National Library of Medicine.)**

BESCHREIBUNG

EINES

AUGEN-SPIEGELS

ZUR UNTERSUCHUNG

DER NETZHAUT IM LEBENDEN AUGE

VON

H. HELMHOLTZ,

PROFESSOR DER PHYSIOLOGIE AN DER UNIVERSITAET ZU KOENIGSBERG.

BERLIN,

A. FÖRSTNER'SCHE VERLAGSBUCHHANDLUNG.

1851.

1-3A

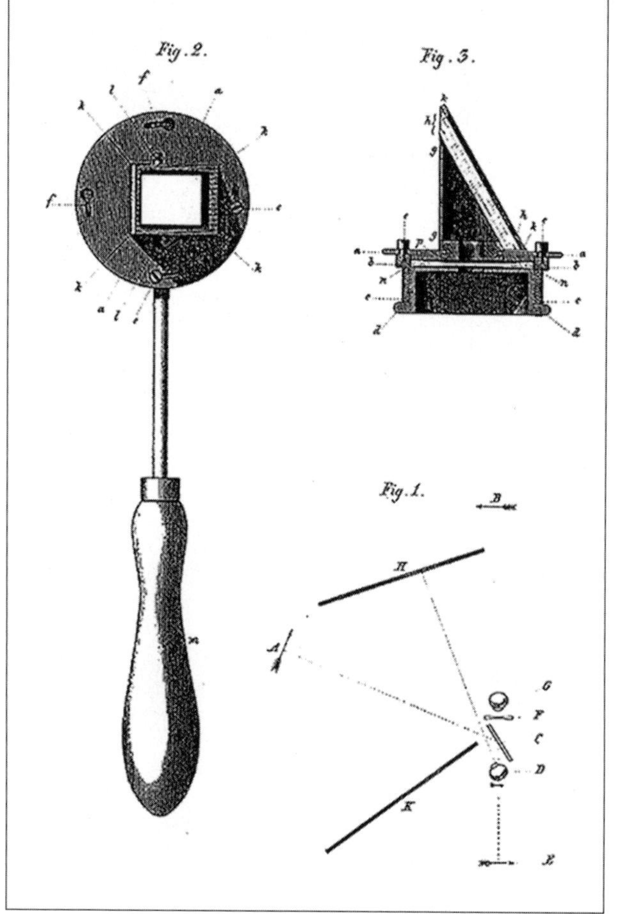

1-3B

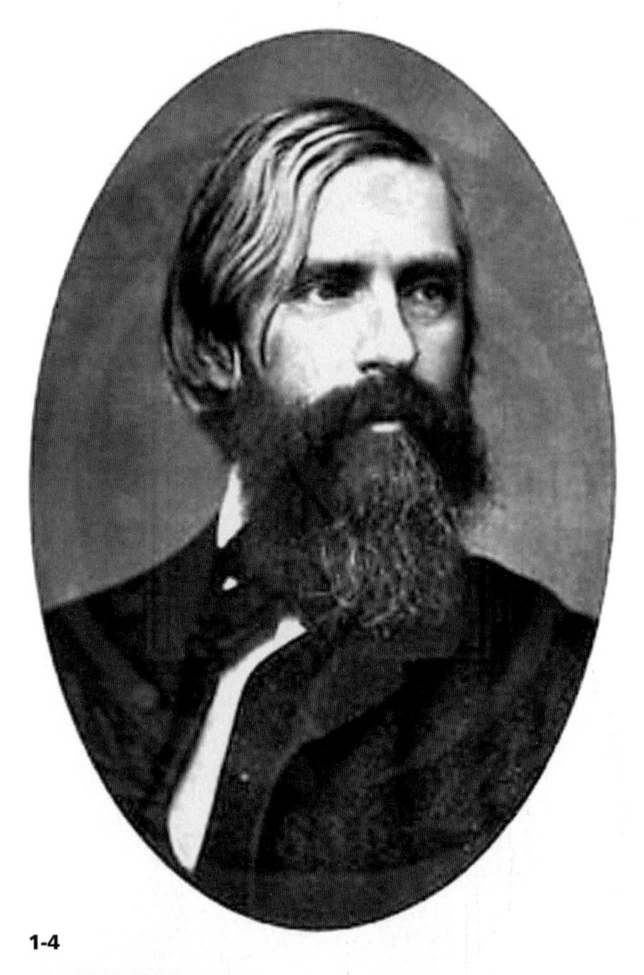
1-4

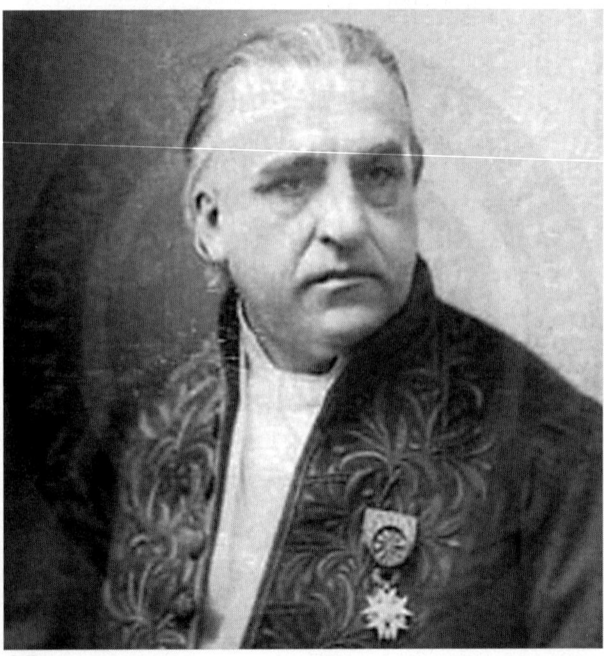
1-5

Although Helmholtz never patented his ophthalmoscope, it soon gained popularity. The term *Augenspiegel* was translated into English as *eye speculum* and became *ophthalmoscope* in France by 1852, in England in 1853, and the United States in 1854.[5]

Refinements in the ophthalmoscope gradually took place. Ruete developed the indirect method of ophthalmoscopy in 1851. In 1885, Dennett introduced a "self-illuminated electric direct ophthalmoscope." ReKoss (1852), Coccius (1853), Loring (1879), and Landolt (1876) all brought modifications of the lighting (including the introduction of oil-burning lamps) to the ophthalmoscope. However, these early pioneers did not fully appreciate the impact and importance of this invention.

Albrecht von Graefe (1828–1870) from Berlin, Germany (often called the "Founder of Ophthalmology") was reportedly one of the first to use the ophthalmoscope invented by Helmholtz for clinical purposes. von Graefe remarked: "Helmholtz has unfolded to us a whole new world."[9] von Graefe used the invention to describe the cupped disc of glaucoma in 1855 and central retinal artery occlusion and "choked disc" in 1861.

Figure 1-4. Albrecht von Graefe (1828–1870) was the son of Karl Ferdinand von Graefe of Berlin. Although he began studying mathematics, he became interested in the natural sciences and medicine. After studying in many universities in Europe (Berlin, Vienna, Prague, Paris, London, Dublin, and Edinburgh), he practiced ophthalmology in Berlin and founded a private institution devoted to treating eyes. He then became the professor of ophthalmology at Berlin's university. He is known for his treatment of glaucoma and describing a surgery for cataracts. He was also the leading authority at that time in diseases of the nerves and brain.[11] (Photograph courtesy of the National Library of Medicine.)

Figure 1-5. The French neurologist Jean-Martin Charcot (1825–1893) organized the clinical service at the Salpêtrière. He reorganized not only clinical neurology and pathology there, but also introduced ophthalmoscopy and established an ophthalmology department (1862–1868). He reported in his lectures on the nervous system: "[It is important] for us, physicians to familiarize

ourselves as much as possible with the regular examination of the fundus of the eye" (1877–1889).[12] (Photograph courtesy of the National Library of Medicine.)

An important neurologist, John Hughlings Jackson was a lifelong enthusiast of ophthalmoscopy. He stated:

The physician is much indebted to Helmholtz as the ophthalmic surgeon is. You cannot investigate cases of cerebral disease methodically unless you use the ophthalmoscope.[13]

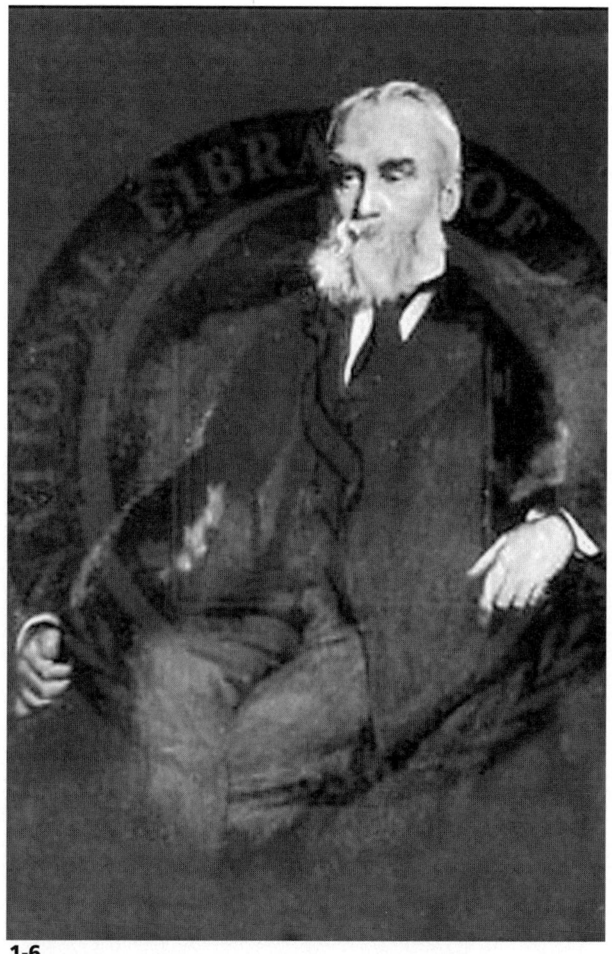

1-6

Figure 1-6. John Hughlings Jackson (1835–1940) is often called the "Father of English Neurology." He practiced at the London Hospital and later the National Hospital for Nervous Diseases. He published extensively on many aspects of neurology. (Photograph courtesy of the National Library of Medicine.)

However, in 1879, Jackson's contemporary, the British neurologist William Gowers, led physicians to realize the importance of systematically viewing the optic disc and retina to diagnose medical and neurologic conditions in his monograph, *A Manual and Atlas of Medical Ophthalmoscopy.* The opening sentence of his book reflects his sentiments:

The ophthalmoscope is of use to the physician because it gives information, often not otherwise obtainable, regarding the existence or nature of disease elsewhere than in the eye.[2]

Figure 1-7. A. **Sir William R. Gowers (1845–1915) was a great clinical neurologist. Born to a poor family in London, he attended Christ Church College School in Oxford and thereafter was apprenticed to a country practitioner. After studying medicine at University Hospital College in London, he became a medical registrar at the National Hospital for the Paralyzed and Epileptic, Queen Square (the hospital to later become famous for neurology and neurologists). Gowers' first book, *A Manual and Atlas of Medical Ophthalmoscopy*, was published in 1879. Thereafter, he published many books and papers, encouraged the participation of women in medicine, and was elected to many honorary societies, including the American Neurologic Association.[14] (Photograph courtesy of the National Library of Medicine.)** B. **Pictured here is the title page from Gowers' book, *A Manual and Atlas of Medical Ophthalmoscopy*, published in 1879.** ***Continued***

1-7A

A

MANUAL AND ATLAS

OF

MEDICAL OPHTHALMOSCOPY

BY

W. R. GOWERS, M.D., F.R.C.P.

ASSISTANT-PROFESSOR OF CLINICAL MEDICINE IN UNIVERSITY COLLEGE,
ASSISTANT-PHYSICIAN TO UNIVERSITY COLLEGE HOSPITAL, AND TO THE NATIONAL HOSPITAL FOR THE PARALYSED AND EPILEPTIC

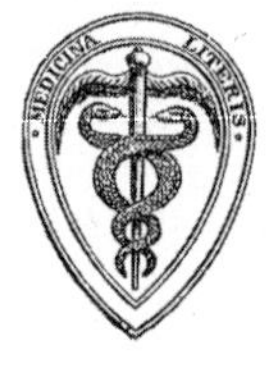

LONDON
J. & A. CHURCHILL, NEW BURLINGTON STREET

1879

1-7B

Figure 1-7. ***Continued.*** **C. This page represents just one of Gowers' many personal drawings used to illustrate the book. He encouraged physicians to draw what they saw. He drew these six discs to demonstrate in each section some important observation. Figure 1 of the plate shows simple congestion of the disc viewed through an indirect lens (the image is upside-down and minimized), and Figure 2 is the same disc viewed with the direct lens through the ophthalmoscope somewhat enlarged. Figure 3 is from a patient with syphilitic neuritis as viewed with the indirect lens (again, image is upside-down and reversed), contrasted with Figure 4, viewing the disc with the direct lens. Figures 5 and 6 are from a patient with a presumed brain tumor, again demonstrating an indirect view and direct view, respectively.**

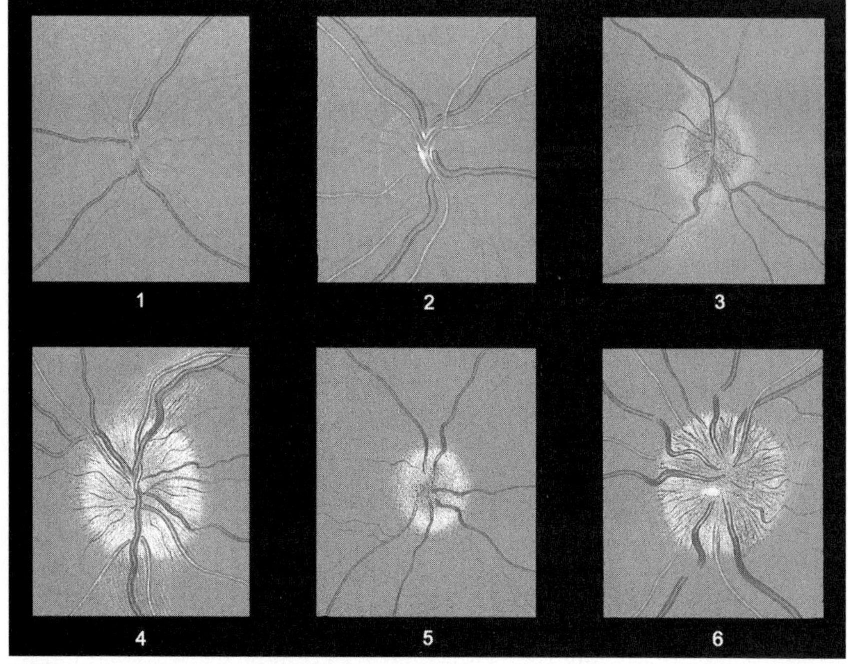

1-7C

Early on, all of the ophthalmoscopes were "reflecting," just like Helmholtz's original. *Reflecting* means that they used an external light source such as a candle, sunlight, or a lamp. After Helmholtz's initial report, inventors made continuous improvements on the ophthalmoscope over the next 50–60 years.

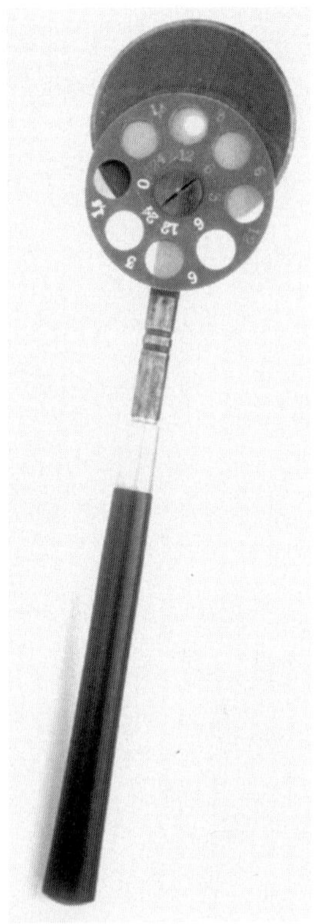

1-8A

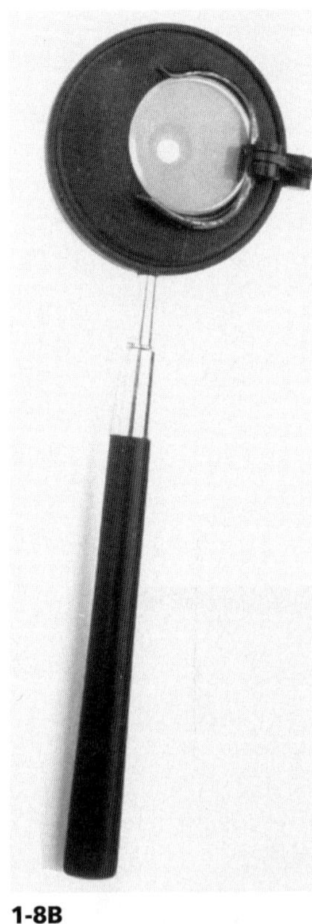

1-8B

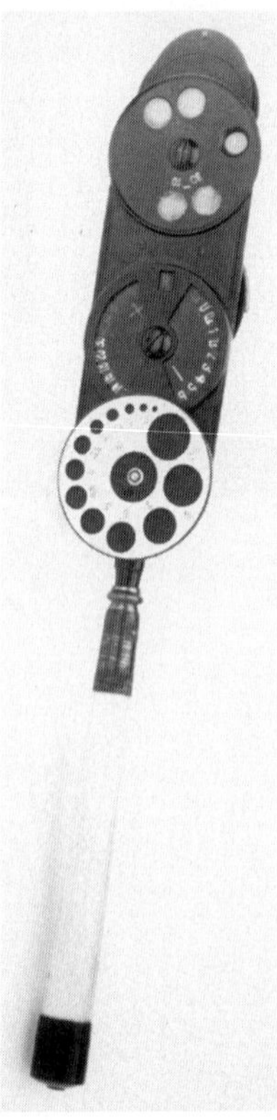

1-9

Figure 1-8. A,B. **An early reflecting ophthalmoscope. The front is shown in** (A) **and the back in** (B)**. This ophthalmoscope is shown with a disc of different lenses, so that changing concave lenses would not be necessary. This disc, known as the *Rekoss disk*, had many variations over the next decades.[5] (Photograph courtesy of Mayo Historical Unit, Mayo Foundation, Rochester, Minnesota.)**

Figure 1-9. Andrew Morton (1883) used a long chain of 29 lenses, which could be rotated by a wheel. The top rotating wheel has four supplemental lenses. The middle disc indicates which lens is in use. The bottom wheel is a pupil gauge for estimating pupillary size.[5] (Printed with permission of Mayo Historical Unit, Mayo Foundation, Rochester, Minnesota.)

By 1913, Rucker reported that there were more than 200 types of reflecting ophthalmoscopes.[5] The direct ophthalmoscope as we know it was not developed until early in the 1900s.

Two inventions that made our modern direct ophthalmoscopes possible were the invention of the electric light in 1878 and the invention of dry-cell batteries in 1910. Although late in the 1800s miniature electrical lamps were used for viewing the inside of the mouth, early lamps gave off considerable heat and were therefore not practical for ophthalmoscopy. An electrician named Preston engineered a small lamp, which illuminated well without much heat.[15] The first U.S.-made ophthalmoscope was credited to Dr. Dennett in 1885, but the cumbersome nature of his invention limited its success.[5] Other early examples were developed by Thomas Reid (Glasgow, 1886), Henry Juler (London, 1886), Wilbur Marple (New York, 1906), David Harrower (Worcester, 1913), and G. S. Crampton (Philadelphia). Finally, Henry DeZeng manufactured the first direct ophthalmoscope with batteries in the handle, and it was he who received the patent in 1908. Two other individuals also deserve mention: Charles May of New York had an ophthalmoscope manufactured by many optical companies, and the May ophthalmoscope was used for years.

The other person, William Noah Allyn, worked for DeZeng, and also knew Dr. Francis Welch, who worked at an electric surgical instrument company. Welch and Allyn formed their own company in 1915. There have been many improvements since that time, designed by Jonas Friedenwald of the Welch Allyn Company and Charles H. Keeler of Keeler Manufacturing in England. For a complete catalog representation of ophthalmoscopes from many countries see the works of Schett[16] and Keeler.[17]

Rucker wrote the following in his history of the ophthalmoscope[5]:

Today's student wants to know what instrument will serve him best . . . and need to know, more than his teachers did . . . and he understands disease processes more clearly than did ophthalmologists of only a generation ago. . . He may regard small dry-cell batteries for his ophthalmoscope as indispensable, without realizing that they were first marketed within my own lifetime, and that for more than 60 years previously, ophthalmoscopists had used light reflected from a nearby lamp.

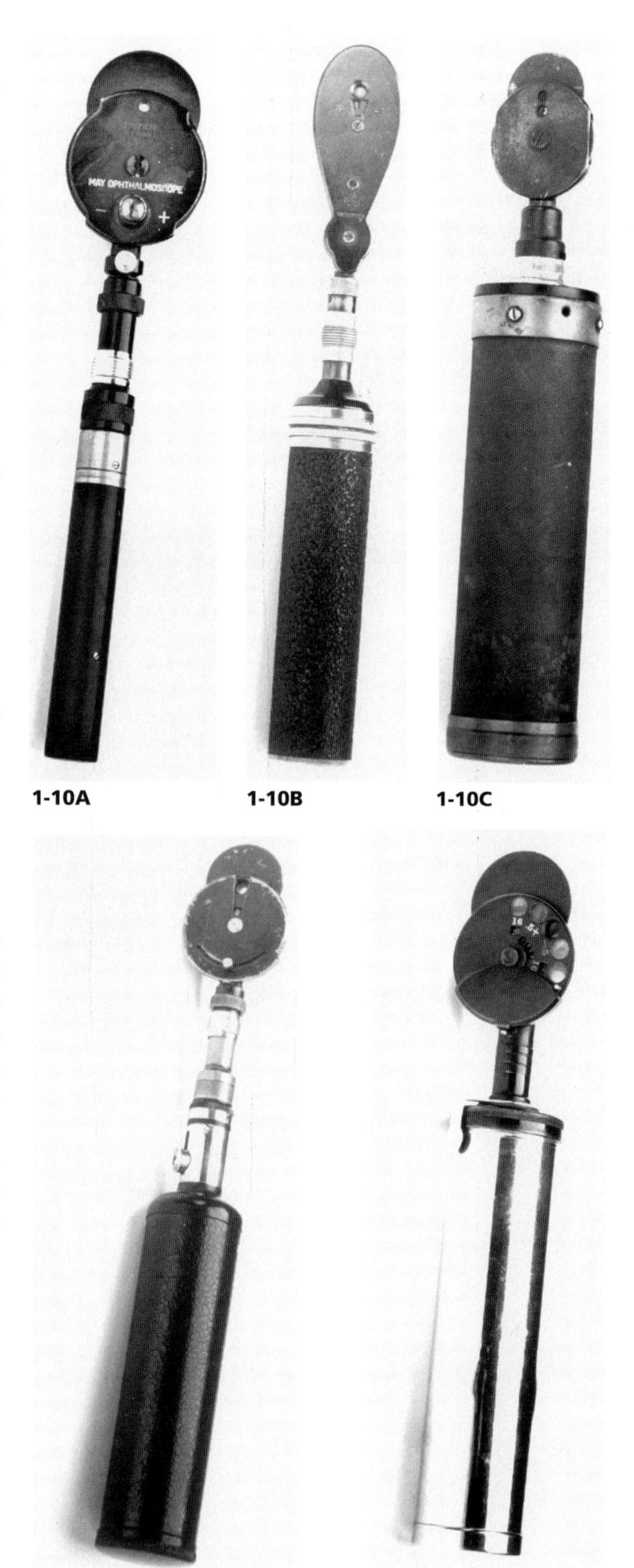

1-10D 1-10E

Figure 1-10. A. **This electric ophthalmoscope, designed by Charles May, used an electric cord (not batteries) and dates from approximately 1930. It was manufactured by the Bausch & Lomb Optical Company. (Photograph courtesy of Mayo Historical Unit, Mayo Foundation, Rochester, Minnesota.)** B. **This battery-powered ophthalmoscope with an unusual shape is called the *Hare* and dates from approximately 1910.[16] (Photograph courtesy of Mayo Historical Unit, Mayo Foundation, Rochester, Minnesota.)** C–E. **These battery-operated ophthalmoscopes date from the 1930s to 1940s.**

The Direct Ophthalmoscope

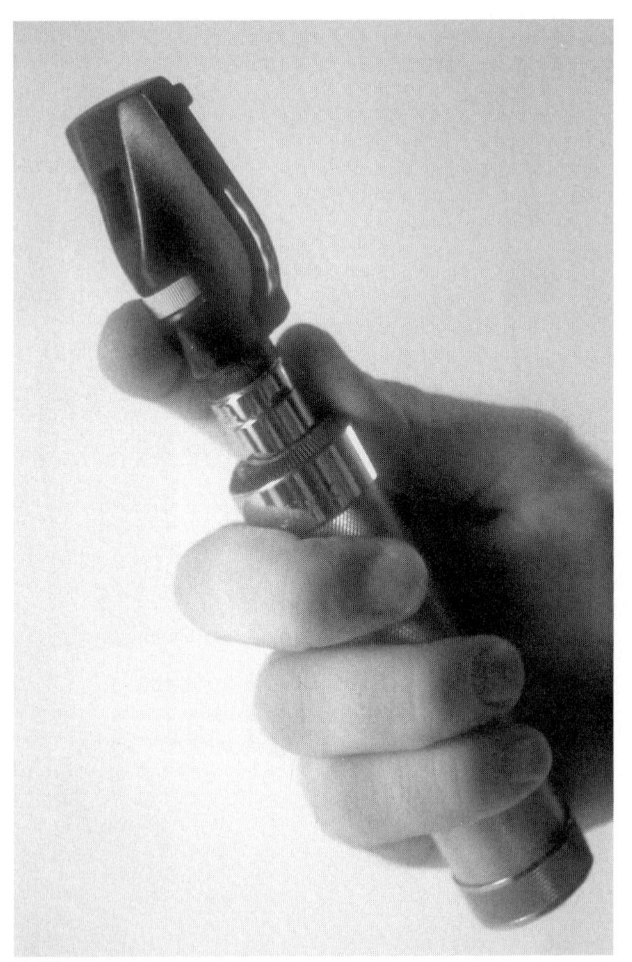

1-11

Figure 1-11. The direct ophthalmoscope.

Do you own your own ophthalmoscope? You should, so that you can practice with your own ophthalmoscope. Becoming knowledgeable about the functions and capabilities of the ophthalmoscope is the first step to successful viewing. The direct ophthalmoscope is basically a light source and a viewing system.

There are many features of the direct ophthalmoscopes of today that we take for granted. First, the light source is constant because of strong batteries, either nickel-cadmium or lithium, which are often rechargeable. The optical systems have improved immensely. The light source is bright, frequently a halogen bulb, with long life and is the brightest portable light available. A rheostat control on the "on" button sets the light intensity and is helpful for extremely photophobic individuals. For the best view of the fundus, however, one should use the brightest possible light source tolerated.

Check the viewing mechanism: Is it clean and clear? Looking to see the optic fundus is difficult enough without dust on the viewing mechanism.

Figure 1-12. A. **Identify the "on" button—notice how you can adjust the amount of light (*black arrow*). Find the aperture-selection dial (*white arrow*) and viewing mechanism (*arrowhead*).** B. **Look at the viewing mechanism. You can see how the principles of viewing through a mirror are not that different from those of Helmholtz's original ophthalmoscope. (Photograph courtesy of the Welch Allyn Company, with permission.)**

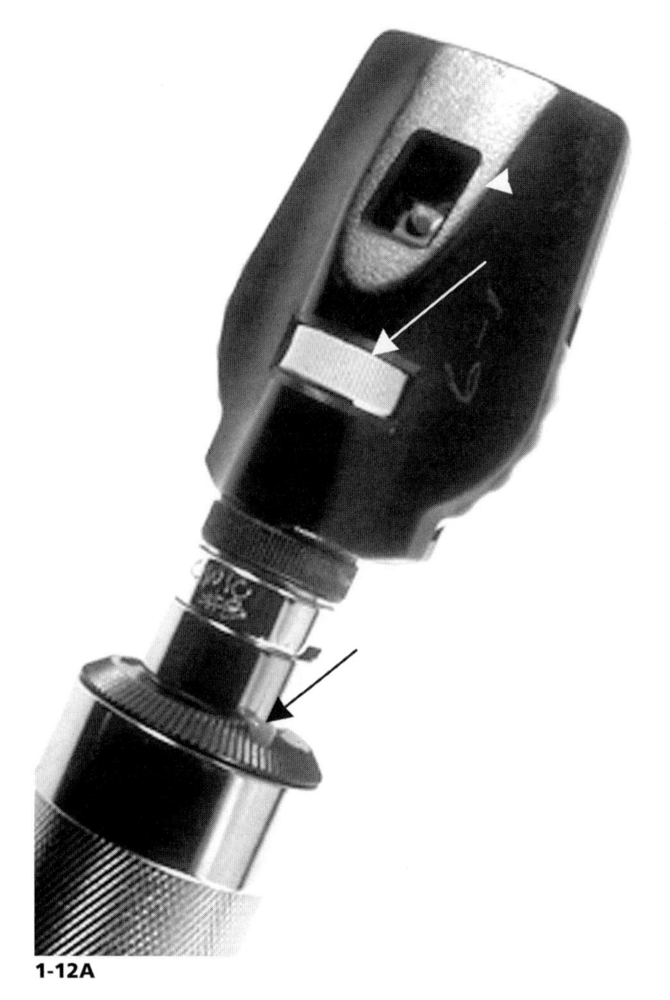

1-12A

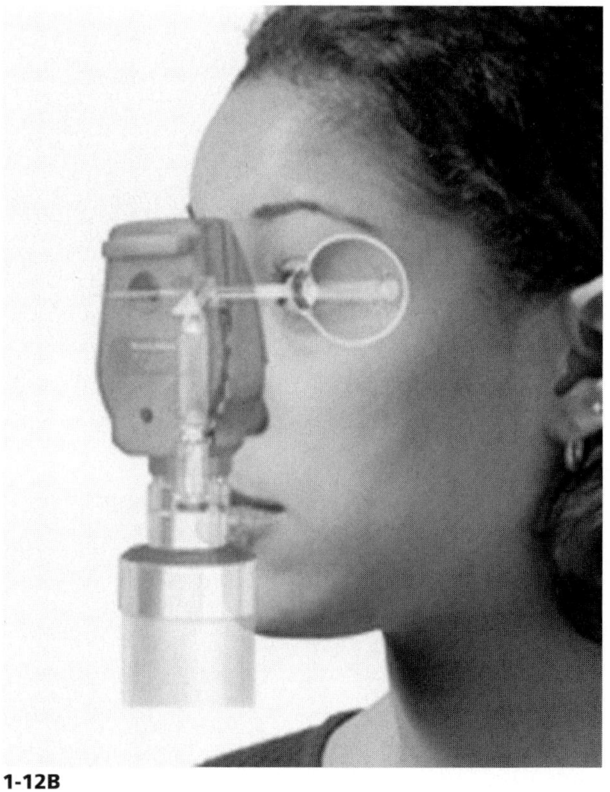

1-12B

Acquaint yourself with the dials of the ophthalmoscope. The aperture-selection dial has several stops for many uses. There are at least two, and sometimes three, aperture sizes. The very smallest aperture is useful in the smallest undilated pupils, usually about 5 degrees. The next smallest size is for larger undilated pupils, usually about 10 degrees.

1-13A

1-13B

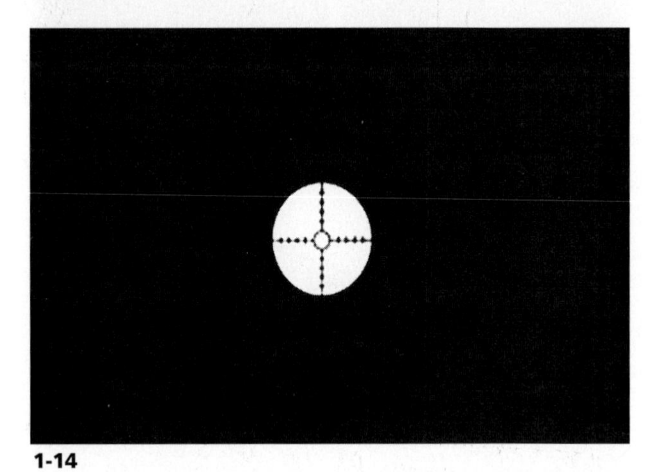

1-14

The largest white aperture should be used in the dilated pupil and in most general examinations of the eye, as it gives the best view of the disc and retina because of wider and brighter illumination.

Figure 1-13. Each different-sized aperture has its own use. The smallest one (A) can be used to view the disc through a smaller pupil. The larger one (B) is best looking through a dilated pupil. Most of the time, you view through the largest aperture.

A fixation device (or bull's eye) with cross hairs is used to measure eccentric fixation. The examiner asks the patient to look at the light. In the normal individual, the macula then should appear in the center of the cross hairs. If the patient is amblyopic with eccentric macular fixation, the macula appears to the side of the cross hairs, and not in the middle of the bull's eye. Often, the cross hairs have small, evenly spaced markings that can be used to measure or locate a lesion.

Figure 1-14. Use the bull's eye with the cross hairs to measure lesions and to view the centricity of the macula. To do this, have the patient look at the light. In the center should be the fovea of the macula.

In many models, a cobalt blue filter is one of the standard apertures.

1-15

Figure 1-15. The cobalt-blue filter is usually one of the standard apertures and can be used with fluorescein dye to view small abrasions or even foreign objects on the cornea. To see the cornea best, use a +20 lens. Even with the best of our current ophthalmoscopes, however, there is considerable chromatic aberration with the +20 lenses, which give rainbow-like colored distortions.

Of what use is the slit-beam aperture? First, view a lesion in the retina with the slit beam. If the beam is not distorted, the lesion is flat. If the lesion is elevated, the beam is raised toward the observer. Depressions such as a macular hole or disc excavation bend the light away from the examiner. The beam can be used to estimate the depth of a lesion. Another use of the slit beam is to sidelight or indirectly illuminate the disc; this method is especially effective in bringing out optic disc drusen or pits of the optic disc.

1-16A

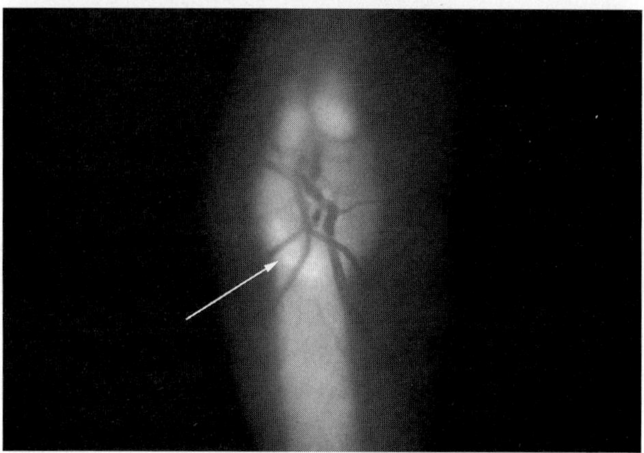
1-16B

Figure 1-16. A,B. **The slit-beam** (A) **allows us to view the disc with indirect lighting—thus illuminating disc drusen** (B)**, for example (*arrow*). In addition, you can use the slit beam to determine if there are drusen buried in the disc.**

Also located in the front of the ophthalmoscope head is a set of filters. Most often, the examiner uses a standard illumination with no filter; this gives the brightest direct light. However, if an opacity (e.g., a cataract) is present, which would produce glare, try the polarized filter for an easier view. The polarized beam eliminates glare from the cornea. The polarized lens works the way polarized sunglasses work to "look through" the glaze of light on a stream when fishing for trout.

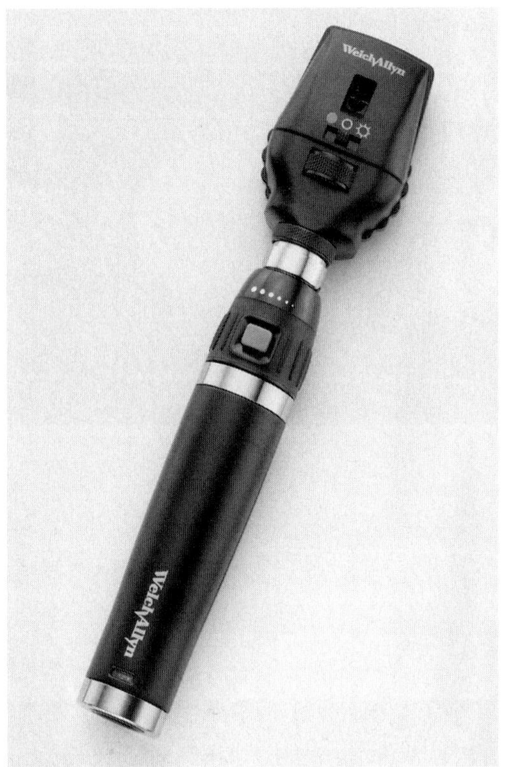

1-17A

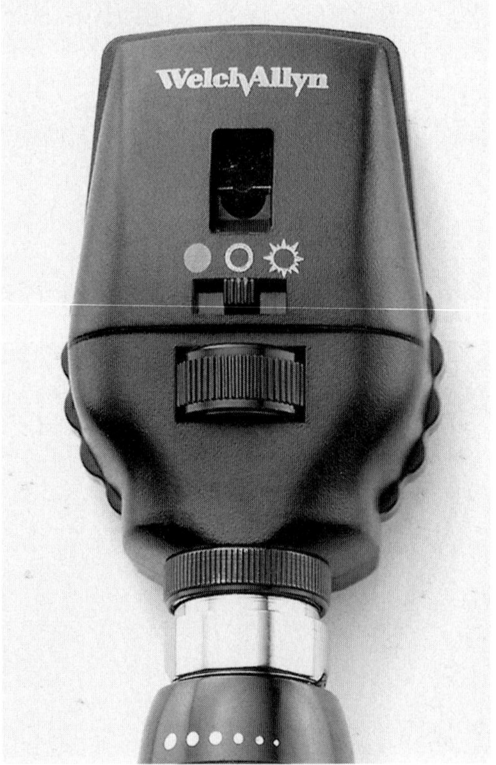

1-17B

Figure 1-17. A,B. **In many models, there are switches for various filters. The solid circle is for the red-free light. The open circle is for regular illumination. The polarizing filter (often designated as a circle with an "X" or a "sunburst") eliminates glare, especially when viewing through a cataract. The red-free light aids in viewing the optic disc and nerve fiber layer. (Photographs courtesy of the Welch Allyn Company.)**

The red-free filter (a green light) is extremely useful. It provides a 450-nm monochromatic light source that blocks long red waves. This filter makes surface lesions easier to see, as the examiner can use this light to illuminate and "see" the transparent nerve fiber layer because the shorter wavelength light reflects off of the non-red inner surface of the retina. This filter is especially useful in identifying nerve fiber–layer defects. The red-free filter is also good for illuminating optic nerve drusen when buried drusen are not appreciated by the standard white light (see also Chapter 3).

Figure 1-18. A–C. **The green light used in** (A) **is a red-free filter designed to block long red waves. It aids in viewing the nerve fiber layer** (B)**. In this photograph, you can see the opaque nerve fiber layer with a loss of the papillomacular bundle owing to trauma. Looking superiorly and inferiorly on the disc, you can see the nerve fiber layer streaming in. In addition, in** (C) **you can view disc drusen more easily—the red-free filter can illuminate drusen (*arrow*) that are missed with conventional white light.**

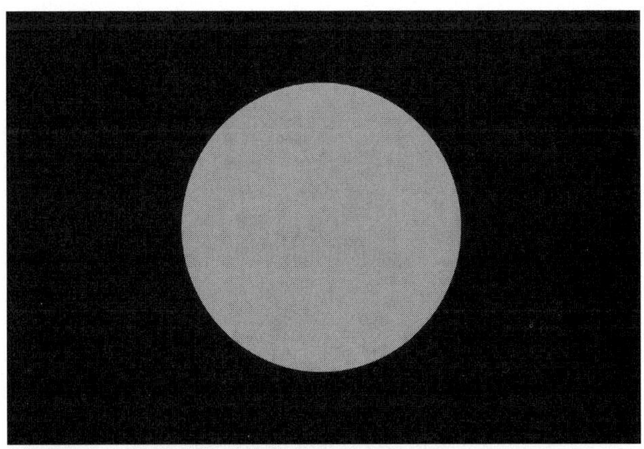

1-18A

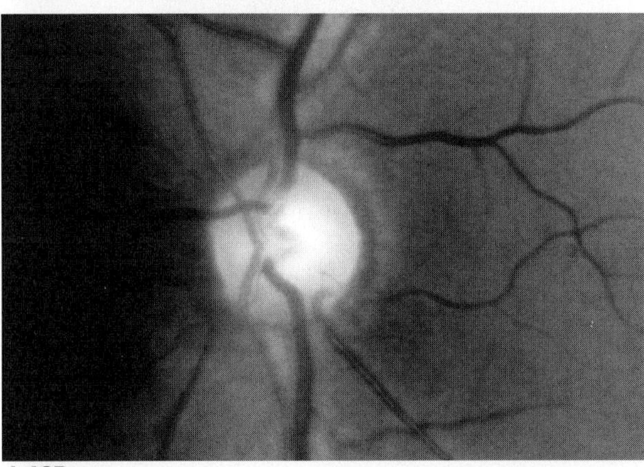

1-18B

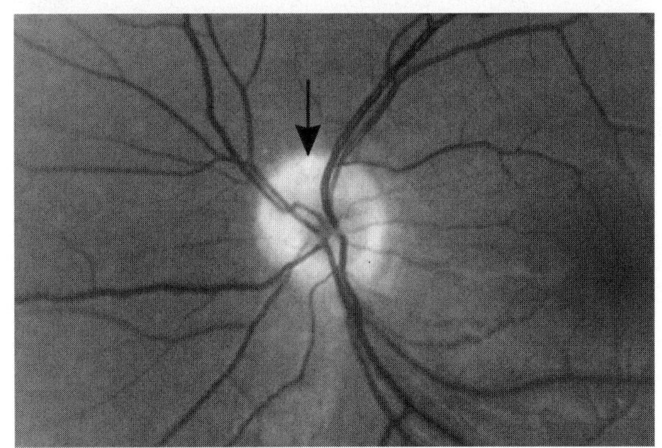

1-18C

Filters can be combined with the different-sized apertures to give the most revealing view. For example, if the examiner wishes to look for optic nerve drusen with a red-free filter through a small, undilated pupil, the choice would be the green light with the smaller aperture or perhaps the slit beam.

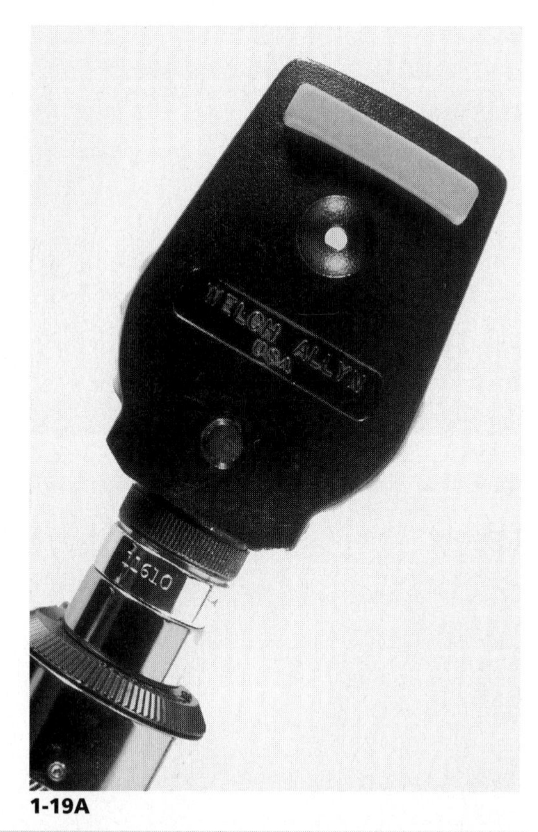

1-19A

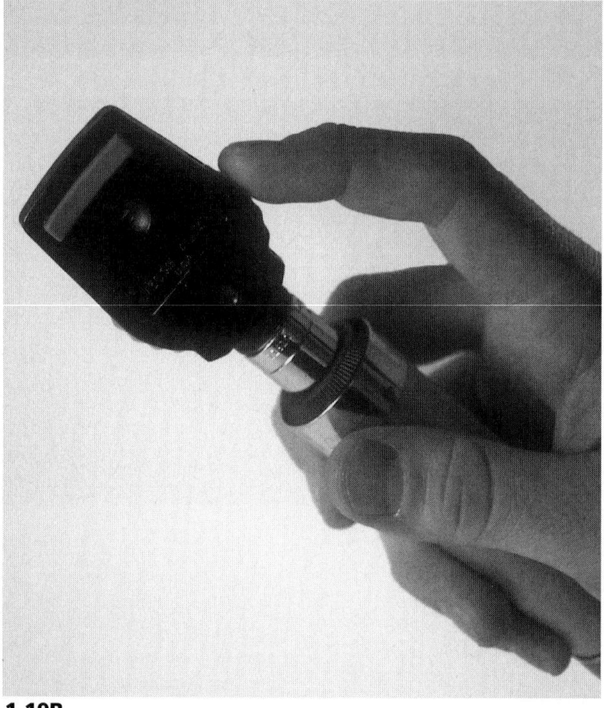

1-19B

Figure 1-19. A. **Notice that the power of the lens you are looking through is set at a red "6." This means that you are viewing through a –6-power lens.** B. **You may change the power of the lens by turning the lens selector dial with your pointer finger. If you are emmetropic (you do not need corrective lenses or you are wearing corrective lens or spectacle), you may wish to start with the "0" setting, whereas if you are myopic (nearsighted), you should start with a red number. If you are hyperopic (farsighted), you should start with the black or green numbers. Also note that the rubber bar in the back of the ophthalmoscope (grey, in this case) can rest against your spectacles, if you choose to wear them.**

Almost all ophthalmoscopes have a lens-selection dial or lens wheel. Some offer up to 68 lenses (–30 to +38) and some only 20 or 28 (–25 to +40). These lens selections represent different powers that can be adjusted both for the examiner's and the patient's refraction. The red numbers are negative-power, concave lenses, for nearsighted individuals or myopes, whereas the black or green numbers are positive-power, convex lenses, for farsighted individuals with hyperopia. If the examiner is *emmetropic* (needs no glasses or is wearing a corrective contact lens or spectacle), the dial should be at zero. The "plus" lens acts like a magnifying glass to make the image bigger. The larger the plus lens, however, the closer the focal point and the larger the image.

If the examiner is myopic and removes the spectacles, the myopic correction (e.g., a –3.00 myope) can be dialed in—a red "3." Similarly, if the examiner is hyperopic (e.g., +3.00), the dial can be set at a black or green "3." If the patient also has a correction, the dial is set at the algebraic sum of the refractive error of the examiner and the patient. See Video 1-19-1, Features of the Ophthalmoscope, on the accompanying CD-Rom.

What You Need to Know before You View the Disc

The patient history and examination allow you to be thinking of what you might expect to see on the disc. Without a history and a basic neuro-eye examination, you will be limited in what you can see.

First, what is the visual acuity in each eye? Check it with a hand-held acuity chart, testing each eye individually. If the patient uses glasses to read, have him or her wear the spectacles. If you don't have an acuity chart, have the patient read the phone book with each eye individually. The acuity of the names in the directory is approximately 20/30. See Video 1-19-2, Checking Visual Acuity, on the accompanying CD-Rom.

Is there a relative afferent pupillary defect (Marcus Gunn pupil)? First, measure the pupil size in darkness and light. Then, perform the swinging flashlight test. If the pupil dilates instead of constricting when you shine light in that eye, there is a relative afferent pupillary defect. A relative afferent pupillary defect is direct evidence that something is wrong with the optic disc. See Video 1-19-3, Looking for a Relative Afferent Pupillary Defect, on the accompanying CD-Rom.

What is the visual field to confrontation? Cover each eye individually and present a different number of fingers in each quadrant. If you detect a visual field defect, you simply bring more information to your examination of the optic disc. Check the central visual field by the method suggested in Video 1-19-4, Checking the Visual Field.

Use of Dilating Drops

In general, it is very helpful to use dilating drops. Although Gowers stated: "In most eyes much can be seen with the pupil undilated, often all that is necessary, and almost always enough to determine whether or not there is more to be learned by examination under atropine,"[2] dilation clearly makes it easier to see the optic disc and retina, and today we have better tolerated dilating drops than in the time of Gowers.

Historically, physicians other than ophthalmologists have been reluctant to use drops in dilating patients' pupils. There are many reasons for this: First, most physicians have rarely or never dilated the pupil and it is not part of their clinical "routine." Second, they do not want to precipitate a glaucoma attack. The evidence that routine use of dilating drops causes glaucoma is slim. Most sources quote an article written in the early 1950s, in which the authors reported three cases, all containing elderly patients, two-thirds of whom had known glaucoma.[18] Later, Harris conducted a study of the effect of cycloplegic agents on intraocular pressure in normal and open-angle glaucoma patients. It was found that only 2% of normal eyes exhibit an increased intraocular pressure with dilating drops, and 23% of patients with open glaucoma exhibited elevation with 1% cyclopentolate; these "responders" were then tested with 0.2% cyclopentolate and 0.5% tropicamide (Mydriacyl), and none of these had increased pressures.[19]

Furthermore, acute angle-closure glaucoma is very uncommon: It accounts for less than 10% of all glaucoma, and the treatment is to send the patient to an ophthalmologist as soon as possible. Finally, the examiner may look at the anterior chamber before dilating the patient to see if it is shallow or deep. By using side-illumination of the cornea and anterior chamber, one can estimate the chamber's depth.

Figure 1-20. A. By using the ophthalmoscope light at a side angle, look to see what shadow you cast. Where there is a deep anterior chamber and a normal angle, you see almost the entire iris without a shadow (*top*). The angle is probably adequate for dilation. When there is a narrow angle, such as seen with angle-closure glaucoma, the iris is in a shadow and the angle may be narrowed (*bottom*). In that case, you may wish to forgo dilation. B. Use the slit beam of the ophthalmoscope—If the angle is open, there is plenty of space between your beam and the iris at the edge of the cornea. The bottom set of arrows shows that there is more space between the slit beam on the cornea and the slit beam on the iris. The top set of arrows shows the two beams. Notice in the normal angle that the slit beam on the iris is also larger because the angle is so much larger. C. However, if the angle is narrow—meaning that the person is at risk for closing the angle due to, for example, glaucoma—there is very little space between the slit beam and the light reflex on the iris. Notice that the cornea (*arrow*) and iris (*arrow*) are very close together.

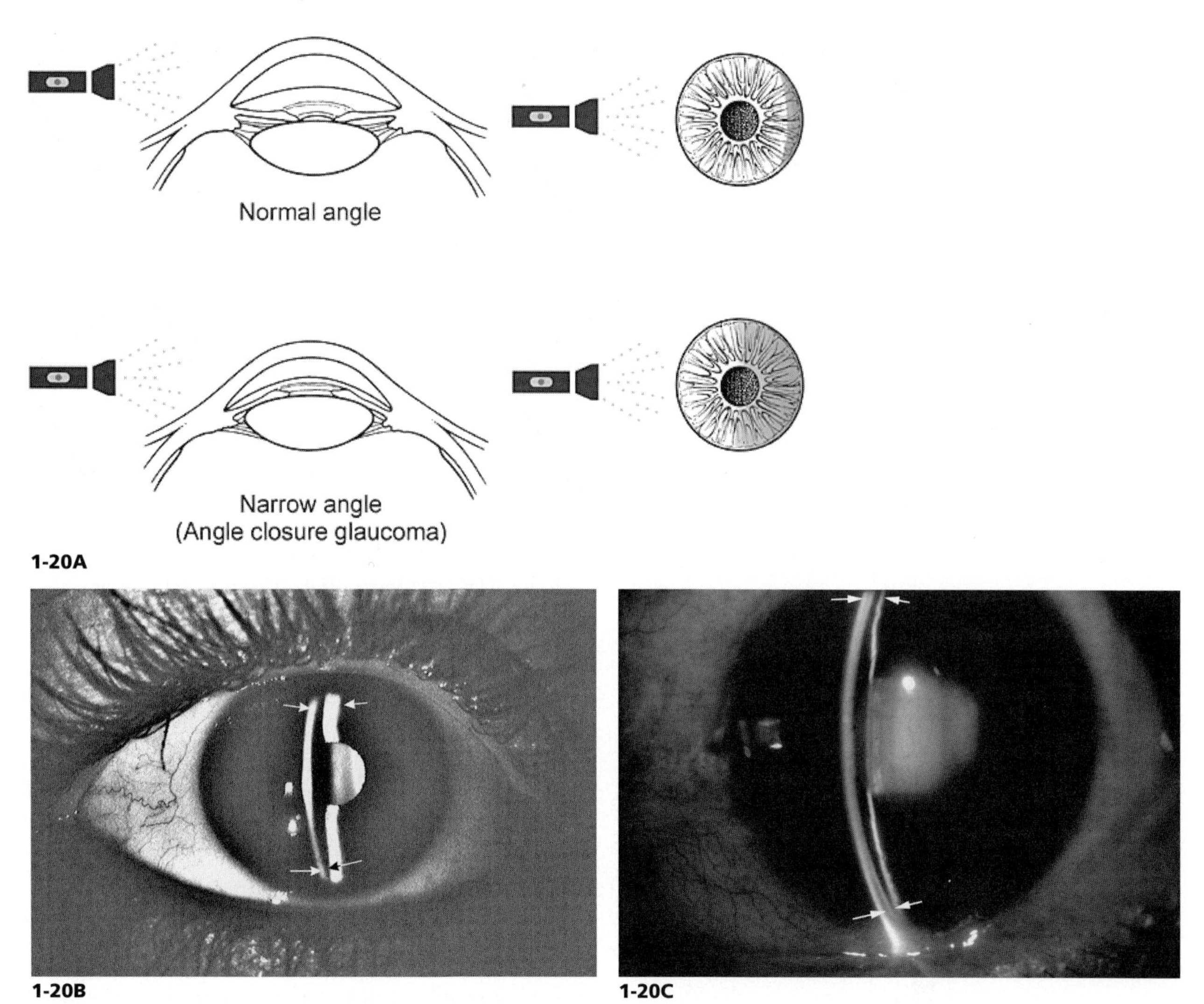

If the anterior chamber is deep, then there is very little risk to dilation. Hyperopic individuals (those wearing glasses that magnify), as well as middle-aged and older individuals, are at slightly higher risk. Furthermore, one can ask the patient if he or she experienced trouble during previous dilations. Ask the patient about symptoms of intermittent angle closure, such as blurring associated with halos around lights and eye discomfort. Refer those individuals with a history of such symptoms for a complete eye examination and intraocular pressure check. If there is any doubt, and you need to see the disc, some have recommended giving acetazolamide 250 mg before dilating the patient. After dilation, 2 drops of pilocarpine 2% solution may bring the pupil down more quickly. Do not use pilocarpine in highly myopic individuals, because retinal detachments have been known to occur after pilocarpine-induced miosis. Many have used other reversing drops, such as dapiprazole hydrochloride (Rēv-Eyes). Tell the patient that, if after the examination there is pain or decreased vision, he or she should come back to check the intraocular pressure. You could also ask the patient's ophthalmologist if it is safe to dilate the patient's eyes.

The other reason neurologists and neurosurgeons are reluctant to dilate the eyes of their patients is because of the concern for missing a "blown" (dilated) pupil owing to herniation from an intracranial mass. Since the advent of computed tomography and magnetic resonance imaging in the 1970s and 1980s, as well as the use of aggressive medical treatments of intracranial pressure with steroids and mannitol, it is rare indeed to have to use the pupil alone to follow a patient's progress or to make a decision to treat intracranial pressure. The overwhelming majority of new patients seen by physicians in an outpatient clinical setting are not candidates for imminent herniation.

Finally, it takes time to dilate the patient. We can get around this obstacle by checking visual acuity and the light reflex, and then instilling the dilating drop at the beginning of the neurologic or general physical examination. By the end of the history and examination, the pupil is dilated enough to see the disc and retina clearly.

The only contraindications to dilation are

- Known narrow-angle glaucoma or chronic glaucoma
- Impending surgical procedure
- Unstable neurologic condition where watching pupil size may be desirable

SPECIFIC TYPES OF DILATING DROPS

Figure 1-21. Dilating drops used routinely for dilation include tropicamide, phenylephrine, and cyclopentolate.

There are many mydriatic agents that can be used based on their chemical characteristics. Tropicamide and phenylephrine (Neo-Synephrine) are most commonly used in offices. One to two drops are placed in the cul-de-sac of the lower lid. This can be repeated in 30 seconds in each eye. Others advocate the use of phenylephrine and hydroxyamphetamine to aid in the examination of the disc, because neither is prone to cause dangerous intraocular pressure elevation in chronic simple glaucoma, and they produce minimal cycloplegia.[20] Dilation usually takes approximately 30 minutes. See Table 1-1 for frequently used dilating agents.

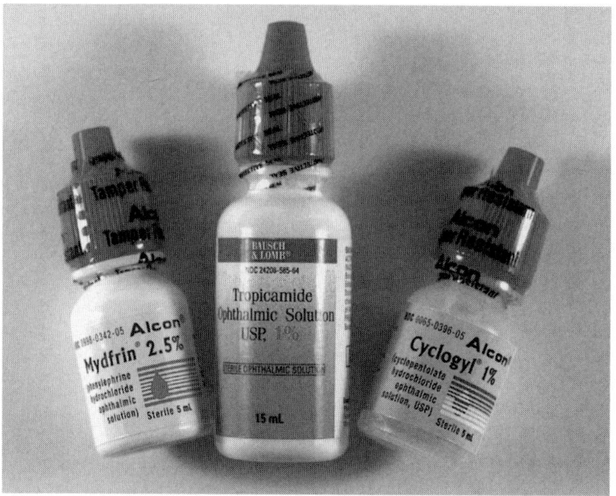

1-21

Table 1-1. Frequently Used Dilating Agents[20]

Agent (trade/generic)	Chemical class	Time to dilation	Length of dilation	Maximum dilation	Effect on accommodation	Side effects	Contraindications	Comments
Sympathomimetics								
Neo-Synephrine/phenylephrine 2.5–10.0%	Alpha agonist	60–90 mins	5–7 hrs	Usually 8 mm, sometimes less in elderly, dark irides less well dilated	Minimal effect on accommodation	Systemic hypertension	Uncontrolled hypertension	Often used with tropicamide
Paredrine/hydroxyamphetamine 1%	Indirect sympathomimetic	45–60 mins	2–6 hrs	Almost as effective as phenylephrine	Mild effect on accommodation	Theoretically, systemic hypertension	Uncontrolled hypertension	More often used as a diagnostic test for postganglionic Horner's syndrome
Anticholinergic/parasympatholytics								
Mydriacyl/tropicamide 0.5–1.0%	Parasympatholytic drug	20–35 mins	2–6 hrs	Excellent mydriasis—8 mm	Moderate—least effect on accommodation of parasympatholytics	—	As with all dilators, glaucoma	Often used in combination with phenylephrine
Cyclogyl/cyclopentolate 0.5–1.0%	Potent parasympatholytic drug	20–60 mins	6–24 hrs	Excellent mydriatic, less so in pigmented eyes	Paralyzes accommodation, used in cycloplegic refraction	Burning; rarely, hallucinations in children; nausea, dizziness, depression	Glaucoma, allergy	Often used in children for a cycloplegic refraction
Atropine	Potent parasympatholytic drug	30–40 mins	10 days	Longest mydriasis	Paralyzes accommodation	Flushing, hallucinations, delirium	Glaucoma	Used for prolonged dilation: iridocyclitis, refractions, occlusion, hyphema
Homatropine 2%	Similar to atropine but much shorter duration	60 mins	3–32 hrs–5 days	Good mydriasis	Paralyzes accommodation	Fewer side effects than atropine	Glaucoma	Used for cycloplegic refractions

Steps to Direct Ophthalmoscopy

First, dim the room light to optimally enlarge the pupils (if they are undilated). If you wear spectacles, you may choose to continue wearing them or take them off and correct your refractive error with the ophthalmoscope lenses. The view is better if you can take off your and the patient's spectacles (because you can get closer). If the patient is highly myopic or highly astigmatic, the examiner may need to view the disc through the patient's spectacles. If the patient is aphakic (i.e., the lens was removed surgically and the patient has thick spectacles), view the fundus without spectacles using a +10 lens. The examiner may continue to wear his or her glasses. Remember that the rubber bar across the back of the ophthalmoscope prevents scratching of your spectacle lenses.

The patient should be comfortable, as should you. By "comfortable," we mean that you and the patient should be at the same head height without straining. Stooping over, holding your breath, and standing on tiptoes all make it difficult to concentrate on the task at hand.

Socially, we have a personal space that, as physicians and health care providers, we are careful not to invade. How close can you get before you or the patient feels uncomfortable? This space varies from person to person, but in general people become uncomfortable when someone is closer than 1 foot from their face. To see the disc, you must get closer than that. How can you overcome the personal space taboo? You should say to the patient, "To be able to thoroughly examine your eye, I need to get very close to your face. Is that okay?" Informing the patient warns him or her and allows him or her to give you permission to move into his or her personal space and "see." Remember that the direct ophthalmoscope must be approximately 1 in. from the patient's eye for you to have the best view.

Obviously, you or your patient may have bad breath at this position. If you are concerned, hold your breath and breathe through your nose. In addition, avoid having your hair touch the patient, which is another invasion of personal space. Take the time to clear a good viewing space and to understand those elements of the close exam that may interfere with your ability to examine or the patient's willingness to be examined. Regardless, you must be up close and personal with the patient to get a good view.

Have the patient fixate on a distant target with the unexamined eye. Point out the target, for example, "Focus on the light switch on that wall [pointing to the wall]." Align yourself with the patient: Your right eye should look into his or her right eye, and your left eye should look into his or her left eye. Looking through the pupil to the fundus is like looking through a keyhole: You have to be close to see anything on the other side, and the closer you are the better. Research has shown that you must be 17 mm in front of the cornea to be in the anterior focal point of the eye,[21] so this is indeed close. If you are afraid of "butting heads," there are two tricks to keep you from getting too close. First, rest your hand with the ophthalmoscope on the cheek of the patient, as this stabilizes the ophthalmoscope on the cheek. Another trick is to place your thumb on the eyebrow of the patient, then resting your forehead on your thumb. This position also stabilizes the ophthalmoscope and, if necessary, you can use your thumb to open the patient's eyelid further.[22]

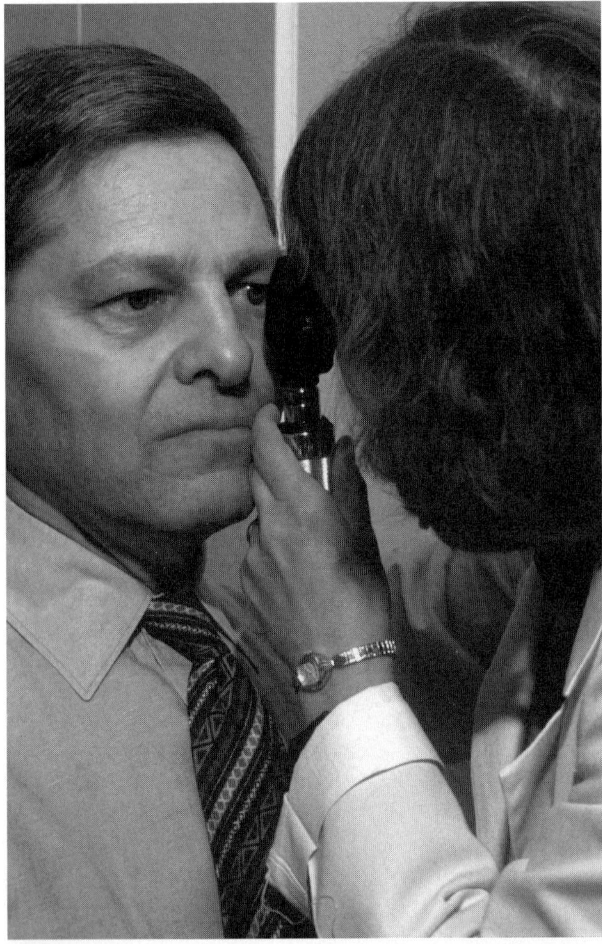

1-22A

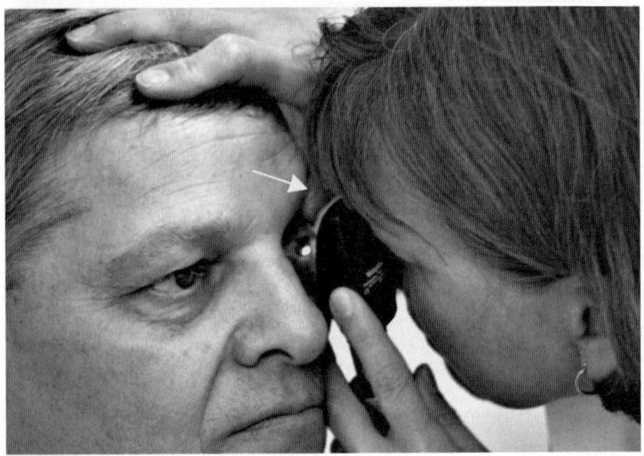

1-22B

Figure 1-22. A. **The examiner is approximately the same height as the patient and looks with her left eye into the patient's left eye.** B. **The examiner rests her finger on the patient's cheek to steady her hand and have the correct distance while she leans the ophthalmoscope up against her thumb on the patient's brow (*arrow*). The other use of the thumb on the brow is to hold up the patient's eyelid. Remember: You have to be close.**

Figure 1-23. A. **Viewing the disc is like viewing through a keyhole: The closer you get, the better you see, and you have to get close. Notice the distance from the patient's eye to the ophthalmoscope. This should be no further than 2 in. from the cornea, and frequently is only 1 in.** B. **If you have one dominant eye and have difficulty ignoring the image from the nonviewing eye, cover it. In this case, the examiner covers her right eye while viewing the patient's left eye.**

- Begin with a look at the cornea and external eye, and then the red reflex of the eye at 4 feet. This is best accomplished by starting with the +20 lens. Changes in the cornea, lens, or vitreous can alter the red reflex, and the lenticular changes owing to cataracts are easily seen.

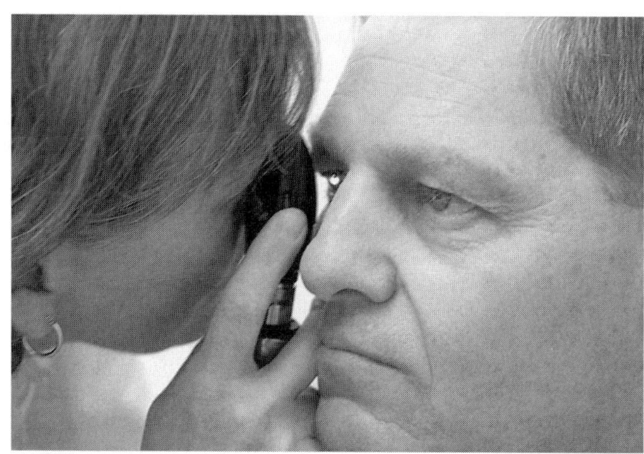

1-23A

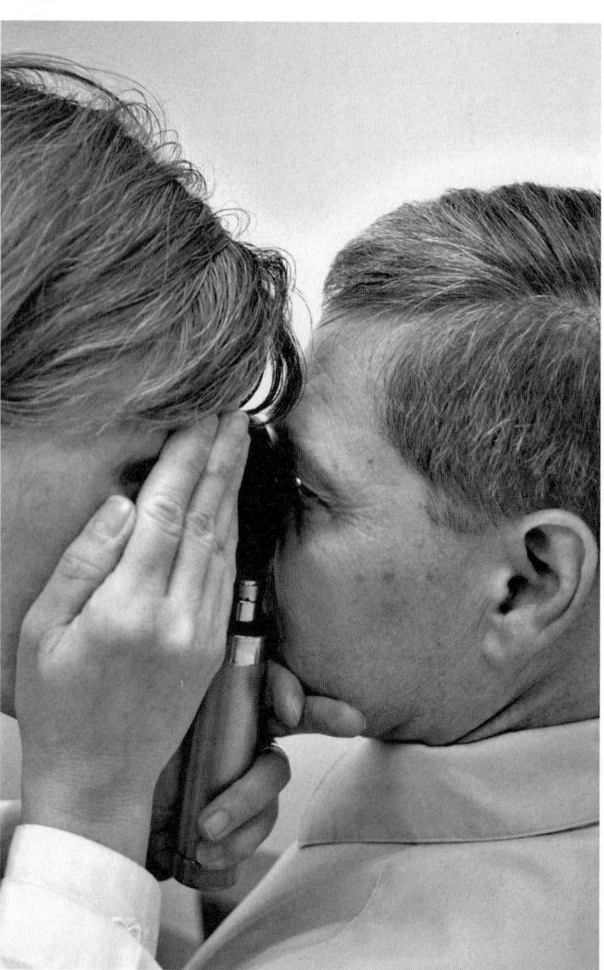

1-23B

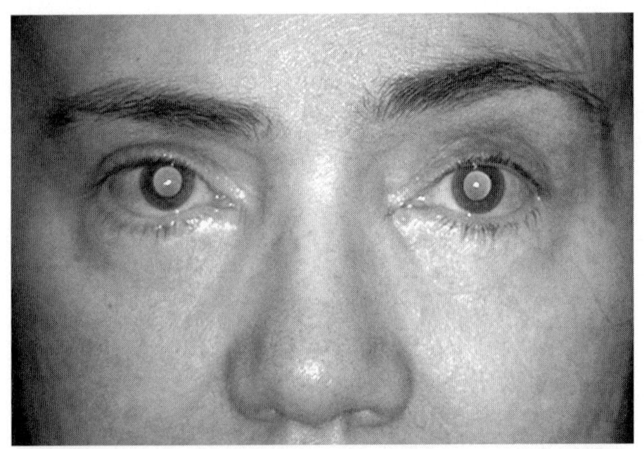

1-24A

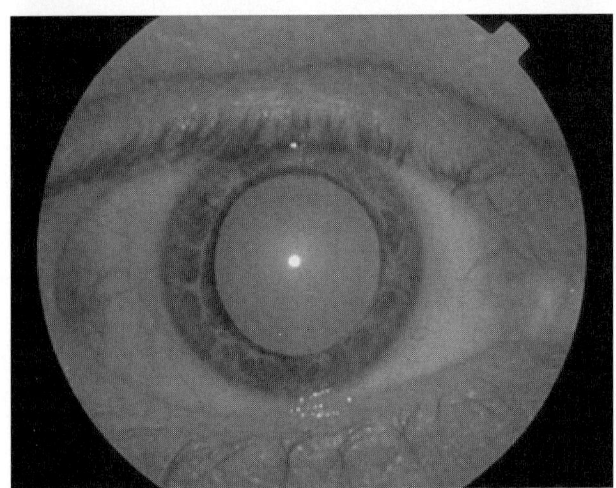

1-24B

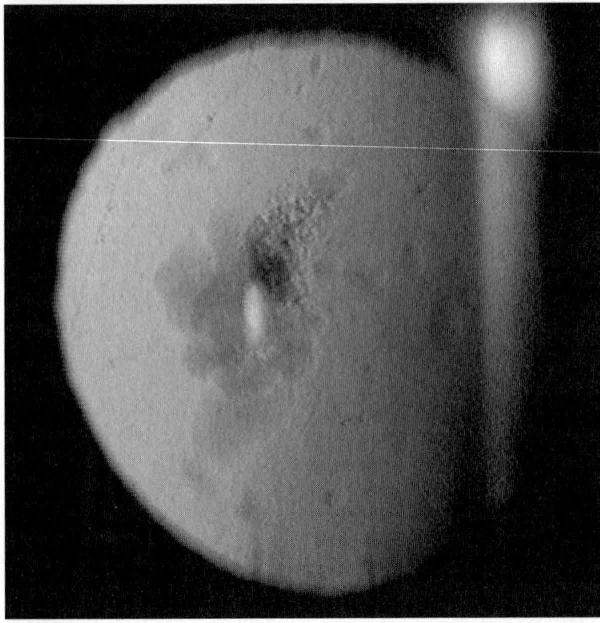

1-24C

Figure 1-24. A. **Look for the red reflex through the viewfinder. Here, you can see that the light is focused centrally on the cornea (see also Figure 1-25C).** B. **Move in on the red reflex of one eye.** C. **View the red reflex for disturbance in the reflex, such as this cataract.**

- Focus on the limbus of the cornea and draw closer to the patient. Continuously peer through the media (cornea, lens, vitreous). The vitreous is more clearly seen with lenses in the +2 to approximately +10 range. Turn the lens "wheel" as you draw closer to focus the light on the retina; you should be approximately 1 in. in front of the patient's eye. The view is magnified approximately 14–15 times if the examiner is emmetropic, slightly more if myopic, and slightly less if hyperopic. The direct ophthalmoscope provides the examiner with approximately a 10-degree view. Vitreous hemorrhages may appear as small black dots, and if the hemorrhage is large, the view of the fundus is obscured, there is no red reflex, and there is no view of the retina (a so-called "eight-ball hemorrhage"). A clue to vitreous change is that they move or float, which is apparent to both patient and examiner.
- Bring the vessels of the retina into view. The retina is focused within the +1 to –1 lenses. Find the optic disc and identify the central retinal artery and vein, as well as their branches. Because the disc is often the focal point of the examination, imagine the disc to be cut vertically into two pieces, giving a temporal half (toward the macula) and a nasal half (away from the macula). Observe the cup inside the disc and estimate the cup-to-disc ratio (see Chapter 2, Figure 2-36).
- Find the macula: It is temporal to the disc. The foveal area is slightly darker than the surrounding retina, and few vessels will be seen. You may see a small spot of yellowish light reflected back at you, which is the foveola, or a minute depression in the center of the fovea that optically reflects the light. Another way to see the macula

is to ask the patient to "look at the light." This also brings the macula and fovea into view.

- By having the patient look to the right, left, up, and down, it is possible to have a more complete view of the peripheral parts of the posterior pole. To do this systematically, follow a single vessel from the disc to periphery. You may need to adjust the focusing dials of the ophthalmoscope, using more positive lens power to better and more clearly view the periphery.

Table 1-2. Settings on Ophthalmoscope for Viewing the Eye*

Part of the eye viewed	Lens setting on ophthalmoscope
Cornea	+20
Lens	+20
Vitreous	+2 to +10
Retina	−1 to +1

*Settings assume that neither examiner nor patient has a refractive error.

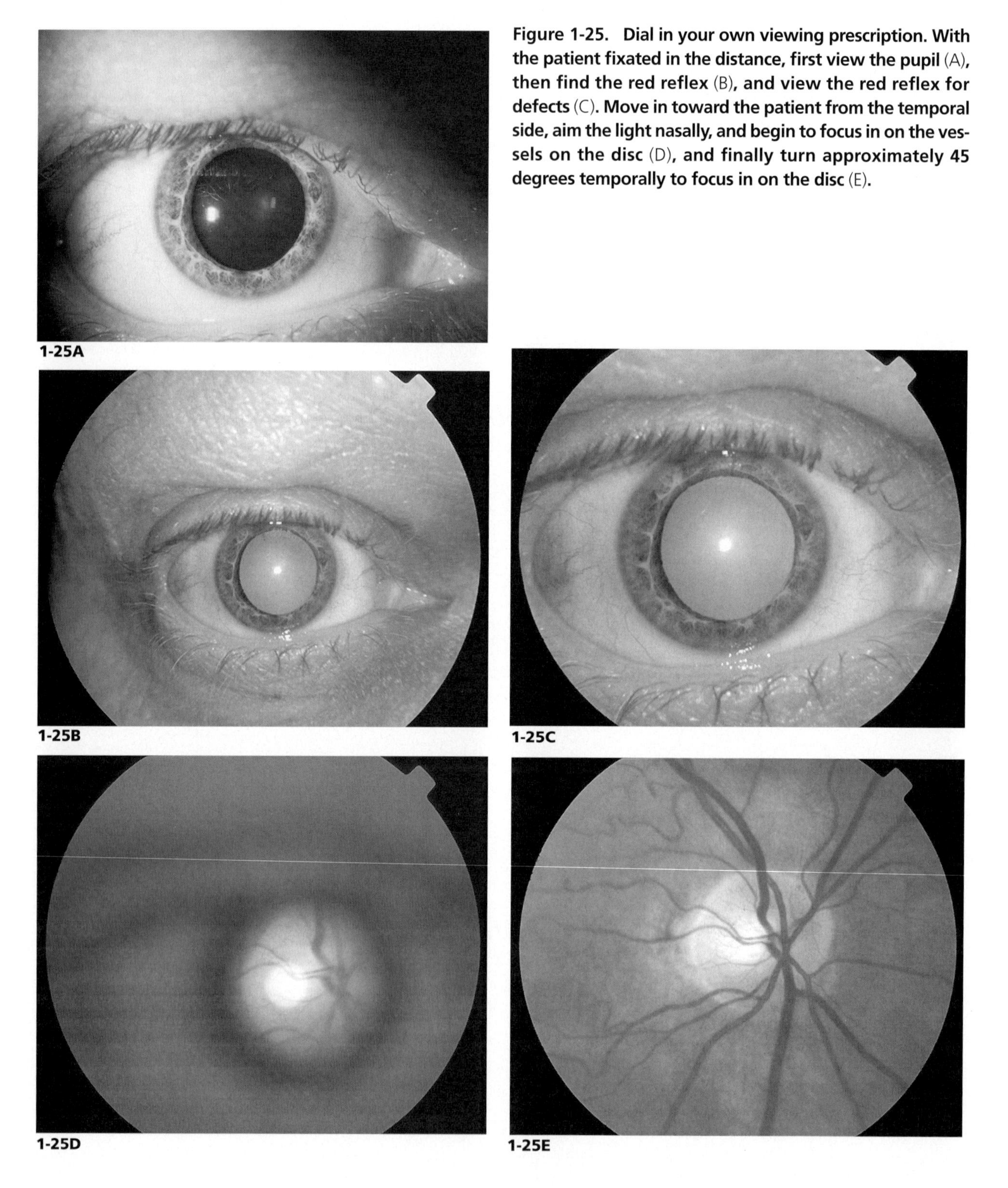

Figure 1-25. Dial in your own viewing prescription. With the patient fixated in the distance, first view the pupil (A), **then find the red reflex** (B), **and view the red reflex for defects** (C). **Move in toward the patient from the temporal side, aim the light nasally, and begin to focus in on the vessels on the disc** (D), **and finally turn approximately 45 degrees temporally to focus in on the disc** (E).

See Video 1-24-1, The Direct Ophthalmoscopic Examination, on the accompanying CD-Rom.

What Gets in the Way of Seeing?

In viewing the optic disc, you can *look* without seeing, or you can *see* and understand what you are seeing.

First, you must be aware of what gets in the way of "seeing." It takes *gumption* to view the optic disc and retina. What is gumption? *Webster's Dictionary* defines gumption as "courage, and initiative, enterprise and boldness." Robert Pirsig writes that "gumption traps" keep people from doing tasks in a high-quality way.[23] His course, *Gumptionology 101*, defined these traps as "an examination of affective, cognitive and psychomotor blocks in the perception of quality relationships." He continued: " These drain off gumption, destroy enthusiasm and leave you so discouraged you want to forget the whole business. I call these things 'gumption traps.' There are hundreds of different kinds of gumption traps, maybe thousands, maybe millions."

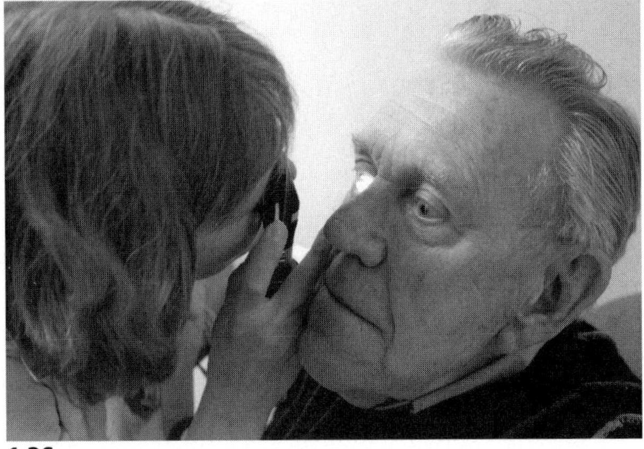

1-26

Figure 1-26. Examine your patient. Examine yourself for gumption blocks—What gets in the way of your seeing in a high-quality way?

WHAT ARE THE "GUMPTION TRAPS" IN VIEWING THE DISC?

- Not having the right equipment
- Weak battery, so the light is not bright enough to see
- Lens is scratched or dusty, so that the view is fuzzy
- Ophthalmoscope is dirty
- Not positioning the patient properly
- Not being at the same level as the patient's eye and having to squat or strain to get close enough to see in
- Not wanting to invade someone's space

- Not wanting to touch the body of the patient with your body
- Not knowing your own or the patient's refraction (i.e., near- or farsighted)
- Not dilating the pupil when necessary
- Not realizing where you are focused (at the disc, at the retina, at the vitreous, at the lens)
- Not being physically close enough to the patient
- Not knowing what to expect
- Not appreciating what is normal
- Not understanding what can get in the way of seeing
- Not having a proper mindset ("I am not good at this")

HOW DO YOU OVERCOME THE "GUMPTION TRAPS"?

Equipment

First, be sure your equipment is kept in good shape. Have your own equipment and do not depend on having equipment provided for you, especially when you are on the wards doing consultations. There are enough other obstacles without having to contend with faulty equipment. Also, check to make sure that the battery is charged and the viewing lens is clean.

Positioning

To minimize distractions, it is important to be comfortable while you are looking. Be sure the patient is positioned at the same height or slightly lower than you are. Take the time to make a good viewing space.

Know Your Refraction

Another trap may be the patient's or your own refractive error. Sometimes astigmatism, high myopia, or hypermetropia lead to a poor view of the disc. In this situation, have the patient continue to wear his or her own spectacles and do the examinations through his or her refraction. If you are the one with the bad refraction, wear your own glasses, as the ophthalmoscope has a rubber rest to sit on your lens.

Dilate the Patient's Pupil

Whenever possible, view the optic disc when the pupil is dilated.

Know Where You Are Focused

Sometimes when looking for the disc, all you see is red or white—the retina or reflected light, respectively. In the first case, if you can get a vessel in view, trace the vessel toward its larger branches: This takes you back to the disc. If all that you see is white, consider the following: First, is the subject viewing in the distance, or focusing on my light? The magnification changes if the patient is viewing your light, so ask him or her to focus at some target in the distance. Second, is there an opacification of the lens that is blocking your view? Check the red reflex again. Third, are you close enough? If you are not, there may be a bright reflection off of the cornea or lens. If you have trouble getting "through" the lens due to early cataract, try the polarizing filter. Another trick is to use the smaller aperture of light: Focusing a smaller light through a small pupil or around an early cataract may get around the reflection.

View with Confidence

Your mindset can be the biggest "gumption trap." Practice "seeing." In this examination technique, practice does make perfect: The more often you "look," the more confidence you acquire, and the better you will "see" in the future. No one is a born ophthalmoscopist. Look for and see specifics—the disc, the cup-to-disc ratio, the optic crescent, the nerve fiber layer, and the vessels.

Know What to Expect

Part of seeing is to know what you are looking for—Do you expect to find something? In any patient, but especially in knowing what to expect with the optic disc, *history* is important. Does the patient report a visual problem? The key questions are the following:

Is it in one eye or both?
How did it start (suddenly or gradually)?
Is pain present?
Are other factors experienced?
What is the pertinent past medical history, family history, social history (smoking, alcohol)?

Be sure you have checked the visual acuity, the pupillary light reflex (looking for a relative afferent pupillary defect), and the visual fields. When you are looking through the ophthalmoscope, expect to see things such as microaneurysms, crossing changes, splinter hemorrhages, and nerve fiber–layer infarcts.

Practice Using the Ophthalmoscope

Helmholtz received many letters reading "Your ophthalmoscope is excellent, but I cannot see anything with it," to which he replied "Practice."[4]

Carefully go through the steps of ophthalmoscopy, with a willing partner at first, so that you begin to feel comfortable with the process and steps. There are also "dummies" (mannequins) that can be used for practice. These have the benefit of not caring whether light is shining for hours on end. Using the dummies, you can test yourself by putting in known "lesions," or slides of various pathologies.

Model eyes with fundus drawings are not a new invention: They were first introduced by Perrin in 1866 and improved on by Landolt in 1876, based on Donders' model.[17] Today, models for practice are sometimes available at medical schools for students to practice ophthalmoscopy.

Other Viewing Techniques

There are other ways to view the optic disc. Because we also look at disc photographs and occasionally a fluorescein angiogram in this book, they are reviewed here.

Photography has recorded the fundus appearance since the early part of the 1900s and regularly since the 1960s. Before this, time-consuming, painstaking drawings served the same purpose. We use photography especially when we are trying to sequentially assess optic disc changes, such as swelling from papilledema or excavation from glaucoma. The alternative to this is intricate and time-consuming drawings to document changes in the optic disc. This is not a viable option. Consider fundus photographs to be the ophthalmologic equivalent of chest x-rays.

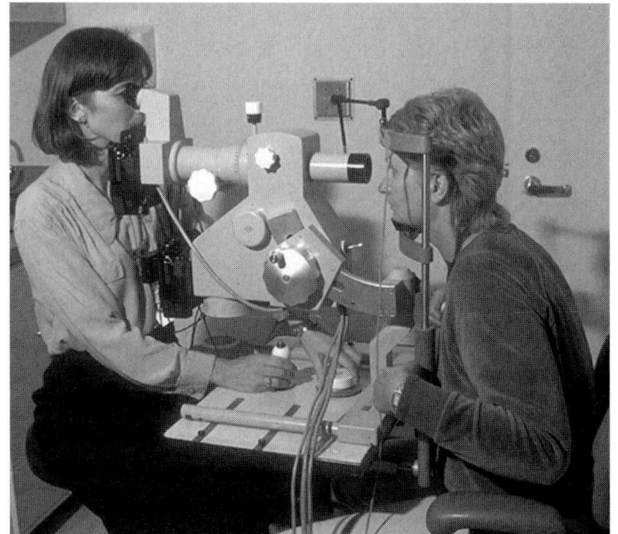

1-27

Figure 1-27. We examine disc photographs throughout this book. They have been, for the most part, taken by a camera that looks like the one shown here.

What should you look for on a fundus photograph? First, identify the right and left eye. The vessels arch toward the macula, and the macula is to the left of the disc in the right eye and toward the right of the disc in the left eye. Also, notice that the macula is just slightly lower than the disc.

You can view fundus photographs in many ways. First, notice the labeling on the photograph. The name and date should be present. Frequently, photographers photograph stereo disc pairs (these are two photographs that are just slightly off-axis, one from the other, to produce a three-dimensional appearance when viewed with both eyes). Disc viewers allow you to look at the stereo disc photographs. In short, the macula is temporal to the disc in either eye.

Various filters can be used in fundus photography, just as with the direct and indirect ophthalmoscopes. For example, a red-free filter can be placed over the camera to enhance the view of the nerve fiber layer. This filters out the long red waves and records the short wavelengths (e.g., blue and green), which optimally reflect off of the nerve fiber layer. Many photography units today use digital technology in still disc photography, video photography, and fluorescein angiography.

Another procedure to be familiar with that is referred to in this book is *fluorescein angiography.* Novotny and Alvis first introduced this procedure in 1960. A nurse or technician administers sodium fluorescein, a dye, through an angiocatheter (3–5 cc) into a vein in the arm. After the injection, the photographer takes photographs at a rate of approximately one per second for 1 minute, then at 1-minute intervals, and finally 10 minutes after injection. Fluorescein angiography is a technique that gives us a lot of information about the state of the fundus blood vessels.

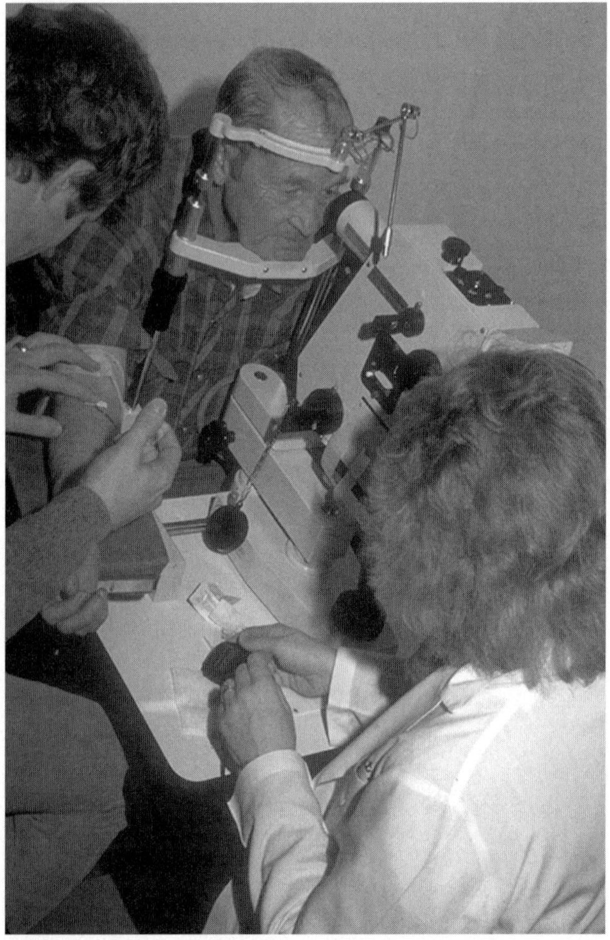

1-28

Figure 1-28. Fluorescein angiography begins by having the nurse or technician place an angiocatheter into an antecubital vein and inject 3–5 cc of sodium fluorescein into the vein. Photographs are then taken by a camera.

The dye reaches the ophthalmic artery after passing through the heart and lungs in 8–14 seconds. There really are two separate vasculatures that are viewed almost simultaneously: the retinal vasculature (central retinal artery as a branch off the ophthalmic artery) and the choroidal vasculature (from the posterior ciliary artery circulation, also branches of the ophthalmic artery). The retinal pigment epithelium partially obscures the choroidal vasculature. The first things to "light up" are the choroid and optic disc. This occurs at 10–15 seconds. The retinal arterioles then illuminate using a red-free light, and the capillary bed and veins become visible at approximately 12–18 seconds (1–3 seconds after the choroidal circulation). We speak of the arterial phase (i.e., the filling of the central retinal artery) and the capillary phase (i.e., the filling of the small vessels, including the choroid). The maximal fluorescence is seen approximately 20–25 seconds after injection. The early venous phase shows laminar flow first in the central retinal vein, and later complete filling in the venous phase (i.e., the complete filling of the veins).

Figure 1-29. A. **Note the red-free photograph taken of each disc (here you see the left disc and fundus) before injection of the dye.** B. **Note the time of appearance of the first dye—in this case, approximately 17 seconds. This is the "arm to retina" time. The first vessels to fill are the ciliary circulation, when present, and almost simultaneously you see the central retinal artery fill.** C. **The other phase to review is the beginning of the venous phase—the veins look "striped" with laminar flow (dye on the edge of the vein, but not in the middle).** D. **The venous phase begins at this point, and all of the vessels are filled.** ***Continued***

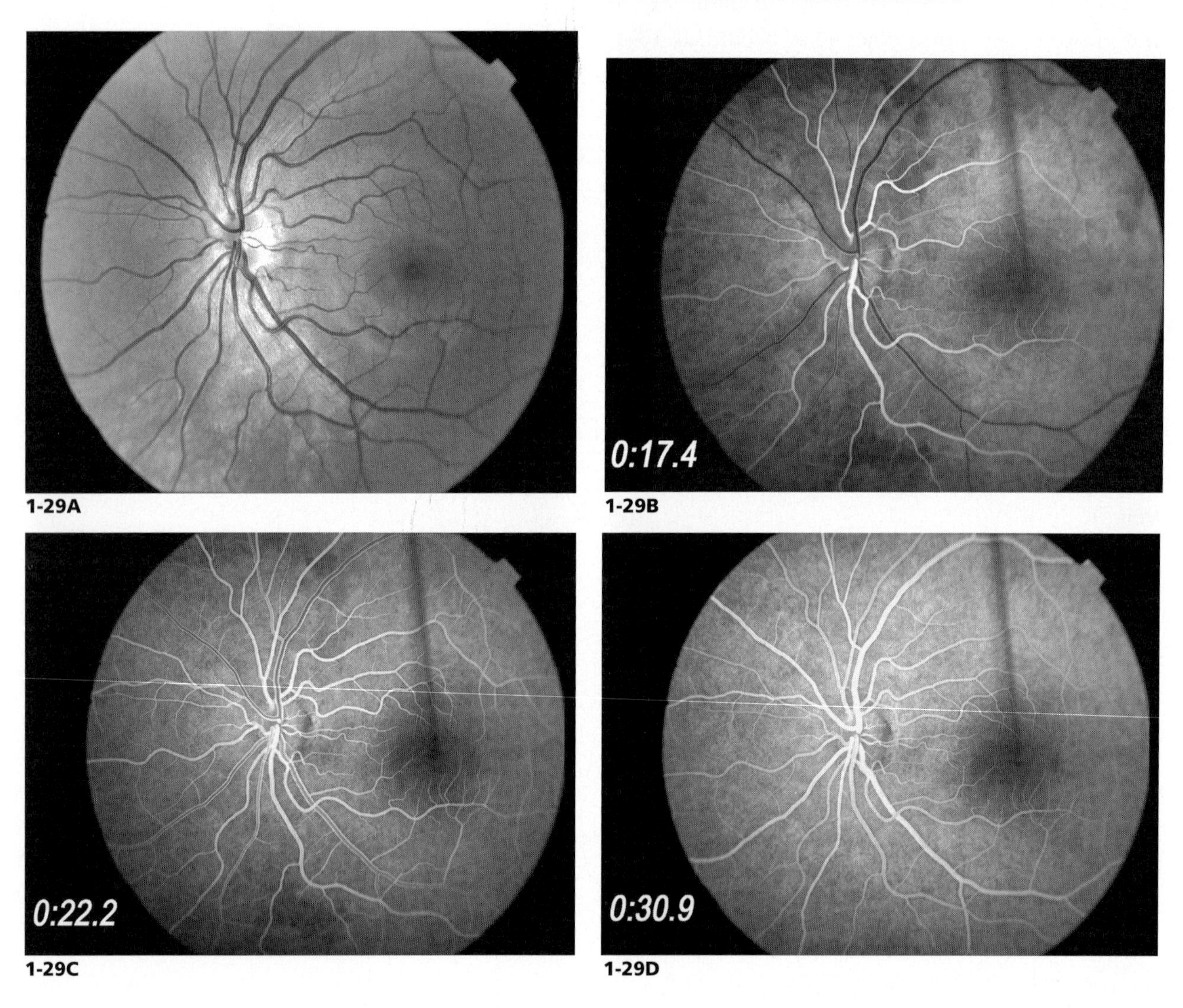

1-29A

1-29B

1-29C

1-29D

Figure 1-29. ***Continued.*** E,F. **A late photograph is taken to be sure there is no disc or retinal staining. The numbers on the photograph indicate how many minutes and seconds have elapsed since introduction of the dye.**

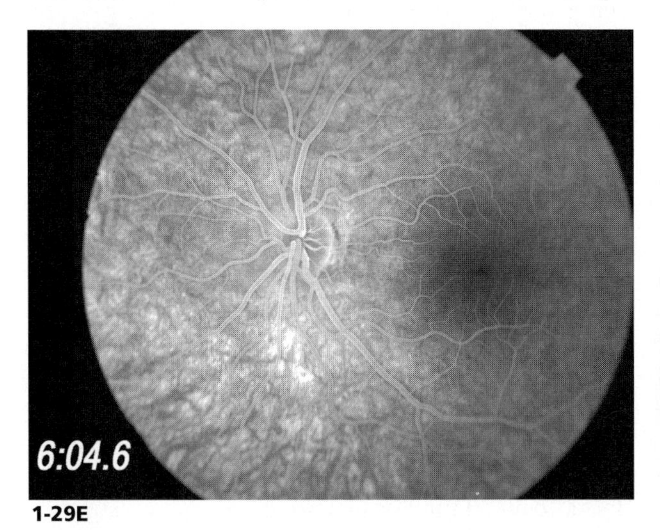

1-29E

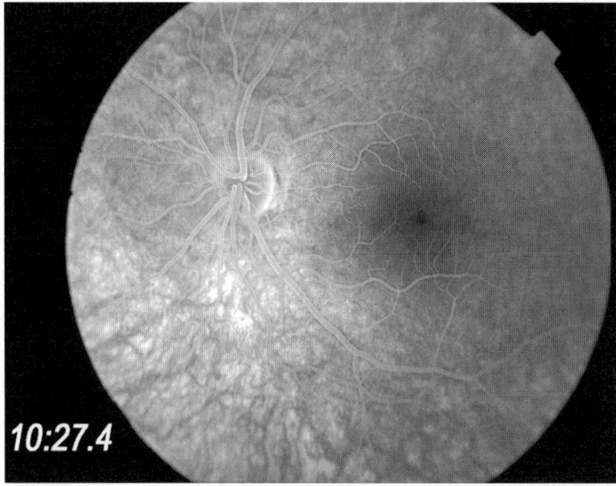

1-29F

Fluorescein angiography can be used to identify many conditions and diseases. It is often used in evaluation of vascular diseases affecting the eye, such as retinal artery occlusion and retinal vein occlusion, and especially in looking for evidence of neovascularization in diseases like diabetes mellitus (see also Chapters 5 and 9). Although fluorescein attaches to some tissues like the sclera and lamina cribrosa, fluorescein does not leak from vessels unless there is a breakdown in the blood retinal barrier or there is some sort of pathology present. Hyperfluorescence means increased fluorescence, and hypofluorescence means decreased fluorescence. Autofluorescence occurs when objects illuminated by the blue light of the camera cause a yellow light to be emitted. Autofluorescence occurs with optic nerve drusen (see Chapter 3).

Hyperfluorescence occurs when there are abnormal retinal or choroidal vessels. Leakage of fluorescein means that the dye has spread beyond the blood vessel into the space around it (extravascular space). If there is a break in a vessel, the dye

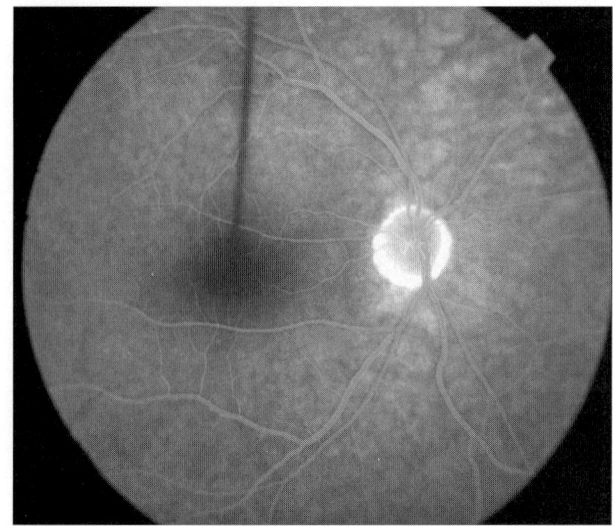

1-30A

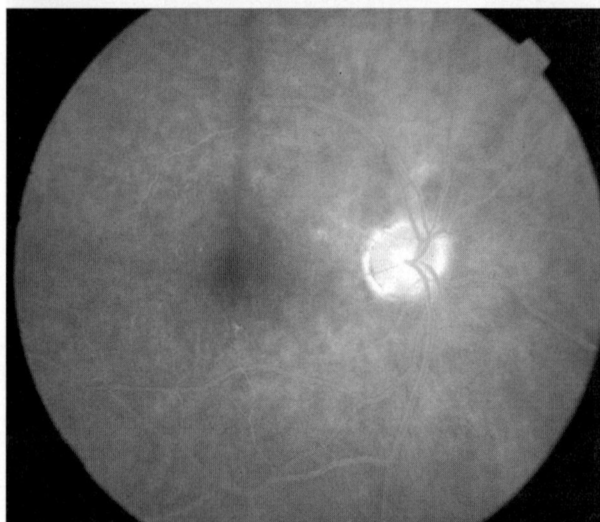

1-30B

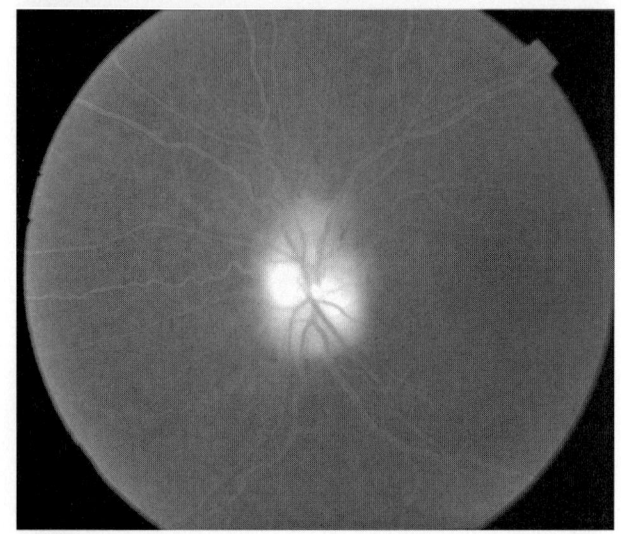

1-30C

accumulates as the study progresses. Examples of leakage are macular edema in diabetes and dye leaking from small capillaries on the disc in papilledema (see Chapter 3, Figure 3-24). Staining is the accumulation of dye on a structure of the eye. The sclera and, to some extent, the disc can stain normally.[24]

Figure 1-30. A. **It is normal to see a thin rim of dye staining around the edge of the disc, but usually not on the disc surface.** B. **Staining is the direct result of leakage from an inflammatory exudate, a scar, or an altered vessel wall. The dye, in other words, gets "hung up." This entire disc is staining.** C. **The term *dye leakage* is used for pathologic conditions within the ocular circulation in which the vessels become permeable to fluorescein. There is a breakdown of the blood-retinal barrier, and dye accumulates beyond the disc margin. The dye "leaks" beyond the disc margin.**

Hypofluorescence can be caused by many processes. It occurs as a result of anything blocking the fluorescent dye. For example, any blood or exudate may block the fluorescence. If you do not see the typical fluorescent pattern and the retinal vessels filling, look for a blockage. If you do not see the typical fluorescent pattern, but you do see the retinal vessels, the blocked pattern lies in the retina or choroid. Besides blood, pigment (melanin), lipid, exudates, and inflammation all can block fluorescence. Look also to see if all of the vessels fill or are slow to fill. We discuss slowly filling vessels in Chapter 5.

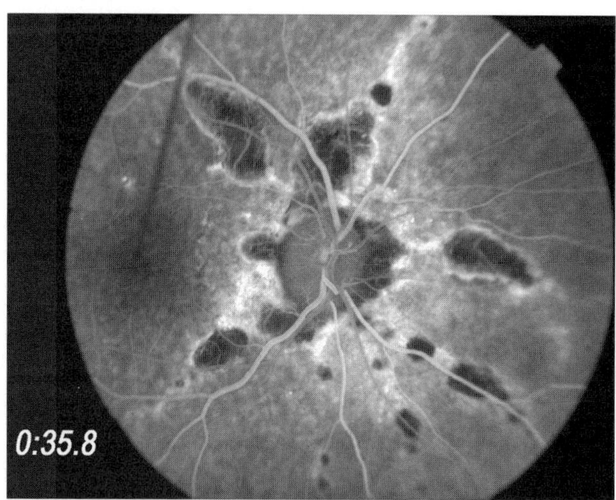

1-31A

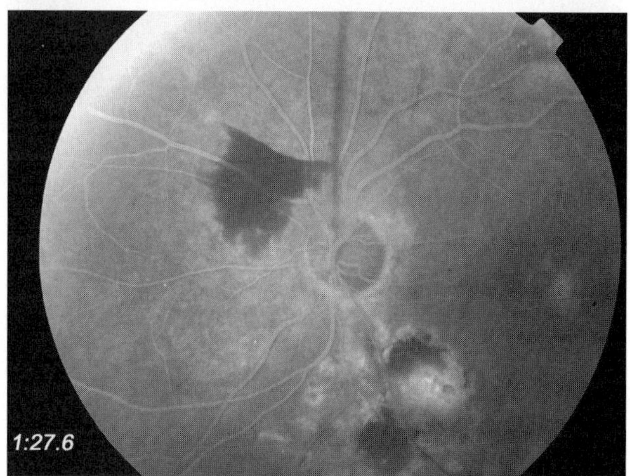

1-31B

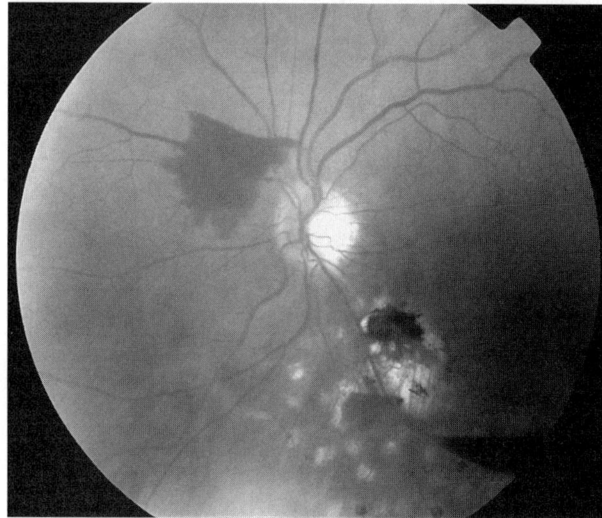

1-31C

Figure 1-31. A. **Here you see angioid streaks from a patient with pseudoxanthoma elasticum. The black areas are the streaks or breaks, and the fluorescein accumulates on the edge of the defect. You can tell the defect is deep within the retinal pigment epithelium and choriocapillaris because the arterial vessel is seen traversing the defect (see the inferior nasal vessel).** B. **Hemorrhages appear black because they block fluorescence of tissue beneath; however, vessels adjacent to the hemorrhage may fluoresce. In this case, the hemorrhage obscures the choroidal and retinal fluorescence.** C. **You can compare the fluorescein with the clinical appearance of the hemorrhage. This patient has multiple laser marks owing to laser treatment of neovascularization.**

The most common side effects of fluorescein angiogram are nausea and vomiting, and these occur in approximately 5–10% of individuals. Almost all patients experience a slight yellow tint to their skin and briefly look "jaundiced." In most, the urine is discolored. Some are allergic to the dye and develop urticaria (1:82). Rarely, anaphylactic shock or severe hypotension has been reported. Severe reactions such as cardiac arrest (1:5,300), respiratory arrest (1:3,800), and seizures (1:13,900) have also been reported. Death (1:221,781) is a rare complication.[25]

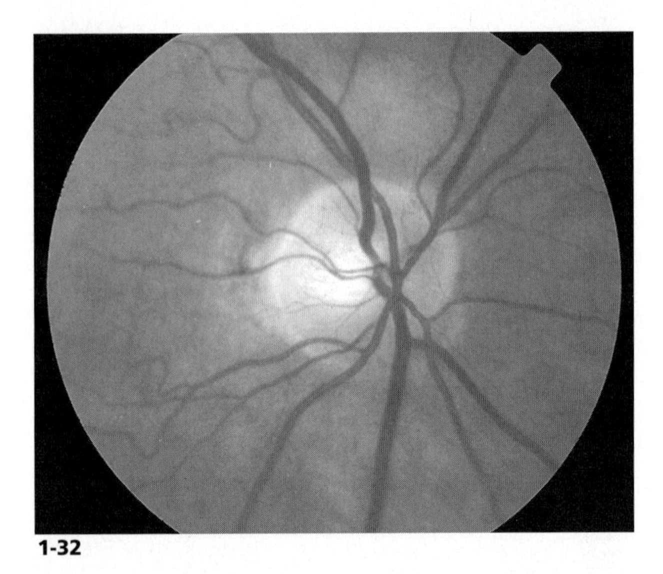

1-32

Practical Viewing Essentials

1. Have your own familiar ophthalmoscope.
2. Place strong, new batteries in the ophthalmoscope.
3. Be sure the ophthalmoscope viewing mechanism is clean.
4. Be familiar with all of the dials of the ophthalmoscope.
5. Know what the use of each dial is.
6. Decide what dilating drops you will routinely use.
7. Know your own refraction.
8. Concentrate on looking at the red reflex, then focus on the vessels.
9. Know what gets in the way of seeing: What are your "gumption blocks"?
10. Know about the uses of fluorescein angiography.
11. Practice, practice, practice viewing the retina, macula, and optic disc.

References

1. Charcot JM. Lectures on the Diseases of the Nervous System. Translated and edited by G Sigerson. New York: Hafner Publishing Company, 1962.
2. Gowers W. A Manual and Atlas of Medical Ophthalmoscopy. London: J & A Churchill, 1879.
3. Nover A. The Ocular Fundus: Methods of Examination and Typical Findings. Philadelphia: Lea and Febiger, 1981.
4. Ravin JG. Sesquicentennial of the ophthalmoscope. Arch Ophthalmol 1999;117:1634–1638.
5. Rucker CW. A History of the Ophthalmoscope. Rochester, MN: Whiting Printers, 1971.
6. Albert DM, Miller WH. Jan Purkinje and the ophthalmoscope. Am J Ophthalmol 1973;76:494–499.
7. McHenry LC. Garrison's History of Neurology. Springfield, IL: Charles C Thomas, 1969;153.
8. Rosen ES, Savir H. Basic Ophthalmoscopy: Ophthalmoscopic Diagnosis in System Disorders. London: Butterworth, 1997.
9. McKendrick JG. The Encyclopedia Britannica (11th ed). New York: 1910;13:248–249.
10. von Helmholtz H. Description of an ophthalmoscope for examining the retina in the living eye. Translated by RW Hollenhorst. In H von Helmholtz (ed), Beschreibung eines Augen-Spiegels zure Untersuchung der Netzhaut im lebenden Augen. Berlin: A Forstner, 1851. Arch Ophthalmol 1951;46: 565–583.
11. McKendrick JG. The Encyclopedia Britannica (11th ed). New York: 1910;12:315.
12. McHenry LC. Garrison's History of Neurology. Springfield, IL: Charles C Thomas, 1969;288.
13. Hughlings Jackson J. Lecture on optic neuritis from intracranial disease. In J Taylor (ed), Selected Writing of John Hughlings Jackson. London: Hodder and Stoughton, 1932.
14. McHenry LC, Gowers W. The beginnings of clinical neurology. In Gowers W (ed), A Manual of Neurologic Diseases. Birmingham: The Classics of Medicine Library, 1981;13–30.
15. Allyn WG. Welch Allyn: An American Success Story. New York: WG Allyn, 1996.
16. Schett A. The Ophthalmoscope. Translated by DL Blanchard. In Hirschberg's History of Ophthalmology. Ostend: JP Wayenborgh, 1996.
17. Keeler CR. The Ophthalmoscope Atlas Monograph. In Hirschberg's History of Ophthalmology. Ostend: JP Wayenborgh, 1997.
18. Gartner S, Billet E. Mydriatic glaucoma. Am J Ophthalmol 1957;43:975–976.
19. Harris LS. Cycloplegic-induced intraocular pressure elevations. Arch Ophthalmol 1968;79:242–246.
20. Mauger TF, Craig EL. Havener's Ocular Pharmacology. St. Louis: Mosby, 1996;53–171.
21. Airaksinen PJ, Tuulonen A, Werner EB. Clinical evaluation of the optic disc and retinal nerve fiber layer. In R Ritch, MB Shields, T Krupin (eds), The Glaucomas. St. Louis: Mosby, 1989;467–494.
22. Luff A, Elkington A. Better use of the ophthalmoscope. Practitioner 1992;236:161–165.
23. Pirsig J. Zen and the Art of Motorcycle Maintenance. New York: Bantam Books, 1974.
24. Mandava N, Guyer DR, Yannuzzi L. Fluorescin angiography. In M Yanoff, JS Duker (eds), Ophthalmology. Philadelphia: Mosby, 1999:8.1–8.6.
25. Yannuzzi LA, Rohrer MA, Tindel LJ, et al. Fluorescein angiography complication survey. Ophthalmology 1986;93:611–617.

2 What Should I Look for in the Normal Fundus?

Know the Range of the Normal Optic Disc

For the efficient use of the ophthalmoscope in medical practice, the student must be familiar with . . . the normal fundus oculi, with the changes in its appearance (congenital, &c) which are of significance, and also with those which are purely ocular significance.

William Gowers[1]

The appearance of the optic papilla in the normal state . . . [is] a well-defined and distinct borders, the cup-shaped depression in its center, finally, the slightly rosy tint which, on the one hand, distinguishes its peripheral portion, and which is due to the presence of the vasae propriae enclosed in the substance of the optic nerve. . . .

Jean-Martin Charcot[2]

It is an unfortunate thing that some investigators do not make allowance for differences in the appearance of the fundus in healthy people. . . those physicians who do not use the ophthalmoscope at all must frequently overlook an important pathological condition altogether.

John Hughlings Jackson[3]

Once you are familiar with the ophthalmoscope and positioning yourself and the patient, how do you know if the disc is normal?

What Are You Looking At?

The *anatomy* of the disc and retina drives the appearance of what you are going to see.

WHAT IS THE OPTIC DISC?

The optic disc is the visible consolidation of the retinal nerve fiber layer into a compact coaxial cable, the optic nerve. We can see all of the optic nerve axons at the optic disc because they pass through a fibrocollagenous structure known as the *lamina cribrosa*. The optic nerve is a cable consisting of 800,000–1.2 million axons that are an extension of the retinal ganglion cells of the retina. The axons travel via the optic nerve, chiasm, and optic tract to the lateral geniculate nucleus, where they synapse. Fibers from the lateral geniculate nucleus go on to the primary visual occipital cortex. The optic nerve is the anterior extension of the brain and is not a peripheral cranial nerve. The axons are covered with oligodendroglia and not Schwann cells. The optic nerves are covered with pia and arachnoid, bathed in cerebrospinal fluid, and surrounded by dura—just like the rest of the brain.

The optic nerve is divided into an intraocular portion (anterior to the scleral canal), a laminar portion (at the lamina cribrosa of the scleral canal), a retrolaminar portion (behind the scleral canal), an intraorbital portion (through the orbit) to the intracanalicular portion (within the bony wall), and an intracranial portion. The optic nerve measures only 1.5 mm in diameter intraocularly, but it becomes 3–4 mm wide after the lamina where the axons acquire a myelin coating just past the lamina cribrosa. What we see when we look into the eye are the optic disc and lamina.

Figure 2-1. Locate the intraocular portion of the optic nerve (in front of the scleral canal). Then notice the laminar portion at the level of the lamina cribrosa. The retrolaminar optic nerve is directly behind the globe, whereas the intraorbital optic nerve travels through the orbit to the bony optic canal (hence, intracanalicular). Finally, the intracranial portion of the optic nerve joins the opposite optic nerve at the chiasm.

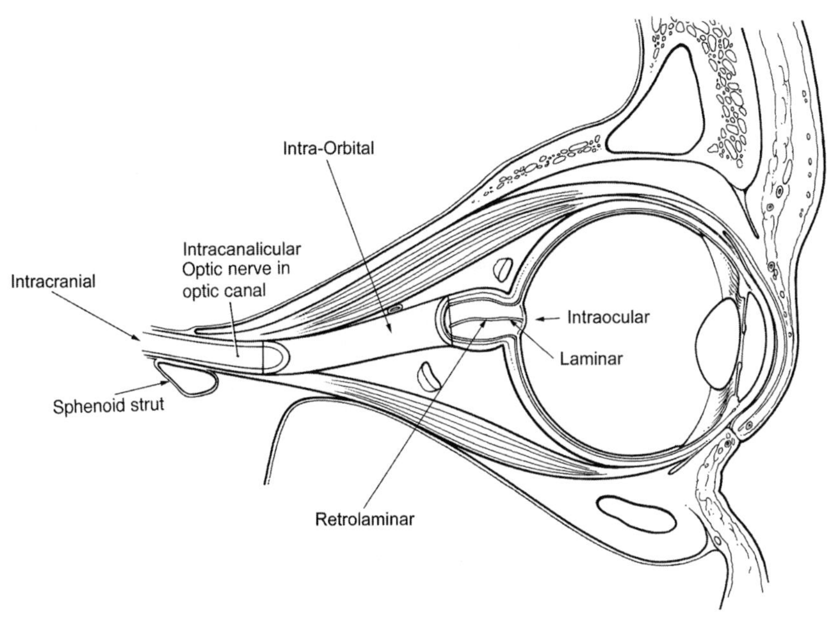

2-1

The optic nerve connects the globe of the eye to the brain. The globe of the eye has a structure that provides the best viewing optics while providing continuous nutrients and oxygen and protection from injury.

Figure 2-2. We need to know the basic disc anatomy to know what we are viewing. First, the dura mater (the covering of the brain) is contiguous with the sclera (the tough fibrous covering of the eye). The cerebrospinal fluid bathes the nerve beneath the dura. The retinal elements are inside the eye and are supported by the retinal pigment epithelium and the choroid. The disc is composed of axons traveling from the retinal ganglion cells through the fibrous lamina cribrosa (which is a connective tissue at the same level as the sclera) in the optic nerve. The blood supply is described in detail later, but this diagram shows the central retinal artery (which supplies the retinal elements) as well as the posterior ciliary artery (which supplies the choroidal elements); both of these arteries are branches from the ophthalmic artery.

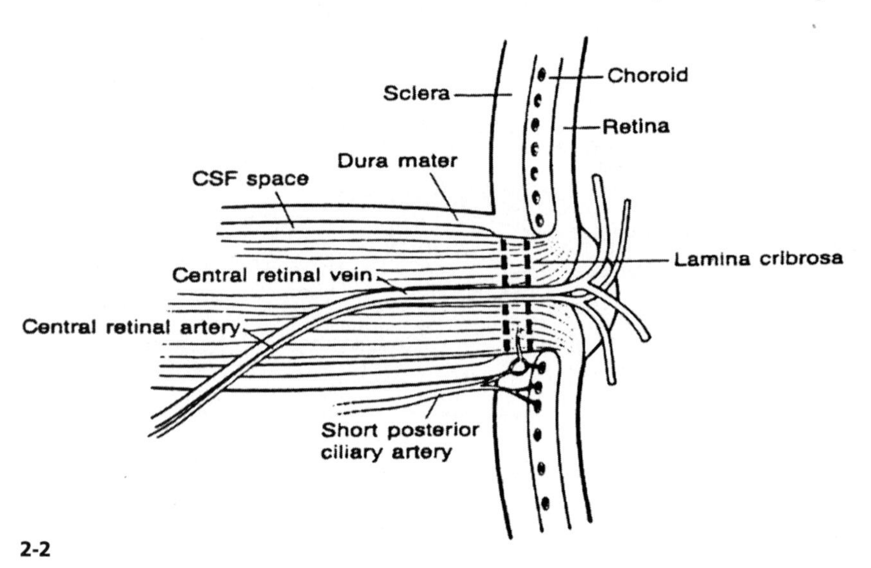

2-2

The optic disc appearance is determined by the size of the globe, the size of the scleral canal, how the nerve is inserted into the globe, the appearance of the lamina cribrosa, how densely the axons are packed, where myelination stops, and what is left behind in normal development.

Figure 2-3. A. The labeled photograph shows the structures that are discussed, including the scleral ring (the white, almost imperceptible ring around the disc), the disc, the cup, the neuroretinal rim, the arteries, and the veins. The lamina is also visible. Notice the cup-to-disc ratio in this eye is approximately 0.7. The cup-to-disc ratio is determined by dividing the diameter of the cup by the diameter of the disc. The cup diameter can be measured either horizontally or vertically and should be roughly roughly equal in both eyes. It may be difficult to identify the margin of the cup. Use the turn or bend of small vessels going over the neuroretinal rim as an indicator of cup margin when in doubt. Also notice that there are two cilioretinal arteries on this disc, located at 8:30 and 6:00 on the disc margin. Even though this is a disc with a large cup, it clearly demonstrates all of the major features that we must attend to when viewing the optic disc. B. Try to identify these structures on the unlabeled photograph.

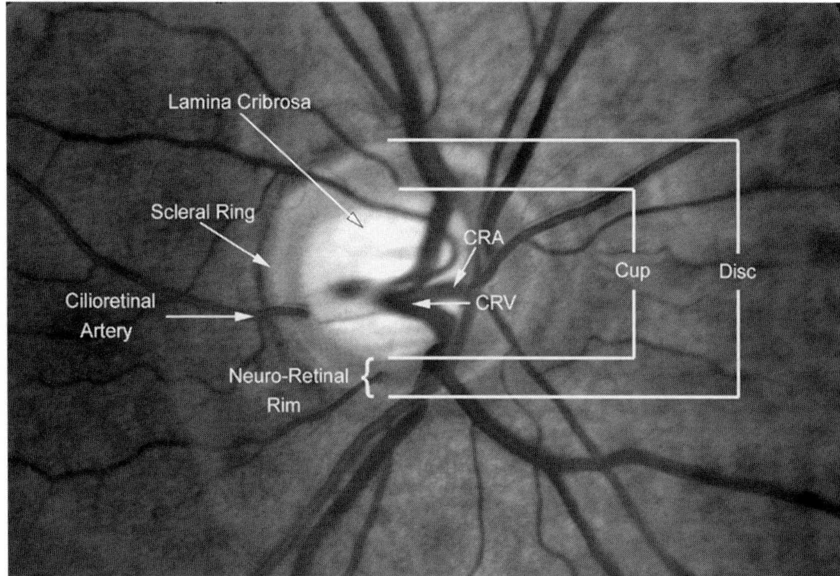

2-3A

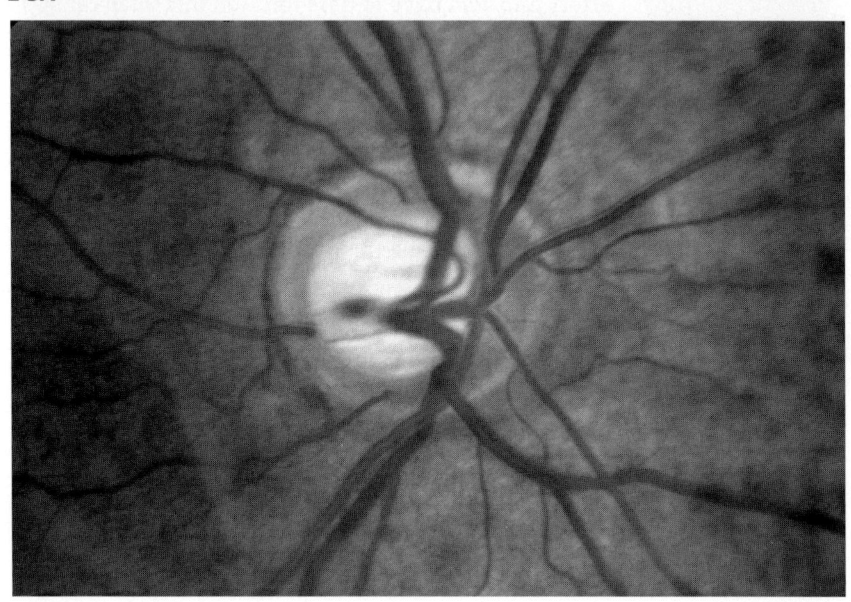

2-3B

SIZE OF THE EYE AND SIZE OF THE SCLERAL CANAL

Whether the globe is short (hyperopic, or farsighted) or long (myopic, or nearsighted) affects the size of the scleral canal and also the configuration of the lamina cribrosa. We all have different-sized scleral canals and lamina cribrosae. Let us look at the two extremes—hyperopia and myopia—so that we can appreciate the wide variations of normal.

Hyperopia is a term for a globe that is foreshortened, resulting in a refractive error. The disc may appear smaller, in part, owing to the refractive error. Small scleral canals are seen in shorter eyes. Therefore, the disc usually has a small or nonexistent cup. There is little or no visible lamina cribrosa. These discs, because they are hyperemic and have no cup, can be confused with pathologic disc swelling (papilledema).

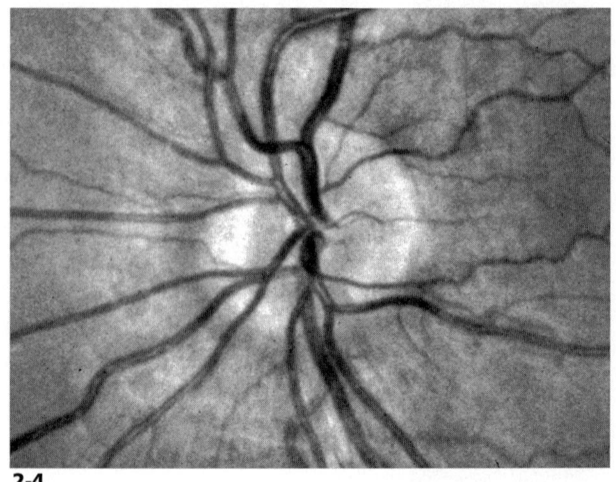

2-4

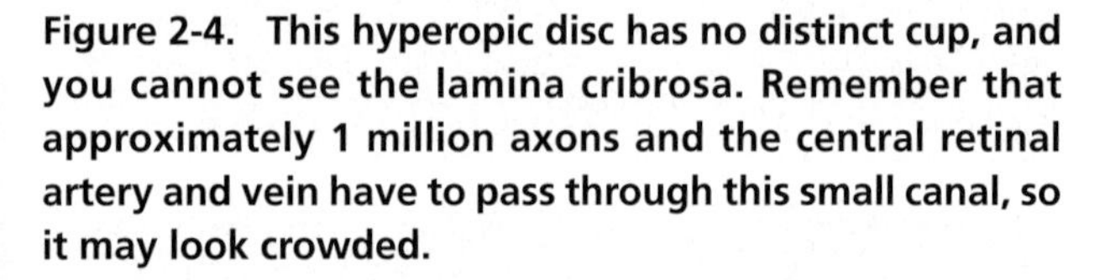

Figure 2-4. This hyperopic disc has no distinct cup, and you cannot see the lamina cribrosa. Remember that approximately 1 million axons and the central retinal artery and vein have to pass through this small canal, so it may look crowded.

Little red discs are related to hyperopic discs in that they are also small and red. H. Stanley Thompson and James J. Corbett coined the term "little red disc" to denote small, hyperemic discs easily and frequently mistaken for papilledema. Little red discs are not always hyperopic discs, but commonly are caused by small scleral canals: The 1 million axons and blood vessels have to squeeze through a tight space. You can recognize them by looking for a small disc that is hyperemic. Sometimes they are even a bit elevated centrally, but there is no axonal swelling.

Figure 2-5. A–C. **Gowers said, "Attention to tint of disc alone is a prolific source of error in ophthalmoscopy."[1] The "little red discs" show a small, crowded disc that can often be mistaken for a pathologically swollen disc.**

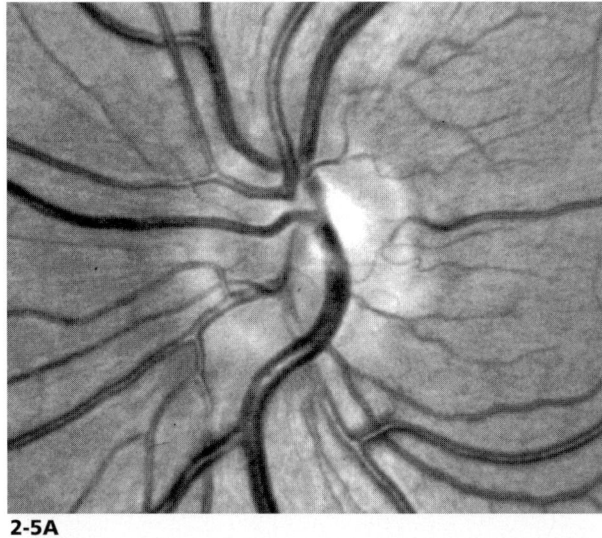

2-5A

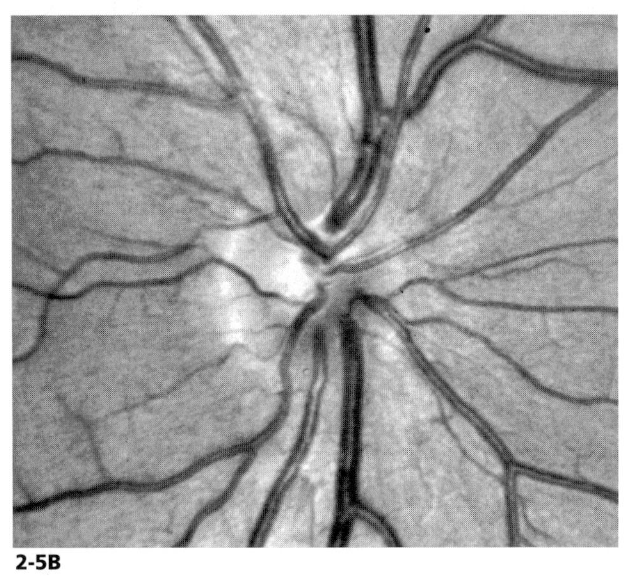

2-5B

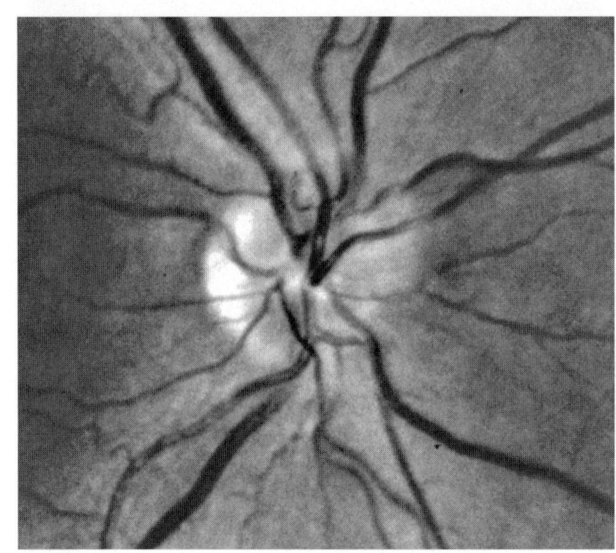

2-5C

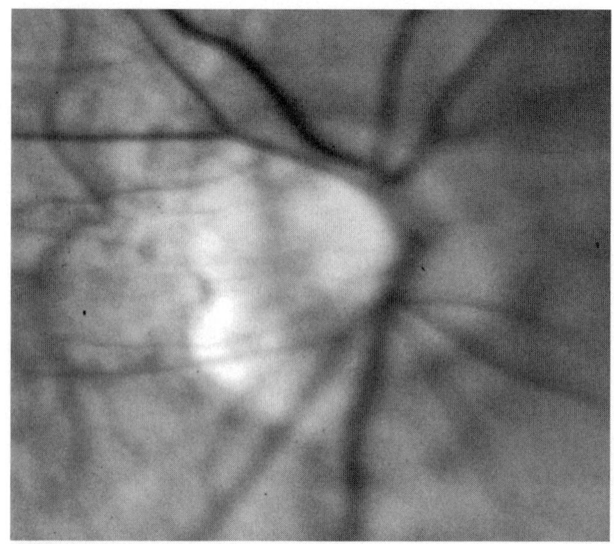

2-6A

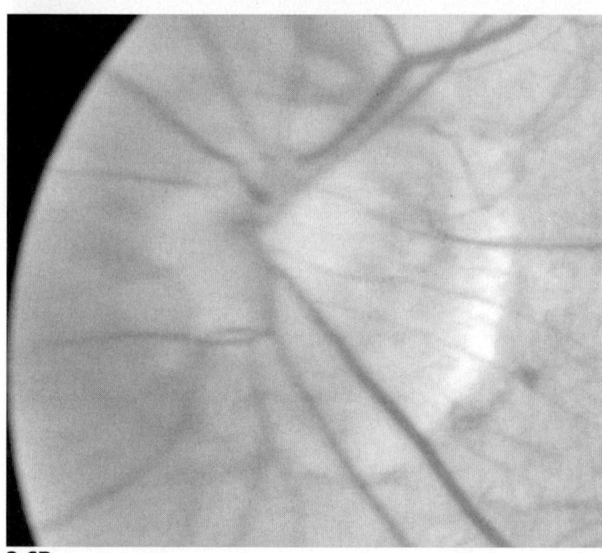

2-6B

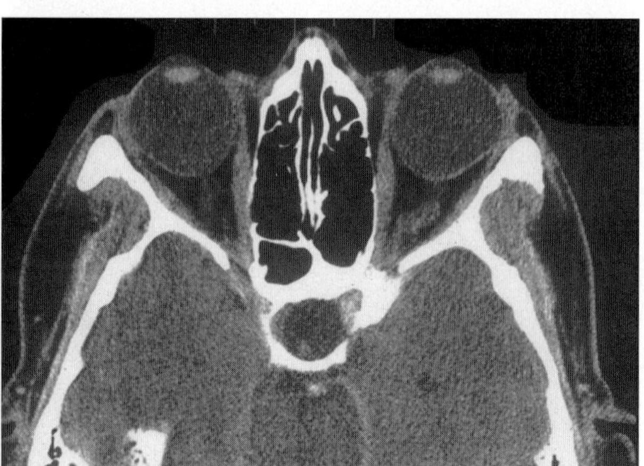

2-7

Myopia is extremely common. It occurs in 25% of the white population aged 12–17 years and 12% of the black population aged 12–17 years in the United States.[4] Although myopia can have profound ophthalmoscopic changes, most myopia is "simple"—that is, there is only a slight or moderate physiologic variation in refraction. Owing to the elongated globe and the larger scleral canal, the retinal, choroidal, and retinal pigment epithelium (RPE) elements fail to extend all the way to the edge of the scleral canal, frequently leading the myopic disc to have a variable scleral temporal crescent. Large physiologic cupping is seen most frequently with myopia because of the larger scleral canal. Estimating the size of the optic cup relative to the optic disc is important (see below). The optic cup size is genetically and racially determined, and directly relates to the size of the scleral canal. Blacks tend to have a broader optic cup than whites.

Figure 2-6. The discs shown here [(A), right eye; (B), left eye] are typical of myopia. Not only is there an enlarged cup, but, because of the large size, there are temporal crescents. The disc appears out of focus because the camera is focused on the retina.

Figure 2-7. CT of myopic globes: Look at the large globes that fill the orbit. This woman's chief complaint was transient visual obscuration whenever she moved her eyes.

Figure 2-8. Examples of high myopia. A. Notice the normal retinal elements are not next to the disc, and there is significant peripapillary atrophy and pigmentation. B. Identify the disc margin—the disc is slightly tilted, and the margin of the retina has pulled away from the disc. There is blotchy pigmentation overlying the exposed sclera. These discs are difficult to envision with the ophthalmoscope alone, so it is better to use the patient's refraction for viewing these cases and to be sure they are dilated.

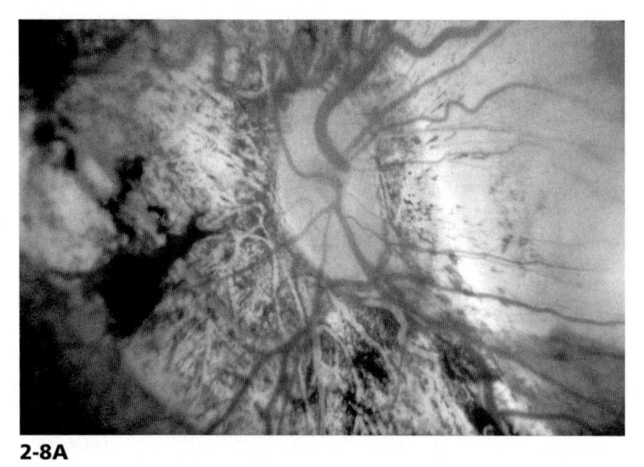

2-8A

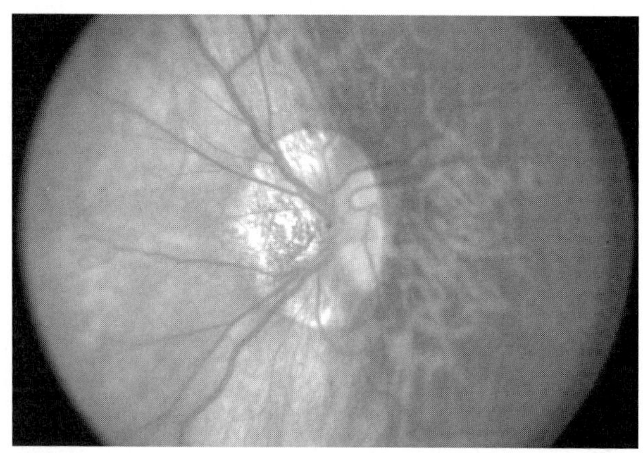

2-8B

Even when the scleral canal is the same size, you may see differences in the cup-to-disc ratio.

Figure 2-9. Although the scleral canal size is similar in these discs, there is a difference in the cup-to-disc ratio. The right cup-to-disc ratio (A) is approximately 0.6 and the left cup-to-disc ratio (B) is approximately 0.3. Whenever you see cup-to-disc asymmetry, you must consider the cause. Although the asymmetry may not be associated with any pathologic condition, the patient's intraocular pressure should be checked for evidence of glaucoma. Glaucoma is one of the most important causes of asymmetry of the cup-to-disc ratio.

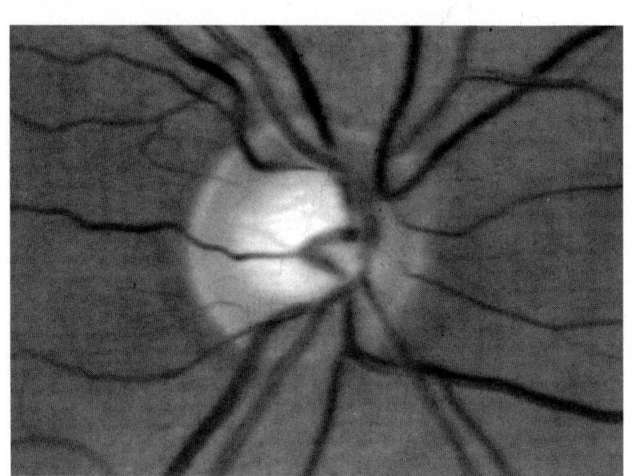

2-9A

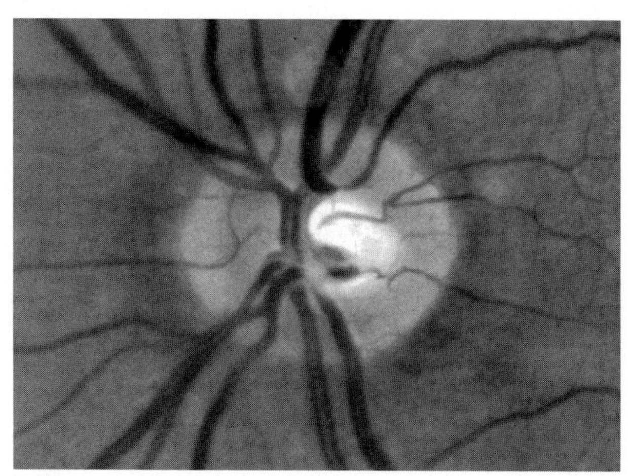

2-9B

A "scleral ring," a white circle variably surrounding the disc, may be seen, and in some the ring is prominent. When the retinal/choroidal elements do not meet the scleral canal, a space develops. This space consists of sclera, pigment, or both, and is called a *temporal crescent.* A temporal crescent can be mistaken for "disc pallor" or as part of the disc. Crescents are present in 25% of people, and most of these (three-fourths) are temporally located, with the rest mainly inferior to the disc (see also the discussion of the tilted disc, Figures 2-13 and 2-14). If the patient is myopic, a temporal crescent is often present and can even be quite large, and more progressive pulling away of the retina from the disc margin is myopic degeneration.

Figure 2-10. A. **Notice how the scleral crescent forms in the diagram.** B. **The left eye of a woman with a scleral crescent temporal to the disc.** C. **This woman has a crescent that extends around the disc. There is pigment in this crescent, and the disc has a nasal tilt. This is a myopic disc. We have circled the disc; arrows point to where the retinal elements have pulled away from the disc.** D. **Another temporal fundus ectasia.**

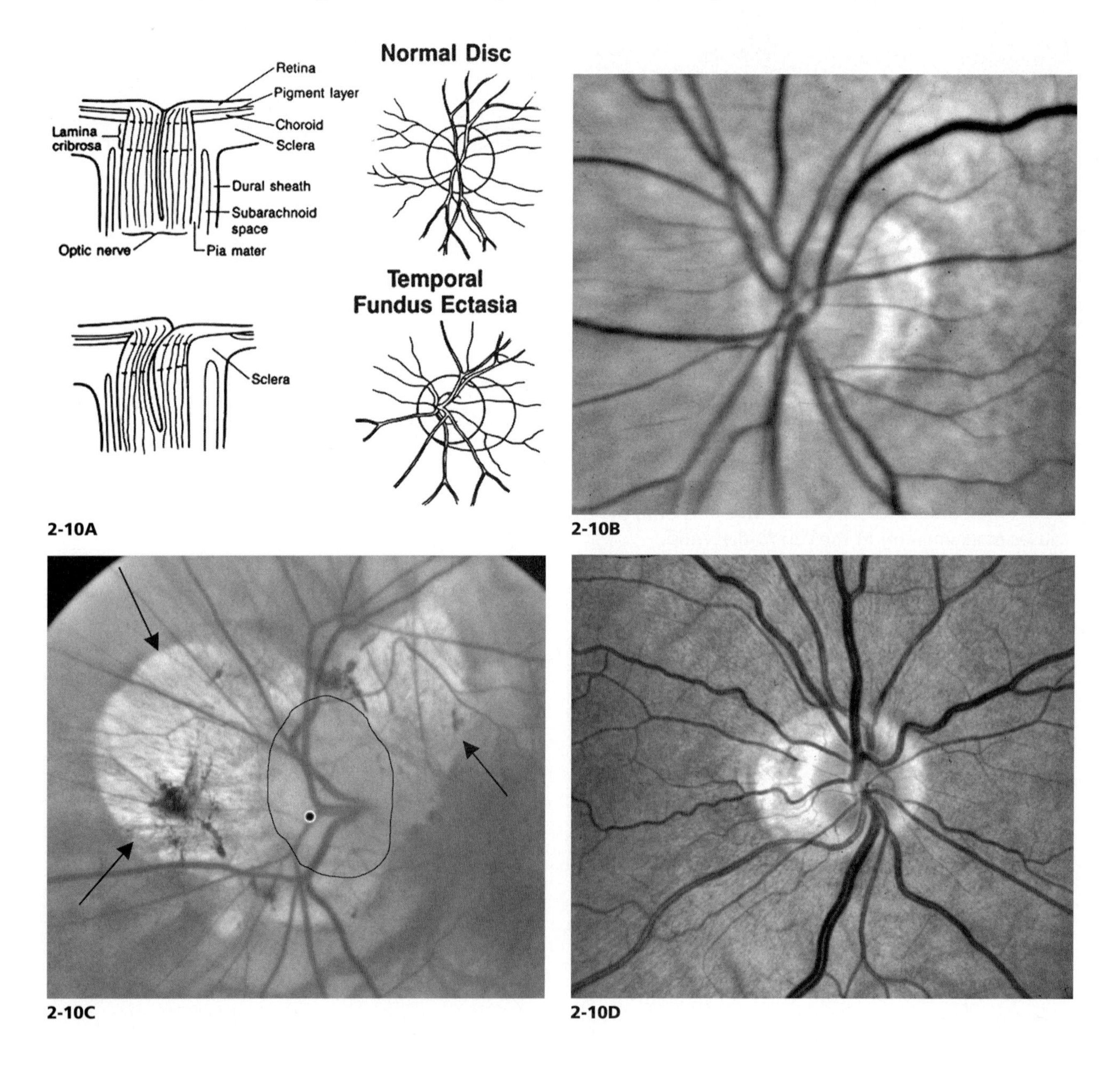

The other element that surrounds the optic nerve as it passes through the scleral canal is the choroid—a richly vascular structure that supplies the deep retina, including the rods, the cones, and the RPE. The choroid or choriocapillaris is red, owing to the rich blood supply. The RPE contains melanin; therefore, some individuals may have visible pigment next to the disc in addition to the white of the sclera. If the RPE is thickened near the optic disc, pigment can be seen around the crescent or around the disc as a normal variant in many people. Notice the pigment around the temporal crescent shown in Figure 2-10C. Furthermore, when there is damage to the retina, the peripapillary area, or both, there may be a pigmented scar.

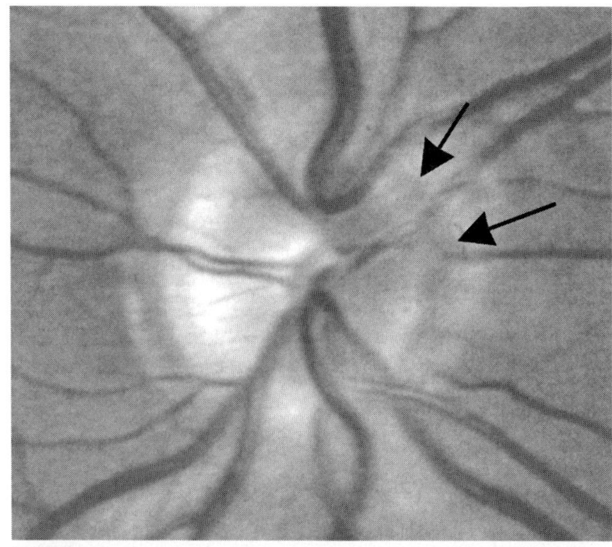

2-11A

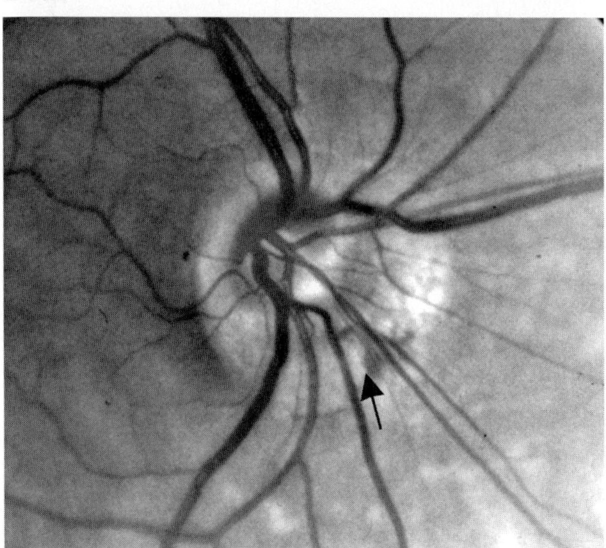

2-11B

Figure 2-11. A. **This disc shows a very small nasal pigmented crescent (*arrows*).** B. **A nasal crescent in a myopic disc with pigment inferiorly (*arrow*).**

Another element that has a profound effect on the appearance of the disc and, as we shall see, the functional anatomy and even disease states, is the lamina cribrosa. The *lamina cribrosa* (Latin: "a thin-layered sieve") is a perforated, fibrocollagenous weave of holes or connective tissue "sieve" support structure that bundles the roughly 1 million axons as they make a right-angled turn from the retina to become the optic nerve. In about one-third of eyes, the lamina cribrosa clearly can be seen. The lamina cribrosa is one of the most important structures related to the optic disc.

The lamina cribrosa is derived from the sclera, with lesser contributions from the pia mater and the perivascular sheaths of the central retinal artery (CRA) and central retinal vein (CRV). The lamina is deep and not well seen in hyperopic eyes, whereas in myopic eyes, the lamina is more completely seen because the disc is broader and shallower.

Figure 2-12. A. **This diagram depicts the connective tissue of the lamina. It houses the central retinal vein and artery in a shared vascular wall. It also shows the "pits" of the lamina through which the nerve fiber layer travels.** B. **In discs with larger cups, you may be able to see the lamina (*arrows* point to small, barely visible indentations of the lamina).** C. **Notice that deep in the cup there are pitlike indentations (*arrows*) of the lamina cribrosa. The lamina is easier to see in discs with a larger cup. The next time you see a large cup, look for laminar dots.**

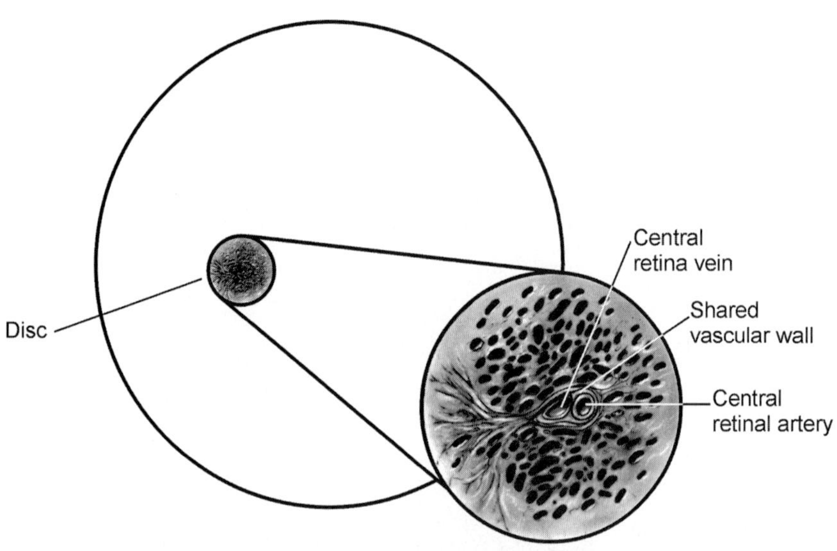

2-12A

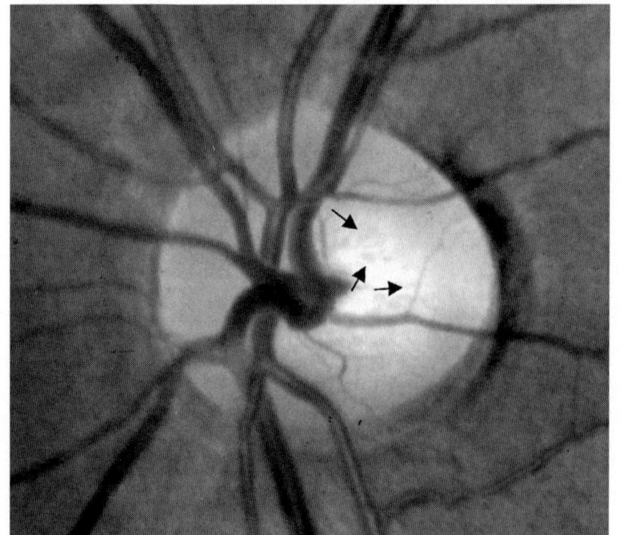

2-12B

2-12C

The optic nerve's exit from the globe lies normally at a nasally acute angle of less than 45 degrees. When there is a more acute (oblique) insertion of the optic nerve to the globe, a tilted disc results. Oblique insertions are very common, occurring in 18% of eyes examined pathologically.[5] Sometimes these are called *dysversions*, because there is an extreme change in the angle of nerve-to-globe insertion. The most common form of tilt is elevation of the superior temporal disc and posterior displacement of the inferior nasal disc. The vessels exit the disc as if spilling from a cornucopia. Tilted discs are associated with situs inversus (the vessels out of the disc run nasally before turning temporally), thinning of the choroid, and RPE leaving a crescent. Many names have been given to this anomaly, including: Fuchs' inferior coloboma, inferior conus, inverse myopia, heterotypical crescent, inversion of the optic disc, and dysversion of the optic disc.[6] Optic disc tilt and crescents can be distinguished from myopic crescents by many factors.

Table 2-1. Distinguishing Myopic from Tilted Optic Disc Crescents

	Myopic crescent	Tilted optic disc
Etiology	Enlargement of the globe with stretching	Related to the embryonic fissure
Location	Almost always temporal	Usually inferior, but can be any direction
Clinical appearance	Temporal flattening of the disc due to stretching; may merge with floor of cup	Sloping to the direction of the defect, does not merge with cup
Refraction	Myopic low and high	Variable—usually myopic astigmatism
Ophthalmic evaluation	Visual field may show enlarged blind spot	Visual field may show bitemporal hemianopia, which is refractive
Vessels	Usually normal	Situs inversus common
Differential diagnosis	Myopic degeneration; enlarged cup-to-disc ratio (can be confused with glaucoma)	Must sometimes be differentiated from intracranial disease due to the visual field defect (e.g., pituitary tumor)
Clinical course	May progress around the disc if myopic degeneration	Not progressive

Source: Adapted and revised from DJ Apple, MF Rabb, PM Walsh. Congenital anomalies of the optic disc. Surv Ophthalmol 1982;27:3–43.

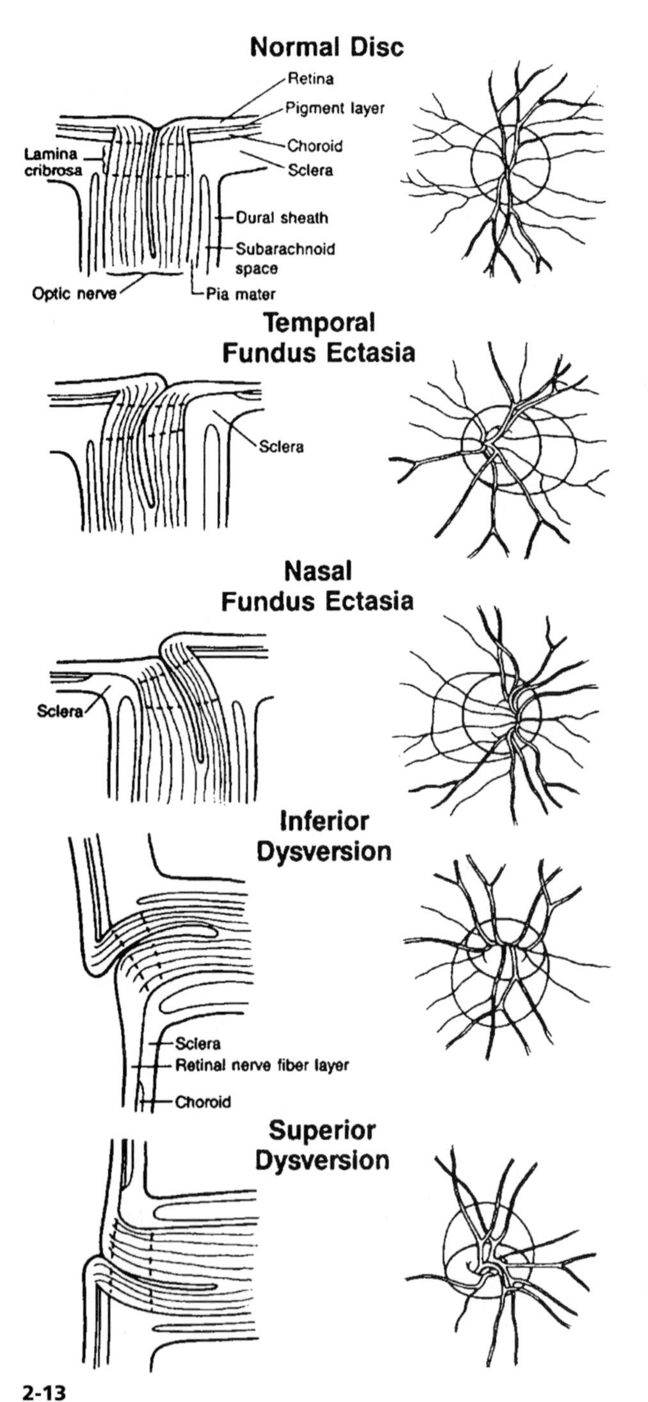

2-13

Figure 2-13. When the optic nerves insert into the globe at an extreme angle, a tilted disc results. A tilted disc is common. Notice that the disc can tilt in almost any direction. Frequently, there is also a change in direction of the vessels, in which the vessels emerge from the optic cup in the direction of the crescent, as if from a cornucopia. These drawings are modifications of work done by von Szily in 1909.

A common disc anomaly, tilted discs, affects approximately 1–2% of people examined.[6] There is equal gender prevalence. Approximately three-fourths of patients have bilaterally tilting discs. Tilted discs are common in patients with hypertelorism. Frequently, the crescents are inferior in location as opposed to myopic crescents, which are temporal to the disc. The crescent may be large or small. The larger the crescent, the more chance of associated myopia; myopia occurs in 90%, and astigmatism is common.[6] Because the superior part of the nerve can look elevated, these defects can be mistaken for papilledema. Vision tends to be normal or only slightly decreased (20/25 to 20/50).

Figure 2-14. A–H (opposite page). **Ophthalmoscopic appearance is of an oval disc (almost football-shaped) from which the vessels may exit inferiorly, superiorly, nasally, and temporally, as if from a cornucopia. The disc may also have hypopigmentation of the ectatic part or a crescent. The direction of the crescent is toward the side of the tilt, as most discs (70%) tilt inferiorly. These discs show temporal** (A,B), **superior** (C,D), **inferior** (E,F), **and nasal** (G,H) **disc dysversion. The temporal dysversion disc in** (B) **is also myopic. Notice that the vessels point to the direction of the dysversion, like a cornucopia. Also notice that there is situs inversus (i.e., the vessels head nasally before heading temporally).**

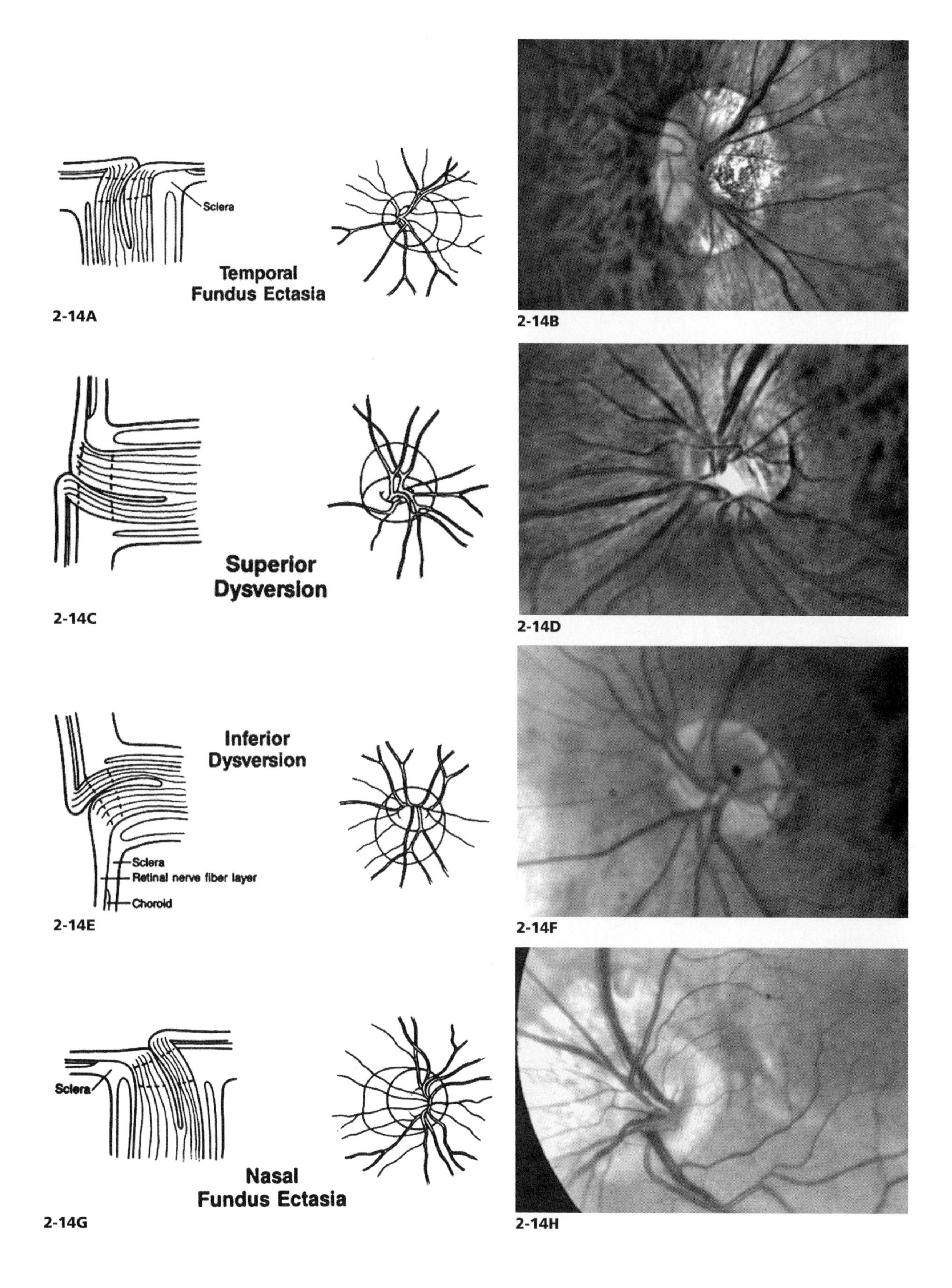

2-14A

2-14B

2-14C

2-14D

2-14E

2-14F

2-14G

2-14H

Figure 2-15. A–C. These discs display bilateral superior dysversion. The computed tomography scan shows the oblique insertion of the optic nerves into the globes. (Photographs courtesy of William Fletcher, M.D., University of Calgary.)

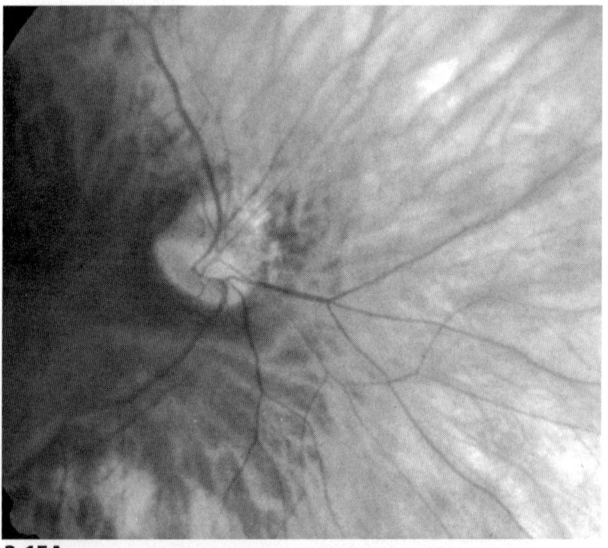

2-15A

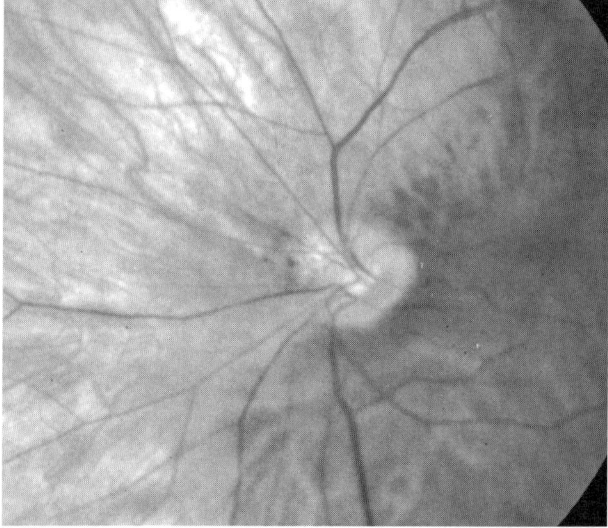

2-15B

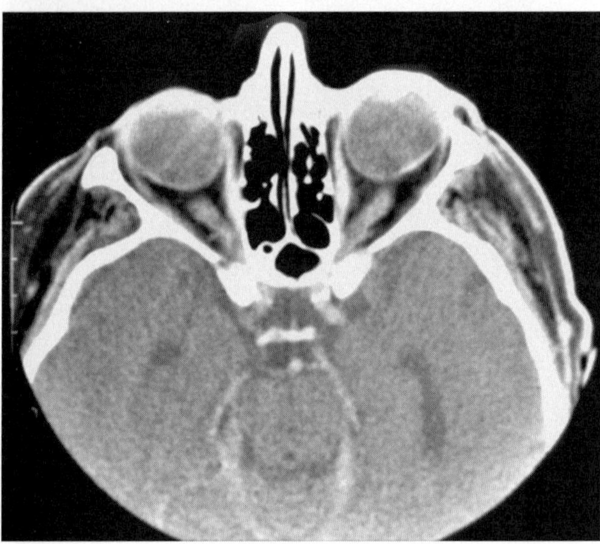

2-15C

Visual field defects are common and occur especially in the superior temporal region (related to the inferior ectasia of the fundus). However, the defect appears like a bitemporal hemianopia defect that does not respect the vertical meridian. The defect can be refracted away with larger targets (e.g., on Goldmann visual fields) or by the use of corrective lenses (e.g., –4.00), which bring targets into focus on the displaced retina (from the tilted disc). Because of this visual field defect, computed tomography or magnetic resonance imaging of the chiasm is commonly obtained.

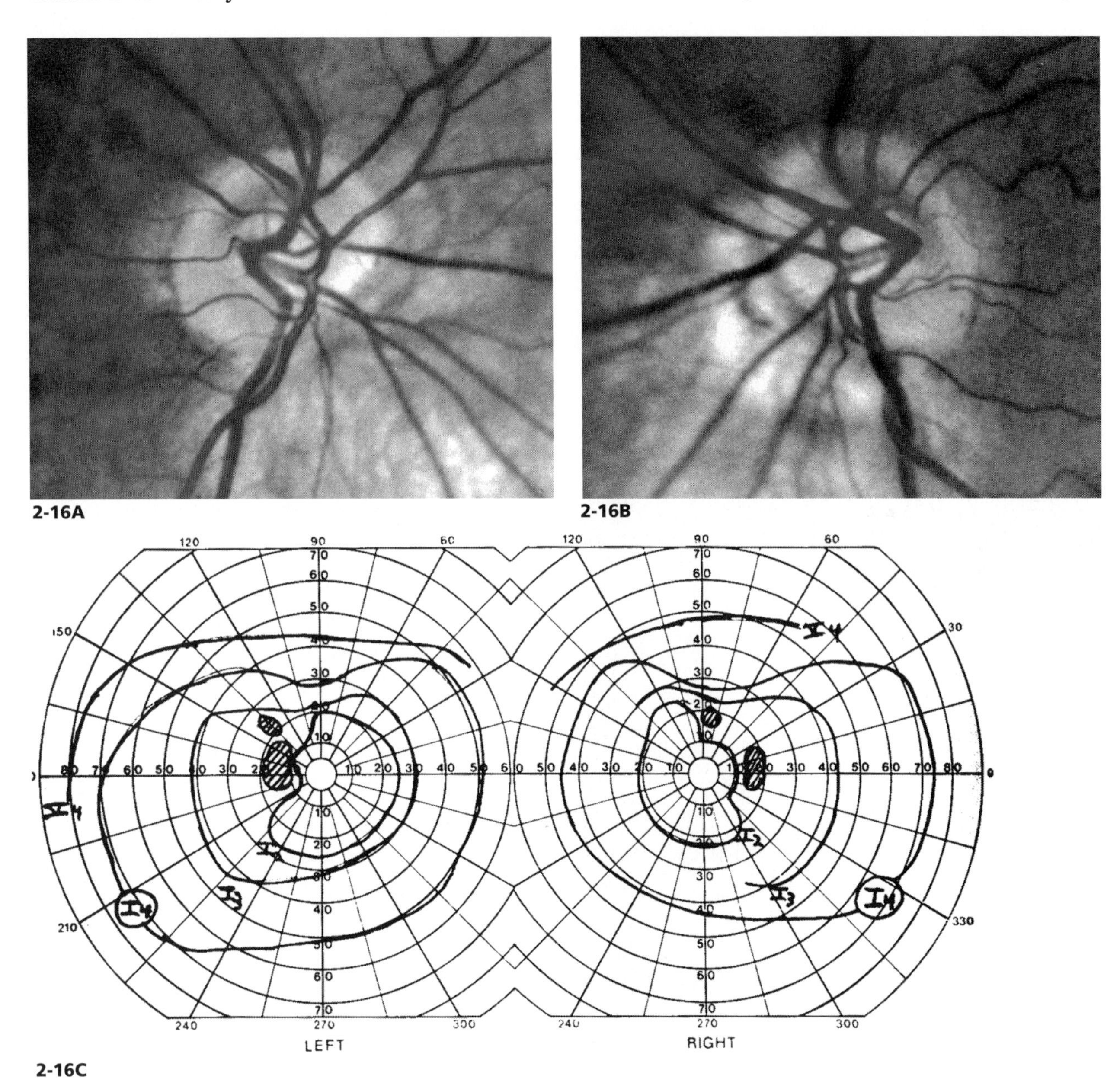

Figure 2-16. A–C. **This man has bilateral nasal dysversion (or tilted discs) in the right eye** (A) **and left eye** (B)**. Note that he has sloping visual field defects temporally** (C) **that could be misconstrued as bitemporal hemianopia, except that the defects are sloping, they do not respect the vertical meridian, and they refract (with plus lenses) away. Although these defects are found on formal visual field testing, they will not be present on visual field testing to standard confrontation testing.**

WHERE THE MYELIN STOPS

Myelin normally stops at the lamina cribrosa during fetal development. *Myelinated nerve fibers* are normal variants that may make the disc look elevated; however, other signs of swelling are absent. Myelination usually stops at the lamina cribrosa after starting at the lateral geniculate body at approximately the 5-month embryo stage. Autopsy studies have shown that myelination of retinal nerve fibers can be present in approximately 1% of people[8] and can be bilateral. They are found on routine examination of the disc.

Gowers wrote

The white patches of opaque nerve fibers are characterised by the partial concealment of the vessels, the feathery edge and by the centre of the disc being commonly unconcealed. When a small patch lies near, but separated from the disc, the resemblance to an inflammatory exudation may be puzzling; the characters of its edge will usually enable its nature to be recognized.[1]

2-17A

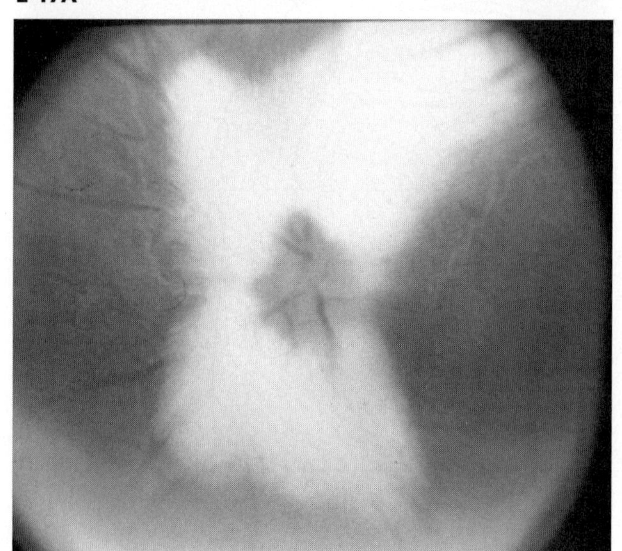

2-17B

Figure 2-17. A,B. **These individuals have myelinated nerve fibers. The myelination may be quite limited and be misconstrued as optic disc pallor** (A), **misinterpreted as nerve fiber layer infarcts** (B), **or misconstrued as papilledema. The key to the diagnosis is the feathery edge. Myelinated nerve fibers at the optic disc appear bright white and feather off at the edges. Look for the feathery edge!**

The myelination obscures the blood vessels. These fibers may be confused with papilledema because the disc can even be slightly elevated. There are many patterns to myelination, but all follow the nerve fiber layer. Myelination may begin at the disc and extend in one direction, it may extend in all directions, or there may be patches of myelination around the disc. Finally, myelination in the retina can appear as white patches that follow the nerve fiber layer in the periphery of the posterior pole (see Chapter 6, White Spots).

Some have speculated that defects within the lamina cribrosa may allow oligodendrocytes to produce myelin. Williams has imagined it to be a race between the oligodendrocyte myelinating to the retina against the formation of the lamina cribrosa. Myelination is therefore seen if the oligodendrocyte beats the formation of the lamina.[9] Myelinated nerve fibers have been known to progress or be acquired in adult life after surgery on the eye.[10,11]

Rarely, myelinated nerve fibers have been reported to disappear as the result of demyelinating disease such as multiple sclerosis, as well as conditions of syphilitic optic neuropathy, retinal artery occlusions, and glaucoma.[12]

WHAT WAS LEFT BEHIND IN DEVELOPMENT ALSO AFFECTS DISC APPEARANCE

A Bergmeister papilla is the product of a normal embryologic structure that has a central vascular core as well as a fibrous/glial sheath; the structure involutes in normal development, but can leave traces of itself in the form of a glial tuft or sheath over the optic nerve. It is part of the hyaloid system.

Of the tissue, Gowers said the following:

Peculiar white films sometimes lie in front of the vessels on the disc, looking like fragments of tissue paper or white gause, and allowing the vessels behind to be dimly seen. These may be left by a pathological process, but they are also frequent as a congenital condition, owing to an undue development at the back of the vitreous. When congenital, the vessels are merely concealed; when pathological they are constricted.[1]

If the papilla incompletely regresses, a glial tuft can be present on the disc. In an autopsy study, almost one-fourth had a glial membrane over the disc.[6] Because the papilla recedes into the cup, some have opined that absent or smaller physiologic cups may be more likely to have remnants of the papilla.[6]

Figure 2-18. The hyaloid system is prominent in the development of the eye. As the hyaloid artery regresses in normal development, the tissue reabsorbs. If, however, the artery is still present, you can see the artery attach to the lens (a Mittendorf dot), and the disc shows an attached ghost artery. There may be glial tissue on the disc or a vascular loop filled with blood reminiscent of that system. See also the discussion of persistent hyperplastic vitreous (in Chapter 11, Viewing the Disc in Children).

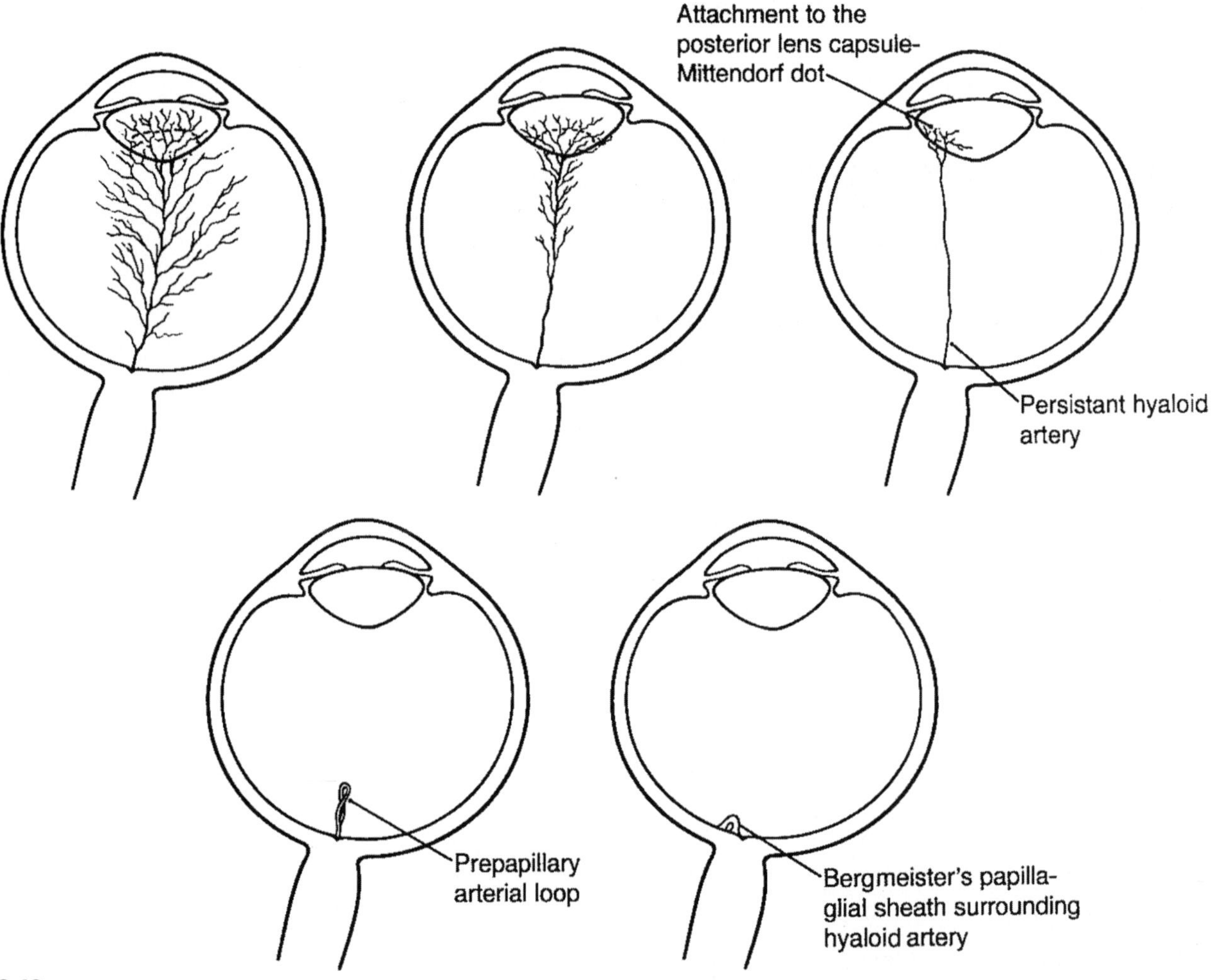

2-18

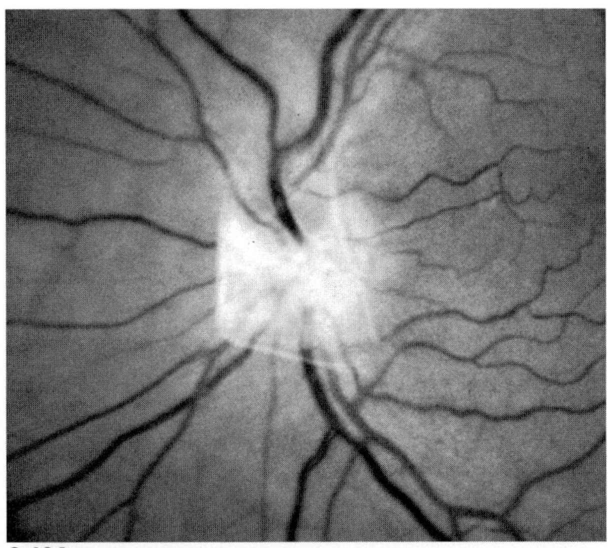
2-19A

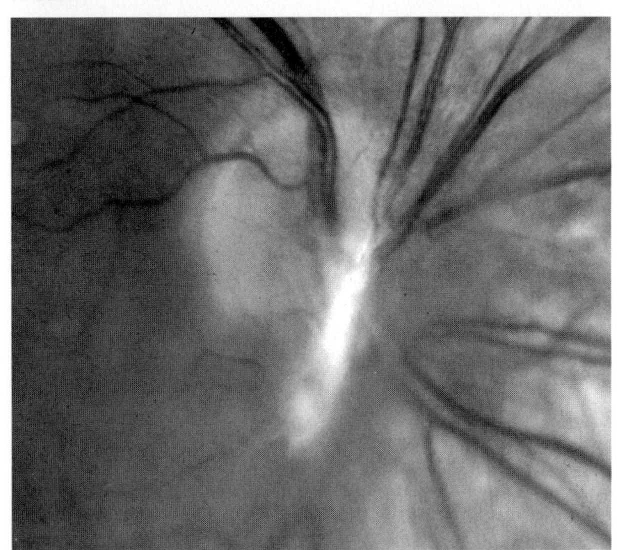
2-19B

Figure 2-19. A. **A glial remnant known as the *Bergmeister papilla* sits on the disc, obscuring the disc detail beneath. This one almost looks square. Notice that the blood vessels look normal.** B. **A white remnant of a ghost vessel protrudes into the vitreous cavity. The visual acuity was normal in** (A), **and the individual in** (B) **had a modest amblyopia.**

Some have speculated that the degree of involution of the papilla may determine the depth of the optic cup.[7] Persistent papillary membranes on the disc or remnants of the hyaloid system lead to glial tissue on the disc that can be mistaken for disc elevation or pallor. Usually the glial tissue obscures any cup, and may give the disc a gray cast and even obscure the vessels as they leave the disc.

There may be vascular loops on the disc as well that can be a remnant from the hyaloid artery. These loops are not generally confused with disc swelling, but can be confusing to observers. Whereas some vessels are loops, others look like extra-tortuous blood vessels. They may be very prominent superiorly on the disc. Dr. William F. Hoyt has called these "congenital pre-papillary arterial convolutions" (*personal communication*).

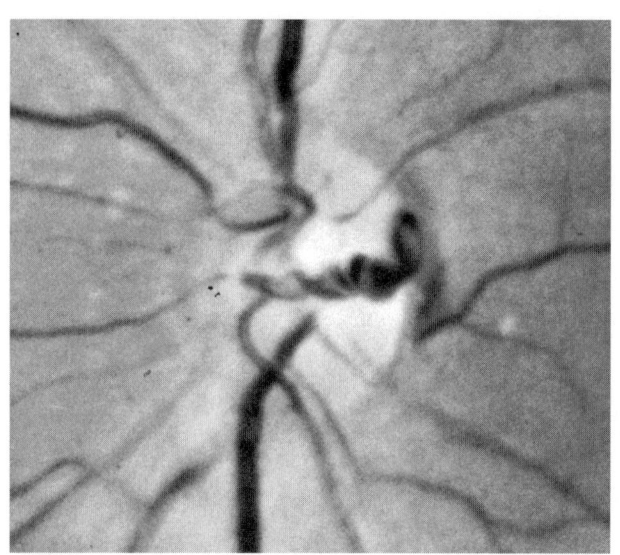

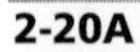

2-20A

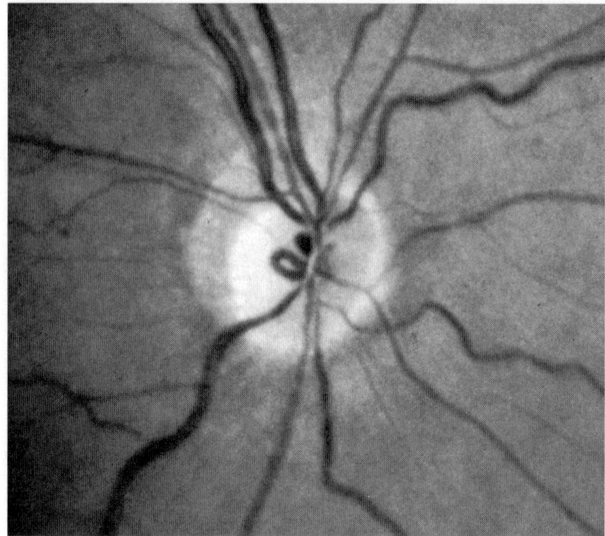

2-20B

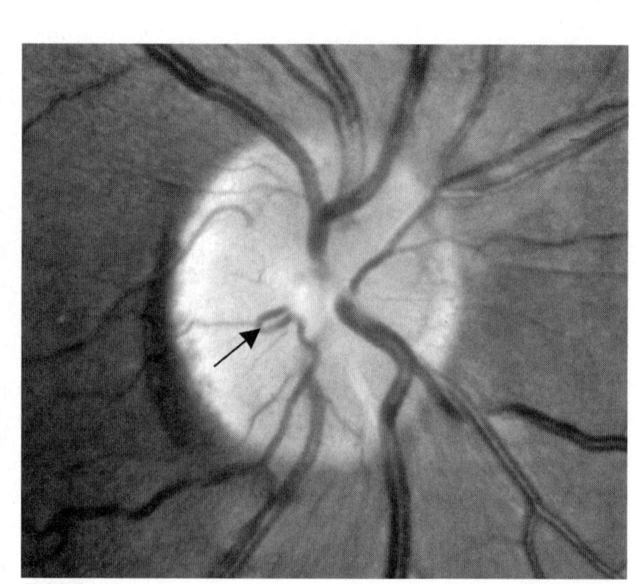

2-20C

Figure 2-20. A–C. **The vascular loop may be visible.** A. **Some have an almost corkscrew appearance projecting into the vitreal cavity.** B. **Some are small and barely visible except with close inspection.** C. **The hyaloid artery seen here comes out from the disc with rudimentary blood supply to the retina (*arrow*).**

WHAT MAKES UP THE APPEARANCE ON THE RETINAL FUNDUS?

The retina itself is completely transparent. So, what we see mainly is the supporting structures *beneath* the retina—the sclera, the choroid, and the RPE. We can also see if we look correctly at the top layer of the retina—the nerve fiber layer—those 1 million axons heading toward the disc.

The retina, an extension of the nervous system, is organized very much like the rest of the sensory system in the brain. Rods and cones are receptive-end organs that transmit to ganglion and bipolar cells. These form the nerve fiber layer, which becomes the optic nerve and tract (similar to the spinothalamic tract) to the lateral geniculate body—the relay station in the thalamus that synapses and conveys information to the primary visual cortex in the occipital lobe.[13]

Just as damage to the sensory or relay nuclei can affect the next cell's function and cause atrophy, pathologic processes within the retina affect vision and the appearance of the optic disc and nerve.

Knowing the layers of the retina is important in determining depths of pathologic lesions that we see. These layers affect the appearance of the lesions we observe because the layers are potential spaces.

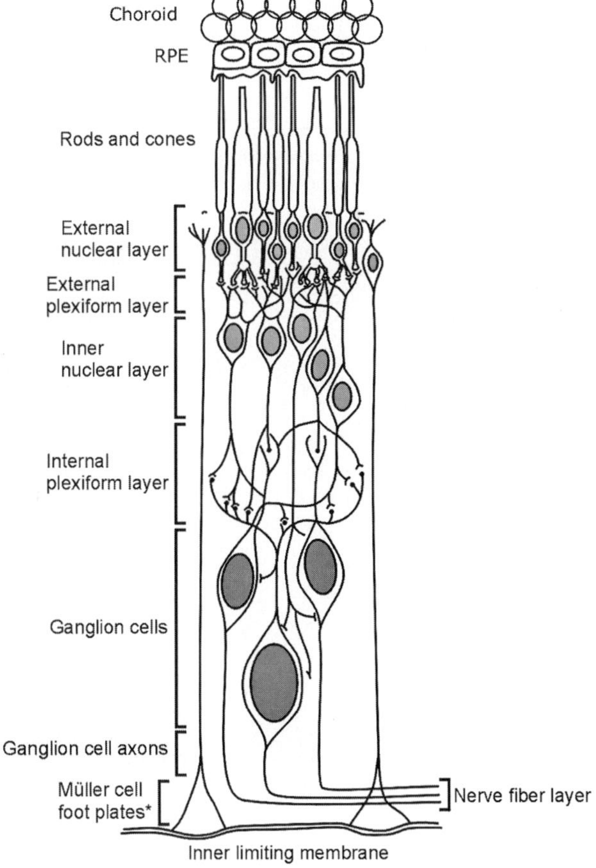

Figure 2-21. Find the following on this diagram: The inner limiting membrane (the footplate from the Müller cell); nerve fiber layer (the axon from the ganglion cell); ganglion cell layer (where the bipolar cells send information); inner plexiform layer (axons of the bipolar cells); inner nuclear layer with bipolar cells (as well as support cells like the Müller cell body, horizontal and amacrine [support] cells); external (outer) plexiform layer (which contains the axons of photoreceptors); external (outer) nuclear layer (which consists of the nuclei of the photoreceptors); external limiting membrane (which consists of attachment sites of the photo receptors and Müller cells [a support cell]); layers of rods and cones; retinal pigment epithelium—the support for the rods and cones; choroid blood supply to the rods and cones.

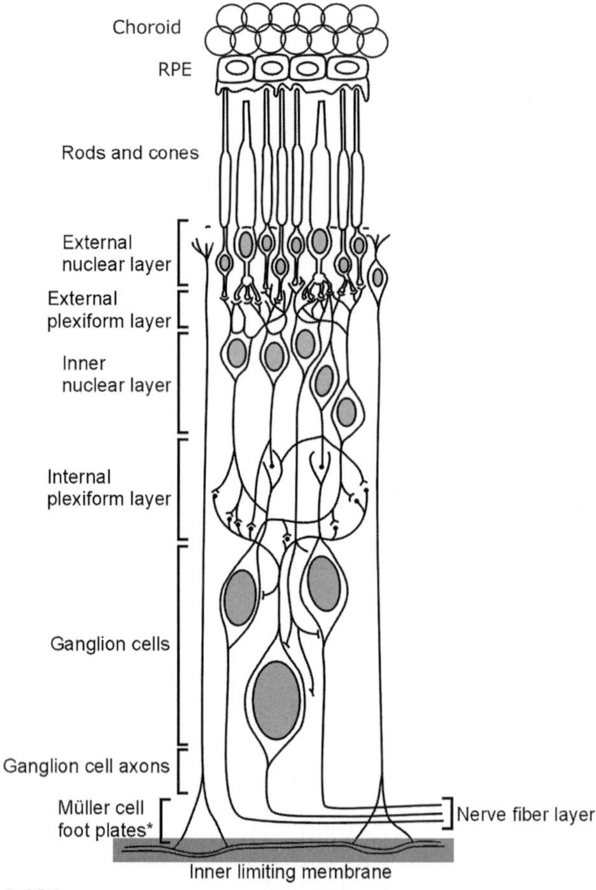

2-22A

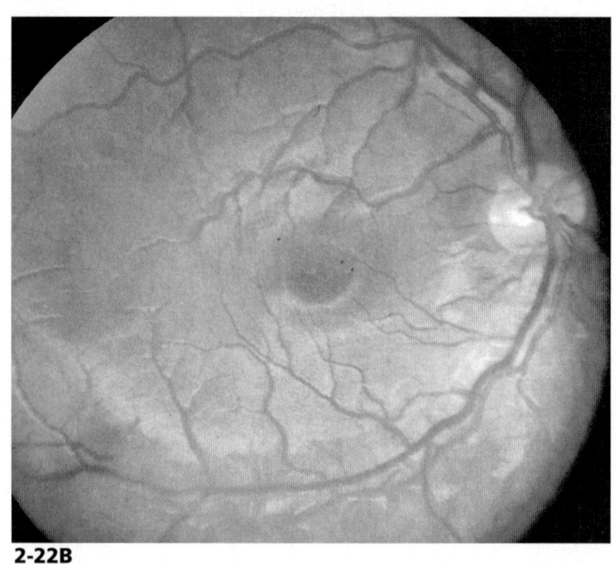

2-22B

IF THE RETINA IS TRANSPARENT, WHAT DO WE SEE WHEN WE VIEW THE FUNDUS?

The internal (or inner) limiting membrane separates the vitreous from the retina. In young, healthy individuals it appears as "retinal sheen" or "wetness" of the retinal surface, like plastic wrap that we use to cover foods. The sheen can be seen most easily temporal to the disc, and can even appear as a ring around the macula. The "glossy reflex" can be seen around major veins and arteries. As individuals age, the sheen becomes less visible. You can eliminate or change this light reflex with a slight change in the angle of the light of the ophthalmoscope.[14]

Figure 2-22. A. **Find the internal (or inner) limiting membrane (*shaded area*).** B. **This 13-year-old boy has typical retinal sheen of the light reflecting off of the internal limiting membrane. In young people, the internal limiting membrane makes the retina look shiny.**

The nerve fiber layer can be seen with practice in many individuals. Some have described the nerve fiber layer as a "sunburst effect"[15] and others as a "horse-hair."[16] Although the nerve fiber layer has been viewed with the red-free light since at least 1925, William Hoyt pointed out the usefulness of routinely viewing the nerve fiber layer to detect glaucoma and other optic neuropathies in which axons are lost.[14] To view the nerve fiber layer, the ophthalmoscope should be fully charged with a bright light. The red-free (green) filter should be used. The pupil needs to be widely dilated. Do not expect to visualize the nerve fiber layer well in blonde or lightly pigmented patients. You may also photograph the nerve fiber layer by using a red-free lens filter.[17]

Although you really cannot see each separate axon, when the axons come together in the peripapillary retina, bundles of nerve fibers can be seen easily, especially superiorly and inferiorly within one to two disc diameters of the disc. This is because the nerve fiber layer is thickest (approximately 200 μm) in the upper and lower portions of the optic nerve. At the temporal border, the nerve fiber layer is much thinner (60 μm).[16] The bundle of nerve axons least easily seen is the papillomacular bundle, because these axons are of smaller caliber, are very close to one another, and come straight to the disc. On the other hand, the loss of the papillomacular fibers tends to highlight the upper and lower bundles.[18]

Get used to viewing the different "bundles" of the nerve fiber layer—superior and inferior to the disc—and the arcuate bundles that stream temporally toward the macular area. These numerous fine fibers serve the nasal visual field, namely, the area of visual field most susceptible to damage from diseases that affect the optic nerve like glaucoma, papilledema, and optic neuritis. The nerve fiber layer overlies the retinal vessels and very slightly opacifies the underlying retinal vessels as they emerge from and enter the optic disc.[19]

Figure 2-23. A. **First, notice where the nerve fiber layer sits in the retina (*shaded area*).** B. **This diagram accentuates how the nerve fibers run into the disc from the retina. This is a left fundus. Appreciate the following: The bundles of fibers into the temporal superior and inferior poles; the long course of fibers entering into the superior temporal and inferior temporal region; the arching of fibers over and under the papillomacular bundle; and the papillomacular bundle.** C. **Next, view the normal nerve fiber layer in this right disc as seen with red-free black and white photography. This disc has a 0.3 cup-to-disc ratio. You can easily see the striations made toward the disc by the nerve fiber layer. (Photograph courtesy of William F. Hoyt, M.D.)**

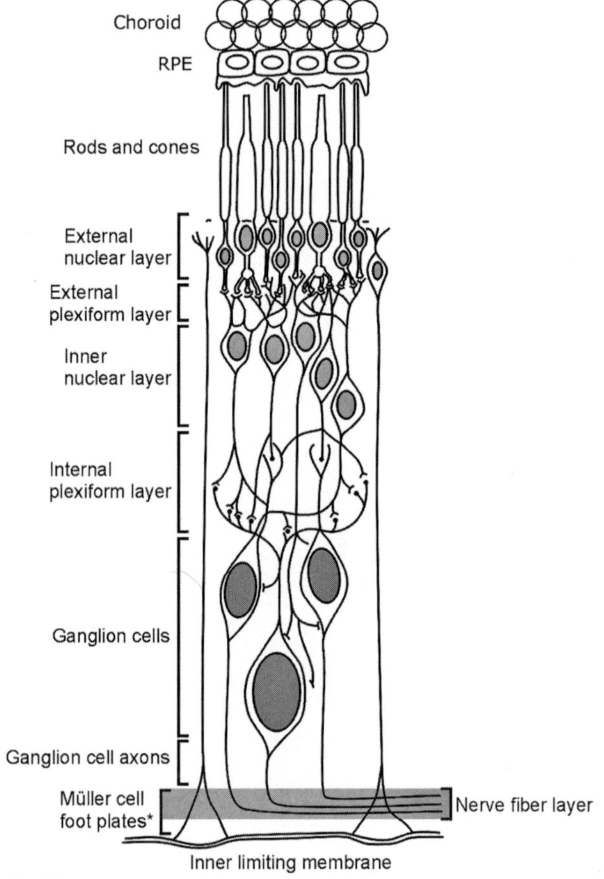

2-23A

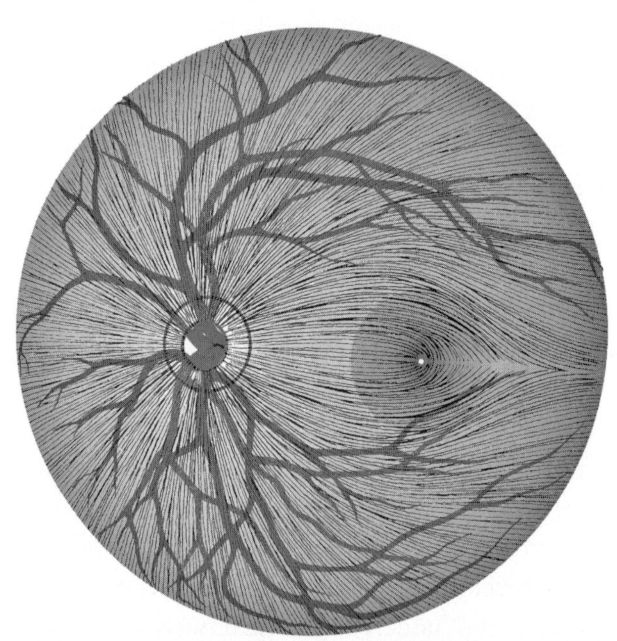

2-23B

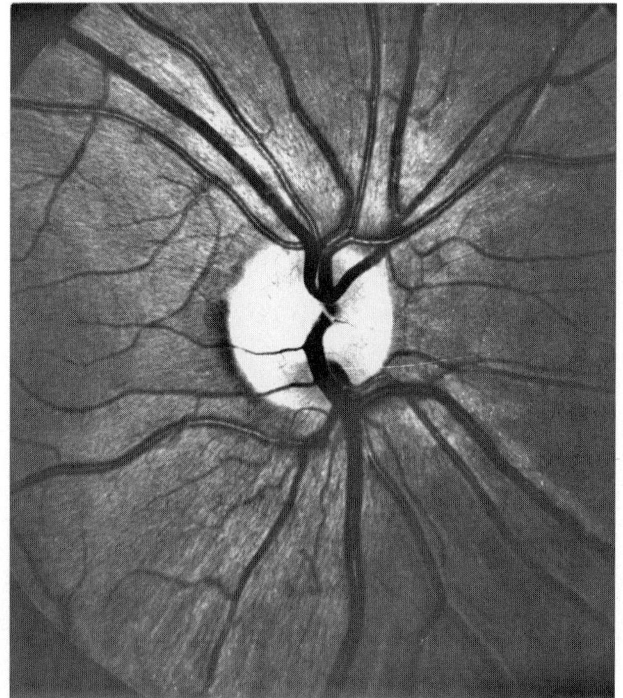

2-23C

WHAT CAUSES THE NERVE FIBER LAYER TO BE MORE EASILY SEEN?

The nerve fiber layer is more visible in someone with a small scleral canal, in which the fibers are jammed together, the disc is small and hyperemic, and there is no cup. This kind of nerve (the little red disc) is most commonly mistaken for disc swelling, as seen in Figure 2-24A–C. The nerve fiber layer can also become more visible when the axons are swollen, such as in anterior ischemic optic neuropathy, papillitis, or papilledema. Other metabolic changes in axonal transport such as nerve fiber layer infarction on the disc or retina (e.g., anterior ischemic optic neuropathy and cotton-wool spots) make the axons thicker and therefore more visible. The other way the nerve fiber layer is more visible is if there is a bundle missing: This provides clear contrast between the nerve fibers and the segment in which the nerve fibers are absent against the backdrop of the deeper red choroid and retinal pigment epithelium.

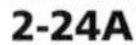

However, within the nerve fiber layer you may be able to observe Gunn's dot with your green (red-free) ophthalmoscope light. These are cell footplates from Müller's cells that slightly bulge out of the nerve fiber layer surface (see Figure 25A–C). Within the layers of the retina are supporting elements like Müller's cells, amacrine cells, and horizontal cells that help with visual processing. These "layers" are generally not observed by the ophthalmoscope.

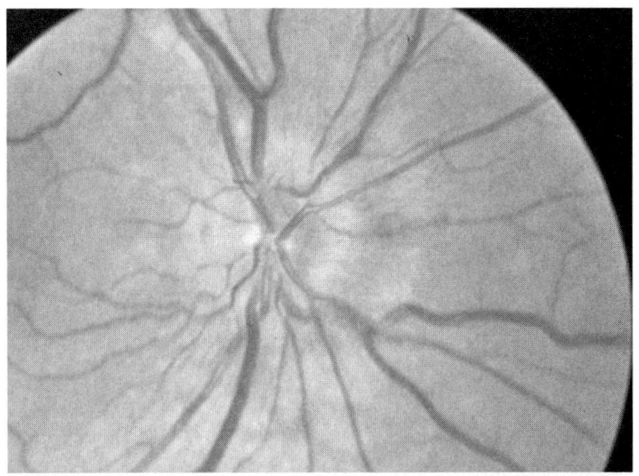

2-24A

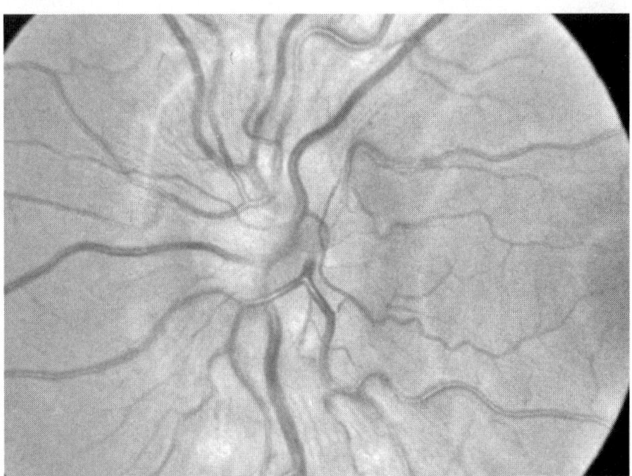

2-24B

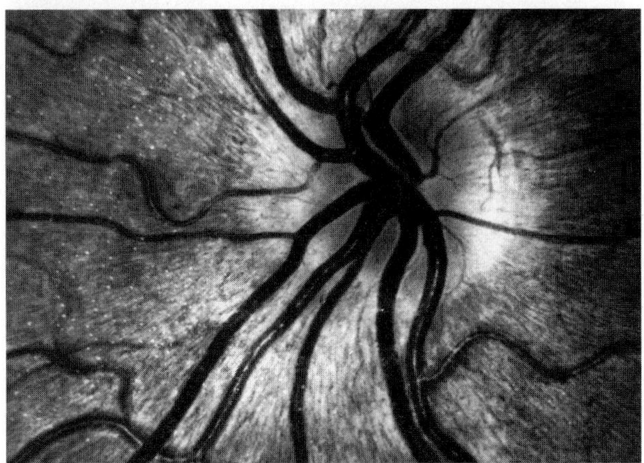

2-24C

Figure 2-24. A. **The nerve fiber layer is seen better in these discs with small scleral canals. The nerve fibers are jammed together, and there is no cup. Look at the disc margin: The elevation and striations are the nerve fiber layer. The disc almost looks elevated, as there are so many nerve fibers on this disc.** B. **This disc is significantly elevated because of the tightly packed nerve fiber layer. You can also appreciate the inner limiting membrane, given the shiny appearance of the retina. There is a lovely sheen off of the limiting membrane.** C. **This black and white photograph of the disc shows no cup, and the nerve fibers appear crowded. The nerve fiber layer is crisply seen. The little speckles are Gunn's dots. (Photograph courtesy of William F. Hoyt, M.D.)**

Figure 2-25. A–C. **The Müller cell foot plates are frequently seen as small bright specks in the nerve fiber layer called *Gunn's dots*.** A. **A close-up black and white photograph of Gunn's dots (*arrows*). (Courtesy of William F. Hoyt, M.D.)** B. **This red-free photograph shows the dots nicely, but they are subtle (*arrows*).** C. **Find the Müller cell foot plates on this diagram—these are Gunn's dots.**

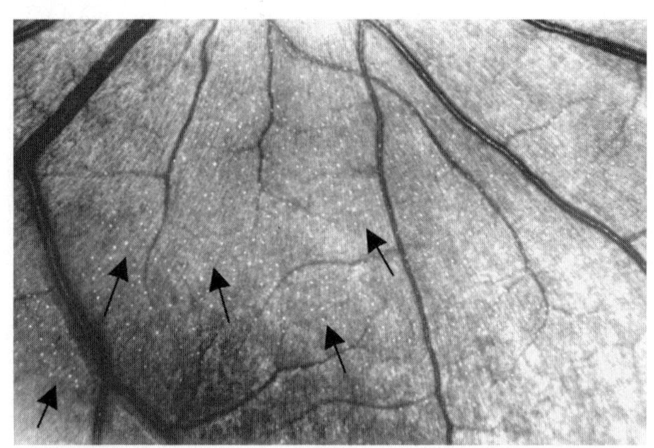

2-25A

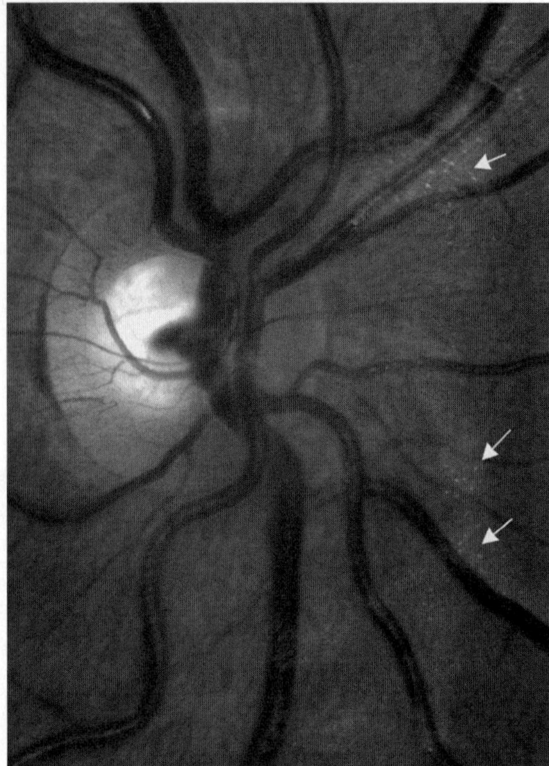

2-25B

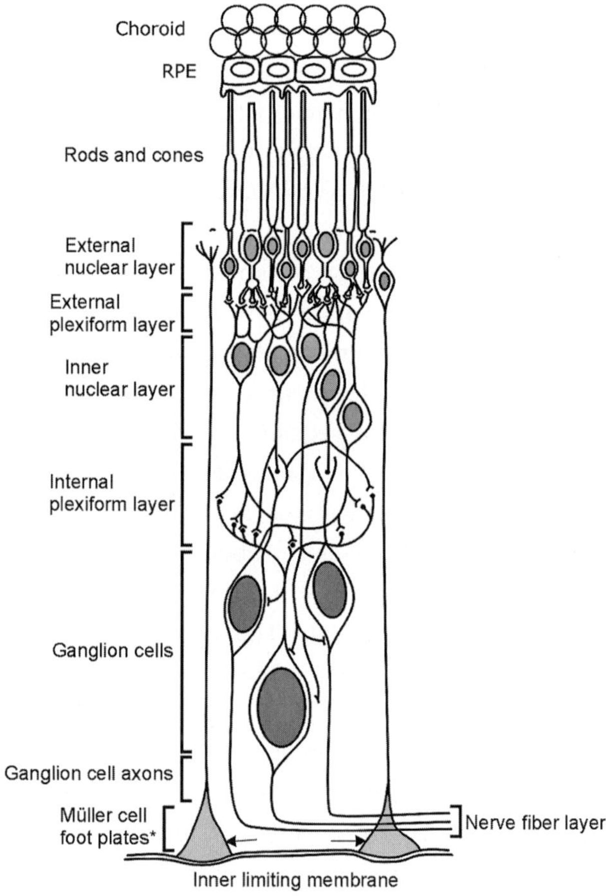

2-25C

The manner in which the spaces of the different layers of the retina affect the appearance of blood and white spots is discussed in Chapters 6 and 7.

Figure 2-26. A. **The usual orange-red color of the fundus is from the retinal pigment epithelium (RPE) and choriocapillaris. The color depends on the color from the blood vessels along with the pigment in the choroidal melanosomes and the RPE.** B. **Notice where the choriocapillaris and RPE are located in the retina (*shaded areas*).**

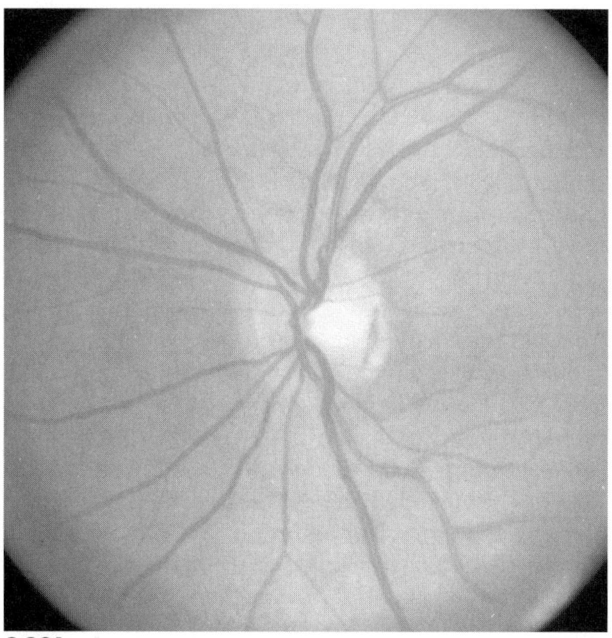

2-26A

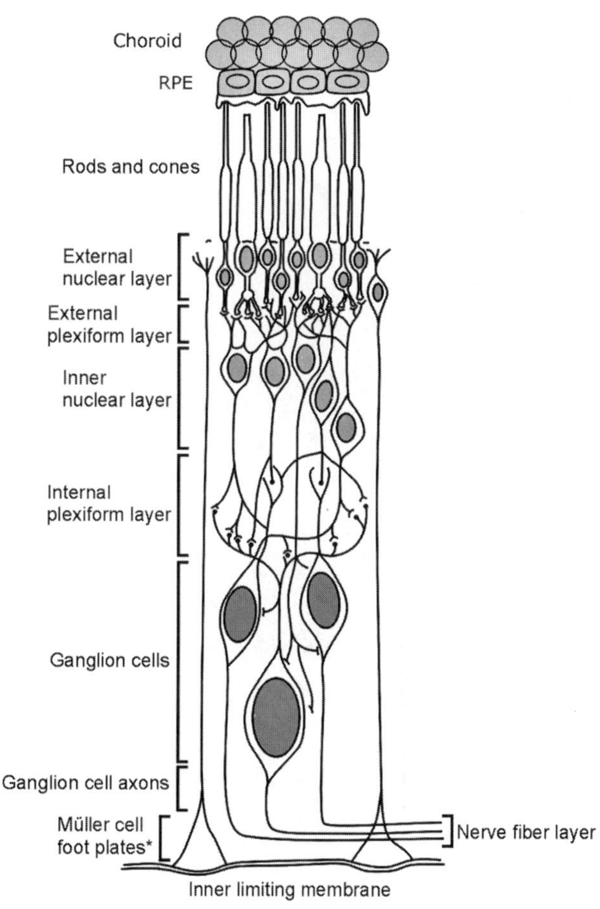

2-26B

The RPE cells and blood vessels (choriocapillaris) give the fundus its color. The color of the fundus depends on color from the blood vessels in the choroid, the pigment in the choroidal melanosomes, as well as pigment in the RPE. In addition, there is yellow pigment, xanthopigment (from the

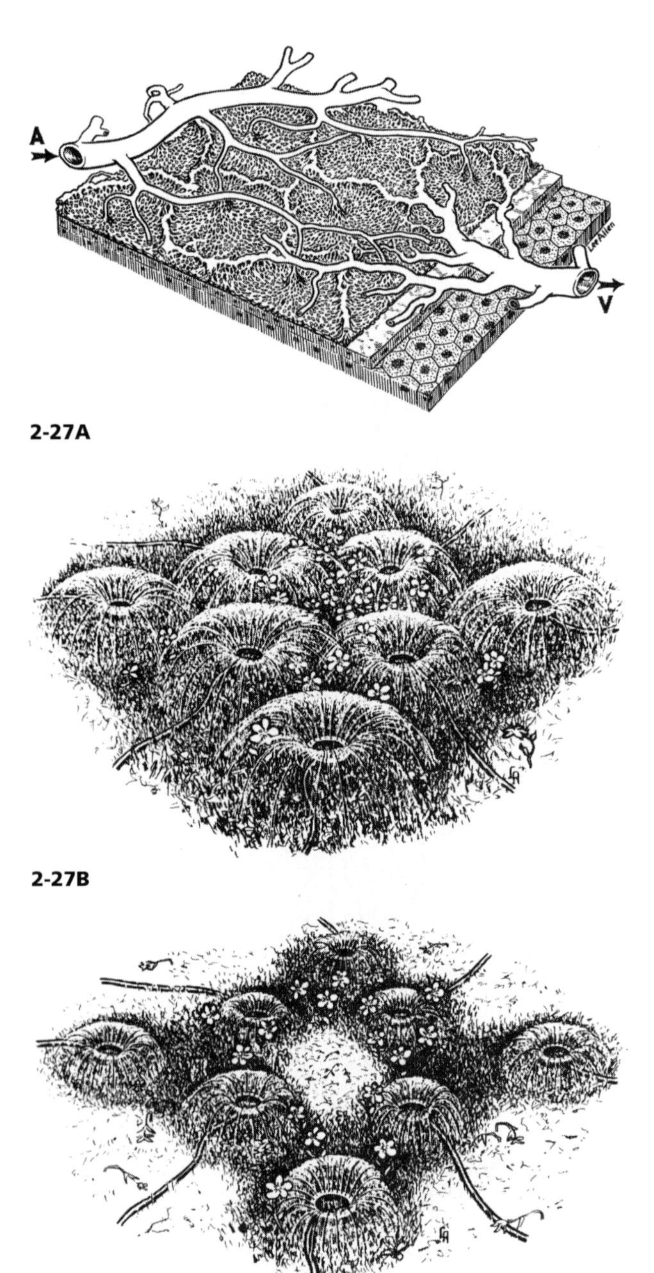

2-27C

carotenoids, lutein and zeaxanthin), which is present in the macula (hence the term *macula lutea*, or *yellow spot*).[20] The yellow pigment is what we see when there is scarcity of black pigment, such as in the albinotic fundus. It is also why the retinal color can take various shades of red, red-brown, and orange (yellow + red of the choriocapillaris). The choriocapillaris is a vascular tissue that receives its arterial supply from the posterior ciliary arteries.

Figure 2-27. A. **The structure (meshlike and arborized-like) of the choriocapillaris. A is the arterial end feeding the choriocapillaris and V is the venous drainage of the choriocapillaris. The top layer is the choroid and choriocapillaris. The middle layer is Bruch's membrane, and the lowest level is the retinal pigment epithelium. (Photograph courtesy of Lee Allen, with permission.)** B. **Lee Allen, graphic artist, and Sohan Hayreh, M.D., Ph.D., from the University of Iowa, visualized the choroid as a sprinkler system coming out throughout the choriocapillaris—feeding the retinal pigment epithelium and inner retinal elements by the vascular network.** C. **When there is damage to the choriocapillaris, the sprinkler system does not completely cover the needs of the inner retinal elements. The "globular nature" of the blood supply of the choroid has been likened to glomerulus of the kidney. "Choroid" is derived from the word chorion, or "placenta-like." (**B **and** C **courtesy of Lee Allen from SS Hayreh. Segmental nature of choroidal vasculature. Br J Ophthalmol 1975;59:631–647, with permission.)**

Together with the RPE, the choroid forms the uvea. *Uvea* comes from the Latin word *uva,* which means a bunch of grapes. The uvea is the pigmented part of the eye that anteriorly becomes the iris and ciliary body. The choroid, or choriocapillaris, is composed of small blood vessels that help to produce the "red reflex" you see when you shine the ophthalmoscope light into the eye at a distance. The red color is oxyhemoglobin in the choroidal vessels. The choriocapillaris feeds and drains the RPE, rods, and cones in a cobblestone pattern.

The RPE is made up of a single layer of cells that contain melanin and provides important metabolic support for the rods and cones. The amount of melanin in RPE cells as well as the choroidal blood supply determine the color of the fundus. Therefore, black patients with heavily pigmented skin have darker fundi, whereas an albino individual has no pigment and all of the choroidal vessels and sclera are seen clearly. Some have little pigment, such as in a fair-haired/fair-skinned individual—the so-called "blonde fundus." Pigmentation can become patchier, clumping around vessels, allowing the choroidal vessels to interdigitate with the RPE layer. This may occur naturally in younger persons or develop as we age. As a result, the *tesselated* or *tigroid fundus* may be more apparent in those who are older.

Most commonly when we look at a fundus, we see a relatively uniform orange-red color. We are really looking at the RPE evenly diffusing or screening the redness of the choroid. We usually only see clearly the retinal vessels like the CRA and CRV. The depth of the red shade is directly related to the amount of pigment an individual has.

Figure 2-28. A. We are used to observing the red-orange color of the normal fundus of an average-pigmented white individual, which comes from the amount of pigment in the retinal pigment epithelium that the individual has and the choriocapillaris. B. Notice how increased pigmentation affects the normal color of the retina. This fundus is from an individual of black descent. C. When there is less pigment, other elements of the eye (e.g., the vortex veins, the choroid, and other vessels) are more visible.

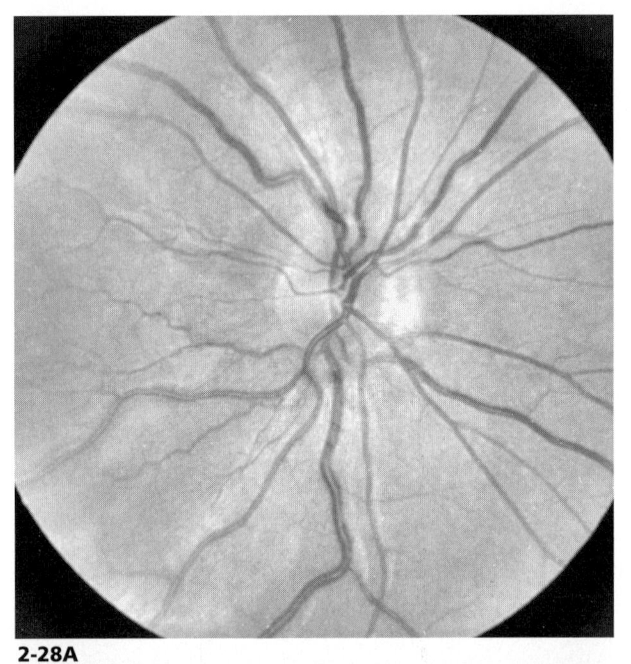

2-28A

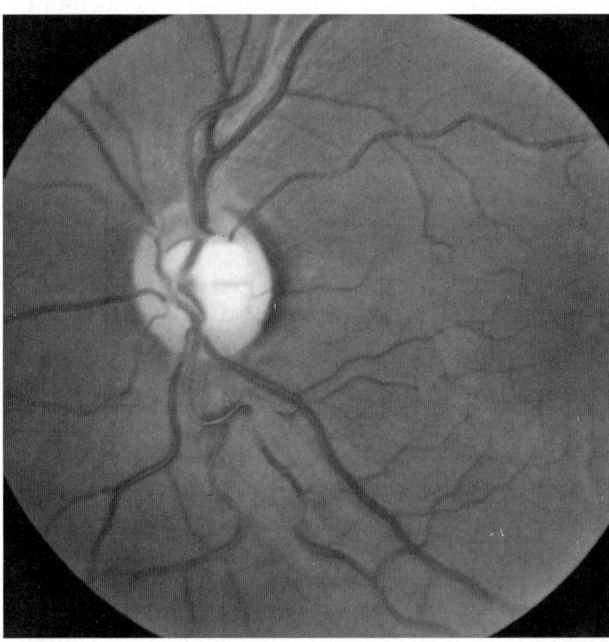

2-28B

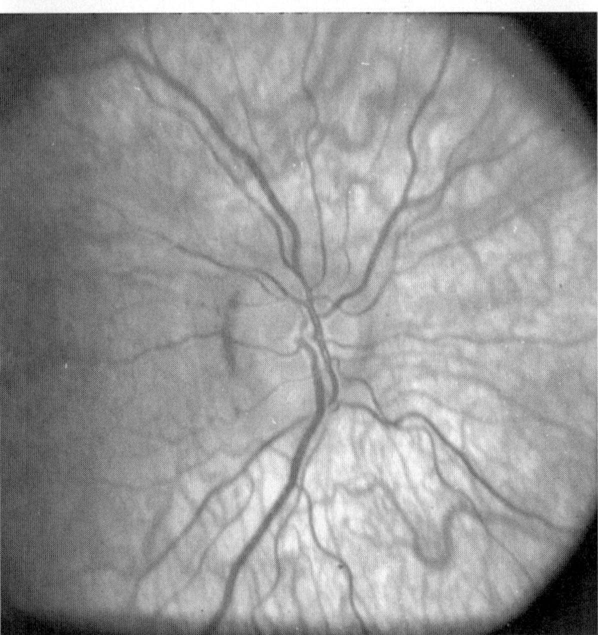

2-28C

Figure 2-29. A–C. **In the tessellated or choroidal fundus, the uniform pigment epithelium screen of the choroid is absent; therefore, we see the pigment of the choroid interspersed between the choroidal vessels in a patchwork pattern. If you are unaware of this pattern, it could be mistaken for "choroiditis" or retinitis pigmentosa. As people age, the fundus becomes more tessellated.**

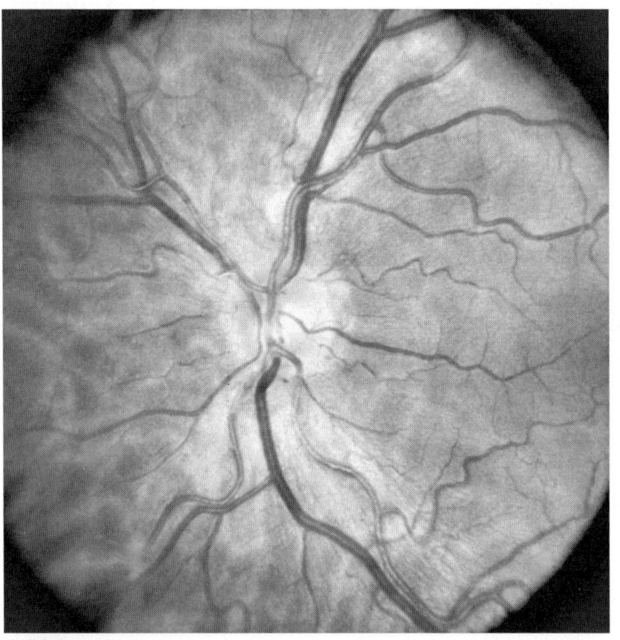

2-29A

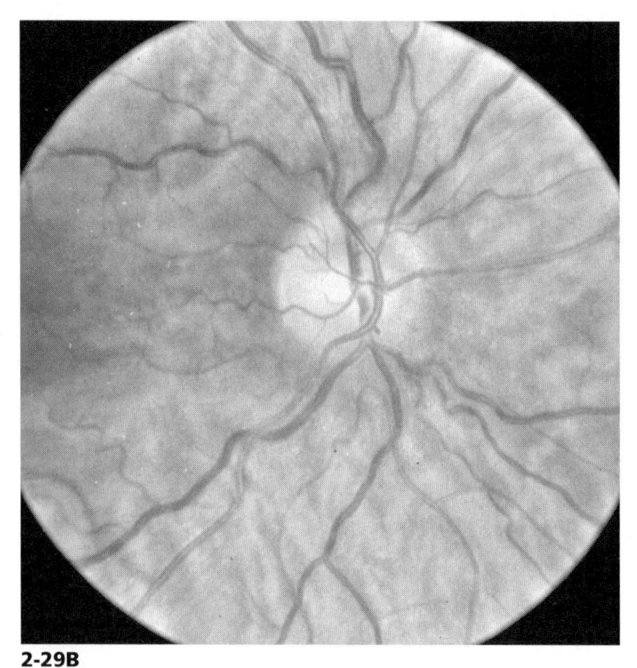

2-29B

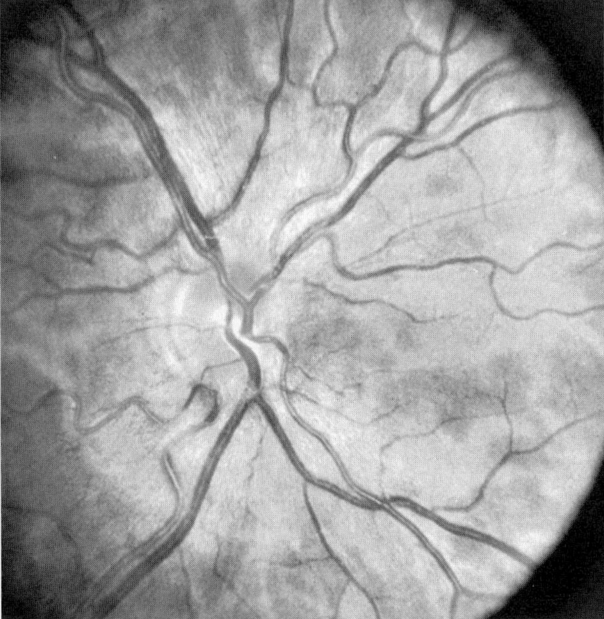

2-29C

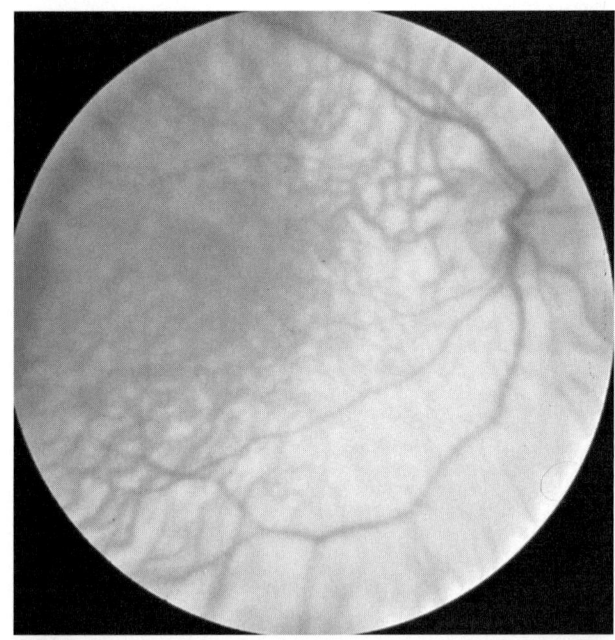

2-30A

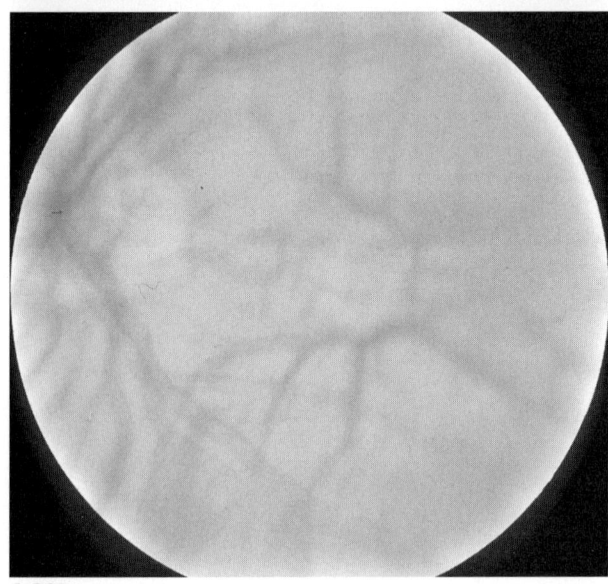

2-30B

Figure 2-30. A. **The albinotic fundus has no pigment in the retinal pigment epithelium or the choroid. What you see are the choroidal vasculature, retinal vasculature, and even the scleral elements. (Photograph courtesy of Michael Brodsky, M.D.)** B. **If you are not used to this view, you may not be able to discern the difference between the retinal circulation and the choroidal circulation. In general, the retinal vessels converge toward the disc, are slightly darker, and demonstrate the light streak, whereas the choroidal vessels never converge on the disc, their color is lighter, the vessels are larger and anastomose with each other, and, finally, they have no light streaks.**

Finally, the outer layer of the eye is the sclera, a tough connective tissue covering the globe, the outer layer of which attaches directly to the dura of the vaginal sheath of the optic nerve. A thin, pale scleral ring surrounds the outer disc. The sclera can be "seen" as white in the retina if, for example, there is a gap in the chorioretinal elements near the disc. The anterior counterpart of the sclera is the cornea, which is clear and protects the rest of the eye.

BLOOD SUPPLY TO THE EYE CONTRIBUTES TO THE APPEARANCE OF THE FUNDUS AND OPTIC NERVE

A brief review of the blood supply to the eye is important.

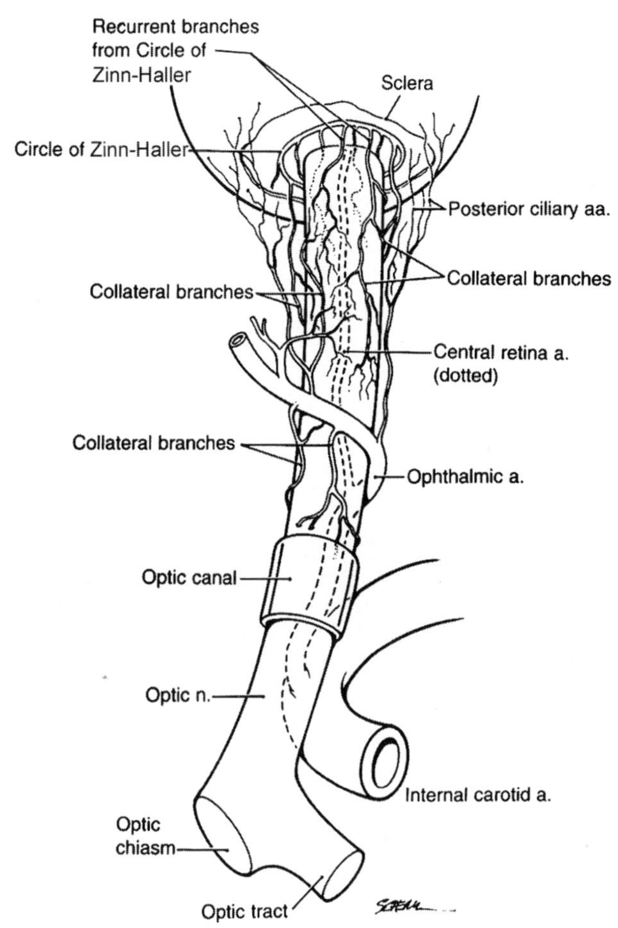

2-31

Figure 2-31. As you can see from this diagram of the blood supply, the eye is supplied by two different systems. Both systems derive blood from the ophthalmic artery, a branch of the internal carotid artery. The choroidal circulation (which includes the choroid and posterior ciliary arteries) is one major blood supply to the eye. These form rich anastomoses with the other choroidal or ciliary arteries to form the circle of Zinn-Haller. The other is the large branch to the retina from the central retinal artery (shown here by *dotted lines*).

Two different arterial networks of blood supply the globe. The choroidal system (which includes the choroid and posterior ciliary arteries) is one major blood supply to the eye. The posterior ciliary arteries (often numbering 15–20, and forming a richly anastomotic network called the *Zinn-Haller arterial circle*) behind the globe perforate the sclera and supply not only the choroid, rods, cones, and sclera, but also the dura, anterior part of the disc, and lamina cribrosa.

The second arterial supply, also a branch of the ophthalmic artery, is the CRA, which pierces the optic nerve 1–2 cm behind the globe and enters the globe through the lamina cribrosa. The CRA supplies the visible retinal elements. Thus, the blood supply of the retina is twofold—by diffusion from the choroidal vessels to the rods and cones and by direct supply to the rest of the layers of the retina from the CRA.

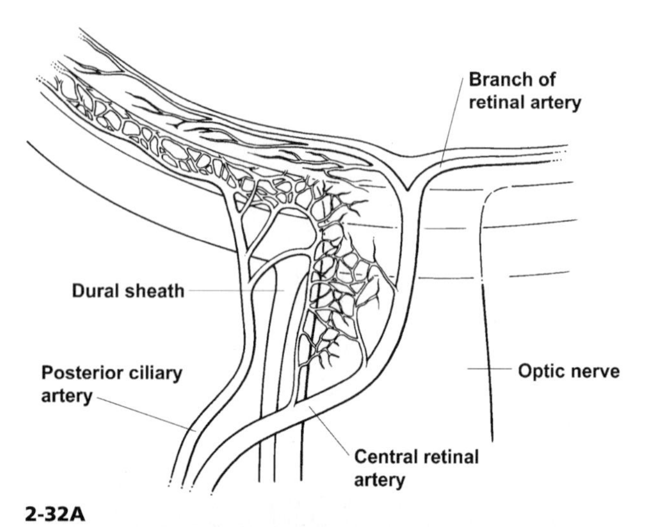

2-32A

Figure 2-32. A. Here you see the short posterior ciliary arteries feeding the choroid and optic disc and lamina cribrosa. The central retinal artery feeds the retina. B. Scanning electron micrographs of the optic nerve and posterior surface of the globe demonstrate the medial and lateral short posterior ciliary arteries alongside the optic nerve. Find the choroid, choroidal vessels, the medial and lateral posterior ciliary arteries, and pial vessels on the optic nerve. C. The lateral and medial ciliary vessels anastomose to form the Zinn-Haller arterial circle (*arrows*) and branches to the optic nerve. (Original photographs B and C courtesy of GA Cioffi, EM van Buskirk. Vasculature of the anterior optic nerve and peripapillary choroid. In The Glaucomas. P Ritch, et al., eds. St. Louis: C.V. Mosby, 1996.)

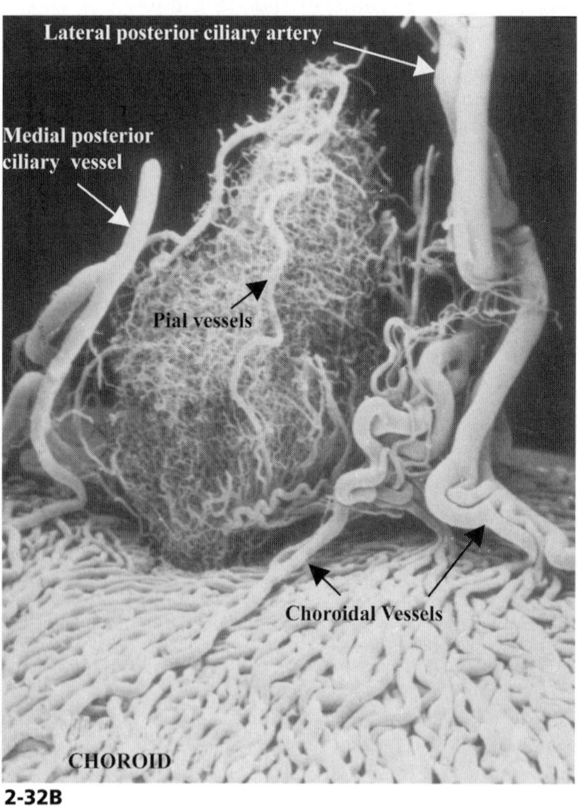

2-32B

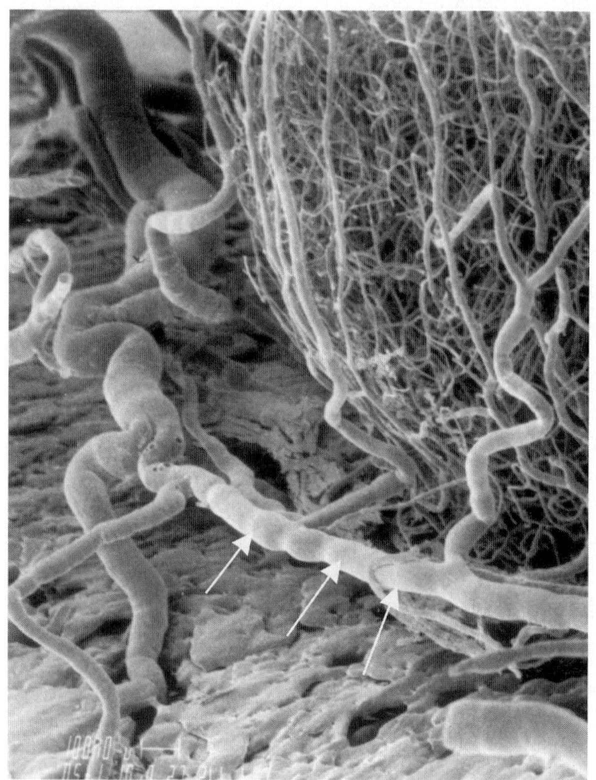

2-32C

The blood supply to the optic disc consists of four parts: The surface nerve fiber layer as an extension of the axons of the retina, the prelaminar area just anterior to the lamina cribrosa (level with the choroid), the lamina cribrosa (level with the sclera), and the retrolaminar region just posterior to the lamina cribrosa.

Table 2-2. Blood Supply to the Disc

Structure	Location	Level	Arterial supply
Surface nerve fibers	Nerve fiber layer	Retina	Arterioles off of the retinal artery
Prelaminar region	Just anterior to the lamina cribrosa	Choroid	Peripapillary choroidal arterioles
Laminar region	Fibrocollagenous structure	Sclera	Posterior ciliary arteriolar branches
Retrolaminar region	Behind the disc	—	Posterior ciliary arteries by way of the pial branches from the peripapillary choroid

Source: Adapted from SS Hayreh. Pathogenesis of optic nerve head changes in glaucoma. Semin Ophthalmol 1986;1:1–13.

Figure 2-33. A. **Scanning electron micrograph (EM) of the optic disc surface as if you are looking into the fundus. The central retinal artery (CRA) and vein (CRV) are obvious, but look at the small capillaries feeding the prelaminar areas by small branches off of the posterior ciliary artery, and small arterioles off of the retinal arteries and by the choroid. You can see in this photograph how very vascular the disc and laminar area is.** B. **This EM view beautifully demonstrates the relationship of the choroidal vessels, the choriocapillaris, and the vessels to the optic nerve. This shows that there is a potential for anastomoses between the choroidal and central retinal artery circulations. You are viewing the junction of the retina and optic nerve from behind the globe. The actual junction is the space between the optic nerve (labeled in the upper right corner) and the choriocapillaris. (Original photographs courtesy of GA Cioffi, EM van Buskirk. Vasculature of the anterior optic nerve and peripapillary choroid. In The Glaucomas. P Ritch, et al., eds. St. Louis: C.V. Mosby, 1996.)**

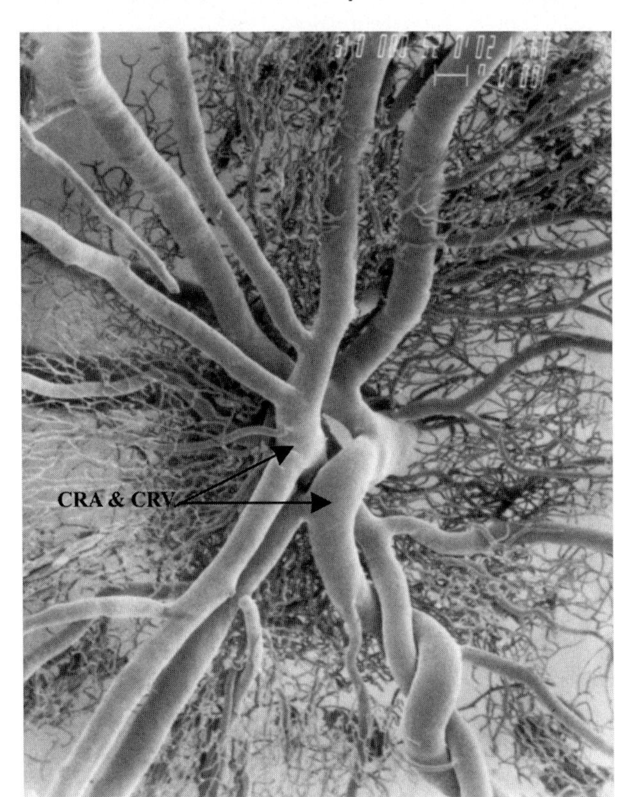

2-33A

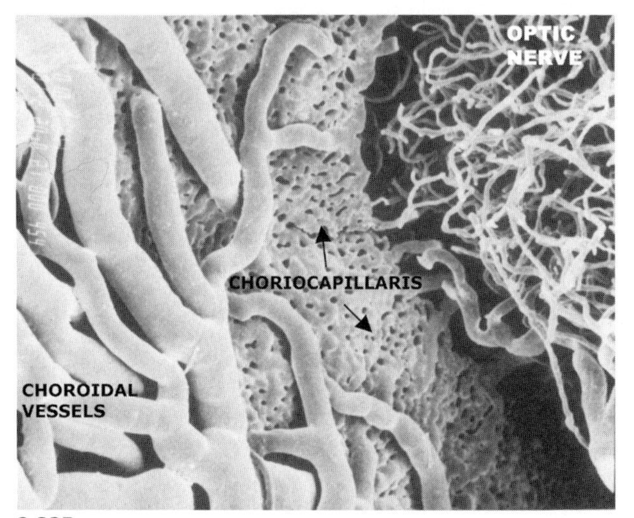

2-33B

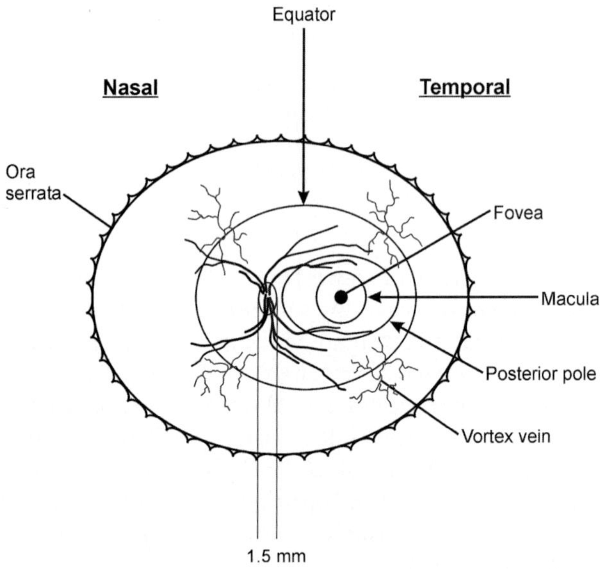

Venous Drainage of the Disc and Retina

Two venous pathways drain blood from the globe. The choriocapillaris drains through the 3–4 posterior vortex veins, which originate in the outer layers of the choroid. They are often seen in myopic or blonde eyes because of the lack of pigment in the retinal pigment epithelium. The vortex veins drain the choroid into veins in the orbit and then into the superior ophthalmic vein, which travels through the superior orbital fissure and the inferior ophthalmic vein through the inferior orbital fissure, both of which drain into the cavernous sinus.

2-34

Figure 2-34. Notice the position of the vortex veins peripherally in the retina.

Figure 2-35. A. **Venous drainage of the disc and retina: The central retinal vein (CRV) drains the retina into the superior ophthalmic vein and then into the cavernous sinus, and into the internal jugular vein via the sigmoid sinus. The choroid drains into veins that become the vortex veins. These, too, drain into the ophthalmic vein, then into the cavernous sinus.** B. **This image shows a prominent vortex vein seen in a blonde fundus.** C. **Fluorescein of vortex vein. Realize that this is a composite of several photographs of the vortex venous drainage. Can you see the disc (*arrow*)? The central retinal vein runs into the disc. The other confluence of veins is into the vortex veins from the choroid. (Reprinted with permission from reference 21.)**

The second venous drainage system is from the retina—the CRV. This vein drains the surface of the retina into the cavernous sinus, also by way of the superior ophthalmic vein, then into the internal jugular vein via the cavernous and inferior petrosal sinus.

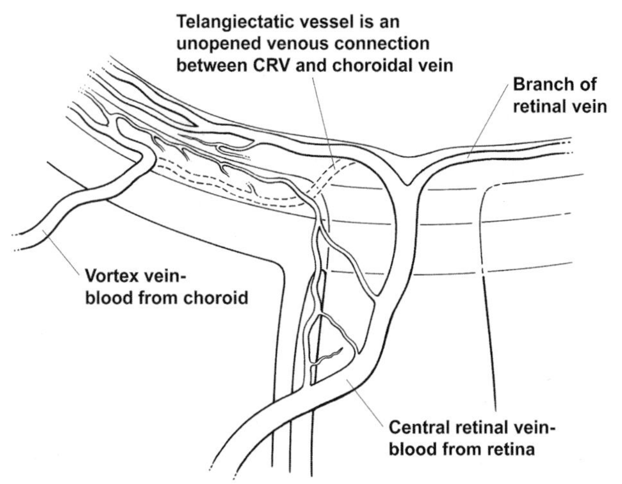

2-35A

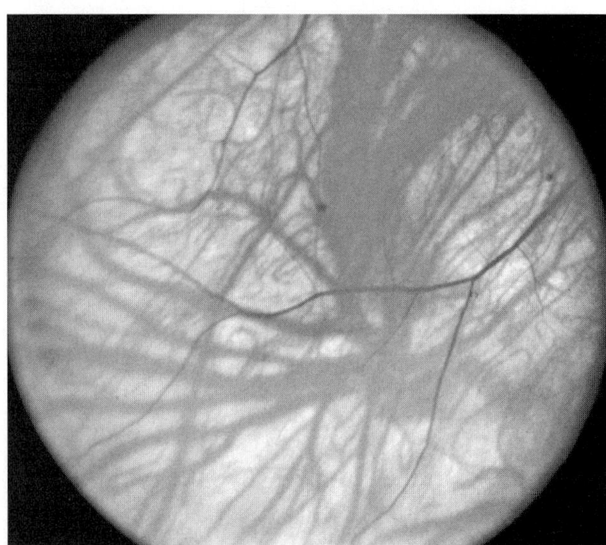

2-35B

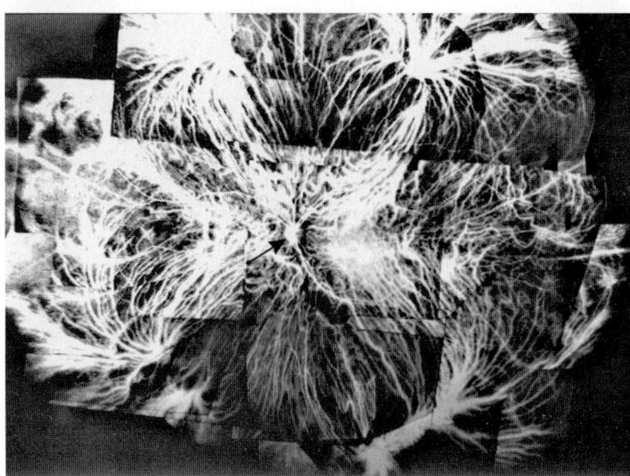

2-35C

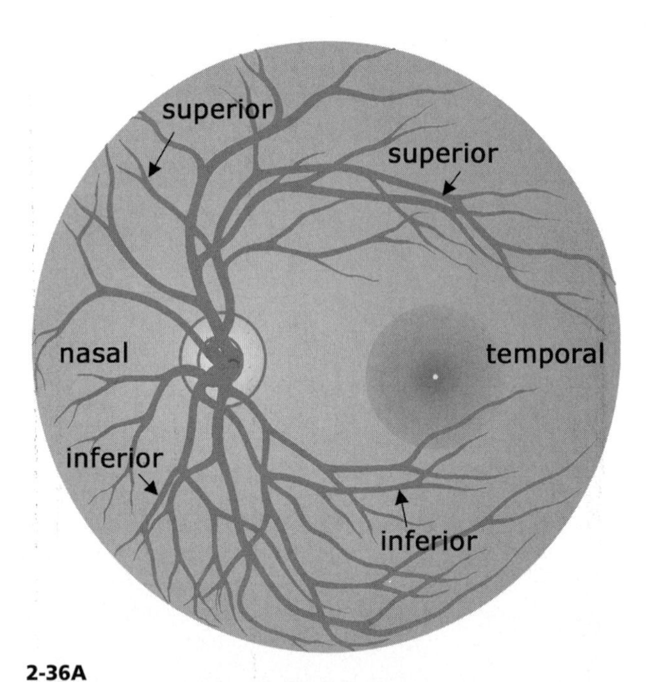

2-36A

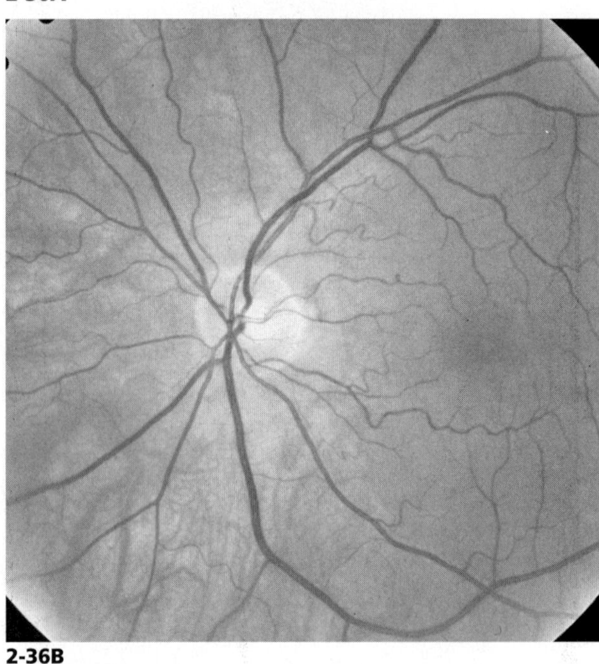

2-36B

Figure 2-36. A. **Notice that the arteries are just slightly smaller than the veins in this diagram. Find the superior temporal, the superior nasal, the inferior temporal, and the inferior nasal arcades.** B. **The color of the arteries is slightly brighter than the vein. Also, the artery has a lighter reflection streak as compared to the veins.**

In general, the artery appears to have a lighter reflection streak on it as compared to the veins. The "light streak" may be either the reflection of the ophthalmoscope's light on the convex vessel wall or a reflection off the internal limiting membrane as it covers the vessels.[15] The veins on the disc have a slightly wider diameter and appear slightly darker in color—more of a wine-red or blue-red—because of the loss of oxyhemoglobin.

When looking at the disc, view the CRA and CRV. The CRA is usually slightly narrower than the CRV. The CRA comes through the subarachnoid space behind the globe and enters the optic nerve. When the CRA pierces the lamina cribrosa, the caliber of the artery becomes smaller because of the loss of the muscular layer as the artery goes more distally in the retina and the loss of the internal elastic membrane. The normal ratio of the width of the artery to the vein is 2:3 to 3:4, with the artery just smaller than the vein. If the vessels are equal in size, the artery may be slightly enlarged or the vein somewhat constricted. When the artery is smaller than two-thirds of the vein, venous distension or arterial constriction could be the problem.

Arteries can branch behind the disc at the lamina cribrosa, at the surface of the disc, or distally off the disc. The retinal arteries emerge just nasal to the veins on the disc. The artery usually divides into superior and inferior branches and further branches temporally and nasally, giving the superior temporal arcade, inferior temporal arcade, superior nasal arcade, and inferior nasal arcade. The branching shows individual variations. In general, the vessels taper as they are traced peripherally. Realize, however, that the distal retinal arteries (unlike the vessels at the optic nerve head) have no collateral circulation.

Sometimes, a posterior ciliary artery emerges next to the disc. These are called *cilioretinal arteries*. A cilioretinal artery is not part of the CRA circulation, but part of the posterior ciliary circulation. The cilioretinal artery (unlike the CRA) maintains its elastic lamina. The cilioretinal artery can supply part of the retina, just like branches of CRA.

At least one cilioretinal artery is seen in up to one-third of all normal fundi. It often looks like a fishhook or a walking stick entering the fundus right at the disc margin. Sometimes it enters from the edge of the disc straight, without such a hook. Cilioretinal arteries may be difficult to distinguish from early (within or behind the lamina cribrosa) branching of the CRA.

The cilioretinal artery usually emerges from the lamina cribrosa temporally. On occasion, a disc may have multiple cilioretinal arteries. Multiple cilioretinal arteries develop during embryogenesis when the hyaloid arterial system fails to form normal central retinal arteries. On occasion, a cilioretinal artery can feed whole large sections of the retina, and there are rare reports of cilioretinal arteries supplying all of the retina as a normal variant.[22] Rarely, if the entire retina is fed by cilioretinal arteries, think about coexisting renal artery disease, the so-called "papillorenal syndrome."[23]

Cilioretinal arteries do not join the CRA, and cilioretinal arteries can supply blood to the macula. This variant may be extremely important in a CRA occlusion; if present, a cilioretinal artery can perfuse the macula and often spare some vision (see Chapter 5, Figure 5-6A–E). Furthermore, in giant cell arteritis, the ciliary circulation is preferentially affected because the elastic lamina is the focus of inflammation, and ciliary circulation does not lose its elastic lamina. In addition to causing arteritic anterior ischemic optic neuropathy, arteritic inflammation of the cilioretinal artery may produce a "tongue" of retinal infarction and central vision loss as the first and only sign of temporal arteritis (see Chapter 5, Figure 5-11E). Finally, the presence of a cilioretinal artery may help to retain the central visual field and visual acuity in chronic optic nerve conditions like glaucoma.[24]

Figure 2-37. A. **Variations in the appearance of cilioretinal arteries. Some emerge on the disc edge, others from the substance of the disc. Notice that there are subtle differences: Number 1 exits the substance of the neuroretinal rim, number 2 is a fishhook off of the neuroretinal rim, and numbers 3 and 4 exit the disc at the very edge of the disc. (Reprinted with permission from G Brown, W Tasman. Congenital Anomalies of the Optic Disc. New York: Grune & Stratton, 1983.)** B. **This diagram shows how the posterior ciliary artery emerges from the side of the disc to form the cilioretinal artery.** ***Continued***

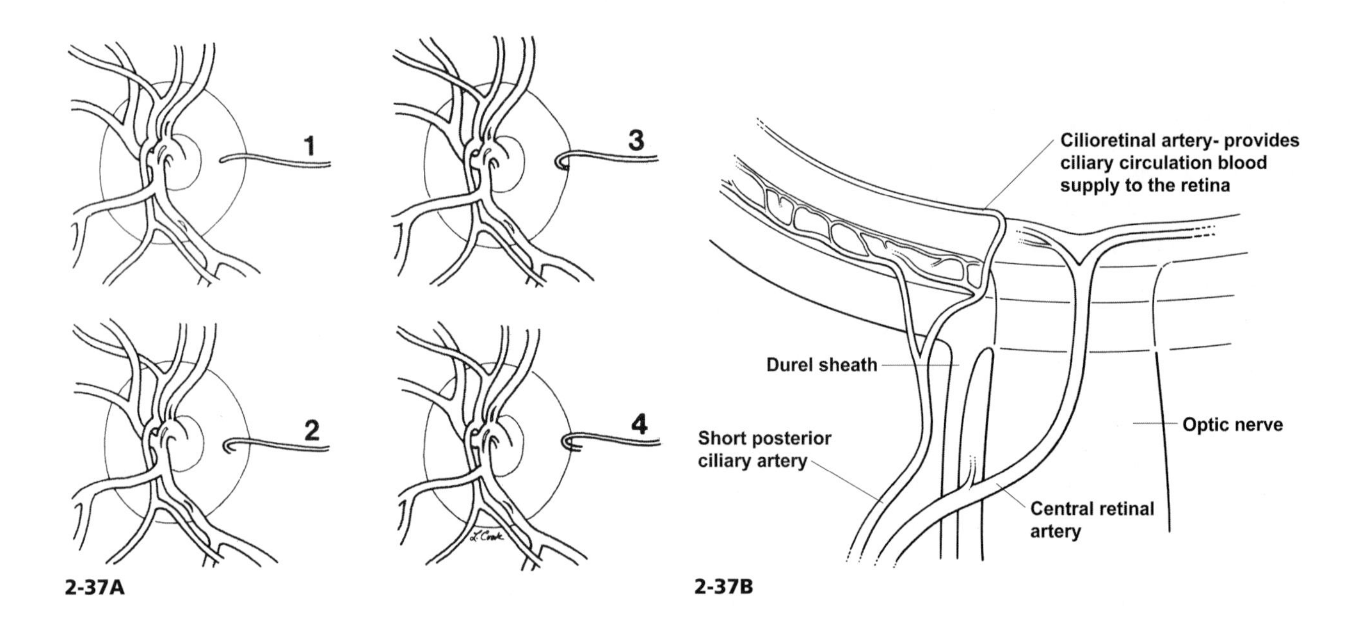

Figure 2-37. ***Continued.*** C. **Most cilioretinal arteries come off the disc temporally. Identify the cilioretinal artery.** D. **Notice the cilioretinal artery's fishhook appearance (*arrow*).** E. **A normal cilioretinal artery (*arrow*).** F. **Fluorescein shows that the cilioretinal artery (inferior branch) fills at the same time as the choroid and before the central retinal artery, showing that this is a cilioretinal artery.**

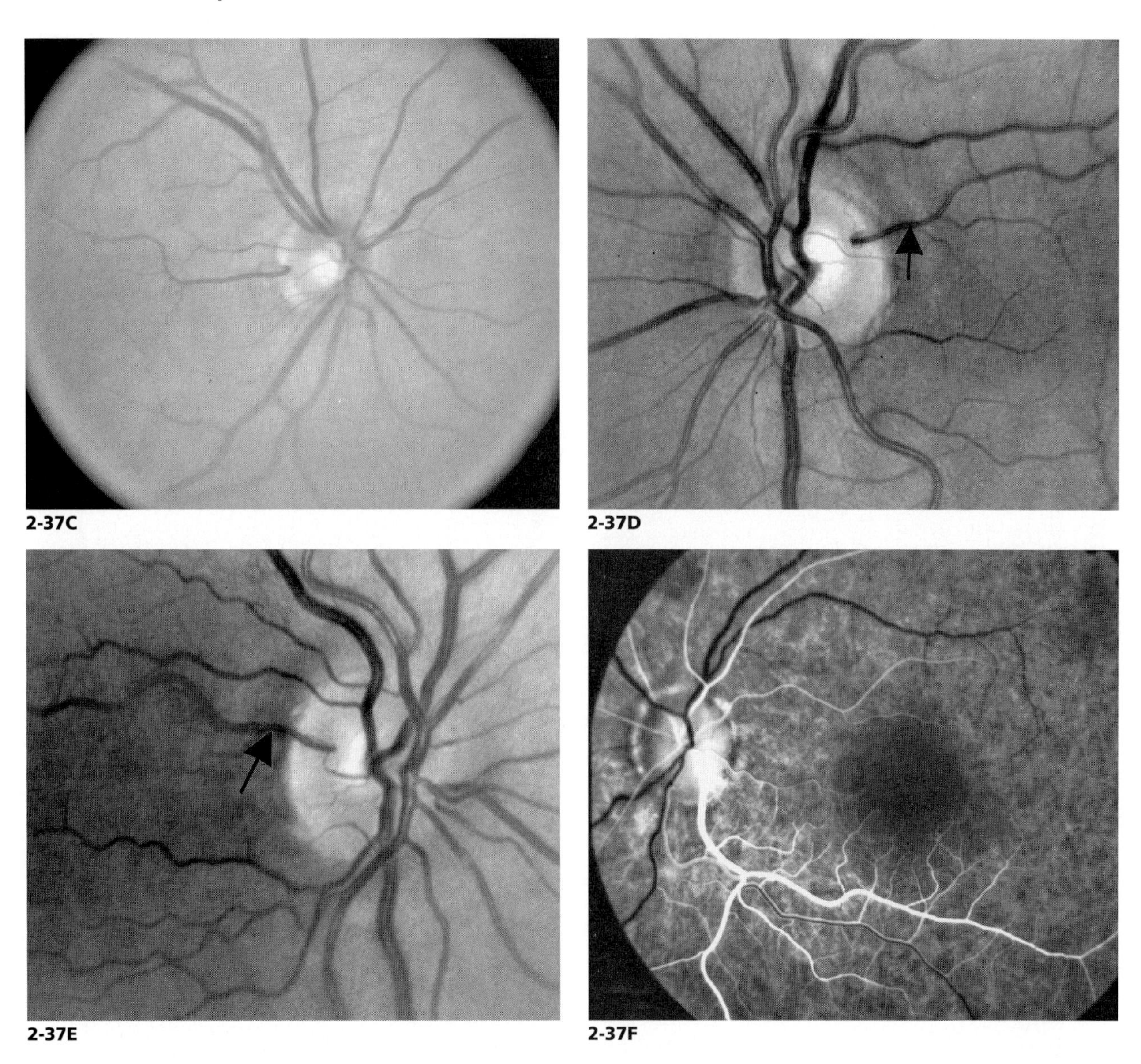

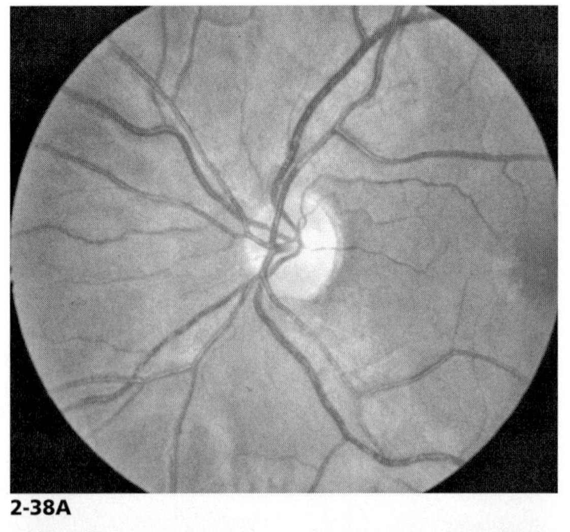

2-38A

Figure 2-38. A. The branching pattern of the retinal arteries and veins is variable. The veins are similarly distributed to the arteries. B. Here you see a trifurcation inferiorly. C. Sometimes the veins and arteries appear to branch behind or within the lamina cribrosa. D. Sometimes there are more than four major arteries and veins emerging on the disc. In this case, there are at least four arteries emerging superiorly. If there is a small scleral canal, these extra vessels add to the crowding of disc tissue. E. Most of the time, arteries and veins project directly to the quadrant that they supply or drain. Occasionally, the temporal retinal arteries and veins take off nasally before heading temporally. This has been called *situs inversus*. It is most often (approximately 80% of the time) seen in tilted discs or fundus ectasia. This disc has a nasal tilt. This pattern can be seen in 1–2% of people.[6]

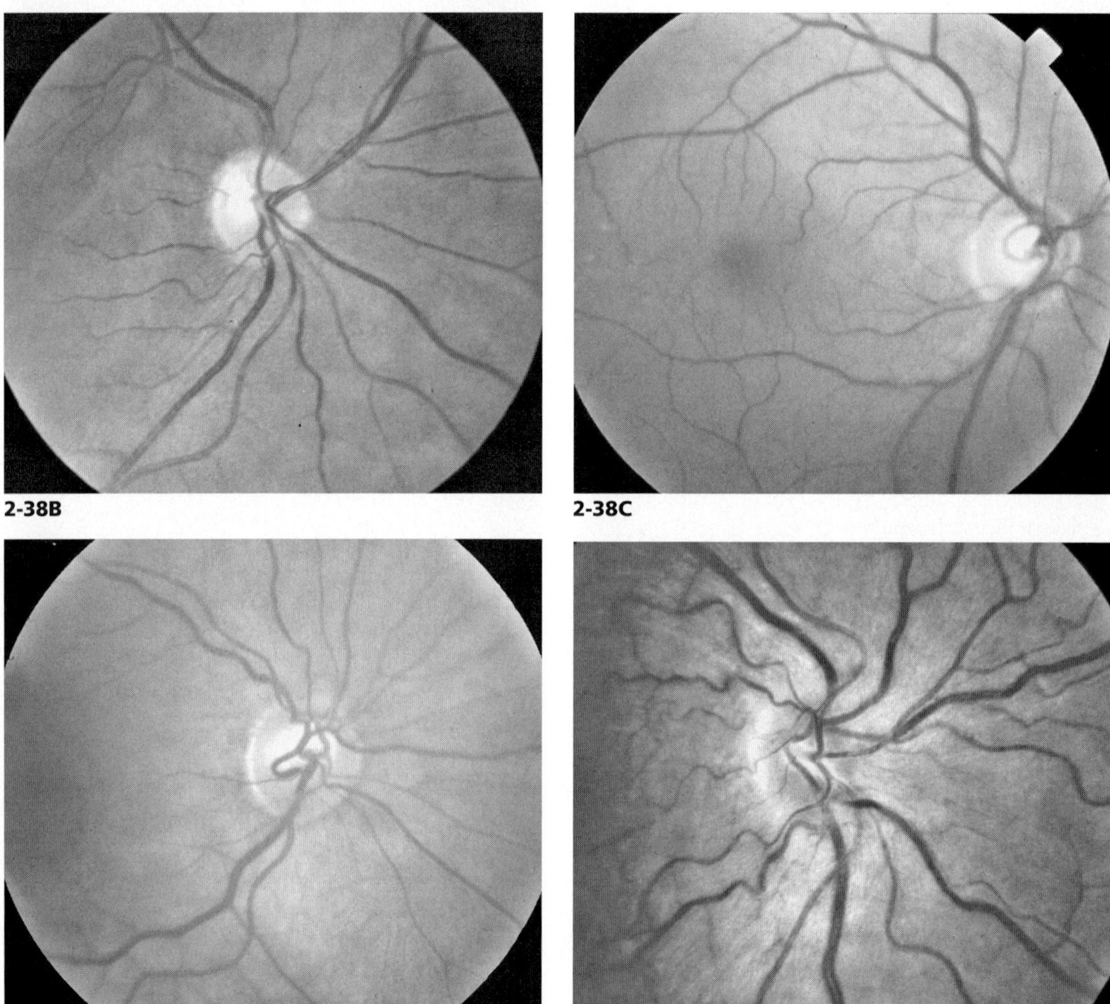

2-38D

2-38E

The branching patterns of the central retinal arteries can be variable. Sometimes you see the branching occurring before the lamina, at the lamina, or above the lamina. There may be just one CRA branching to four quadrants, or there may be variable combinations.

The retinal veins are similarly distributed and drain into the CRV. Usually the superior and inferior retinal veins join the CRV somewhere around the lamina cribrosa. If the venous pressure is increased, the veins dilate. As they dilate, they elongate and become tortuous. In general, the vein dips *below* the artery at any artery/vein crossing, but occasionally it humps up over an arteriole.

MACULA CONTRIBUTES TO FUNDUS APPEARANCE

The macula is a horizontally oval depression located temporally, approximately one and a half to two disc diameters temporal to and slightly inferior to the temporal margin of the disc. In the center of the macula is the fovea, the most central portion of which is foveola. The foveola is comprised purely of cones and is avascular. Sometimes you see a yellow spot in the fovea; this is due to the pigment lutein, which is responsible for the name *macula lutea*. The layers present in the retina are altered in the macula, with the foveolar ganglion cells and their nerve fiber layer laterally displaced. No ganglion cell or other nuclear or support cells overlie the fovea (see the anatomic diagram of the macula, Chapter 10, Figure 10-4B). There are no retinal blood vessels in the macula, so it is sometimes called an *avascular* region. The color of the macula comes from the choriocapillaris, which, without the overlying layers of the RPE, is easily seen. This makes the color of the macula slightly darker. Cones have a one-to-one relationship with ganglion cells in the fovea.

Sometimes a circumferential macular-retinal light reflex is apparent, in the shape of a ring. This is best seen with the indirect method of ophthalmoscopy and is more often appreciated in younger individuals. In the center of the darker area is a bright "foveal reflex," which appears to flicker *above* the retina. The reflex moves opposite to the movement of the ophthalmoscope light. This appearance is due to the reflection of light off of the parabola-shaped foveola with light rays focusing above the retina. Look for the fovea reflex.

The axons from the macula radiate out spoke-like from the fovea to reach supporting cells like the amacrine cells and bipolar cells around the macula. These axon fibers reside in Henle's layer. Exudative inflammatory change in the macula in Henle's layer assumes a "star-like" pattern owing to the arrangement of the axons (see Chapter 10, Figures 10-18 and 10-19).

Nasal
Temporal
Foveola
Fovea
Macula

2-39A

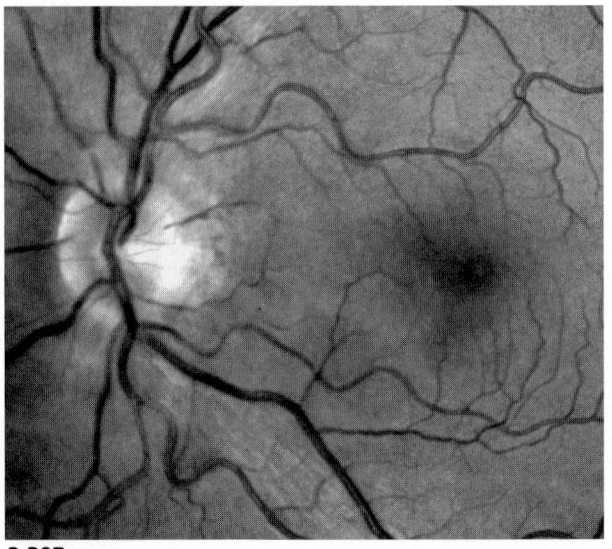

2-39B

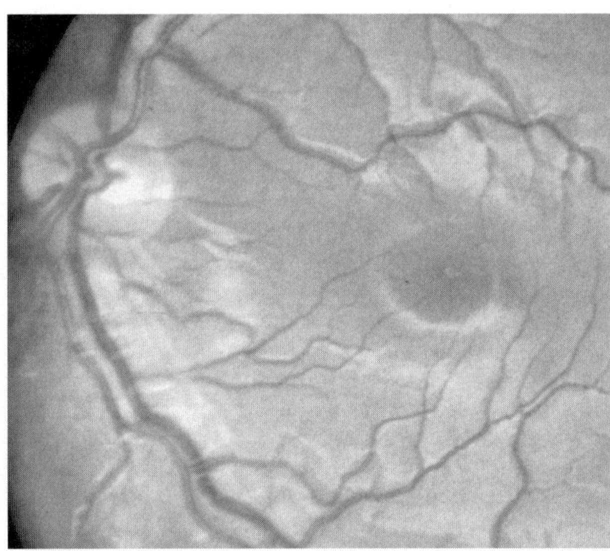

2-39C

Figure 2-39. A. **Notice that in this diagram, the fovea lies in the center of the macula.** B. **Notice that the macula is just slightly lower than the disc.** C. **You may occasionally also see a prominent light reflex around the macular area.**

When You View the Optic Disc, What Should You Notice in Everyone?

Table 2-3. Features to Consider When Examining with the Direct Ophthalmoscope

Part of anatomy	Features
Disc	Size and shape
	Color
	Optic cup
	Estimate the cup-to-disc ratio
	Nerve fiber layer
	Neuroretinal rim
	Peripapillary disc
Blood vessels	Arteries and veins on the disc and peripherally
	Venous pulsations on the disc
Retina	Color
	Amount of pigment
	Abnormalities (spots—red or white; scars, folds, wrinkles)
Macula	Foveal light reflex
	Abnormalities: pigment, cherry-red spot

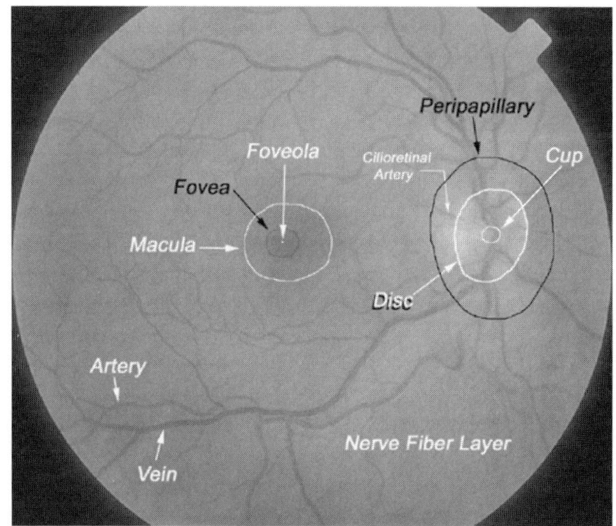

2-40A

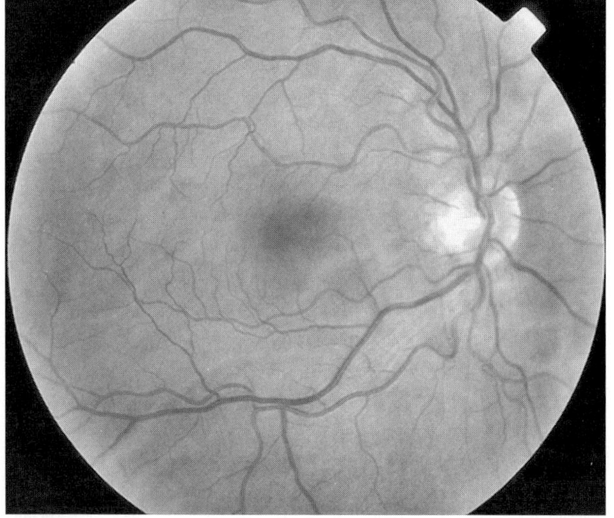

2-40B

Figure 2-40. A. **Diagram of features to consider when examining with the direct ophthalmoscope.** B. **Now try to identify all of the aforementioned features on this unlabeled fundus photograph.**

Because the optic disc is a distinctive orienting landmark, look for it first. Sometimes, if the pupil is not dilated, only a retinal vessel is visible; if this is the case, follow the vessel as it enlarges until you find the disc.

SIZE OF THE DISC

First, take note of the shape and size of the disc. Normal discs are round or slightly vertically oval. The actual size is only approximately 1.5–1.7 mm in diameter and 2.1–2.7 mm^2 in area. With the 15× magnification of the direct ophthalmoscope, it may appear to be approximately 1 cm. The size of the optic disc and the optic cup is directly related to the size of the scleral canal.

One technique (described and copyrighted by Gross) for determining whether the disc is small or large is to shine the small aperture of the direct ophthalmoscope onto the retina. This 5- degree aperture produces a spot with a diameter of approximately 1.5 mm or an area of 1.77 mm^2. Therefore, the disc is only a little bigger than the spot of light.[25]

If the disc looks large, the patient may be myopic, or it may be a large disc. If the disc is small, the patient may be hyperopic, or you may consider other causes of small discs. See the section on big discs/little discs in Chapter 11.

You may wish to divide the disc into quadrants using imaginary vertical (nasal and temporal) and horizontal (superior and inferior) lines. The temporal margin of the optic disc is usually sharper and more clearly seen than the nasal margin. Vessels are seen to course from the nasal center of the disc both superiorly and inferiorly, draping temporally and nasally.

Gowers wrote the following regarding viewing of the optic disc:

One . . . which give(s) rise to special trouble . . . is . . . the colour of the optic disc. It has been well remarked that the tint of the optic disc may vary as much as the tint of the cheek. It is always redder in the young than in the old. In the latter the redness has often a grey tint mingled with it. In rare cases, in young persons, the tint may be scarcely lighter than that of the adjacent choroid.

WHAT GIVES THE DISC COLOR?

The color of the disc is usually yellowish with a pink blush. The blush is produced by fine capillaries, which are plentiful on the disc surface. The yellowish tint is produced by the background lamina cribrosa. The axons themselves are colorless, because the axons usually do not acquire their myelin coat until they pass through the lamina cribrosa.

Figure 2-41. A. **The diagram outlines a coronal outline of the disc. Notice the lamina cribrosa, sclera, retinal pigment epithelium (RPE), retina, and nerve fiber layer. Remember that the color of the fundus is directly related to the choroids and RPE.** B. **The color of the disc is related to the size of the disc, the size of the cup, and whether you look on the temporal or nasal aspect. Sometimes the temporal aspect looks less pink.**

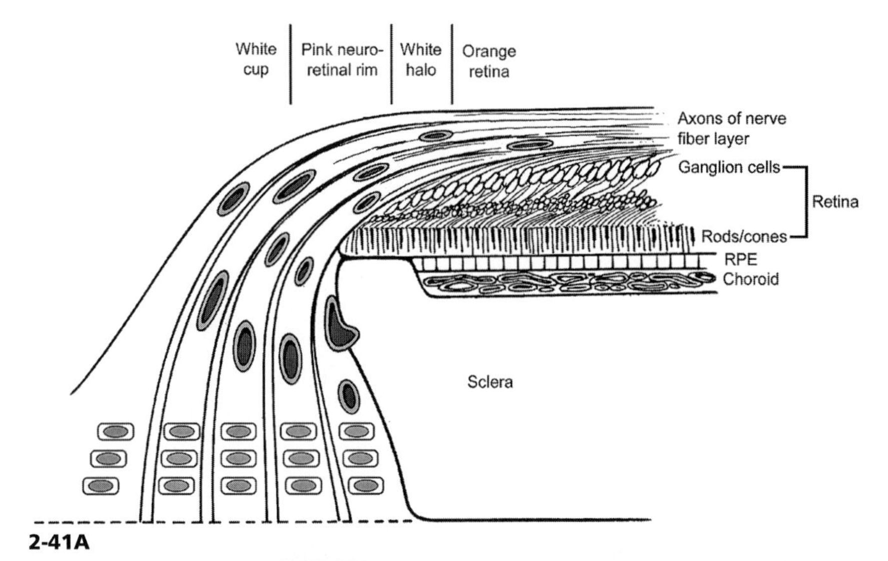

2-41A

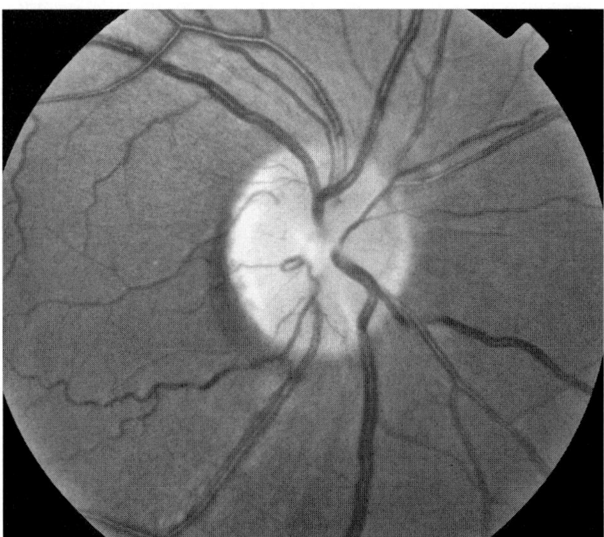

2-41B

The size of the disc, in part, determines the normal color of disc: Bigger discs may have more lamina cribrosa present and appear paler, whereas smaller discs appear pinker because less lamina is seen and the small blood vessels on the disc surface impart a pinker tinge. In addition, the size of the cup may cause the disc to look paler. The disc normally appears pinker on the nasal half because there are more axons pouring into the disc.

PROBLEM OF TEMPORAL PALLOR

On the temporal half of the disc, the axons are smaller in diameter and spread over a larger surface area, giving the temporal disc a paler color. Thus, one must be cautious about declaring discs to have "temporal pallor." Furthermore, unless pallor is unilateral or there is evidence of loss of visual function (e.g., a relative afferent pupillary defect, change in central visual field loss or color vision), or both, disc pallor, no matter where it is located, should not be equated with atrophy. As discussed in the chapter on disc pallor (Chapter 4), atrophy denotes irreversible loss of optic nerve (axons) tissue and function, whereas pallor may or may not be associated with a change in function. The tint of the disc is also affected by the color of the surrounding fundus. For example, a darkly pigmented fundus may make the disc appear to be "paler" than it really is, whereas a blonde fundus may make the disc look pinker than normal.

View the optic cup. One can estimate the cup size in the horizontal and the vertical plane. The cup-to-disc ratio is often roughly assessed by looking at the color difference between the cup and the neuroretinal rim, but true size of the cup should be made by the disc contour because the cup is actually a depression. Ophthalmologists and optometrists view the cup with an indirect, three-dimensional, slit-lamp viewing technique. For most medical practitioners, however, an estimation of the cup size should be attempted every time you look at the disc. Both tint and vascular clues are helpful. Look to see where the vessels dive into the cup—this can give you an idea of where the cup begins. Vertical cup enlargement may be a more accurate predictor of glaucoma than horizontal cup-to-disc ratio.[26]

Estimate the size of the cup-to-disc ratio. This is done by comparing the cup size to the total disc size.

NORMAL CUP-TO-DISC RATIOS

The direct method of ophthalmoscopy may underestimate the size of the optic cup, whereas the indirect method of ophthalmoscopy may overestimate the size of the cup.

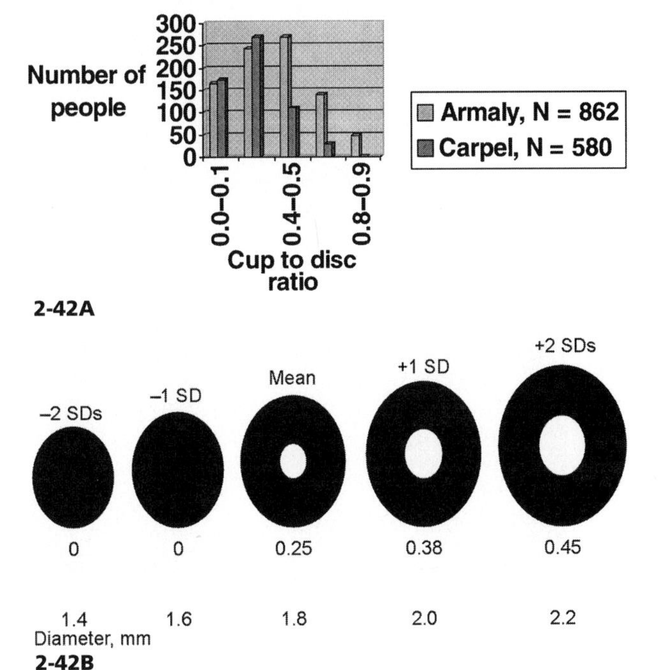

Figure 2-42. A. **Cup-to-disc ratios in the population. (From references 27 and 28.)** B. **These are optic disc sizes and cup-to-disc ratios in a population. The mean cup-to-disc ratio was 0.25. The diameter of the disc enlarged as the cup-to-disc ratio enlarged. (Diagram adapted from reference 5, with permission.)**

The cup-to-disc ratio increases very slightly with age.[15]

Figure 2-43. A. No cup-to-disc ratio. B. Cup-to-disc ratio is 0.1. C. Cup-to-disc ratio is 0.3. D. Cup-to-disc ratio is 0.5. E. Cup-to-disc ratio is 0.7. F. Cup-to-disc ratio is 0.9. This very large cup-to-disc ratio should alert you to at least think about glaucoma.

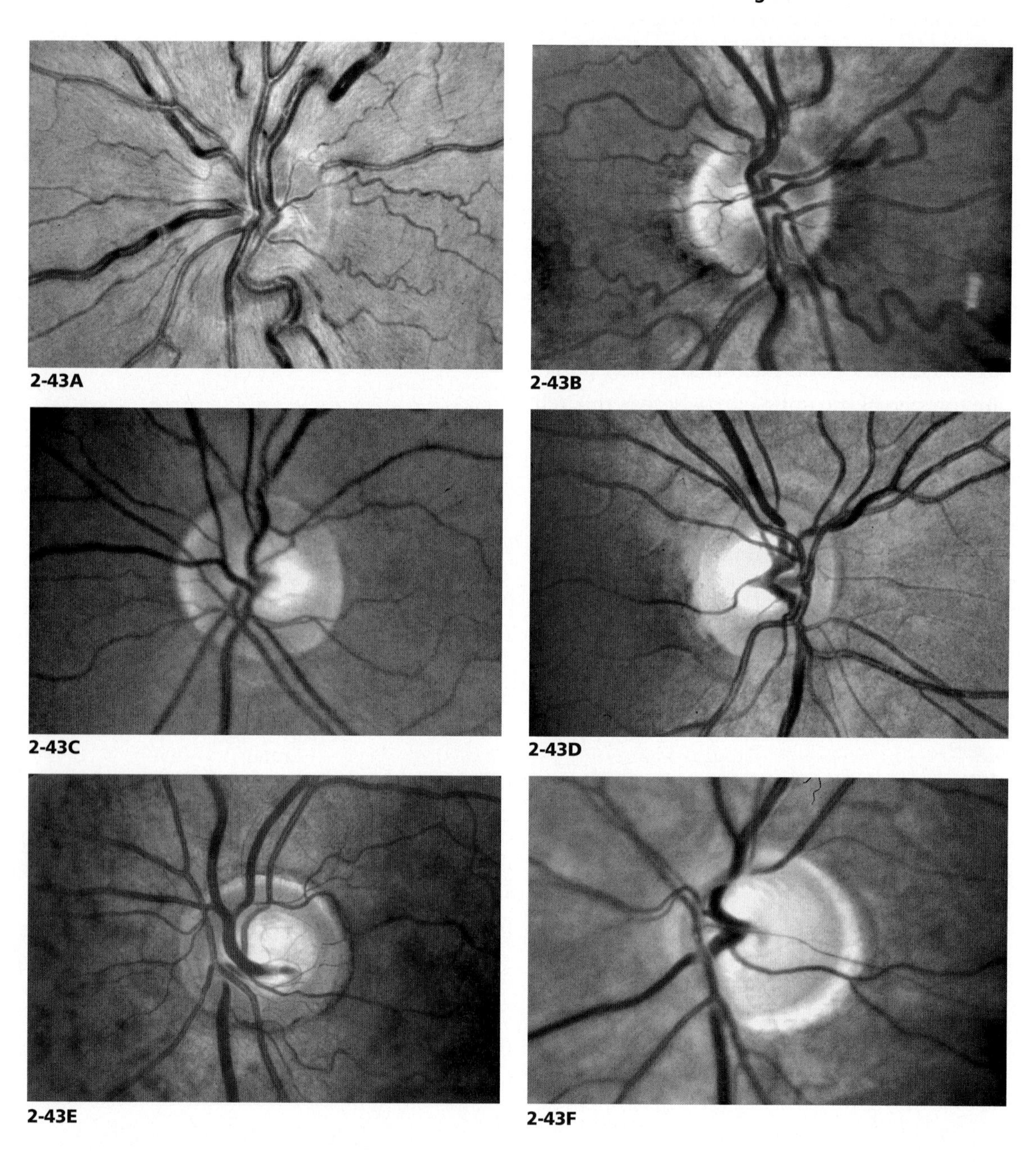

When should you suspect an abnormal ratio, such as in glaucoma? In general, a vertical cup-to-disc ratio over 0.6 is approximately 90% specific and 84% sensitive for glaucoma in one study.[26] Refer the patient for an ophthalmoscopic examination and intraocular pressure check at this point. Aside from the appearance of the disc, an ophthalmologist would evaluate the visual field and intraocular pressure as well.[26]

The other feature to assess is the neuroretinal rim. The neuroretinal rim is the nerve fiber layer from the edge of the disc to the point at which the cup deepens. The neuroretinal rim can be assessed by looking at the vessels on the disc. Do they make a sudden dive or do they make a gentle bend into the cup? The neuroretinal rim is helpful in that if there is atrophy or elevation or swelling, you will see it here. In glaucoma, the neuroretinal rim progressively narrows and is lost. Furthermore, notching of the neuroretinal rim may be another sign of glaucoma or of microvascular events in the past.

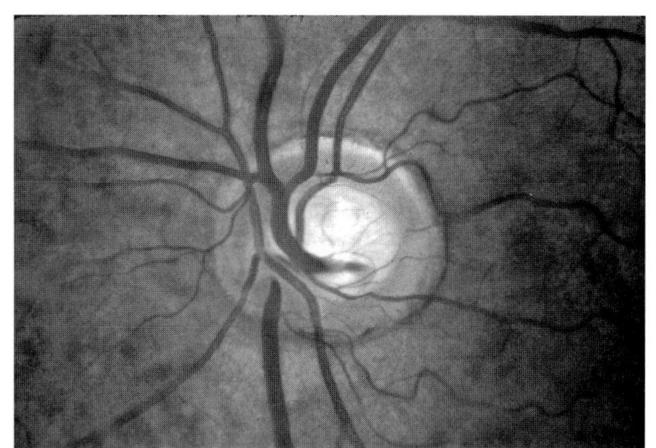

2-44A

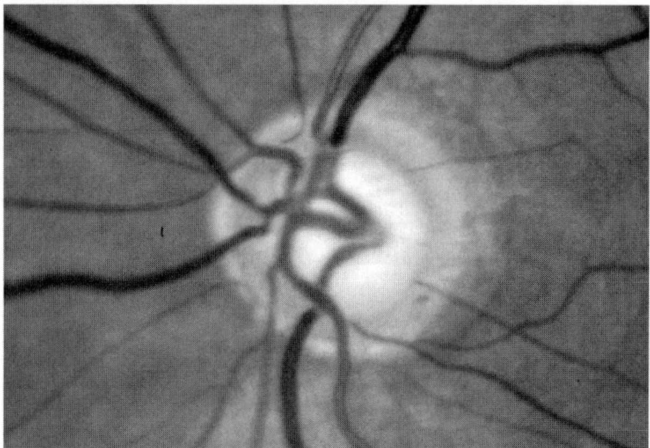

2-44B

Figure 2-44. A. **Look carefully at the neuroretinal rim. How do the vessels bend into the cup? Is there atrophy? Is there narrowing or cupping?** B. **These neuroretinal rims are healthy appearing. The cup-to-disc ratio is approximately 0.6 in each.**

Figure 2-45. A,B. **The peripapillary disc area should be viewed. The peripapillary area is the area surrounding the optic disc. Whereas a peripapillary temporal crescent may be a physiologic variant, atrophy and pigmentary changes in the same area also occur with glaucoma, following papilledema, disc drusen, and infectious/inflammatory processes. The nasal peripapillary area shows sclera owing to the tilted disc** (B).

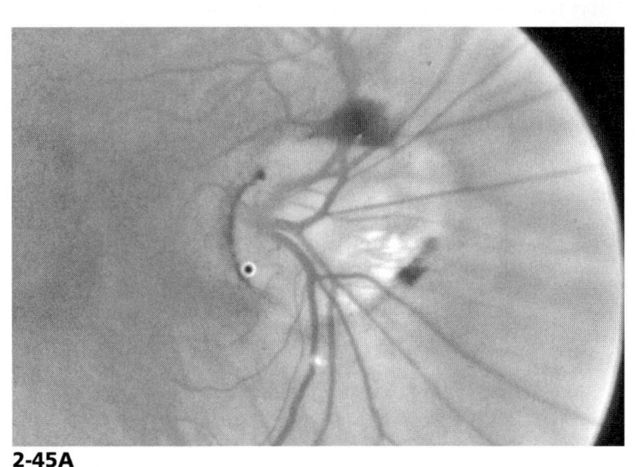

2-45A

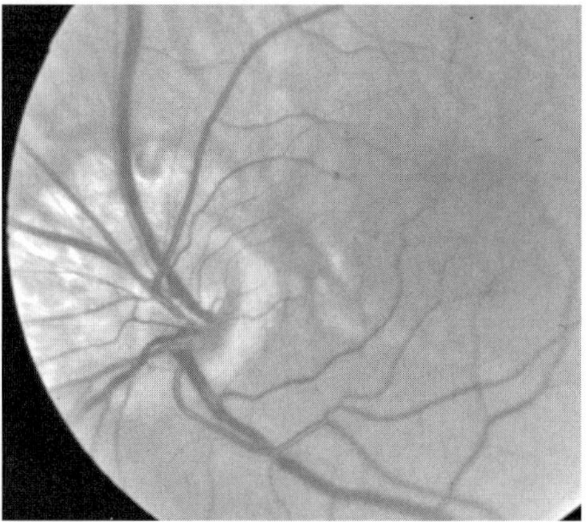

2-45B

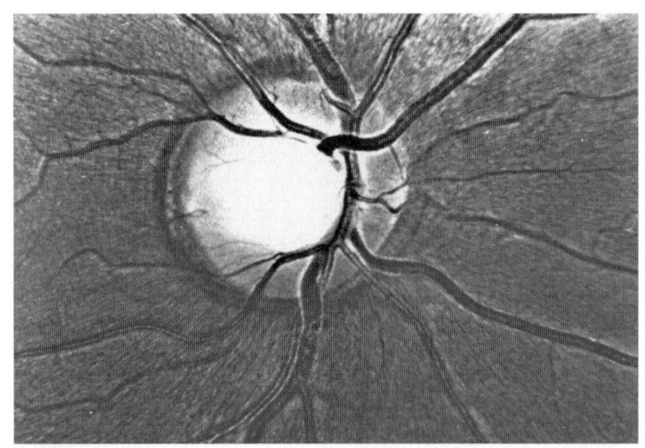

2-46A

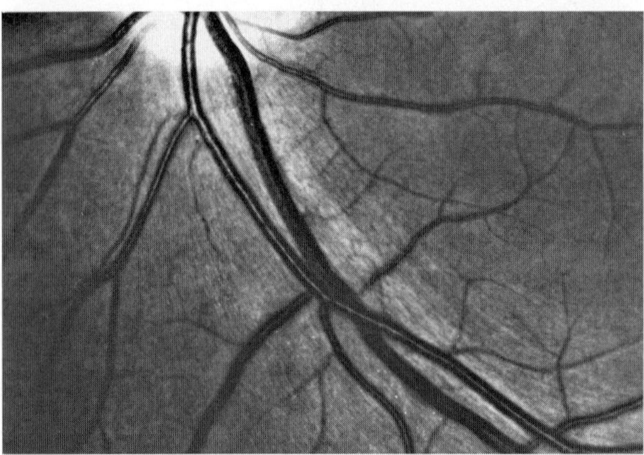

2-46B

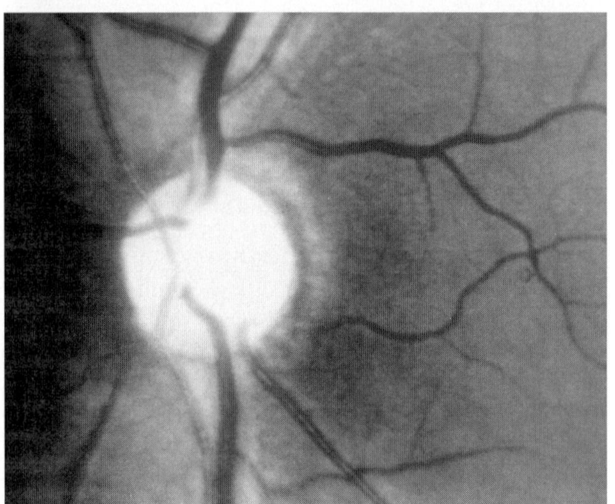

2-46C

Notice also the nerve fiber layer: The nerve fibers (axons) entering the disc commonly may be seen, especially in darkly pigmented patients, and less well in blondes. To view the nerve fiber layer on the disc, use the green light (i.e., red-free light). In glaucoma and other optic neuropathies, there may be clearly detectable bands of loss of nerve fibers at the disc and peripapillary area with this technique.

Figure 2-46. A. **Notice the nerve fiber striations in this black and white photograph. (Courtesy of William F Hoyt, M.D.)** B. **This red-free photograph shows the major inferior bundle of the nerve fiber layer. (Photograph courtesy of William F. Hoyt, M.D.)** C. **Using the red-free light (green light), look at the nerve fiber layer. Here you can see the nerve fibers traversing into the superior and inferior aspect of the disc. There is dropout of the nerve fiber layer nasally and temporally owing to chiasmal injury and bow-tie atrophy (see Chapter 4).**

Finally, look at the blood vessels. View the CRA and CRV at the disc. Note the branching pattern. As one moves away from the disc, the vessels tend to bifurcate. The venous vessels in anomalous optic discs frequently trifurcate or quadrifurcate on the disc and are tortuous. The clean superior and inferior vessel distribution is frequently replaced by a spokes-of-a-wheel appearance.

Do the arteries and veins extend temporally and nasally? Do the vessels appear nasally and then turn temporally like in situs inversus?

Figure 2-47. A. **Notice the normal width of the vessels. Obviously, there are pathologic reasons as to why arteries may be narrowed or veins distended (see Retina, Chapter 9). Do you see the cilioretinal artery?** B. **Notice that the central retinal artery exits the disc and promptly trifurcates to feed the retina (*arrows*).** C. **Note the unusual branching pattern to the optic disc vessels.**

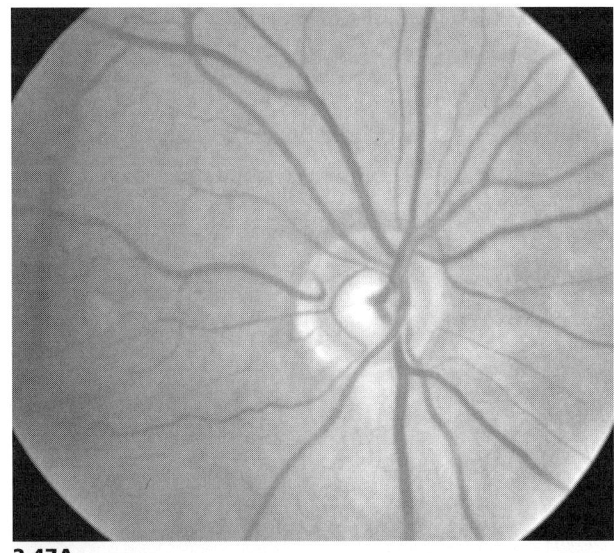

2-47A

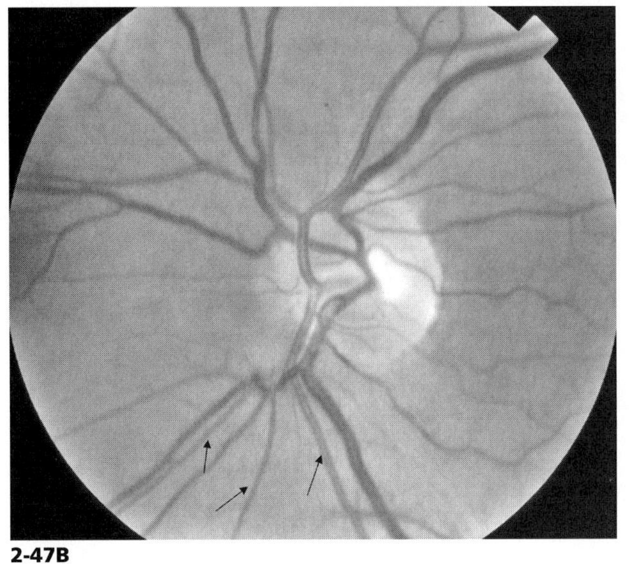

2-47B

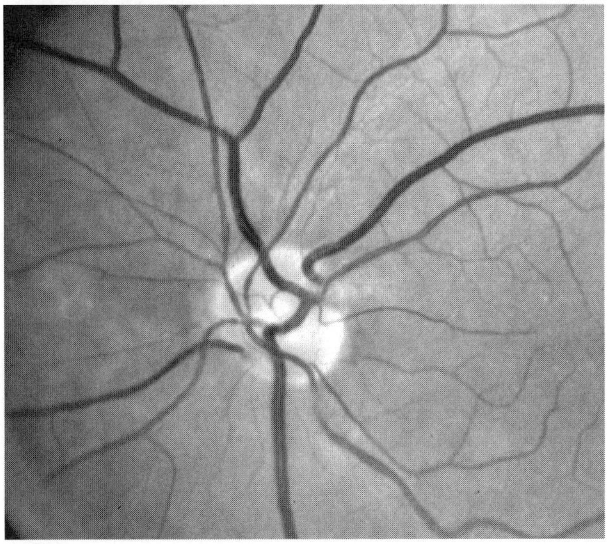

2-47C

Look at the relationship between the arteries and veins. In general, when arteries cross over veins, the veins do not change size or caliber at the crossing. When pathologic crossing changes occur, we traditionally think of changes due to hypertension. Review the section on hypertension, if you see crossing changes (see Chapter 9 on Retina).

Congenital tortuosity of the retinal vessels involving arteries, veins, or both can be a normal variant. Rarely, these vessels have been reported in patients with coarctation of the aorta. They can also be confused with the tortuosity seen with Leber's optic neuropathy (see Chapter 3, Leber's Optic Neuropathy). Finally, they could be confused with opticociliary shunt vessels (see Chapter 5 on Retinochoroidal Collaterals).

Figure 2-48. A–C. **Congenital tortuosity is frequently a benign variant of normal. However, tortuosity has been associated with coarctation of the aorta.** A,B. **Typical congenital tortuosity of the vessels.** C. **Another case of crowded discs with congenitally tortuous vessels. You can see the light reflexes reflecting off the inner limiting membrane nicely (see also Figure 2-24B).**

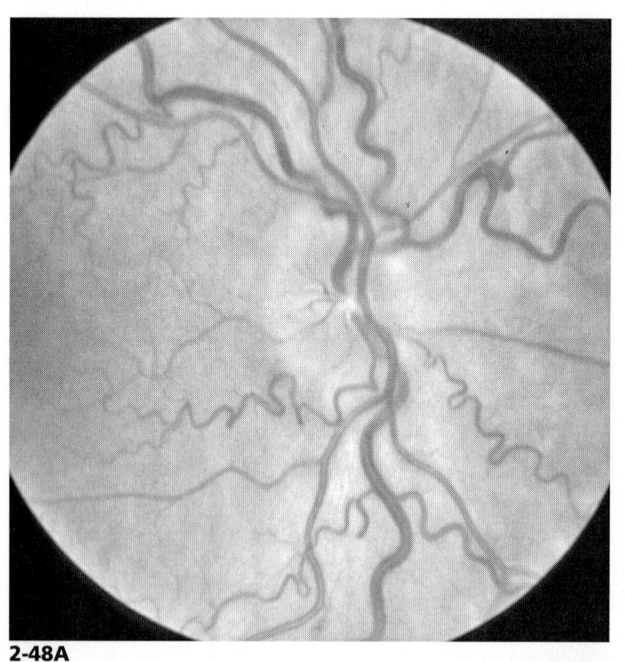

2-48A

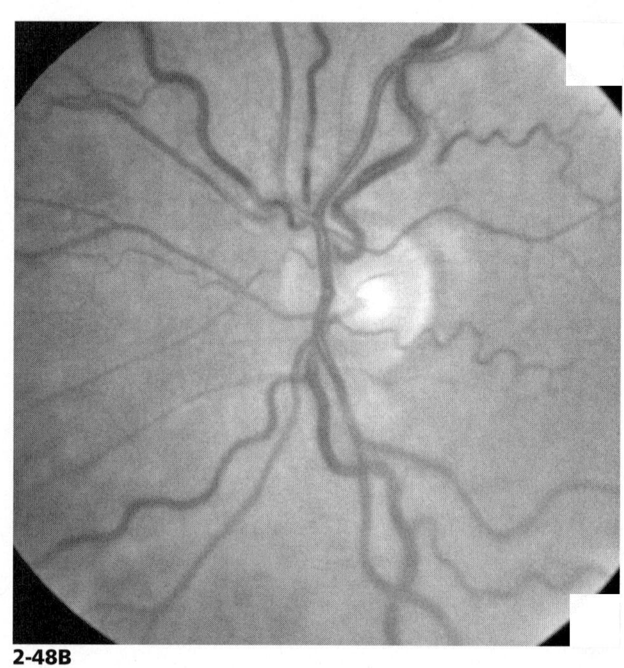

2-48B

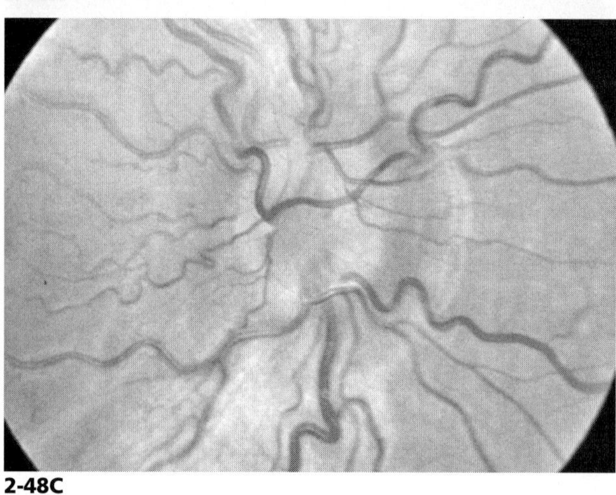

2-48C

Is there CRA pulsation? The CRA does not visibly pulsate normally.

Table 2-4. Causes of Central Retinal Artery Pulsation

Increased intraocular pressure
Occlusion of the central retinal artery or ophthalmic artery
Increased intraorbital pressure
Widened pulse pressure, such as in aortic insufficiency

However, the veins do pulse; look for spontaneous venous pulsations (SVP). SVP can be seen in the large trunks of veins at the level of the disc margin. They are normally present and seen in 37–90% of people, depending on the experience of the examiner and the shape of the disc.[29] SVP are useful when they are known to be present and then are lost.

SVP is thought to occur because there is a common wall at the level of the lamina cribrosa (see Figure 2-12A), where arterial pulse is easily transmitted to the thinner-walled venous vessel. Others have suggested that because the CRV pressure is higher than the intraocular pressure, there is a momentary collapse of the vein during systole as the choroidal vessels fill and increase the intraocular pressure slightly to collapse the vein.[30] In one study by Walsh et al.,[30] 10 subjects whose intracranial pressures were measured by the lumbar puncture method were subjected to a Queckenstedt test, in which pressure was exerted over the jugular veins, and the intracranial pressure rose. They noted that SVP was obliterated at 204.2 ± 25.5 mm of water and returned at 201.6 ± 25.1 mm of water. They concluded that SVP vanishes with elevated intracranial pressure.

Levin confirmed that venous pulsations were present in patients without increased intracranial pressure, so that if you see the pulse, an elevated pressure is unlikely. However, he found that 20% of normal-pressured individuals had no SVP. They

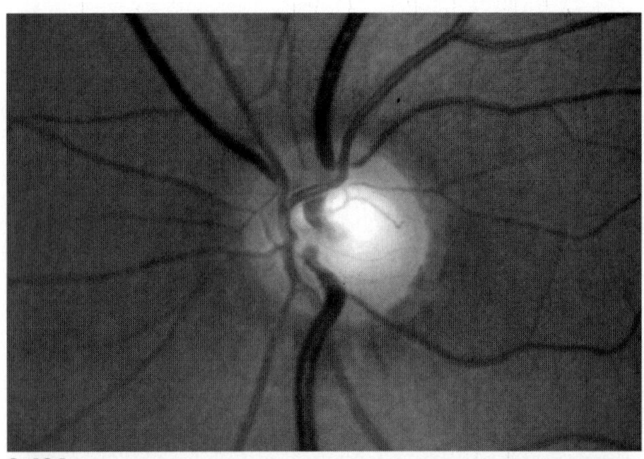

2-49A

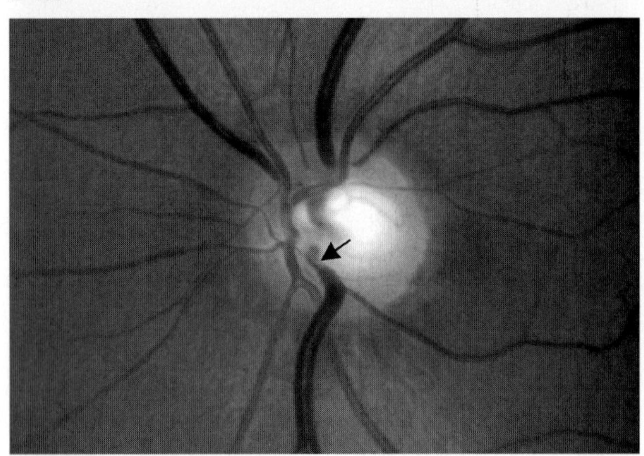

2-49B

concluded that the absence of SVP is not a helpful sign for increased pressure.[31]

In a more recent study, Hedges et al. studied 194 healthy eyes. They found that the best disc configurations in which to see venous pulsations were discs with clearly visible cups and discs where the veins draped over the edge of the neuroretinal rim. In 70% of healthy eyes they were able to view pulsations. The most difficult discs in which to view venous pulsations include those with absent cups, congenitally full discs, and discs in which the veins are obscured by the artery. In the Hedges study, only 6% of these discs had SVP.[32]

Caution must be used, however, in interpreting that venous pulsations mean normal intracranial pressure, because in healthy individuals SVP may not be seen and, occasionally, in pathologically increased intracranial pressure, SVP may still be present. In 1938, Pines declared the test "of no clinical significance."[33] Nevertheless, SVP may be helpful when examining someone for intracranial pressure, noting whether they are present or absent. See Video 2.V.1, Venous Pulsations, on the accompanying CD-Rom.

Figure 2-49. A. **The inferior retinal vein as it comes over the disc is a good place to look for the pulse.** B. **Notice there is a small divot in the vein where the pulse occurs (*arrow*).**

VIEW THE RETINA AND MACULA

Notice the color of the retina: normal, albino, blonde, tesselated. Look for any abnormalities.

In the past, ophthalmologists would normally make a detailed drawing of an optic disc and fundus. Now, the examiner fills in the appropriate abnormalities on a template. It is not a bad idea to get into the habit of drawing the disc features. Sometimes, it may save you time and avoid a lengthy discussion of the findings. Remember that you can also photograph the disc.

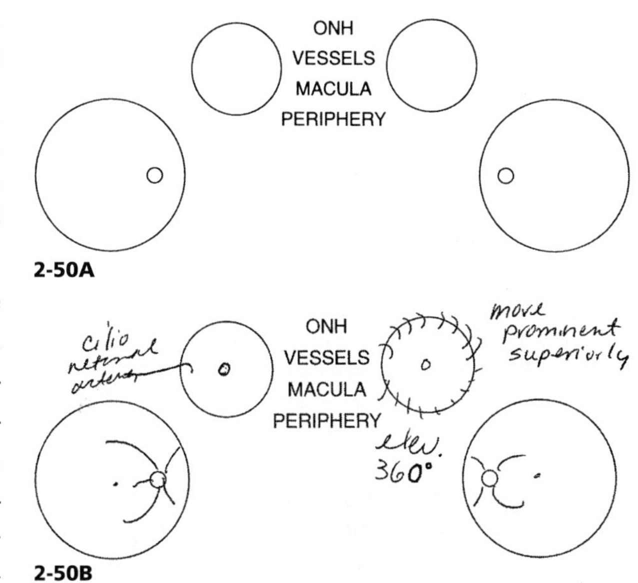

Figure 2-50. A. **This is just one template from a work-up sheet showing a circle at the top to represent the disc and the retina below. Draw and record your results. When you are forced to draw what you see, your viewing skills become more keen. (ONH = optic nerve head.)** B. **Here is an example: the right disc has a small cup-to-disc ratio of 0.1; there is a cilioretinal artery. The left disc is swollen 360 degrees but more prominent superiorly.**

A busy practitioner, however, may not have time for a detailed examination. The following information is helpful. First, the disc is flat (or elevated, or swollen) with normal color (or pallor, swelling, hemorrhages, etc.). The cup-to-disc ratio is 0.3 (or 0.1, 0.6, 0.9). The neuroretinal rim is intact, and the peripapillary area is normal. Venous pulsations are present (or not). Arteries/veins are normal (or there is arteriolar narrowing; venous engorgement, crossing changes [nicking]). The macula is normal (or abnormal—describe). No other retinal or optic disc lesions were seen (e.g., emboli, cotton-wool spots, hemorrhage).

See Video 2.V.2, Tour of the Fundus, on the accompanying CD-Rom. View a tour of the fundus of the eye. Identify the disc, and superior and inferior nasal and temporal arcades. View the macula.

Practical Viewing Essentials

1. Make viewing the optic disc, the peripapillary area, and the macula part of your examination routine.
2. Look for the cup-to-disc ratio.
3. View the nerve fiber layer with a red-free light.
4. Note the size, caliber, shape, and color of the blood vessels.
5. Is there a cilioretinal artery present?
6. Look for venous pulsations.
7. Know what normal variants look like.
8. Try drawing what you see.
9. Keep practicing with your direct ophthalmoscope.

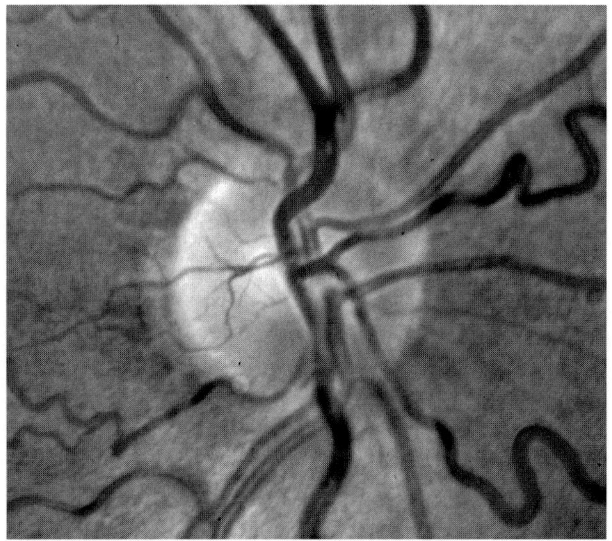

2-51

References

1. Gowers W. A Manual and Atlas of Medical Ophthalmoscopy. London: J & A Churchill, 1879.
2. Charcot JM. Lectures on the Diseases of the Nervous System. Translated and edited by G Sigerson. New York: Hafner Publishing Company, 1962.
3. Taylor J. Selected Writings of John Hughlings Jackson. London: Hodder and Stoughton, 1932.
4. Fong DS, Pruett RC. Systemic associations with myopia. In DM Albert, FA Jakobiec (eds), Principles and Practice of Ophthalmology. Philadelphia: WB Saunders, 1994;3142–3151.
5. Quigley HA, Brown AE, Morrison JD, Drance SM. The size and shape of the optic disc in normal human eyes. Arch Ophthalmol 1990;108:51–57.
6. Brown G, Tasman W. Congenital Anomalies of the Optic Disc. New York: Grune & Stratton, 1983.
7. Apple DJ, Rabb MF, Walsh PM. Congenital anomalies of the optic disc. Surv Ophthalmol 1982;27:3–41.
8. Straatsma BR, Foos RY, Heckenlively JR, Taylor GN. Myelinated retinal nerve fibers. Am J Ophthalmol 1981;91:25–38.
9. Williams TD. Medullated retinal nerve fibers: speculations on their cause and presentation of cases. Am J Optom Physiol Opt 1986;63:142–151.
10. Jean-Louis G, Katz BJ, Warner JEA, et al. Acquired and progressive retinal nerve fiber layer myelination in an adolescent. Am J Ophthalmol 2000;30:361–362.
11. Aaby A, Kushner BJ. Acquired and progressive myelinated nerve fibers. Arch Ophthalmol 1985;103:542–544.
12. Brodsky MC, Baker RS, Hamed LM. Pediatric Neuro-ophthalmology. New York: Springer, 1996.
13. Cogan DG. Neurology of the Visual System. Springfield, IL: Thomas, 1966;7.
14. Hoyt WF, Frisén L, Newman NM. Fundoscopy of nerve fiber layer defects in glaucoma. Invest Ophthalmol Vis Sci 1973;12:814–829.
15. Chester EM. The Ocular Fundus in Systemic Disease. Chicago: Year Book, 1973.
16. Airaksinen PJ, Tuulonen A, Werner EB. Clinical evaluation of the optic disc and retinal nerve fiber layer. In R Ritch, MB Shields, T Krupin (eds), The Glaucomas. St. Louis: Mosby, 1989;467–494.
17. Miller NR, George TW. Monochromatic (red free) photography and ophthalmoscopy of the peripapillary retinal nerve fiber layer. In JL Smith (ed), Neuro-ophthalmology Focus. New York: Massey, 1979;50–51.
18. Salzmann M. The Anatomy and Histology of the Human Eyeball in the Normal State. Translated by EVL Brown. Chicago: Photopress, 1912;76–79.
19. Frisén L. Ophthalmoscopic evaluation of the retinal nerve fiber layer in neuro-ophthalmologic disease. In JL Smith (ed), Neuro-ophthalmology Focus. New York: Massey, 1979;53–67.
20. Rapp LM, Maple SS, Choi JH. Lutein and zeaxanthin concentrations in rod outer segment membranes from perifoveal and peripheral human retina. Invest Ophthalmol Vis Sci 2000;41:1200–1209.
21. Takahashi K, Muraoka K, Kishi S, Shimizu K. Watershed zone in the human peripheral choroid. Ophthalmology 1996;103(2):336–342.
22. Barroso LHL, Hoyt WF, Narahara M. Can the arterial supply of the retina in man be exclusively cilioretinal? J Neuroophthalmol 1994;14:87–90.
23. Parsa CF, Silva ED, Sundin OH, et al. Redefining papillorenal syndrome: an underdiagnosed cause of ocular and renal morbidity. Ophthalmology 2001; 108:738–749.
24. Lee SS, Schwartz B. Role of the temporal cilioretinal artery in retaining central visual field in open-angle glaucoma. Ophthalmology 1992;99:696–699.
25. Airaksinen PJ, Tuulonen A, Werner EB. Clinical evaluation of the optic disc and retinal nerve fiber layer. In R Ritch, MB Shields, T Krupin (eds), The Glaucomas. St. Louis: Mosby, 1996.
26. Garway-Heath DF, Ruben ST, Viswanathan A, Hitchings RA. Vertical cup/disc ratio in relation to optic disc size: its value in the assessment of the glaucoma suspect. Br J Ophthalmol 1998;82(10):1118–1124.
27. Carpel EF, Engstrom PF. The normal cup-disk ratio. Am J Ophthalmol 1981;91:588–597.
28. Armaly MF. The optic cup in the normal eye. Am J Ophthalmol 1969;68:401–407.
29. Lorentzen SE. Incidence of spontaneous venous pulsation in the retina. Acta Ophthalmol (Copenh) 1970;48:765–770.
30. Walsh TH, Garden J, Gallagher B. Relationship of retinal venous pulse to intracranial pressure. In JL Smith (ed), Neuro-Ophthalmology. St. Louis: Mosby, 1968;288–292.
31. Levin BE. The clinical significance of spontaneous pulsations of the retinal vein. Arch Neurol 1978;35: 37–40.
32. Hedges TR Jr, Baron EM, Hedges TR 3rd, Sinclair SH. The retinal venous pulse. Its relation to optic disc characteristics and choroidal pulse. Ophthalmology 1994;101:542–547.
33. Pines N. Some clinical notes on the nature of the retinal venous pulse. Br J Ophthalmol 1938;22:470–482.

3 Is Swelling Present in the Disc?

With respect to the choked papilla nothing can be more simple. The papilla, in fact, then exhibits a tumefaction, a swelling, manifest at the first glance. The borders, ill-defined besides, are, as it were, effaced by an exudation apparently spread both over the papilla and around it. This exudation is of a reddish-grey colour. Here and there the central vessels are, to all appearance, interrupted. This phenomenon, very marked as regards the veins, is less evident with respect to the arteries, which are small in comparison. The capillaries are well-developed, at least at a certain period. This assemblage of the phenomena is already very striking . . .

Jean-Martin Charcot[1]

[Papilledema] is found in most cases to result, not merely from vascular congestion and oedema, but from changes in the nerve fibers and connective tissue . . .

William Gowers[2]

The big question every practitioner faces is "Is the disc swollen?" Why is this important? First, a swollen optic disc is a direct indicator that there could be increased intracranial pressure. Second, a swollen disc could indicate that there is a systemic condition that needs immediate attention. A swollen disc could be the sign of vascular disease, inflammation, or a tumor of the disc. There are many factors that provide clues as to whether the disc is swollen as a result of cerebrospinal fluid–increased pressure, systemic disease, inflammation, or ischemia. First, we need to determine if the disc has true swelling.

Is It Really Swollen?—Mimics of Disc Swelling

HYPEROPIA

Hyperopic discs can be elevated because there is a narrowed scleral canal and a foreshortened globe. Through the narrowed scleral canal and lamina cribrosa, more than 1 million axons must pass; this leads to crowding and elevation that can be mistaken for true disc swelling. One clue to hyperopic disc recognition (or any anomalous disc, for that matter) is the recognition of early-branching retinal vessels. Furthermore, the vessels will seem to come from the center of the disc, and there may be abnormal vasculature such as trifurcations of vessels. The disc may be slightly hyperemic, but there is no venous engorgement, hemorrhages, or exudates.

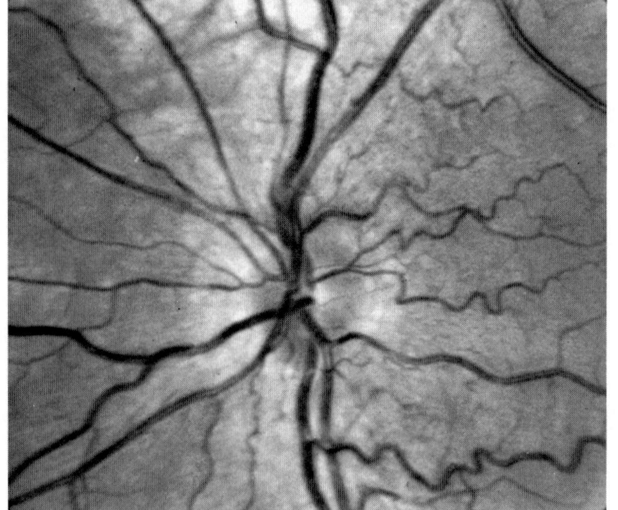

3-1

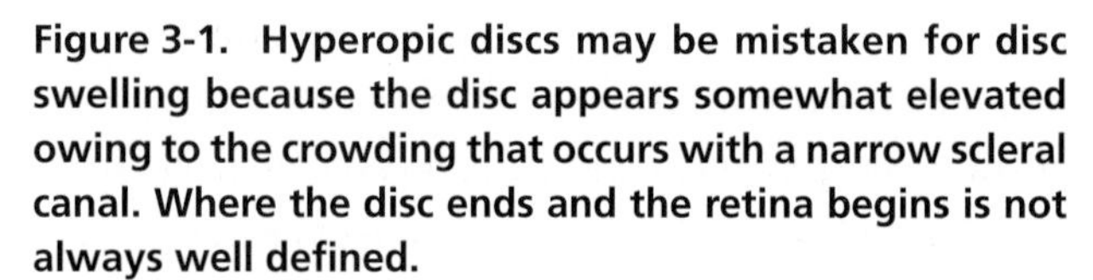

Figure 3-1. Hyperopic discs may be mistaken for disc swelling because the disc appears somewhat elevated owing to the crowding that occurs with a narrow scleral canal. Where the disc ends and the retina begins is not always well defined.

LITTLE RED DISCS

The error in diagnosing little red discs as papilledema is due to the dependence placed on hyperemia as a sign of disc swelling. Gowers admonished: "Attention to tint of the disc alone is a prolific source of error in ophthalmoscopy."[2] The little red disc may be elevated, but the elevation is central and not peripheral. There is little or no cup.

Figure 3-2. A,B. **The little red disc is often mistaken for papilledema. The disc appears elevated and hyperemic, but the veins are not engorged. Notice the tortuosity of the arteries and veins occasionally seen with little red discs.**

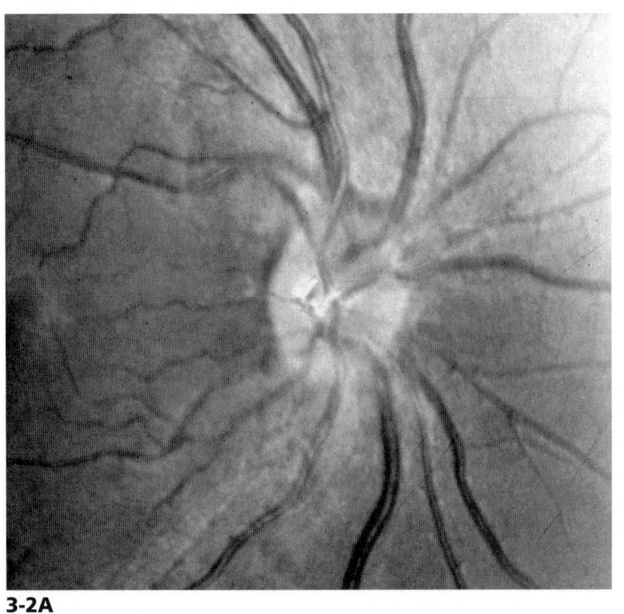

3-2A

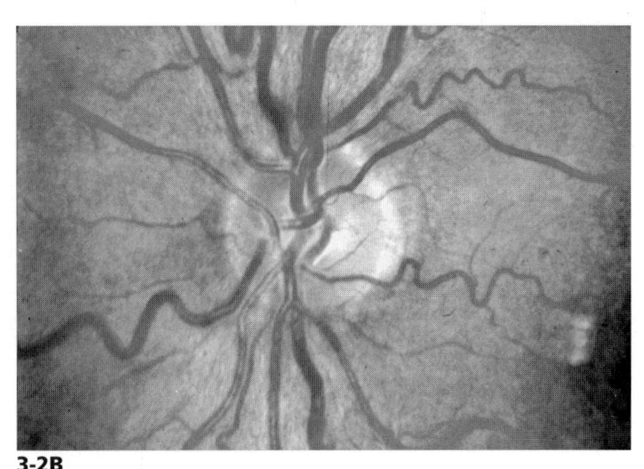

3-2B

PERSISTENT MEMBRANES ON THE DISC

The features that separate persistent membranes of the disc from true papilledema include the lack of venous or capillary dilation and lack of hemorrhages and exudates, and no cup is seen owing to obscuration of the disc. Vision is usually normal, although some degree of amblyopia may be present.

Figure 3-3. Persistent membranes left behind in development can be mistaken for papilledema, but notice that there is no obscuration of the vessels at the disc margin.

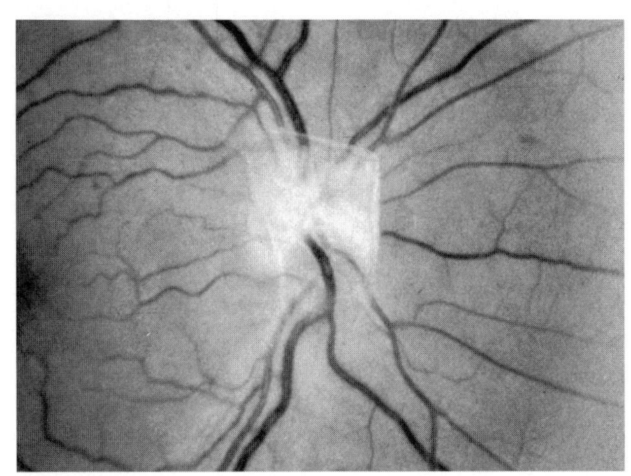

3-3

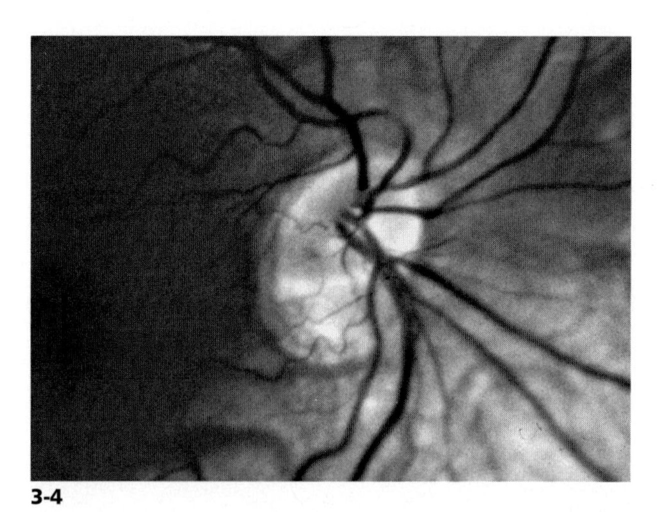

3-4

TILTED DISCS

Tilted discs, normal variants of discs caused by oblique insertion of the optic nerve to the globe, can be, and frequently are, mistaken for papilledema. Because the superior portion of the nerve in a disc that is tilted inferiorly is slightly elevated, these variant discs can be mistaken for early or slight papilledema.

Figure 3-4. Tilted discs may be mistaken for papilledema because one of the edges is elevated. However, look for the other features of a tilted disc. The superior aspect of the disc is elevated and tilted. This disc exhibits a nasal inferior tilt.

MYELINATED NERVE FIBERS

Myelinated nerve fibers can be confused with papilledema. Note the feathery edge.

Figure 3-5. Myelinated nerve fibers are frequently confused with papilledema. Seeing the feathery edge concealing the disc should provide the clue. A. **Myelinated nerve fibers make this disc look elevated and the margins blurred.** B. **These myelinated fibers make the margin of the disc look blurred.**

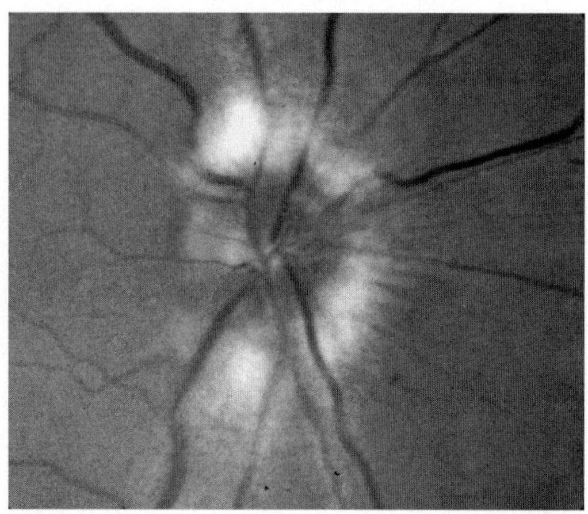

3-5A

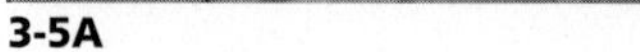

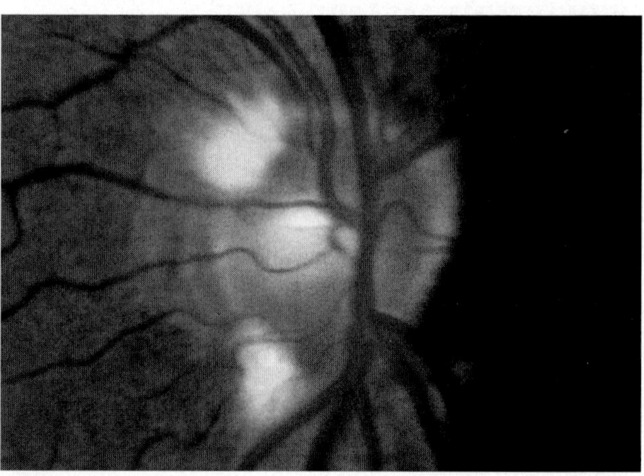

3-5B

DISC DRUSEN

Anomalously elevated optic discs with *disc drusen* are most frequently mistaken for papilledema. One must differentiate optic nerve drusen from retinal drusen. Although the name is the same, the histopathology and source are completely different. Retinal drusen, as is discussed later, are really byproducts of the retinal pigment epithelium deposited on Bruch's membrane (see Retinal Drusen, Chapter 6, Figure 6-16).

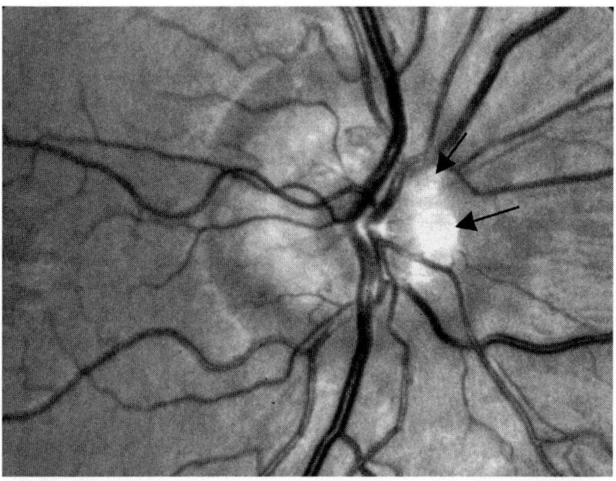

3-6A

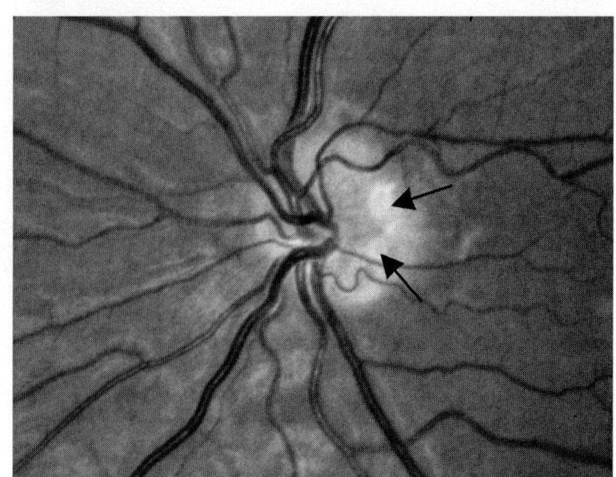

3-6B

Figure 3-6. A,B. **Optic disc drusen are autosomally dominant–inherited disc anomalies that can look like papilledema because the disc is elevated and the margins are blurred. The combination of disc drusen and headache is the most common reason for mistaking anomalous disc swelling for papilledema. The arrows point to visible calcified drusen.**

Optic nerve drusen, also called *hyaline bodies of the optic disc*, are congenital, refractile bodies that may be buried in the disc but with time become visible. The drusen are mainly mucoprotein structures with acid mucopolysaccharides, and smaller quantities of amino acids and iron. They stain positive for calcium and amino acids and negative for amyloid.[3] Disc drusen occur in 0.34% of all people according to Lorentzen, who studied thousands of Danish people for this condition.[4] In an autopsy study, drusen were found in 15 of 737 cadavers' eyes.[5] Drusen are more common in whites than in blacks and are bilateral in approximately 75% of patients, but may be strikingly asymmetric. The youngest case of optic disc drusen reported in the literature is 3.8 years.[6]

Figure 3-7. A. *Drusen* is the German word for crystals. A single crystal is a *druse*, and a rock filled with crystals is a *geode*. Optic disc drusen look like the crystals in a geode. B. The crystals present in rocks resemble drusen on the disc.

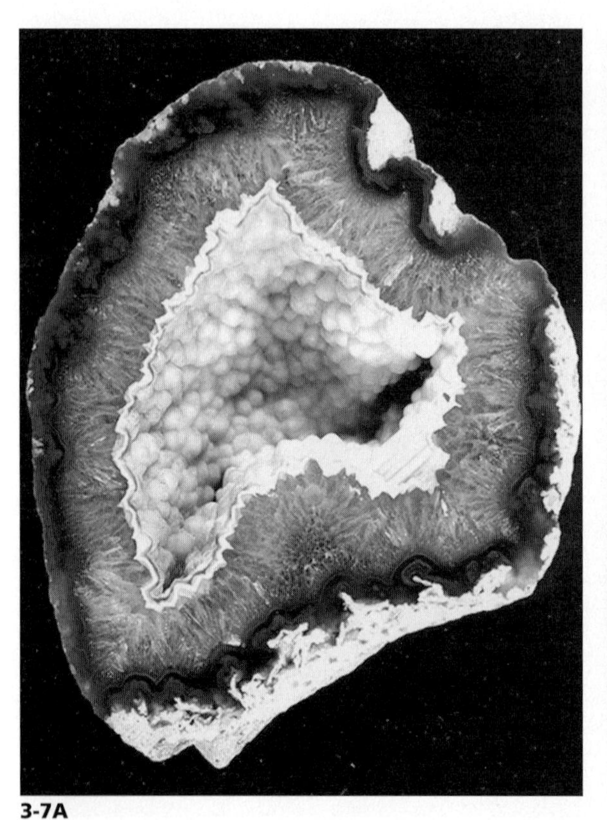

3-7A

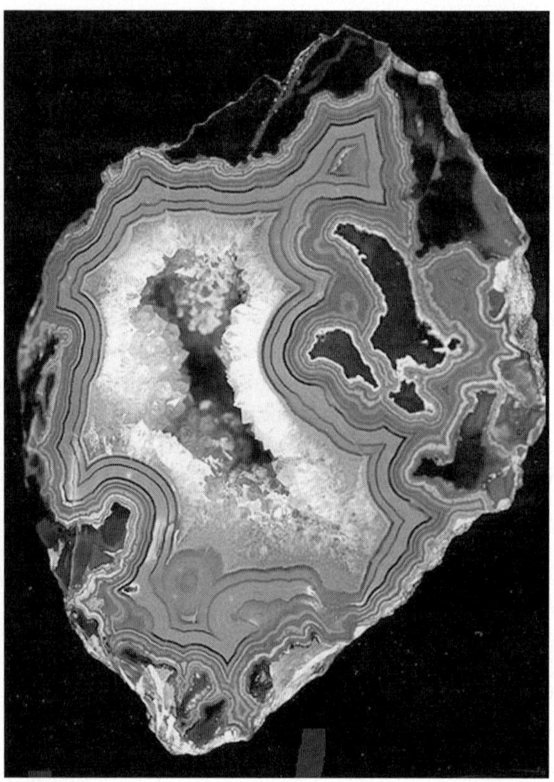

3-7B

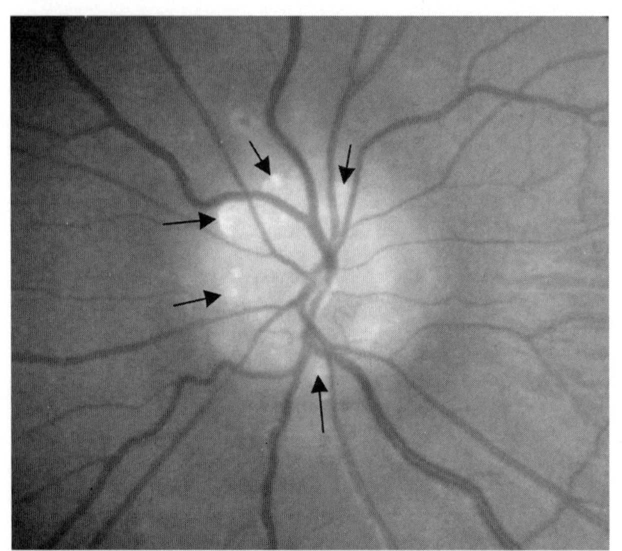

3-8

Figure 3-8. Drusen appear to be small, white crystalline, or yellowish-white, grain-like or round globules, often glistening, seen in the center of the disc or at the disc margin. They may appear singly or in clusters. They are often seen on the nasal edge. The arrows point to some of the drusen on this disc.

Figure 3-9. The associated small scleral canal causing axonal crowding may mechanically interfere with axonal transport, causing the axons to degenerate into drusen or hyaline bodies.[7]

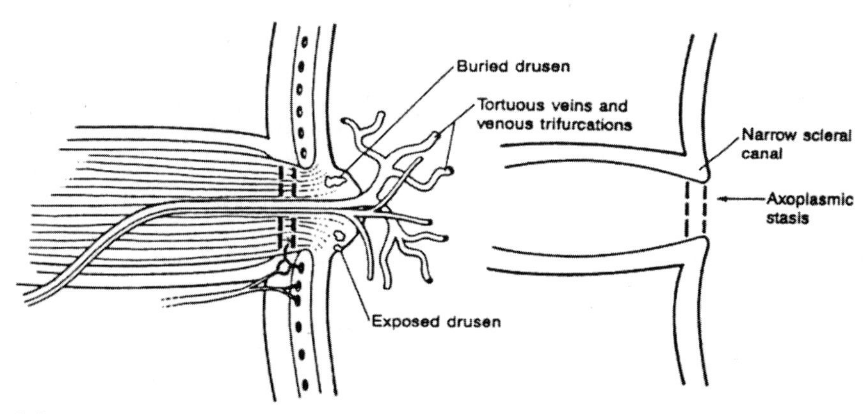

3-9

Drusen may be the *result* of axonal degeneration, rather than its cause.[7] Optic nerve drusen signify a "chronic, low-grade optic neuropathy measured over decades."[8] Antcliff et al. examined relatives of families with drusen. They found anomalous vasculature in more than one-half of the eyes evaluated; also, approximately one-half of the members of the family had no visible cup. This study would indicate that optic disc drusen may be an inherited disc dysplasia along with an abnormality of blood vessel supply.[9]

Although many patients with disc drusen are identified during a routine eye examination or are referred with the diagnosis of headache and presumed papilledema, some patients with drusen present with frequent transient visual obscurations.[6] Children with buried drusen (or underdeveloped drusen) are often referred with suspected papilledema.[10] Occasionally, episodes of transient monocular blindness occur in drusen: Thus, drusen should be in the differential diagnosis of amaurosis fugax. Progressive vision loss frequently occurs, and if patients are aware of vision loss, it may be stepwise. This stepwise progression of vision loss suggests an ischemic mechanism.

Figure 3-10. Typical visual field defects in optic disc drusen—Goldmann visual field. Optic nerve drusen are associated with visual field loss in some patients. As in glaucoma, the visual acuity is normal. The visual field defects are usually nerve fiber bundle defects, enlargement of the blind spot, and field constriction (sometimes severe). Interestingly, the Goldmann visual field defect does not always correlate with the position of the drusen. The visual field of this patient showed complex nerve fiber bundle defects in the eye with the drusen (left eye).

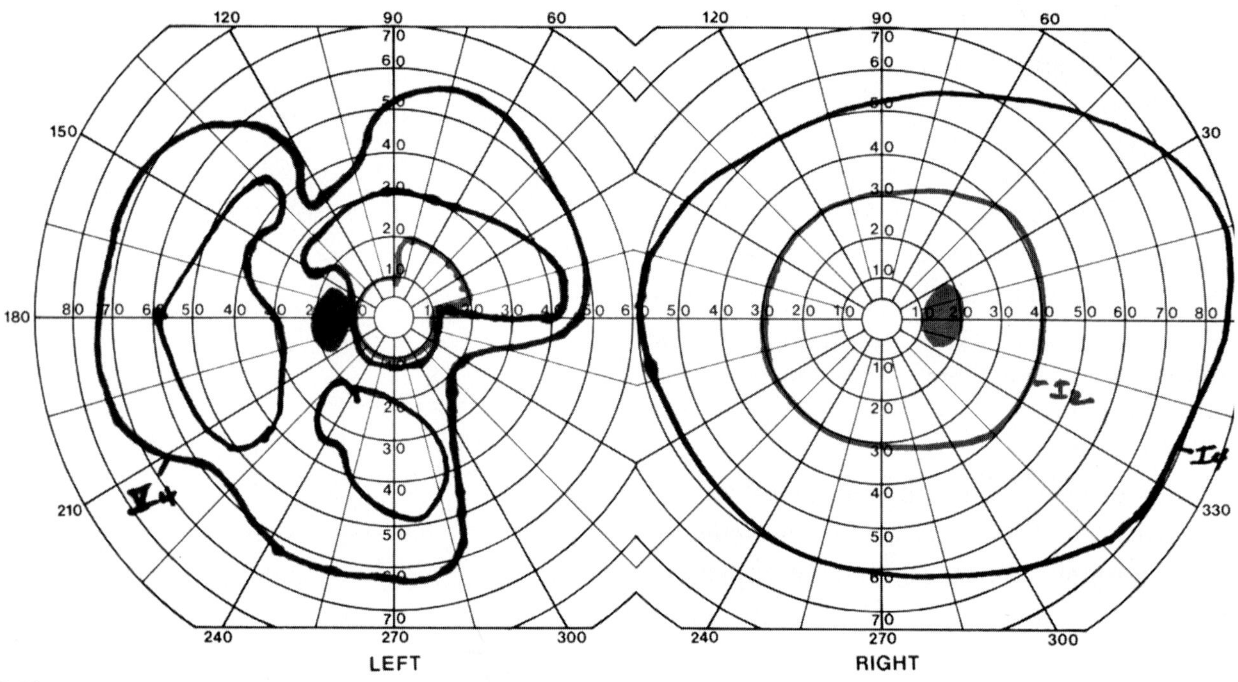

3-10

There are two types of optic disc drusen: The first type is *visible drusen*, in which the glistening drusen are seen on the disc with the direct ophthalmoscope by direct visualization, by using the red-free filter (green light), or by transillumination with the slit lamp.

Figure 3-11. A,B. **Visible drusen exhibit glistening particles easily visible on the disc with the direct ophthalmoscope.**

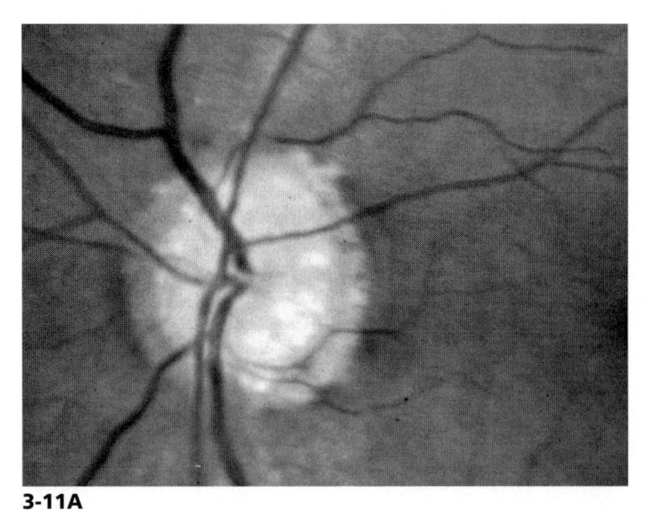

3-11A

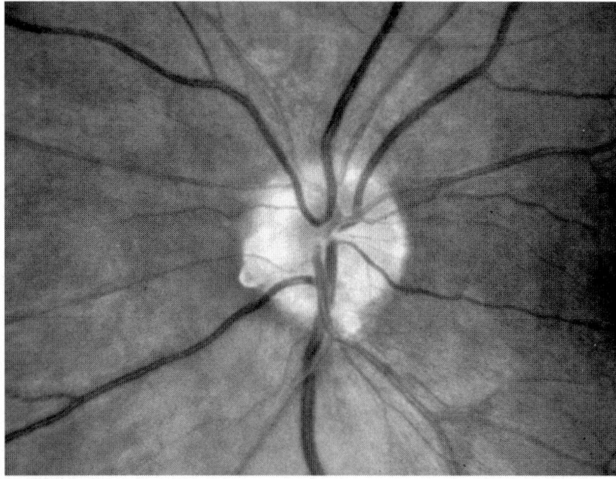

3-11B

Figure 3-12. If you are having trouble determining whether optic disc drusen (*arrows*) are present, use a red-free (green) filter (A) **or the slit beam to side-illuminate the disc** (B).

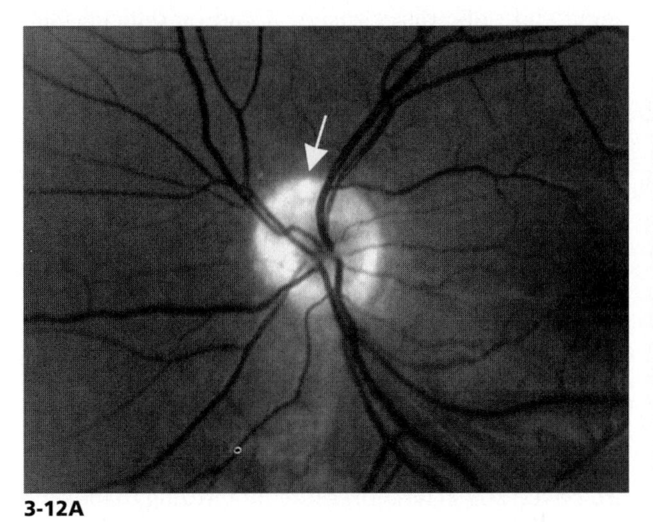

3-12A

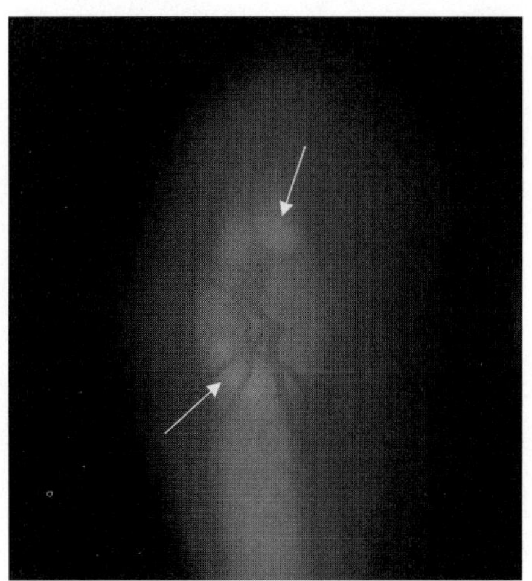

3-12B

The second type is *buried drusen*, in which the disc is elevated without visible refractile bodies being visible. Buried drusen are more likely to be seen in young people. If you see suspect drusen in a youngster, look at the parents. Drusen become visible or increasingly apparent (or "emerge") as individuals age. Buried drusen mimic papilledema so closely that frequently neuroimaging and an extensive evaluation are done before the diagnosis of drusen is correctly made.

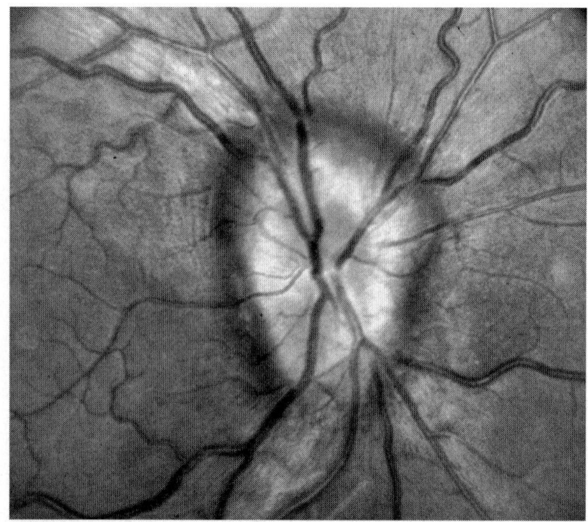

3-13A

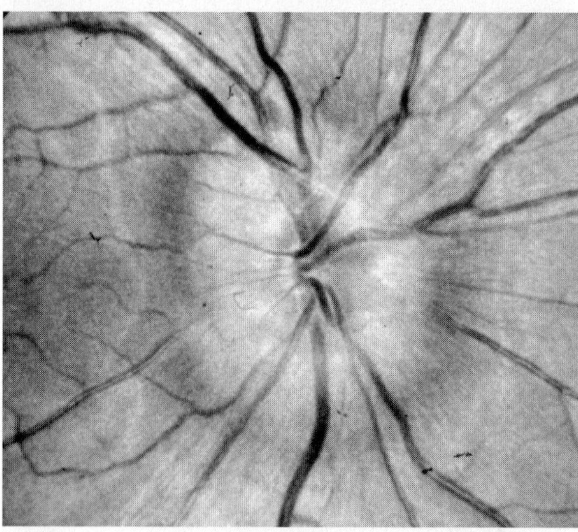

3-13B

Figure 3-13. A,B. **Buried drusen of the disc make the disc look elevated and irregular and are frequently confused with papilledema. Notice that the vessels are plainly seen from where they emerge to the outer edge of the disc.**

Do not confuse optic nerve drusen with superficial drusen-like bodies associated with chronic atrophic papilledema. The drusen-like bodies in papilledema do not mineralize and resolve as the nerve becomes more atrophic. The drusen-like bodies are also caused by a blockage of axoplasmic transport at the optic nerve head. Further confusion can occur because papilledema from increased intracranial pressure has been reported in association with true optic nerve drusen. Thus, drusen do not "protect" against the development of papilledema.

How do you tell the difference between papilledema and optic disc drusen? It can be difficult (see Table 3-1). Sometimes, simply viewing the disc is not enough to make the diagnosis, and further evaluation with fluorescein angiography, orbital ultrasonography, or computed tomography (CT) scanning may be necessary. A fluorescein angiogram can be useful. First, drusen typically autofluoresce. Drusen show early hyperfluorescence of the disc and late focal fluorescence ("staining") of the optic disc. There is no leakage of major vessels (which would be present in papilledema).[11] If there is still confusion after further ophthalmologic evaluation, a lumbar puncture or prolonged spinal fluid pressure monitoring to look for increased intracranial pressure may be necessary.

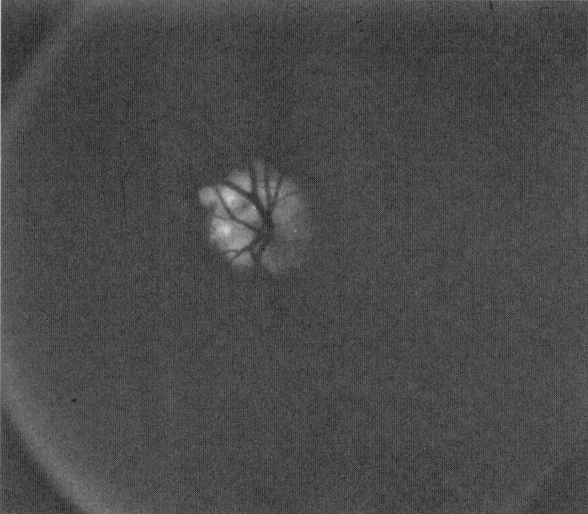

3-14

Figure 3-14. Drusen exhibit autofluorescence. Autofluorescence occurs when a blue light (the excitation light) is shined on the fundus and a disc with drusen; the drusen change the blue wavelength to green and emit the green light that passes through a blue emission filter and is "seen" by the film. B-mode ultrasound is more sensitive than autofluorescence for detecting drusen of the disc and is more available.

Figure 3-15. A. B-scan ultrasound is excellent at detecting buried and not-so-buried drusen. In fact, B-scan echography, when compared with CT and preinjection photography (red-free photographs), was superior.[12] In the right-hand figure, you can see the optic nerve and globe. In the left-hand figure, the gain is turned down and you can appreciate the drusen (*arrow*). B-scan ultrasonography can detect other concomitant optic nerve disorders, such as papilledema and optic neuritis.[13] (Photograph courtesy of Roger Harrie, M.D.) B. CT scans can also detect drusen. Look at the insertion of the optic nerve into the globe. Often a patient has had a scan for presumed papilledema—be sure to look for disc drusen on the scan. In this case, drusen are present bilaterally (*arrows*).

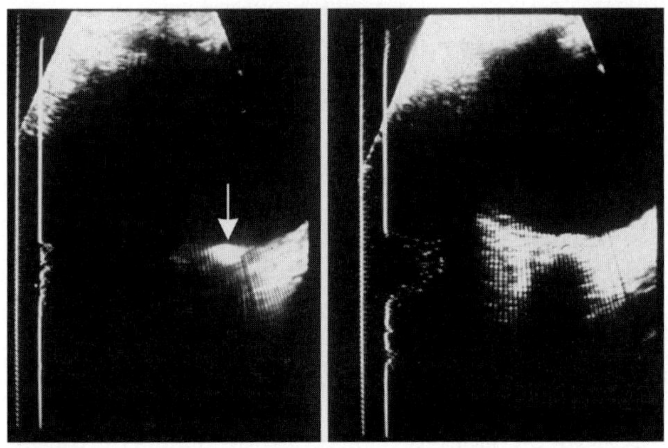

3-15A

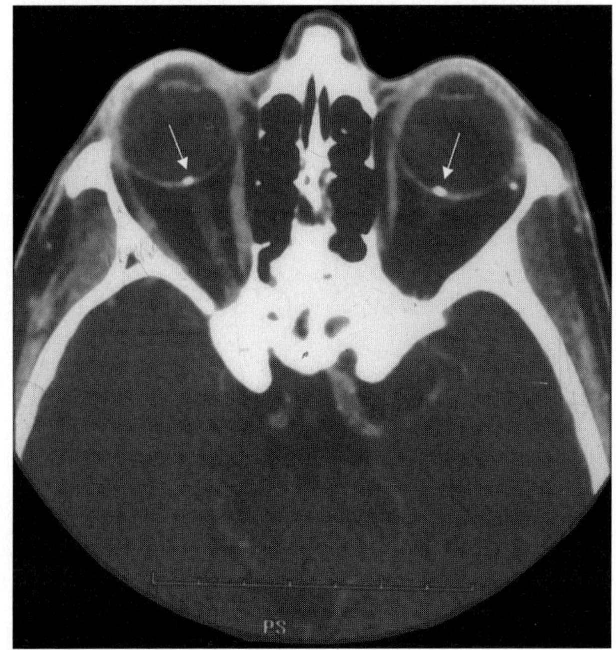

3-15B

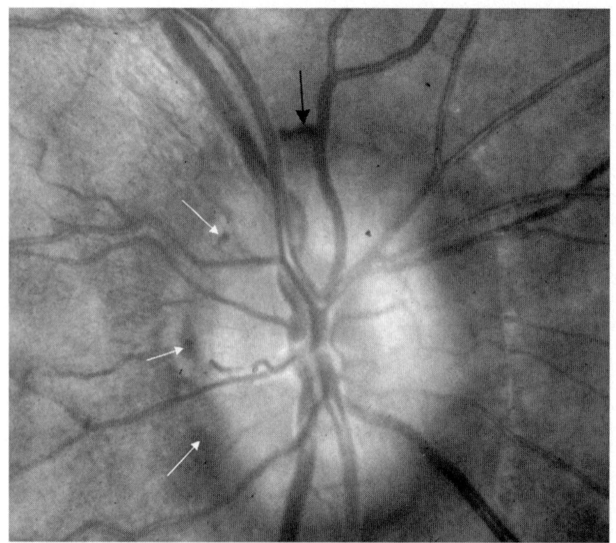

3-16A

Figure 3-16. Hemorrhages of the optic disc associated with optic disc drusen. A. **A small subretinal hemorrhage at 12:00 (*black arrow*). Also note sites of previous hemorrhage at 8, 9, and 10:00 (*small white arrows*).** B. **Subretinal hemorrhages at 12:00 and along the nasal margin of the disc (*arrows*).** C. **Superficial hemorrhage on the disc as a result of the vitreous face pulling away from the disc with drusen. Note that there is a hemorrhage in the vitreous (*top arrow*). The bottom arrow points to blood in the vitreous.**

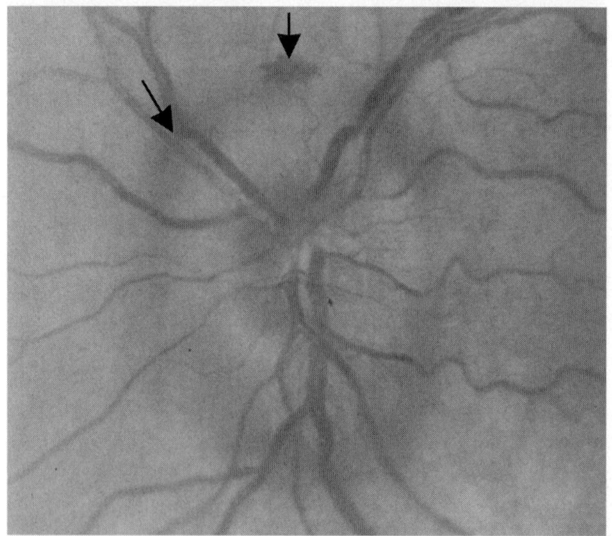

3-16B

3-16C

Drusen may be associated with intraretinal or subretinal hemorrhages around the disc. Look for splinter hemorrhages along the disc: These are linear and follow the nerve fiber layer. Splinter hemorrhages are usually single, compared to multiple hemorrhages seen in papilledema. Deep subretinal hemorrhages can occur in the immediate peripapillary area. Although these hemorrhages do occur in severe papilledema, they are not common in the less severe grades of swelling. Deep subretinal hemorrhages disrupt the retinal pigment epithelium, leading to secondary pigmentary changes seen surrounding the disc with drusen. A third kind of hemorrhage seen with drusen is the development of neovascular peripapillary subretinal hemorrhage.

Figure 3-17. Although hemorrhages are more common, anterior ischemic optic neuropathy (AION) is a common vascular event associated with drusen. In this case, the patient experiences fairly abrupt onset of painless vision loss, often in the morning. The examiner finds a truly swollen, usually pallid optic disc. Drusen are identified as the cause after the swelling subsides, or occasionally they are identified with B-scan ultrasonography while the disc is acutely swollen. The vision loss with drusen is disc-related and usually permanent. Other, much less common, vascular events include branch or central retinal artery occlusions and retinal vein occlusions.

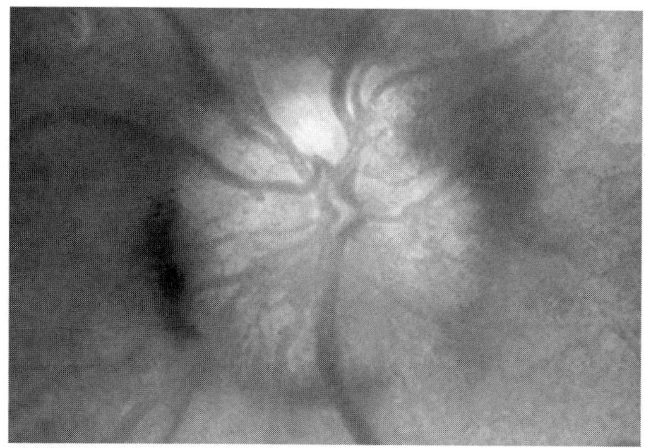

3-17

Drusen are seen infrequently with other conditions such as retinitis pigmentosa, microphthalmos, and angioid streaks. Retinitis pigmentosa, early on, can be associated with disc elevation, and a careful look for narrowing of the retinal arterioles and peripheral bone spicule formation is helpful.[14] If retinitis pigmentosa is suspected, order an electroretinogram. Angioid streaks are seen with drusen, but are also a feature of pseudoxanthoma elasticum (see Chapter 9).[15] Migraine is frequently mentioned as a drusen association; however, migraine is so common that this almost certainly reflects that the headache prompted the doctor to do an ophthalmoscopic evaluation.

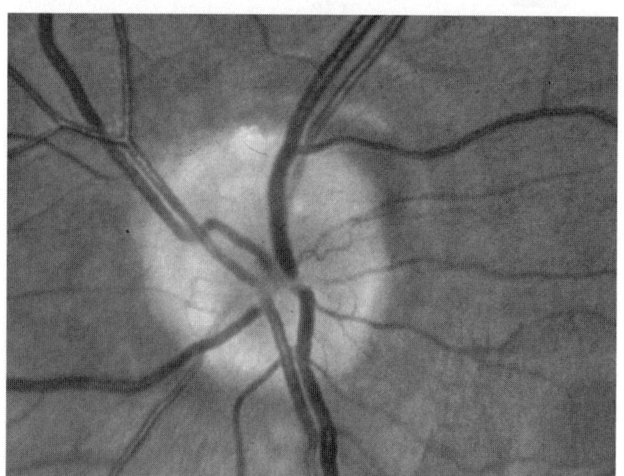

3-18A

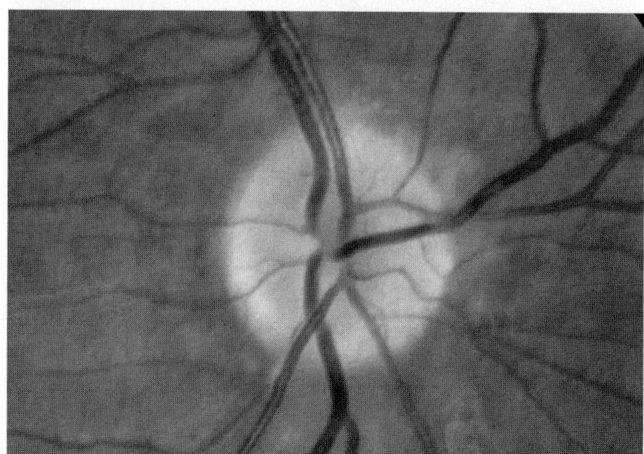

3-18B

Figure 3-18. A,B. **Drusen can be associated with papilledema. Don't be misled: Sometimes patients have drusen and papilledema. This woman presented with headache and disc swelling. A magnetic resonance image (MRI) was normal, but ultrasonography of the orbit revealed bilateral drusen. A lumbar puncture showed intracranial pressure of more than 300 mm H_2O. She was later diagnosed with idiopathic intracranial hypertension.**

The Swollen Optic Disc

3-19A

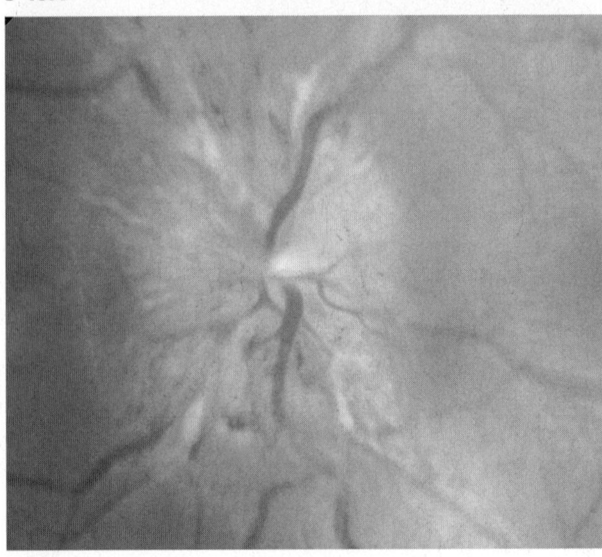

3-19B

Figure 3-19. A,B. **True disc swelling due to increased intracranial pressure.**

Many people are confused by the terminology used to designate disc swelling: *Swollen disc*, *disc edema*, *papilledema*, *papillitis*, *choked disc*, and *elevated optic nerve* are terms used interchangeably. The important concept here is that a disc can swell as a result of many inciting events. The disc can respond to pathologic processes in only so many ways.

Swollen disc: This broad term encompasses axonal distention and disc elevation. Causes of disc swelling include increased intracranial pressure, inflammation, ischemia and compression of the optic nerve, hypotony, toxicity, and a congenitally narrow scleral canal.

Disc edema: True edema of the optic nerve is where there is histologic evidence of not only swollen axons, but increased fluid around the axons. In experimental models of optic disc swelling, there is primarily axonal swelling and little actual fluid (edema). *Disc edema* is a term that loosely and inaccurately encompasses all forms of swelling of the disc.

Papilledema: A swollen disc owing to increased intracranial pressure.

Papillitis: A term used to denote inflammation of the optic disc, such as is seen in syphilis, or inflammation seen with the anterior form of optic neuritis.

Choked disc: An English translation by Clifford Albutt of the German term *Staaungspapilla*[16] that is used to denote any form of optic disc swelling: Literally, *choked disc* refers to axoplasmic stasis at the level of the lamina cribrosa in which the scleral canal is too narrow to accommodate the distended axons, hence "choked." Congenital "choking" is really a hyperopic disc or an anomalously elevated disc, whereas acquired choke is more often true swelling. The term *choked disc* has about as much specificity as *swollen disc* or *disc edema*.

Neuroretinitis: Neuroretinitis is usually seen with a prominent macular star (e.g., optic disc edema with macular star). The term denotes an inflammatory optic disc swelling owing to parainfectious or infectious damage of the optic nerve and retina. Thus, not only is the disc swollen, but changes in the retina are present.

Optic neuritis: Years ago, *optic neuritis* was the term used by Gowers and others to denote *all* causes of swelling of the optic disc. Now, optic neuritis refers to a nerve affected by inflammation, demyelination, or degeneration. Anterior optic neuritis shows swelling anterior to the lamina cribrosa, whereas retrobulbar optic neuritis denotes inflammation, demyelination, and degeneration behind the lamina cribrosa not visible with the ophthalmoscope. In retrobulbar optic neuritis, there is usually no disc swelling.

WHAT CAUSES THE DISC TO SWELL?—MECHANISM OF DISC SWELLING

Tso and Hayreh experimentally demonstrated in the monkey that axoplasmic stasis caused optic disc swelling whether the swelling was from papilledema (caused by high-dose radiation to the brain and inflated intracranial balloon) or ocular hypotension (ciliary body destruction). After the disc became swollen, tritiated leucine was injected into the vitreous cavity. The leucine was incorporated, by way of the protein-making RNA in the ganglion cell, into axoplasm. The investigators traced axoplasmic flow with radiophotographs and showed that stasis of axoplasm occurred at the retrolaminar portion of the lamina cribrosa.[17] These studies confirmed earlier studies of Weiss and Hiscoe,[18] and later Wirtschafter et al.,[19] that showed that tying a ligature around the optic nerve caused axoplasmic stasis and optic disc edema.

Figure 3-20. This figure demonstrates that the mechanism of swelling is similar, no matter what the underlying cause. A. **The normal ganglion cell has unimpeded axoplasmic flow through the lamina cribrosa. Intracranial pressure (ICP) and intraocular pressure (IOP) are also normal.** B. **Axoplasmic flow is impeded when IOP is lower than ICP—a pressure gradient.** C. **If ICP is high and IOP is normal, a pressure gradient is produced and the axoplasm is static at the lamina cribrosa.** D,E. **Both irreversible and reversible toxic metabolic effects cause damage to mitochondria, and axoplasmic flow, which requires energy, becomes dammed up.** F. **Inflammation also acts to slow axoplasmic flow focally and results in disc swelling.**

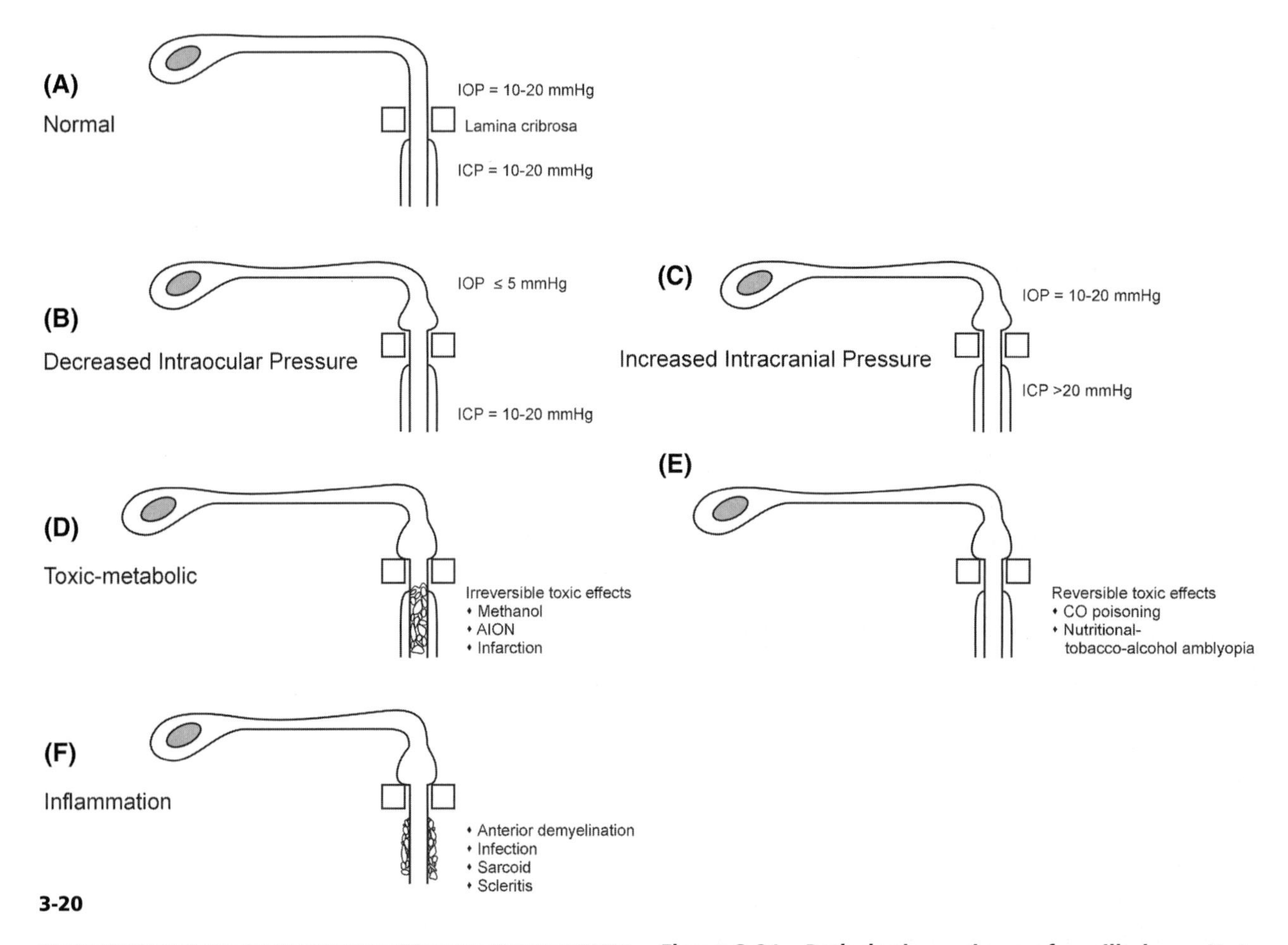

3-20

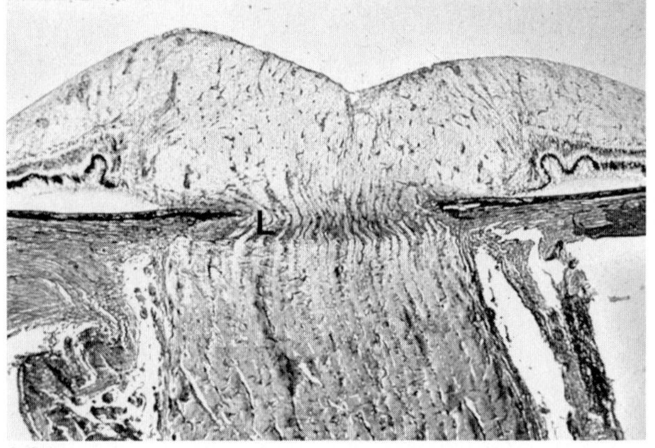

3-21

Figure 3-21. Pathologic specimen of papilledema. Note that you can see the "damming up" of axoplasm at the level of the lamina cribrosa (L). The axons make a right-angle turn from the retina to pass through the lamina cribrosa. The axons are swollen anterior to the lamina cribrosa, leading to the heaped-up disc. The swelling is worse on the nasal aspect and lifts the retina up somewhat, as described by Samuels.[20]

Clearly, swelling of the optic disc has a basic and common mechanism whether it is owing to increased intracranial pressure, ischemia, poisoning from methanol or carbon monoxide, ocular hypotension, or even a small scleral canal. Damming up of the axoplasmic flow at the level of the lamina cribrosa causes physical swelling of axons, and it is the axoplasmic swelling that causes "edema" of the disc. True interstitial edema fluid is not responsible for the increased disc volume and elevation. It is the swelling of the axons that causes disc swelling: This is why the "cup" is preserved until late in papilledema. The cup is axon free and gradually fills with swollen axoplasm as the axoplasmic stasis persists. That is also why a disc with atrophy cannot swell—if axons have been lost, there is no swelling.

Papilledema or swelling of the optic disc owing to increased intracranial pressure is caused by axoplasmic stasis caused by the pressure differential between the intraocular pressure and the intracranial pressure at the level of the lamina cribrosa.

Vascular changes occur in true disc swelling. The swollen axons reduce the space required by capillary blood vessels; this leads to dilation of the capillaries and stasis of venous drainage from the disc. Retinal veins are engorged and become elongated and tortuous. The telangiectatic capillary network over the optic disc becomes dilated and hyperemic, and frequently looks like a hairnet with multiple knotted microaneurysmal dilations. Some people have called this hairnet the *caput medusae* (literally, the head of the mythical creature Medusa). Retinochoroidal vessels begin to form to provide alternative venous drainage via the choroidal vortex veins. Focal areas of ischemia may produce nerve fiber layer infarcts. Hemorrhages occur both on the disc and in the peripapillary nerve fiber layer, as well as in the subretinal space. Any process that produces axoplasmic stasis has the

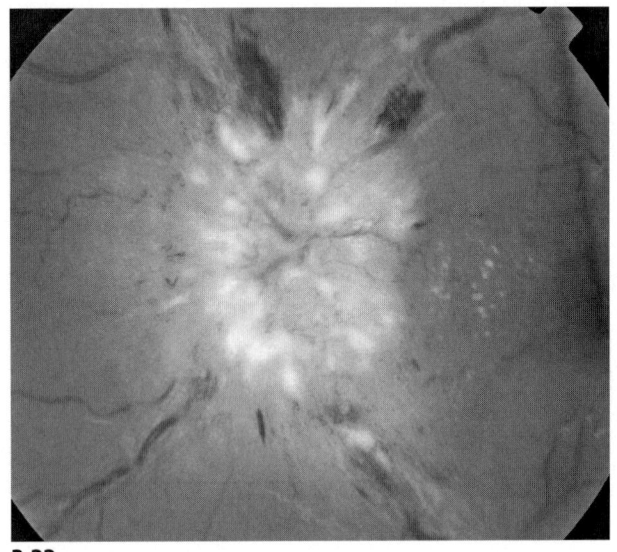
3-22

potential to produce similar changes. Thus, the appearance of swelling alone is not diagnostic of the cause of disc swelling.

Because a disc may swell in a number of different clinical settings, what features give you clues that the disc is swollen owing to a pathologic process and not as the result of pseudoswelling (e.g., anomalous optic discs, drusen, tilted optic disc, hyperopia, little red discs)? What are the findings of bona fide disc swelling, whether from papilledema or another process?

Figure 3-22. This disc exhibits features of true disc swelling: hyperemia, swelling of axons (blurred disc margin), elevation, hemorrhage, dilation of the veins, cotton-wool spots, and hemorrhage.

First, *hyperemia* that is caused by dilation of the disc capillaries is frequently used to denote papilledema. Gowers attached significance to hyperemia in three conditions:

Abnormal redness of the disc does occur as a morbid state, and, although in itself a sign of little value, it derives importance from certain concomitant conditions. It is significant (a) when it possesses special characters to be immediately described; (b) when developed under observation; and (c) when it is notably greater in one eye than in the other.[2]

The primary element pathologically of a swollen optic disc is *swelling of axons* in the peripapillary nerve fiber layer that causes blurred disc margin. *Blurring* is something that takes practice looking for. Remember that you are looking for nerve fiber layer swelling. The place to look for earliest blurring is the lower pole, then the upper pole, and then the nasal aspect of the disc. The temporal margin is the last to blur. The texture of the nerve fiber layer is shaggy and relatively opaque. According to Hayreh,[21] the earliest sign of papilledema in the experimental animal is "swelling"; in fact, swelling precedes hyperemia by almost 24 hours.[21] *Blurred disc margin* alone can be seen with anomalous elevation, but in anomalous discs the vessels crossing the disc tissue are not obscured by swelling. Blurring owing to true disc swelling and papilledema first occurs superiorly and inferiorly on the margin of the disc, because that is where the nerve fibers are thickest, and any swelling of the axons causes coarsening of the axons and "blurring" there first. Furthermore, the blurring begins to obscure the blood vessels at the disc margin. To see blurring, look at the superior and inferior disc: Does the edge of the disc appear distinct, or is there some opacity or graying of the nerve fiber layer? What do the vessels look like at the disc margin?

The third finding of pathologically swollen optic nerves is disc *elevation*. With swelling of the optic disc, elevation of the disc occurs peripherally before it is seen centrally, and the swollen disc may take on the appearance of a "red blood cell," erythrocyte, or volcano. This is because the cup, if present, is maintained until very late. To see minor elevation, move your head and ophthalmoscope slightly from the disc to retina: Is there a change in elevation? Use the slit beam on the ophthalmoscope and note whether it is straight or there is bending (bending indicates elevation). Hoyt admonishes us: "Disc elevation in itself does not mean papilledema!"[22]

A fourth finding is *hemorrhage*. Usually, peripapillary retinal nerve fiber layer hemorrhage and occasional subretinal circumpapillary hemorrhage are seen. Single perivascular splinter hemorrhages at the disc margin can be important. Hemorrhages seen with papilledema include several types, including the splinter hemorrhages. *Dilation*, elongation, and tortuosity of the retinal veins occur as venous outflow is retarded. Exudates or cotton-wool spots (nerve fiber layer infarcts) may appear along with hemorrhages.

Also look for small retinal folds or striae—concentric, circumferential wrinkles—that may be present with severe swelling of the disc (*Paton's lines*). These concentric wrinkles are owing to displacement of retinal elements. This displacement is in part responsible for the enlarged blind spot seen on visual field testing. The blind spot enlargement is due more to elevation of the peripapillary retina than to lateral displacement. After swelling resolves, the folds may or may not disappear; frequently, the enlarged blind spot remains owing to the displacement of those retinal elements.

On a historical note, Leslie Paton was a pathologist who, with Gordon Holmes in the early part of the twentieth century, examined 39 patients clinically by ophthalmoscopy and later by autopsy and histologic sections of optic nerves displaying papilledema. In their seminal work, Paton and Holmes describe what came to be known as *Paton's lines* thusly: "As the disc swells lateral wards it displaces the retina either raising it up from the pigment layer, or throwing it into a series of folds which run concentric with the edge of the disc."[23]

Look for venous pulsations. Another early sign of papilledema may be the loss of spontaneous venous pulsations. Although loss of spontaneous venous pulsations is not an absolute indication of increased intracranial pressure, it can be a helpful sign. A patient in the emergency room, for example, with severe headaches may present a diagnostic dilemma. The presence of bounding venous pulsations may allow you to diagnose migraine. Conversely, absent venous pulsations with an acute headache may signal increased intracranial pressure. Although certainly not the most important part of diagnosing papilledema, you should get used to looking for pulsations (see 2-V-1, Venous Pulsations, on the accompanying CD-Rom).

Putting it all together, there is not one single sign that denotes true disc swelling or papilledema—there are many. In your mind, get in the habit of viewing the optic disc for these features. Getting used to looking at swollen discs takes practice. Once you begin to look, you will see.

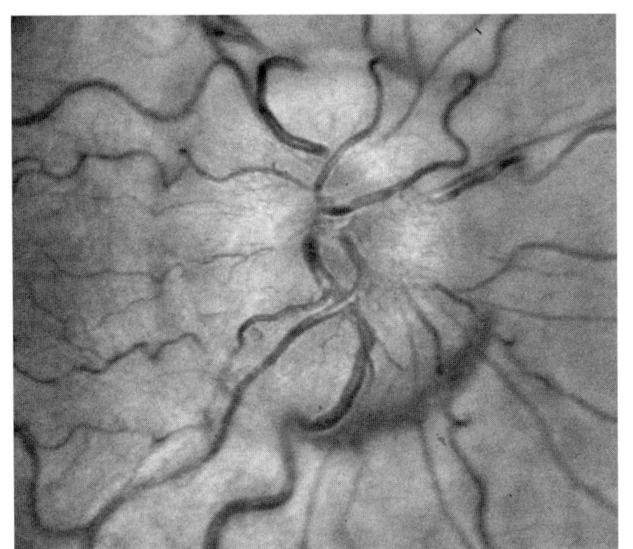
3-23A

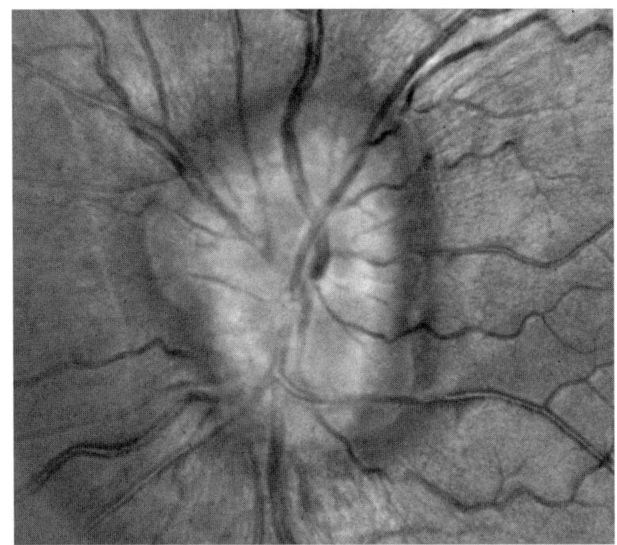
3-23B

Table 3-1. Features That Distinguish between Pathologic Disc Swelling and Pseudoswelling

Characteristic	Papilledema and other causes of true disc swelling (see also Figure 3-23A)	Pseudopapilledema or pseudoswelling (see also Figure 3-23B)
Disc and cup	Physiologic cup is present until late.	Physiologic cup is absent.
Vessels	Vessels arise normally in the disc with a normal pattern; veins may be engorged; capillaries leak on fluorescein; may see retinochoroidal collaterals.	Vessels arise from the apex of the disc; early branching with trifurcations on the disc, frequent cilioretinal artery; vessels bifurcate above the retinal plane; vessels and veins not engorged; no leakage of fluorescein from vessel, but may have focal fluorescence.
Peripapillary area	Swollen axons obscure the peripapillary area and blood vessels.	Disc margin irregular, pigment changes around the disc; often see a peripapillary ring of light; blood vessels not obscured.
Color	Hyperemia with capillary dilation; *caput medusae*.	Absent capillary telangiectasia; disc color varies from pale to hyperemic.
Elevation	Diffuse elevation of the disc.	Elevation irregular; refractile bodies (drusen).
Hemorrhages	Peripapillary nerve fiber layer hemorrhage or subretinal hemorrhage.	Occasionally see peripapillary subretinal hemorrhage or rare superficial hemorrhages.
Exudates	Exudates if the papilledema is chronic; late superficial tiny pseudodrusen.	No exudates.
Folds	Small concentric folds around the disc (Paton's lines); or horizontal retinal/chorioretinal folds.	No folds.
Red-free filter	No drusen.	Drusen may be found.
Venous pulsations	Absent spontaneous venous pulsations.	Spontaneous venous pulsations present.
Genetic influence	Not familial.	Frequently familial—drusen autosomal dominant.

Source: Data from RA Hitchings, JJ Corbett, J Winkelman, NJ Schatz. Hemorrhages with optic nerve drusen. Arch Neurol 1976;33:675–677; MC Brodsky, RS Baker, LM Hamed. Pediatric Neuro-ophthalmology. New York: Springer, 1996.

What can you do if, after going through the checklist, you still don't know if it is real disc swelling or pseudoswelling?

First, check the history. Go over the findings of real papilledema. Other tests may be helpful—check the visual field. Is it normal? Does it show enlargement of the blind spot? Fluorescein angiography may also be helpful in determining whether there is true disc swelling. The nerve in a swollen disc turns white from late disc staining.

Figure 3-24. Fluorescein angiography can be helpful in discerning whether true disc swelling exists. A. Red-free photograph of the right disc before fluorescein injection. B. Red-free photograph of the left disc. Notice that from 11:00 to 6:00 there is a subretinal hemorrhage, which looks black on this red-free photograph. C. Left disc with early laminar flow stage—see the striped flow in the vein. One characteristic of true papilledema early on is the capillary dilation (*caput medusae*) directly on the disc. D. Later, there is leakage of dye of the left disc, making the disc look larger. Notice the subretinal hemorrhage now blocks normal fluorescence of the choroid. E. Even later, there is staining of the disc and dye leakage beyond the disc margin.

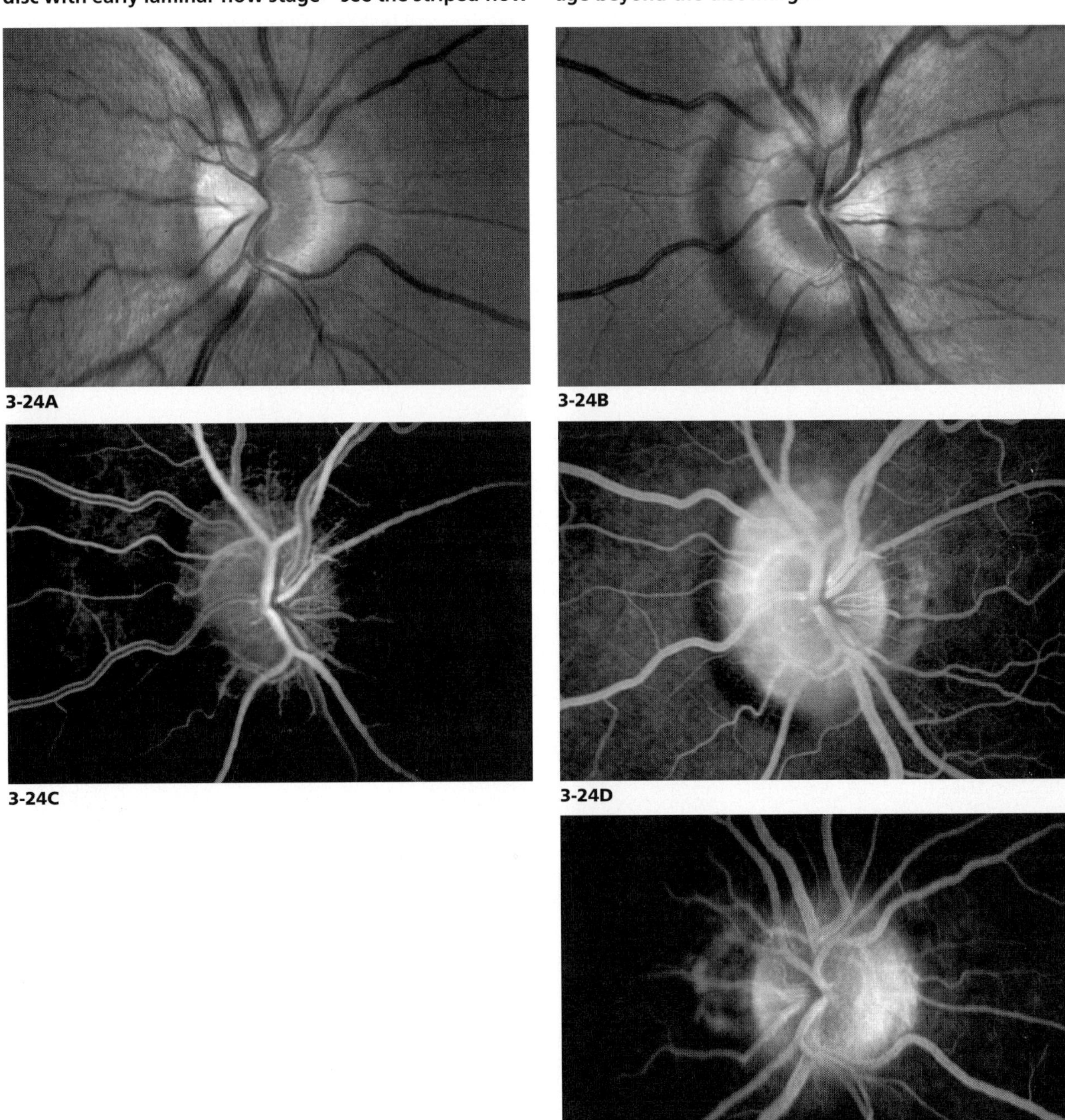

3-24E

Figure 3-25. A. **The right disc does not convincingly show disc swelling. This patient has idiopathic intracranial hypertension with asymmetric papilledema. The fluorescein angiogram helps to diagnose that both discs are swollen. Use the fluorescein angiogram if you are not sure if there is papilledema.** B. **The left disc shows more swelling. A fluorescein angiogram shows staining and leakage on the right** (C) **and left** (D), **confirming disc swelling due to papilledema.**

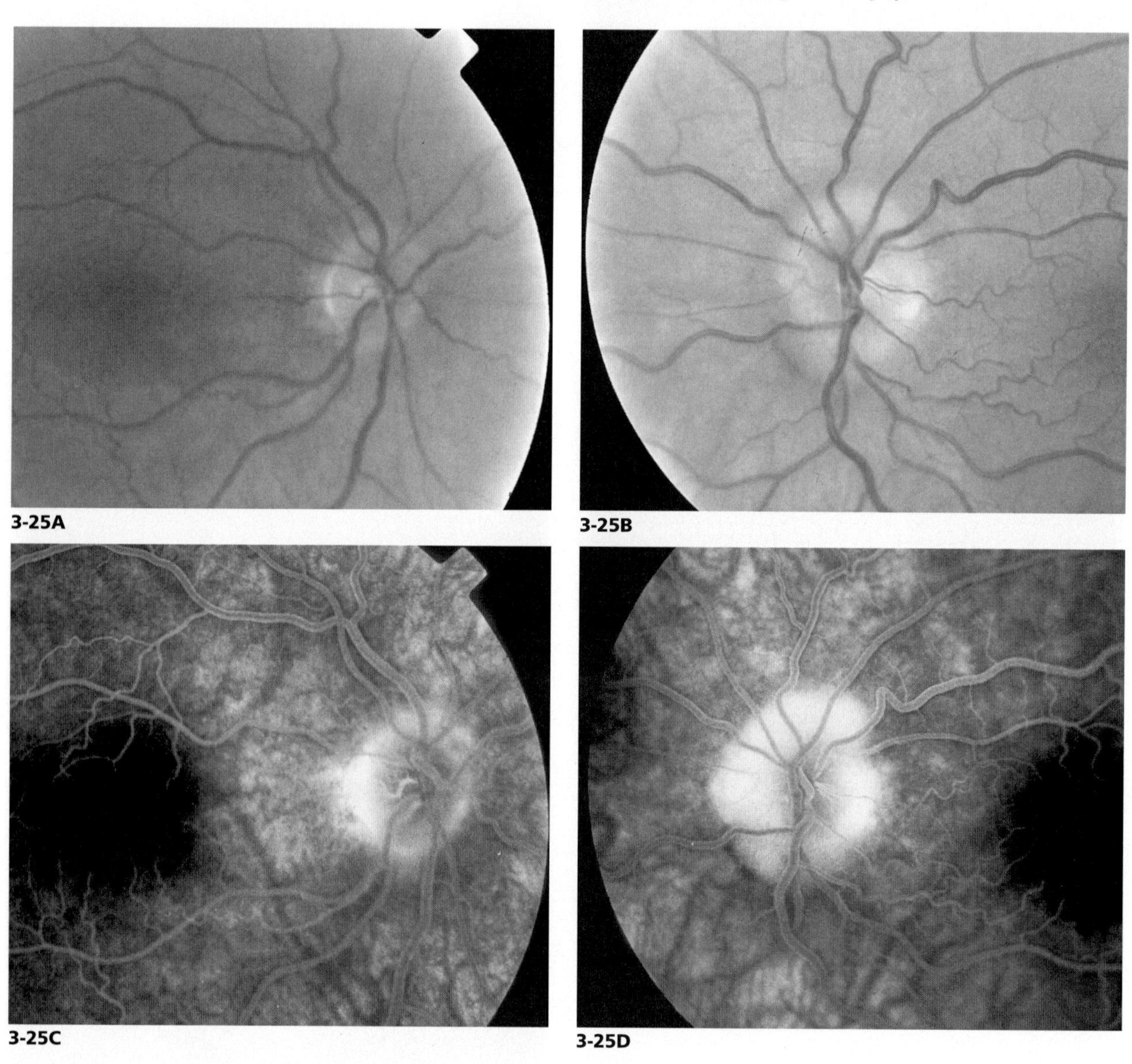

B-scan ultrasonography may be helpful. The ultrasonography may show a calcified druse that was buried. A "30-degree test" is a standardized way of telling whether there is extra fluid behind the optic nerve. The ultrasonographer measures the optic nerve while the patient is looking straight ahead and then measures the optic nerve size when the patient looks 30 degrees in one direction. If there is compressible fluid, the optic nerve changes size (because of the fluid shift), indicating that there is extra fluid around the optic nerve. A negative test shows no change in the optic nerve size.

One can image the brain and orbit with CT, MRI, or both, to see if there is a cause of disc swelling such as a tumor in the brain, venous occlusion, or enhancing optic nerve lesions. Look for the findings of papilledema or increased intracranial pressure on MRI (see Figure 3-51A–E). Finally, and usually more reliably, a lumbar puncture that measures opening pressure may tell you that there is high pressure giving early disc swelling.

Once you know that you have bona fide disc swelling, how are you going to figure out what has caused the swelling? The evaluation of a person with a swollen disc must begin with a careful history because the appearance of the swelling alone does not give you the diagnosis—the history and the examination do. The following is a list of historical features you want to know:

Who is the patient?
Is he or she a child, middle aged, or elderly?
Was the vision disturbed?
When did the vision begin to become disturbed?
How did the disturbance start?
Is it permanent or intermittent?
How long does it last?
Does the eye hurt?
Is there headache?

What other diseases or conditions does the patient have (e.g., hypertension, diabetes)?
Are there environmental factors (e.g., smoking, alcohol, or toxins)? See Table 3-2.

How does the examination help? In papilledema, both discs are usually swollen and the visual acuity is most frequently normal until *late*, whereas swelling owing to inflammatory, compressive vascular, and demyelinating causes has a profound effect on the visual acuity, and usually only one eye is affected at a time. Similarly, visual field examination also helps in the diagnosis because there are frequently specific visual field defects seen in association with various processes that make the disc swell.

Table 3-2. Historical Information to Obtain from Patients with Swollen Discs

Question	Papilledema	Inflammatory/ papillitis	Demyelinating	Ischemic	Compressive	Toxic/metabolic	Hereditary (Leber's)
Age of patient	Any age	Any age	Younger	Older	Any age	Any age; older	Younger
Gender	Either	Either	Women >men	Either	Either	Men >women	Men >women
Family history	None	None	Usually none	None	None	None	Can be present
Risk factors	Tumor, obesity, hypercoagulable state	Flulike illness, environmental risk (e.g., cats, ticks), history of diabetes	Northern latitudes	Hypertension, diabetes, smoking	History of neurofibromatosis	Environmental exposure: alcohol, methanol, tobacco, carbon monoxide	Can be precipitated by oxidative stress (e.g., fever)
Onset	Often insidious	Subacute	Subacute to acute: 1–10 days	Often acute, wake up with symptoms in a.m.	Insidious	Insidious	Insidious, acute
Symptom	Transient visual obscurations	Decreased central vision, both eyes	Decreased central vision, one eye	Decreased vision, one eye	Slow decrease in vision in usually one eye	Decreased central vision, both eyes	Decreased central vision in one eye, followed by the second eye in wks to mos
Time course of the symptom	Brief (secs to mins)	Continuous	Continuous	Continuous	Continuous	Continuous	Continuous
Pain with eye movement	Usually none <20%	Often pain with eye movement	Usually pain with eye movement >90%	Painless unless arteritic	Painless	Painless	Painless
Headache	Often the presenting complaint	May have headache	Usually no headache	Headache with arteritic form	No headache	No headache	No headache
Pulsatile tinnitus or other noises	Present	Absent	Absent	Absent	Absent	Absent	Absent

Table 3-3. Physical Findings in Evaluating the Swollen Disc

Physical finding	Papilledema	Inflammatory/papillitis	Demyelinating	Ischemic	Compressive	Toxic/metabolic	Hereditary (Leber's)
Visual acuity	Usually normal	Usually affected bilaterally	Usually affected unilaterally	Usually affected unilaterally	Usually unilaterally decreased, can be normal	Usually affected bilaterally	Sequential or bilateral
Relative afferent pupillary defect	Variable	May be none because bilateral	Present	Present	Present	May be none	May be none
Visual field	Enlarged blind spot	Any field defect; constriction	Central scotoma, altitudinal, constriction	Altitudinal and constriction, central defect	Visual constriction	Central scotoma	Central scotoma
Bilateral/unilateral	Usually bilateral (but can be asymmetrical)	Usually bilateral, can be unilateral	Usually unilateral	Usually unilateral	Unilateral	Bilateral	Bilateral
External appearance (conjunctivae, orbit)	Normal	May see conjunctival erythema, proptosis	Normal	Normal	Proptosis, enophthalmos	Normal	Normal
Appearance of the disc—acute	Hyperemia, elevation, margins obscured, cup preserved until late, venous engorgement	Hyperemia, more sloping elevation, margins obscured, more exudation and inflammatory opacities, vessels may be sheathed	Swelling is variable (30%), rarely see hemorrhages	Swelling is pallid, segmental swelling may be present	Swelling is variable, retinochoroid vessels seen, choroidal folds	Disc is hyperemic	Nerve is elevated, hyperemic; vessels tortuous
Appearance of the disc—chronic	If elevated, gliosis, small glistening pseudodrusen, may see "high-water mark," gliotic changes around vessels	May be normal, pallor	Pallor diffuse	Pallor diffuse or segmental	Pallor	Pallor—especially temporally with loss of nerve fiber layer	Pallor diffuse; begins temporally and becomes generalized
Presence of spontaneous venous pulsation	Absent	Present	Present	Present	Absent or present	Present	Present

IS THE SWELLING UNILATERAL OR BILATERAL?—CAUSES OF DISC SWELLING

Table 3-4. Causes of Disc Swelling

Usually unilateral, but can be bilateral	Usually bilateral, but can be unilateral
Optic neuritis	Papilledema
Diabetic papillitis	Infiltration
AION	Infections
Compression	Leber's (often sequential)
Sarcoid	Toxic
Retinal vein occlusion	Malignant hypertension
Vascular fistulas	Neuroretinitis

Bilateral Disc Swelling

Remember that unilateral causes of disc swelling can produce bilateral swelling.

Papilledema

Papilledema is optic disc swelling owing to increased intracranial pressure. The swelling of papilledema has characteristics including disc elevation, hyperemia, blurring of the nerve fiber layer, obscuration of the major vessels, and variable nerve fiber layer infarcts and hemorrhages. The cause of papilledema is stasis of axoplasmic flow from increased intracranial pressure.

WHAT CAUSES INTRACRANIAL HYPERTENSION?

Table 3-5. Causes of Increased Intracranial Pressure

Etiology of increased intracranial pressure	Examples
Adding anything to the intracranial cavity	Tumor, abscess, enlarged ventricle
Increased CSF production	Choroid plexus papilloma
Obstructing CSF outflow	Status-post subarachnoid hemorrhage; venous thrombosis; meningitis
Swelling of the brain (brain edema)	Ischemia, venous thrombosis
Blockage of CSF flow	Hydrocephalus
Increased blood volume	Venous hypertension

CSF = cerebrospinal fluid.

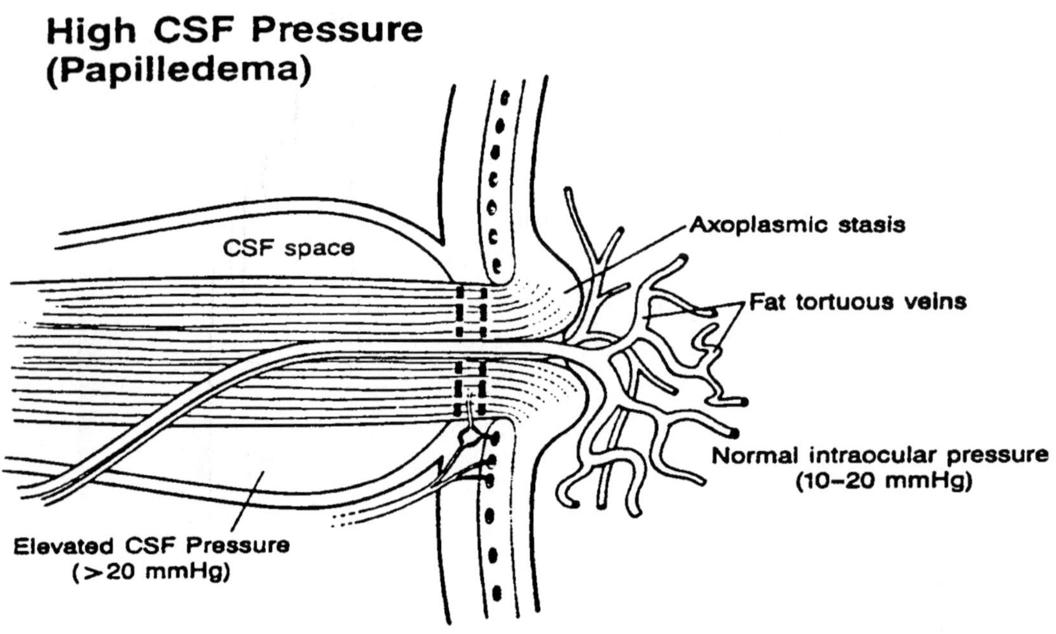

Figure 3-26. Papilledema by convention is disc swelling owing to increased intracranial pressure. The swelling is produced by the intracranial pressure, creating axoplasmic stasis.

Although intracranial hypertension of whatever cause can lead to papilledema, not all discs swell with intracranial hypertension. Cogan noted that there are many factors that must be present for a disc to swell. First, the optic nerve and sheath must be in direct communication with the fluid intracranial contents. If there is blockage of the transduction of intracranial pressure by a mass at the optic foramen (such as in Foster Kennedy syndrome) or adhesions around the optic nerve, papilledema is not present. Second, the state of the optic disc at the time of increased intracranial pressure is important; there must be enough nerve tissue to swell. That is, if there is already severe atrophy with axonal loss, swelling cannot occur. In addition, small hyperopic discs swell more easily than myopic ones because hyperopic discs are already crowded, with less room for more axonal stasis. Next, is the intracranial pressure itself intermittently elevated? If so, swelling may be less likely to occur. In addition, the height of pressure itself may be important.[24]

PAPILLEDEMA: ELEVATION

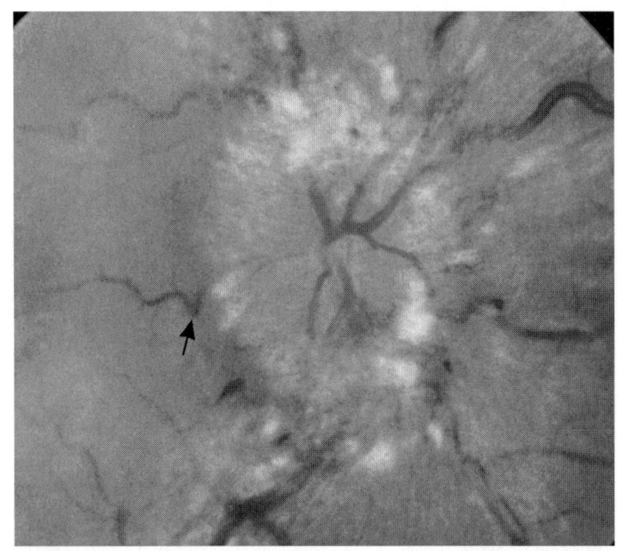

Figure 3-27. This optic disc is elevated from papilledema owing to idiopathic intracranial hypertension. Notice the camera is focused on the retina and the top of the disc is somewhat out of focus because of the elevation of the disc. The arrow points to a vessel that is moving up the disc, giving another clue that the disc is elevated.

3-27

PAPILLEDEMA: BLURRED DISC MARGIN

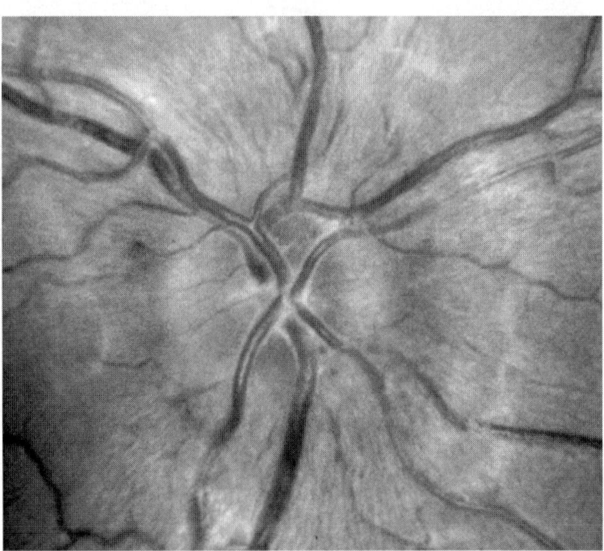

Figure 3-28. Blurring of the disc margins occurs when there is axoplasmic stasis. No distinct margin can be seen. In this case, all of the margins are blurred owing to papilledema. If the swelling of the nerve fiber layer and blurring of the disc margin are abnormal, the retinal vessels at the disc's edge will be somewhat obscured or there will be a slight opacity over the vessels. In this disc, it is difficult to tell where the disc ends and the retina begins. The swelling is from papilledema developing due to a malignant glioblastoma.

3-28

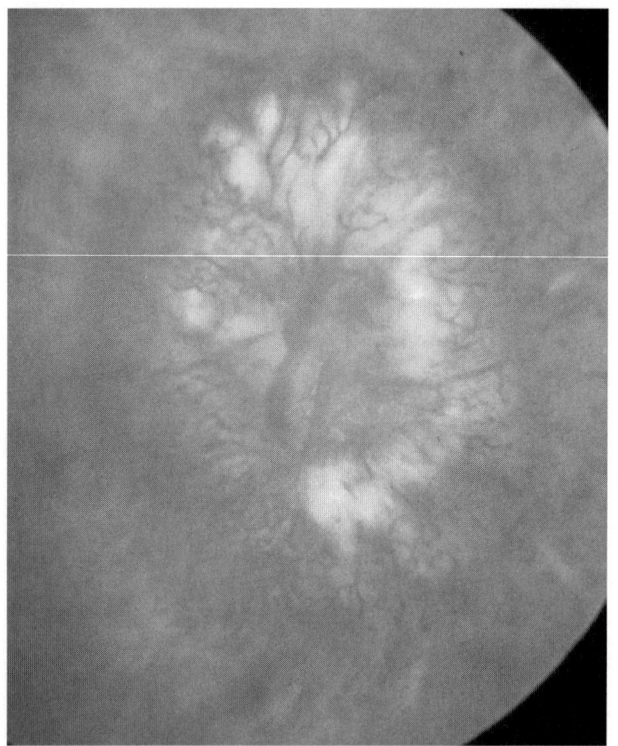

3-29

PAPILLEDEMA: THE CUP IS THE LAST TO GO

Figure 3-29. The cup, provided there is a cup in the first place, is the last part of the disc to appear swollen in papilledema. In other words, the cup is the last part of the disc to elevate. Because the cup is often small or absent in anomalous discs, look carefully for the cup—is there a small or absent cup? In the case shown here, despite major swelling, the veins are distended and the cup is still somewhat visible.

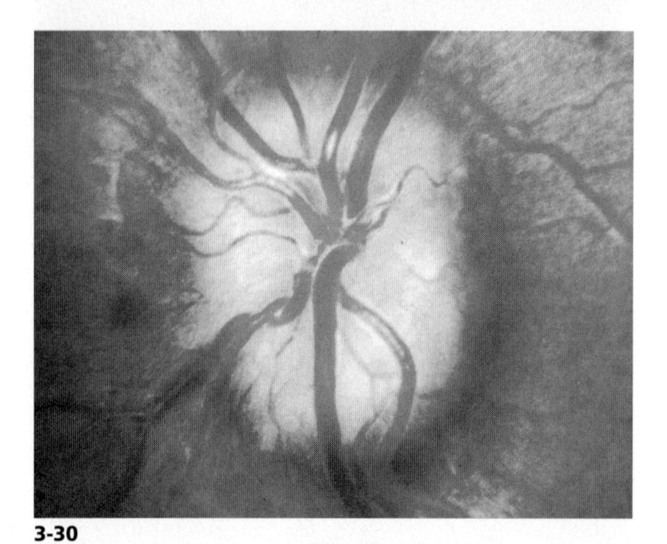

3-30

PAPILLEDEMA: ENGORGED VEINS

Figure 3-30. Look at the veins. Are they enlarged, engorged? Tortuosity of the veins alone is not a helpful sign of papilledema.

PAPILLEDEMA: DILATED CAPILLARIES ON THE DISC

Figure 3-31. A. A fine net of capillaries can frequently be seen in chronic disc swelling. From this fine "hairnet," or *caput medusae*, retinochoroidal connections can be made. You can appreciate the small, dilated vessels on the top of the disc. Also, notice how elevated this disc is—the retina is in focus below. In (B), the arrows point to the fine retinochoroidal connections.

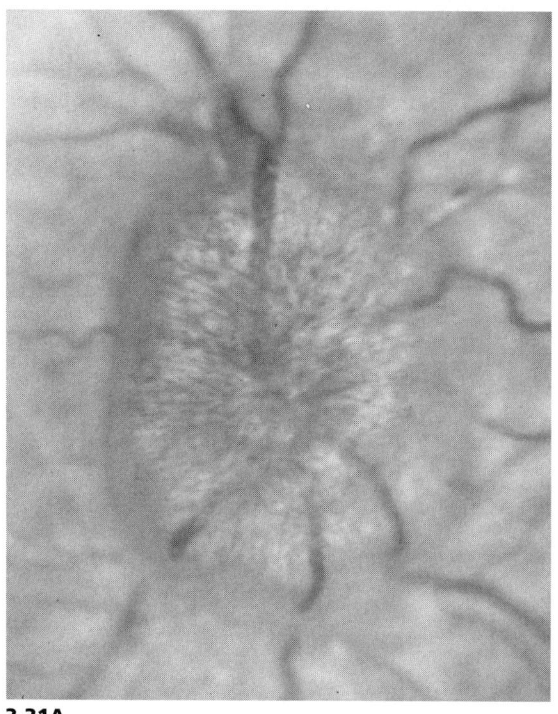

3-31A

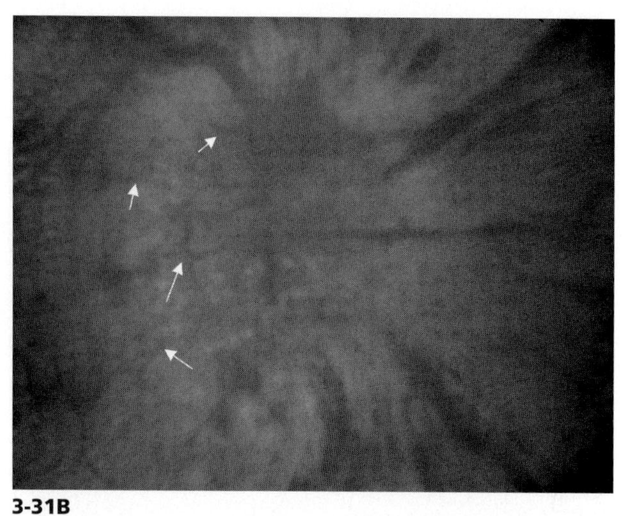

3-31B

PAPILLEDEMA: HEMORRHAGES

Figure 3-32. Are there disc hemorrhages? Remember that a hemorrhage alone does not make the diagnosis of papilledema, because splinter and deep subretinal hemorrhages can accompany disc drusen and intraocular hypertension, and may occur with fits of coughing, vomiting, or sneezing.[25] Hemorrhages seen with papilledema are of several types, including splinter (along the nerve fiber layer), peripheral dot-blot, preretinal, vitreous, and subretinal. Here you see nerve fiber layer hemorrhages extending from the disc due to papilledema. In this case, there are splinter (*white arrow*), subretinal (*white arrowheads*), and a blot of confluent splinter hemorrhages (*black arrow*).

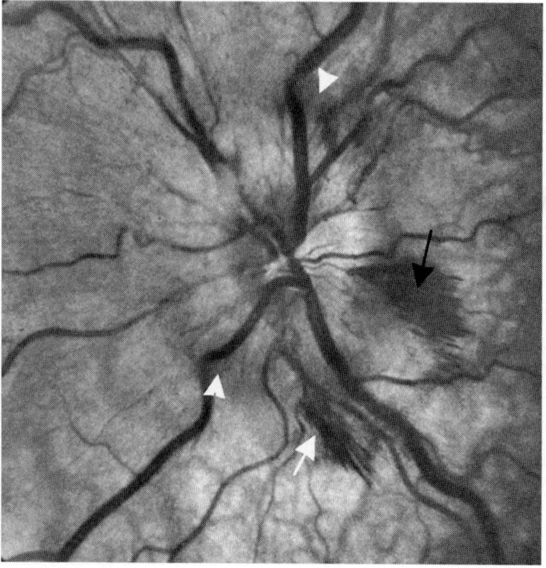

3-32

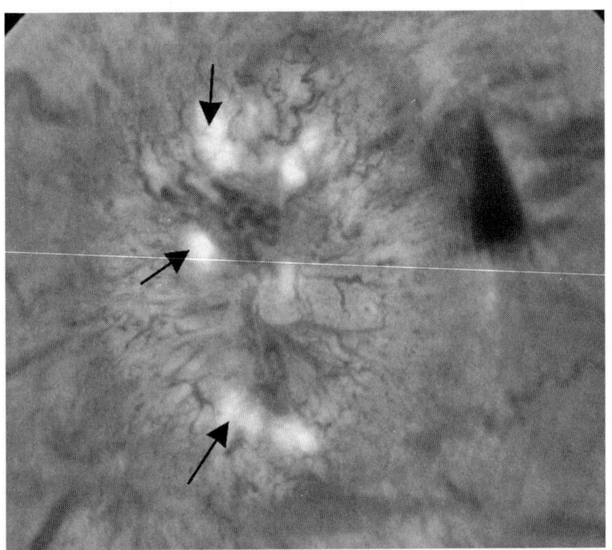
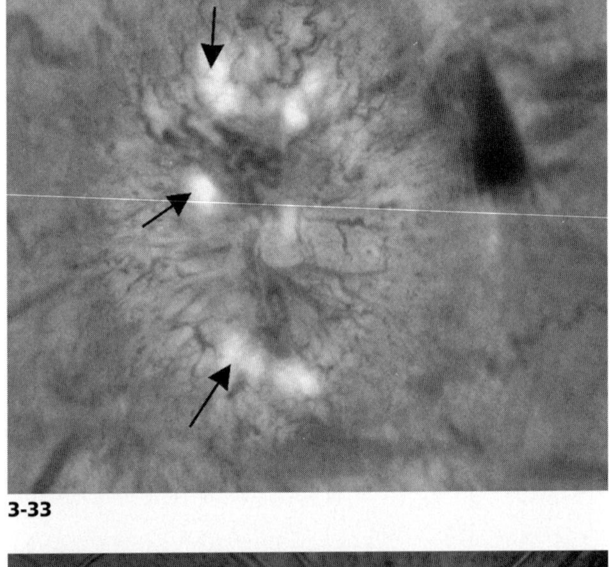

3-33

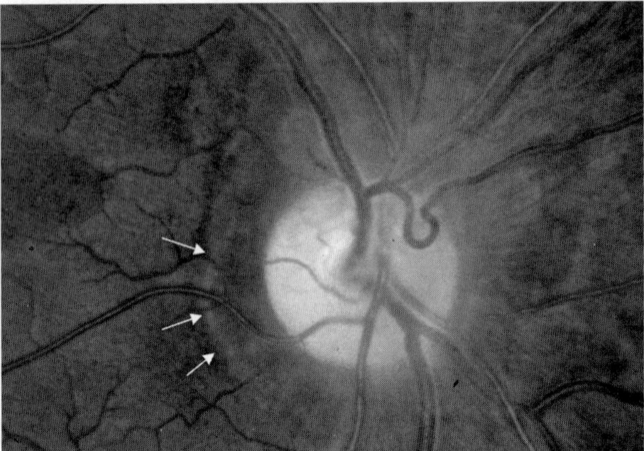

3-34

Figure 3-33. Exudates (*arrows*) may appear with papilledema. These are in the form of pseudodrusen, or hard exudates on the surface of the disc. Although they may look like drusen, they vanish when the papilledema is gone (unlike true optic disc drusen). Finally, cotton-wool spots (nerve fiber layer infarcts) can be seen with papilledema.

Figure 3-34. Look for evidence of previous swelling, such as "high-water marks." Sometimes as the swelling recedes, these stay behind as a sign of previous swelling. See the intraretinal "high water mark" (lipoproteinaceous deposits) of previously severe swelling in this patient (*arrows*).

Figure 3-35. A,B. Look for subtle retinal striae temporally. Small retinal striae (folds, ripples) just temporal to the disc (*arrows*) are suggestive of papilledema. These are called *Paton's lines*. These lines are found in up to one-third of discs with confirmed papilledema. You see them best when you direct the ophthalmoscopic beam to one side and transilluminate the temporal aspect of the disc and retina. The striae are extremely subtle, but you may see them if you look for them.

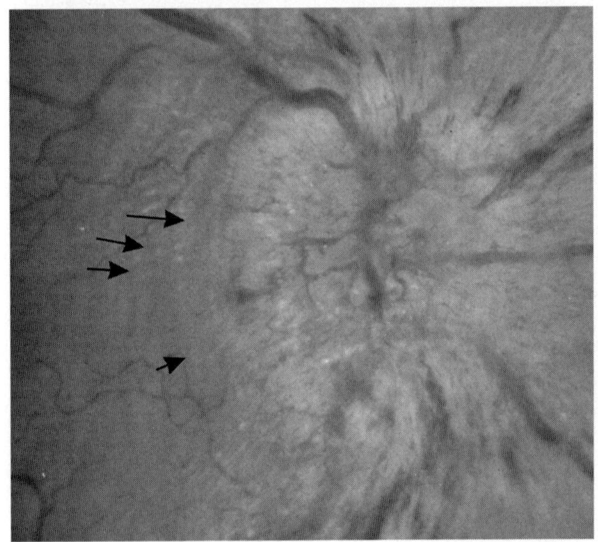

3-35A

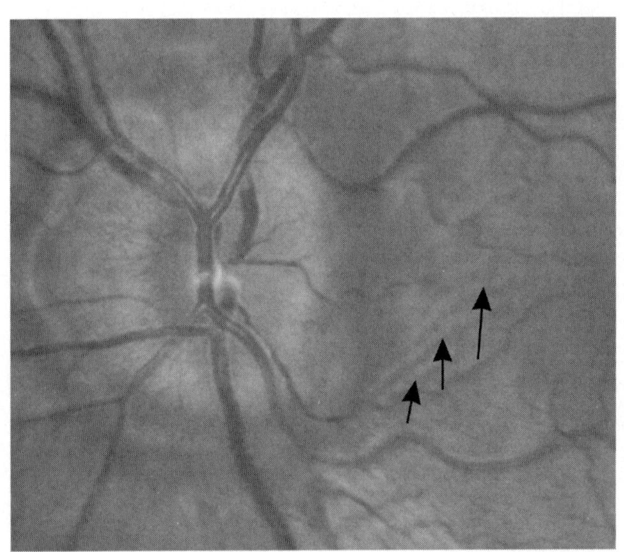

3-35B

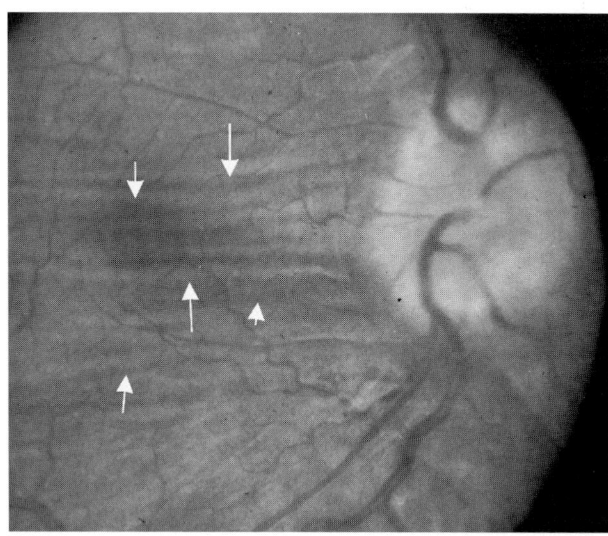
3-36

Figure 3-36. Look for horizontal folds. Chorioretinal folds may be caused by a mass indenting the globe, but, on occasion, these folds can be seen with papilledema. The folds are nicely represented here (*arrows*).

How Quickly Can Papilledema Develop?

In general, papilledema may develop within 1–7 days of increased intracranial pressure.[26–28] However, Cushing found he could produce papilledema in dogs experimentally within hours of acute increases of intracranial pressure.[16] The speed with which cerebrospinal fluid pressure increases is also directly related to the severity of papilledema.[27] This means that in acute concussive, nonhemorrhagic head trauma, you are not likely to see papilledema right away because brain swelling may not be initially present. This also means that chronic conditions, such as a slowly growing brain tumor, may or may not be associated with papilledema. In subarachnoid hemorrhage, however, in which the pressure immediately rises, papilledema is visible earlier (but still requiring many hours to days).[29]

Selhorst et al. found that papilledema occurred in only 3.5% of patients who experience closed head injury with 3 or more days of intracranial pressure elevation. They studied with intracranial pressure monitoring nine patients with pressures from 20–60 mm Hg with acute head trauma. Six patients had no papilledema, with intracranial pressures of more than 60 mm Hg for 3 days. Selhorst et al. concluded that it takes a while to develop papilledema.[30] If one carefully looks for disc swelling in patients with acute increased intracranial pressure (measured by monitoring) from trauma or spontaneous hemorrhage, one finds that the papilledema (disc swelling owing to intracranial hypertension) does not acutely appear. Steffen et al. found that, of 37 patients with acute intracranial hypertension, only one patient developed blurring of the disc margin on the sixth day of continuously monitored intracranial hypertension, and three had only venous congestion by that time. The majority of patients had no acute changes seen. Steffen et al. concluded that in their patients, papilledema took 5–6 days to develop and that the development of papilledema is a relatively slow process.[31] In our experience, we would agree with the Selhorst and Steffen studies: It takes some time to develop papilledema.

GRADING PAPILLEDEMA

We grade papilledema to tell us how severe it is. Many grading classifications have been suggested. Except in very chronic papilledema, it is very difficult to say with any precision how long any disc swelling has been present on the basis of appearance alone. Hence the terms *vintage* or *early papilledema* have little meaning.

Hughlings Jackson discussed "stages" of disc swelling:

The onset—The disc is redder (and more coarsely red), slightly swollen, and therefore prominent. Its edge is indistinct, and the arteries are slightly obscured from the swelling. The veins are large, dark and tortuous. . . . Second Stage—In this condition the disc is quite lost in a patch, which is about two or three times the diameter of the normal disc. The arteries are not traceable, or only faintly here and there, in the patch, which from great swelling is much raised above the neighbouring fundus. The veins are very large and tortuous, and are more or less obscured in the patch, and seem to "knuckle" over its edge. There are scattered blotches of effused blood on and beyond the patch, especially near its margin. There are often, also, near the edge, small shapeless white patches, sometimes edged with blood. Occasionally there are, especially near the macula lutea, brilliant white spots.[32]

Measuring and Grading Papilledema

Some advocate measuring the amount of elevation of the disc swelling. We can speak of two *diopters of elevation.* How is this done? First, focus the ophthalmoscope on the top of the disc and note the number in diopters at the back of the ophthalmoscope. To do this, start with a plus lens and slowly decrease the plus until you are focused on the top of the disc. Then, bring the retina into focus by dialing more minus—bring the retinal vessels into focus. The difference between the initial diopter and the final diopter gives the diopters of elevation. Although this measurement may be helpful in following someone with disc swelling, the height of elevation alone does not give you prognostic or predictive information. The most common error in measuring diopters according to Cogan is that the observer's own or the patient's own ocular accommodation takes over and, as a result, one fails to use the highest plus lens in focusing either on the top of the disc or retina.[33] In general, a three-diopter difference between the retina and top of the disc indicates approximately 1 mm in elevation.[34] Because of many examiners' abilities to accommodate, this method of grading is rarely used.

Others have graded papilledema as follows: "Early" (without hemorrhages), "Acute or Fully Developed" (i.e., hemorrhages and infarcts), "Chronic" (No hemorrhages or exudates), "Vintage" (i.e., small drusen-like figures on the disc that disappear when the swelling is gone; swelling present in different grades for years), and "Chronic Atrophic" (the end result of uncorrected papilledema).[28] This method mixes temporal and descriptive terminology and is not very helpful.

Lars Frisén has provided the most sensible and reproducible grading scheme (see Table 3-6.) His scheme relies heavily on how much of the disc is swollen and the extent of obscuration of the blood vessels.

Table 3-6. Grades of Papilledema

Stage	Characteristics
0	Normal disc with blurring of nasal and temporal disc; no obscuration of the vessel and the cup is maintained (see Figure 3-37).
1	C-shaped blurring of the nasal, superior, and inferior borders. Usually the temporal margin is normal (see Figure 3-38A–C).
2	360-degree elevation of the disc margin (see Figure 3-39).
3	Elevation of the entire disc with partial obscuration of one or more retinal vessels at the disc margin (see Figure 3-40A–C).
4	Complete obliteration of the cup and complete obscuration of at least some vessels on the surface of the disc. There may be small, dilated telangiectatic capillaries on the disc (see Figure 3-41A and B).
5	Dome-shaped appearance with all vessels being obscured (sometimes called "champagne cork" swelling) (see Figure 3-42A–C).

Source: Adapted from L Frisén. Swelling of the optic nerve head: a staging scheme. J Neurol Neurosurg Psych 1982;45:13–18.

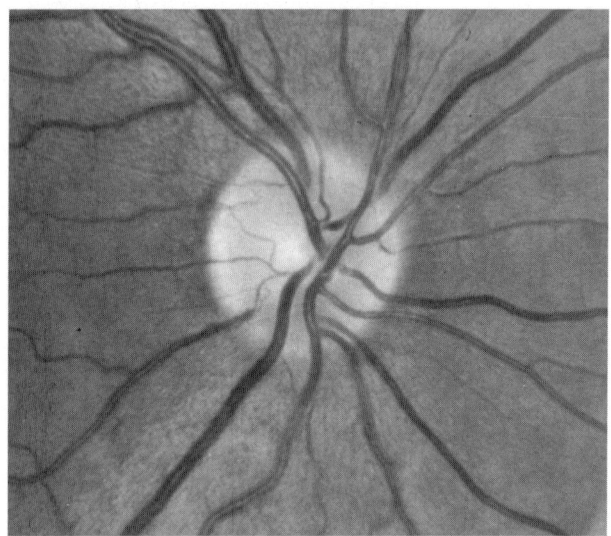

3-37

Figure 3-37. Photograph of papilledema stage 0. This woman has documented increased intracranial pressure of 340 mm CSF owing to idiopathic intracranial pressure. Very little, if any, disc swelling is seen. There is no obscuration of vessels.

Figure 3-38. A–C. **Photographs of papilledema stage 1. C-shaped blurring and elevation of the nasal, superior, and inferior borders. The temporal margin is normal.** B. **Notice the chorioretinal folds (*arrows*) toward the macula (M).**

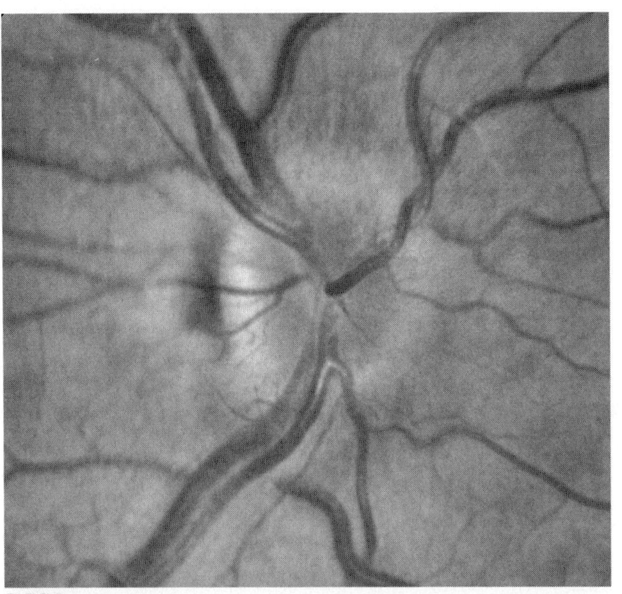

3-38A

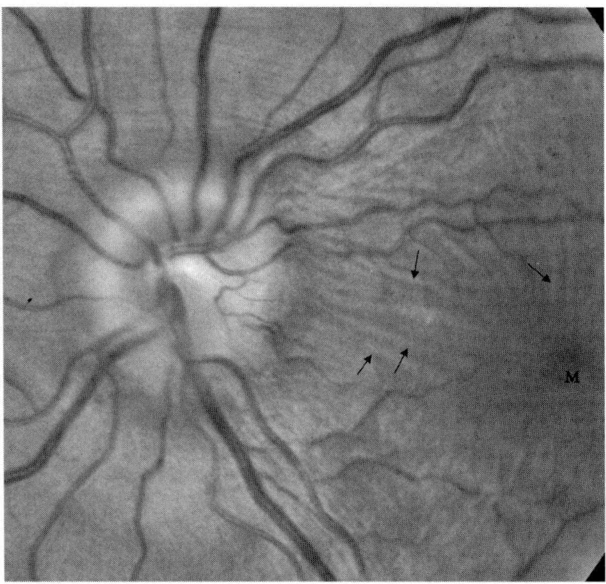

3-38B

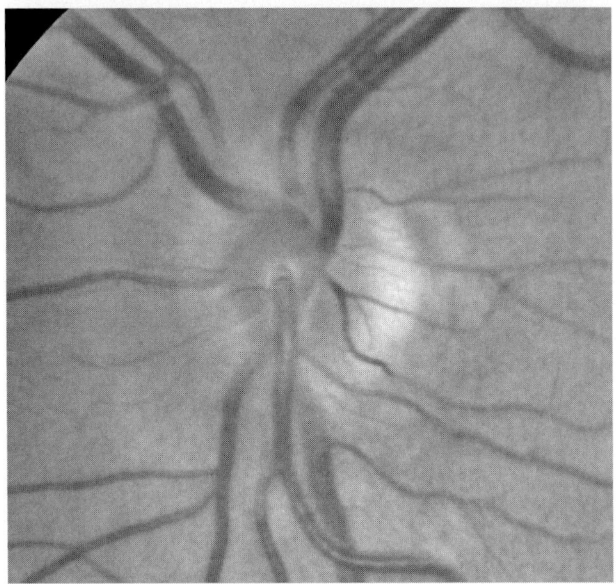

3-38C

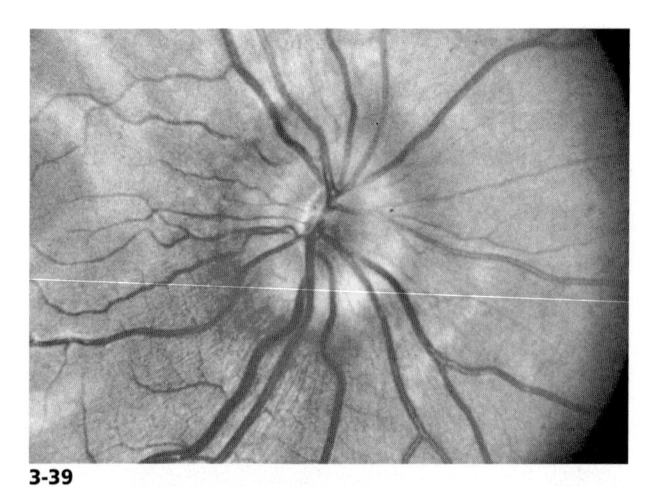

3-39

Figure 3-39. Photograph of stage 2 papilledema. Elevation of 360 degrees of disc margin. The vessels are not obscured.

Figure 3-40. A–C. Photographs of stage 3 papilledema. Elevation of the entire disc with partial obscuration of the retinal vessels at the disc margin.

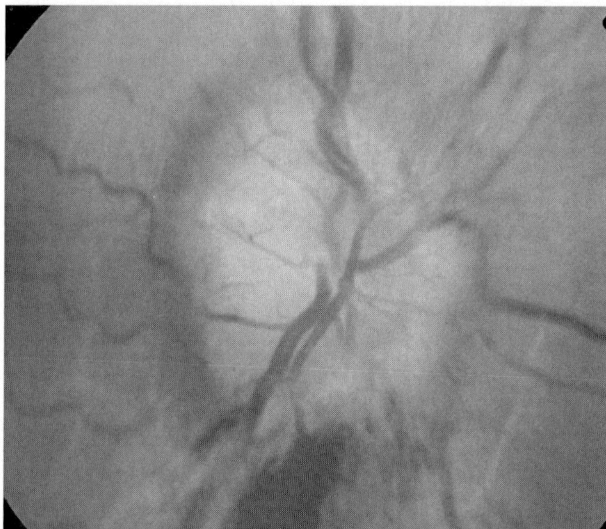

3-40A

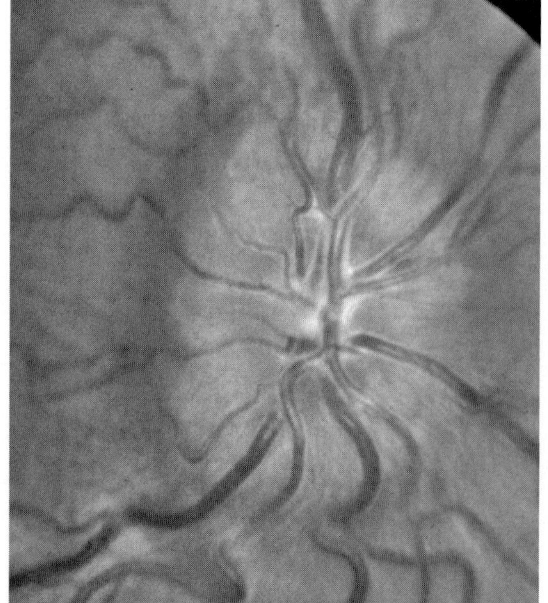

3-40B

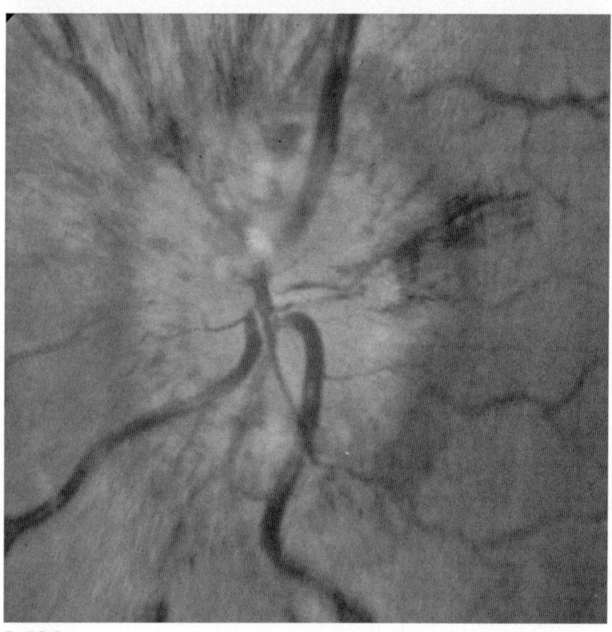

3-40C

Figure 3-41. A,B. **Photographs of stage 4 papilledema. Complete obliteration of the cup as well as the blood vessels.**

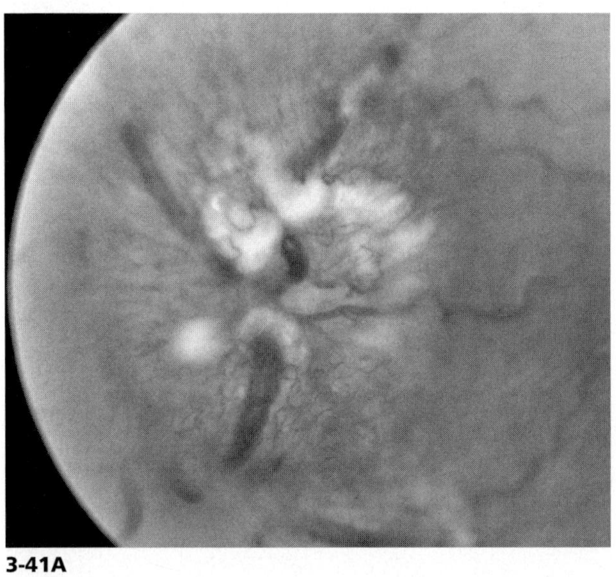

3-41A

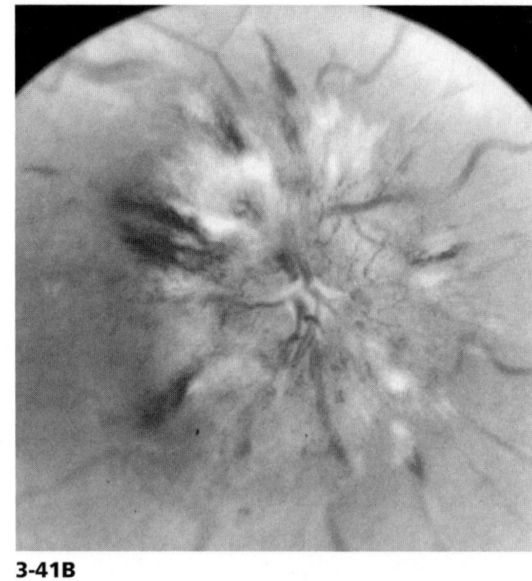

3-41B

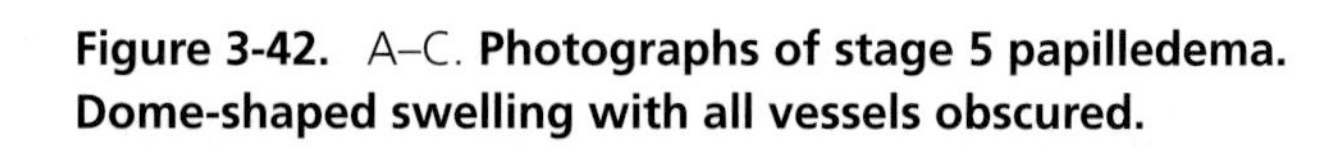

Figure 3-42. A–C. **Photographs of stage 5 papilledema. Dome-shaped swelling with all vessels obscured.**

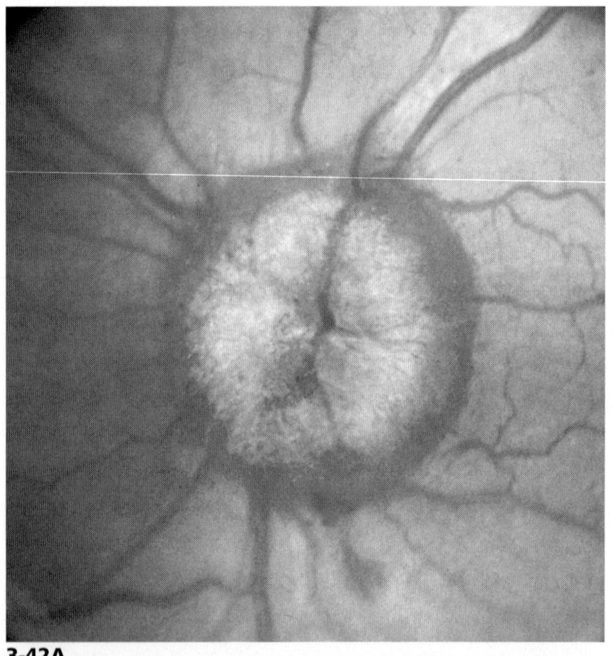

3-42A

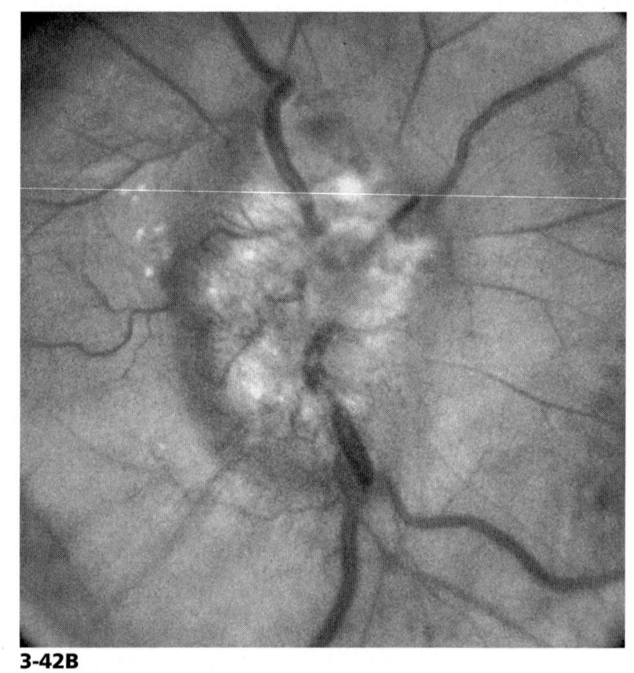

3-42B

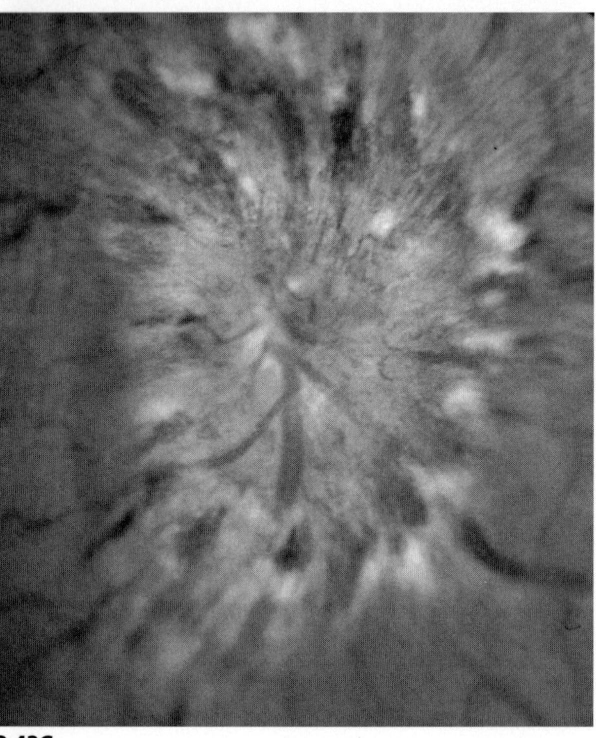

3-42C

Make a Drawing of What You See

Drawing what you see of the disc swelling helps in many ways. First, it forces you to better observe the characteristics of the disc swelling. Furthermore, it serves as a benchmark for what the disc looked like at one point in time to compare with another point. A photograph is also helpful to document the swelling.

WHAT HAPPENS TO UNCORRECTED PAPILLEDEMA?

Although occasional patients can continue to have swelling for years with little or no vision loss, if papilledema persists untreated, atrophy to some degree eventually ensues. First, sheathing of the veins may occur. The hyperemia and redness diminish as pallor develops. Sometimes, drusen-like structures are present, and although they may resemble drusen, in time, with atrophy or with decreased pressures, they resolve (unlike optic nerve drusen, which remain). Sometimes lipid deposits form around the macula, forming a "macular star" exudate. Finally, the disc is flat and grey-white or tallow colored, with sheathing of the blood vessel and atrophy. Significant vision loss has occurred owing to the loss of axons.

Figure 3-43. A,B. **This man has idiopathic intracranial hypertension. Watch how his papilledema gradually resolves within 2 weeks after an optic nerve sheath decompression onset. There is grade 3 swelling, with small hemorrhages on the disc. The vessels are not obscured.** C,D. **Twelve days later, the swelling is more improved (grade 2) on the left side (the side of the decompression).** ***Continued***

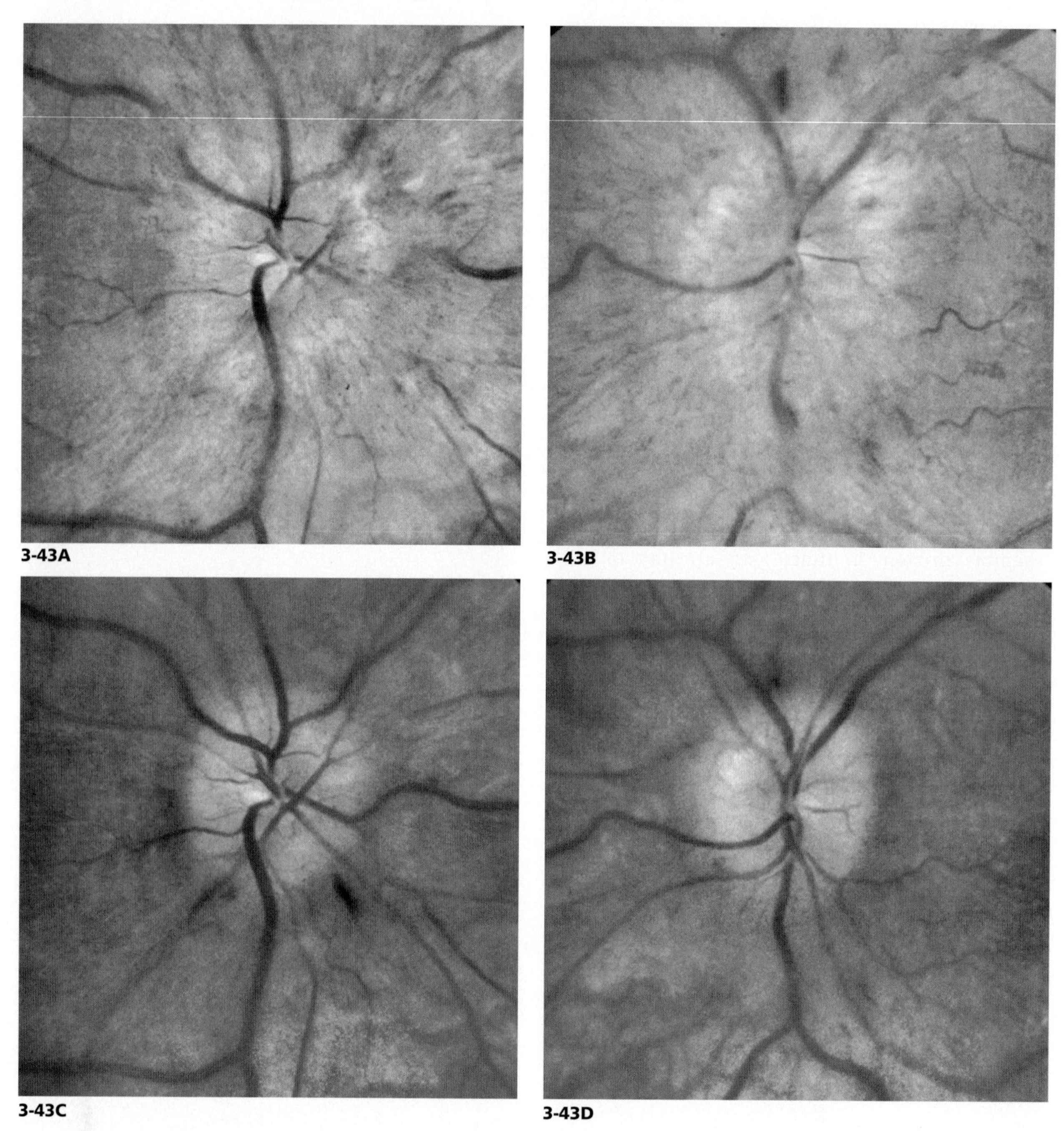

3-43A **3-43B** **3-43C** **3-43D**

Figure 3-43. ***Continued.*** E,F. Three months later, both discs are much less swollen (grade 0). There is some pallor to the left disc.

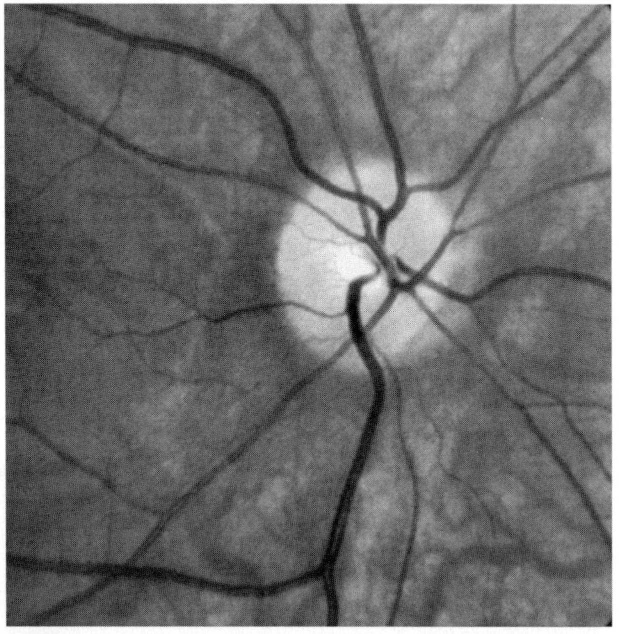

3-43E

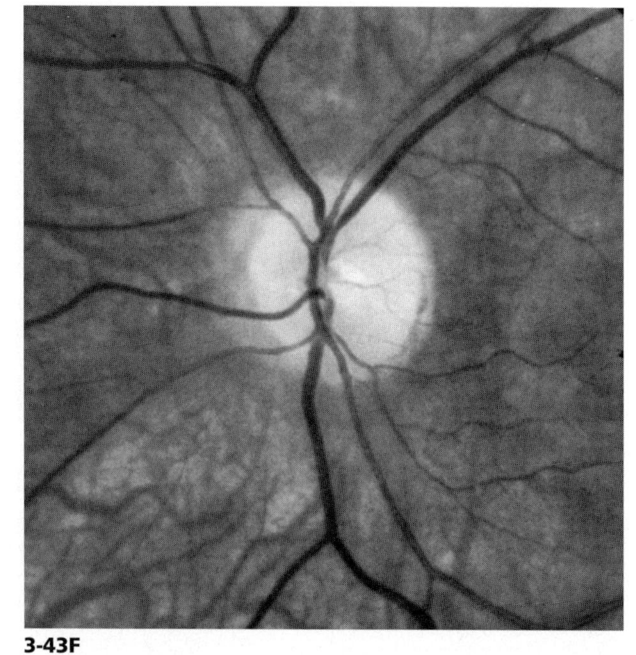

3-43F

Figure 3-44. A. This woman has idiopathic intracranial hypertension with chronic papilledema (grade 4). B. Her papilledema disappeared on use of steroids and acetazolamide, and later recurred as soon as the medications were stopped. Her visual fields were constricted. Not only did she have elevated intracranial pressure, but she also had elevated intraocular pressure—witness her large cups, especially when the swelling is diminished. You can also see the "high-water marks" of her swelling (*arrows*). This case also shows how the cup is "filled in" with papilledema and preserved until late.

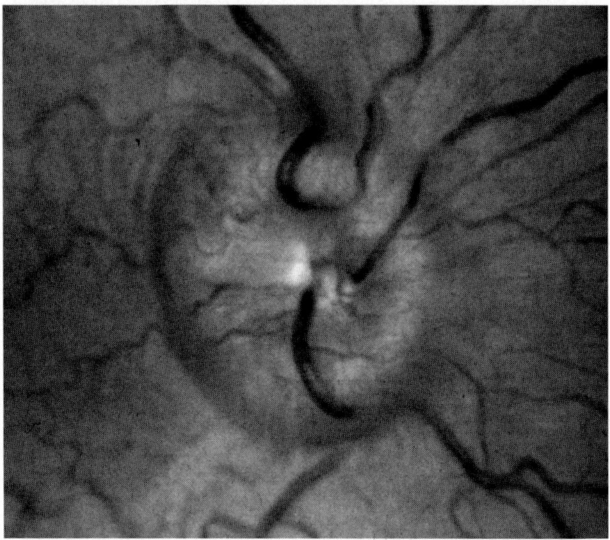

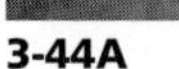

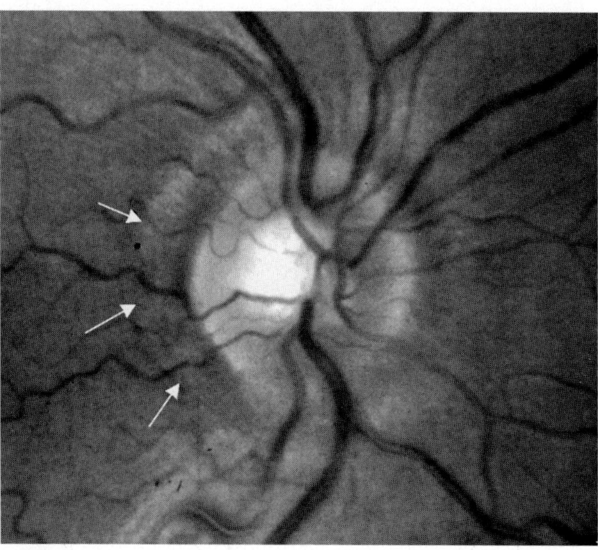

3-44B

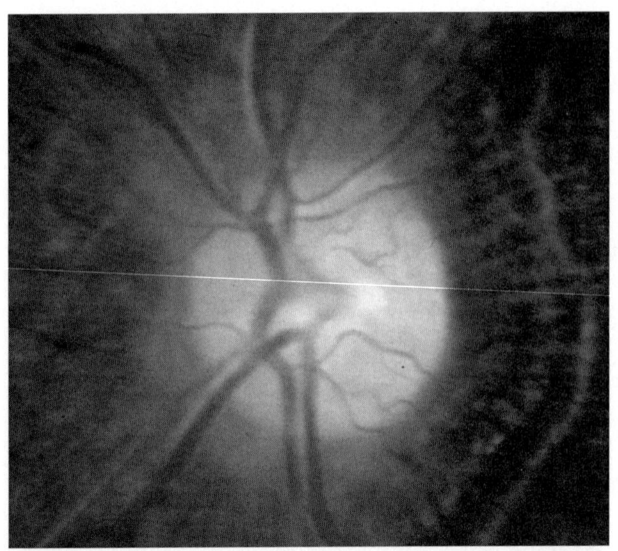

3-45A

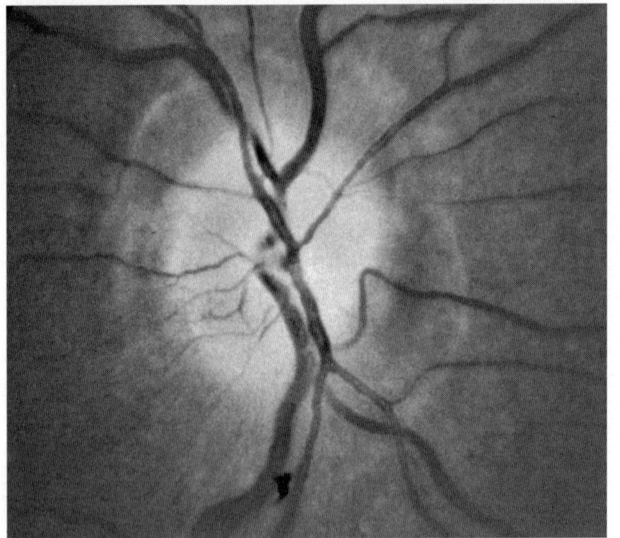

3-45B

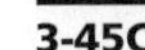

3-45C

Figure 3-45. A. **This woman with idiopathic intracranial hypertension has severe atrophy after papilledema. You can appreciate the gliotic sheathing of the veins, the veil-like pallor, and the "high-water mark."** B. **Chronic atrophic papilledema owing to idiopathic intracranial hypertension. Notice the "high-water mark" here, also. Look also for changes in the pigment epithelium next to the disc; you might see a dark or light ring that could alert you to the possibility that the nerve was swollen at one time.** C. **You can appreciate the "high-water mark," as well as the gliosis of the blood vessels. Multiple concentric intraretinal "high-water mark" lipoprotein rings and a Bergmeister papillary glial veil are present.**

WHAT ARE SYMPTOMS OF PAPILLEDEMA?

Papilledema of whatever cause has some characteristic symptoms. The most frequent visual symptom is *transient visual obscuration*. Patients with idiopathic intracranial hypertension (pseudotumor cerebri) with papilledema describe these as "a rheostat being turned down for several seconds" and then immediately or slowly returning. Sometimes, the obscuration can last up to 1 minute. It can be so dramatic that patients will describe going blind in one eye for a period of time, making the examiner consider arterial occlusions or amaurosis fugax. Although frequently unilateral, bilateral obscurations are common. Other ways of describing these phenomena include blackouts, grayouts, or whiteouts, occurring most commonly with a change of posture; going from recumbent to sitting or sitting to standing or bending over may provoke the transient visual obscuration.

In pseudotumor cases, gaze-evoked blindness in papilledema has also been reported.[36] Other visual phenomena reported include green lights, pulsating halos, black spots, and visual blurring.[37,38]

The most common nonvisual symptom associated with all papilledema is headache. The pain itself is most frequently holocranial and commonly called the worst headache of a patient's life. The headaches are usually not episodic, but continuous, and also may be aggravated by a Valsalva maneuver. There may be superimposed migrainous phenomena, such as sound and light sensitivity, as well as nausea and vomiting. Distinguishing features include pain behind and in the eye, pain on eye movement, and radicular pain in the neck and shoulders (note that the patient may not give this history unless you directly ask for it). Radicular pain is caused by stretching of the dura of dilated root sleeves from increased cerebrospinal fluid pressure.

A very important symptom that is frequently not mentioned spontaneously is pulsatile tinnitus. Patients with increased intracranial pressure report "noises in their heads"—whooshing or swishing sounds, high-frequency noises like buzzing, "wind-like" sounds, or sounds like a river running. This symptom can be so bothersome that it may be the presenting complaint in patients with idiopathic intracranial hypertension, especially to otolaryngologists. Furthermore, these pulsations may be audible simply by using a stethoscope, and have even been reported to be audible without one.[39] The cause of the tinnitus is also thought to be the turbulent flow though the venous sinuses and the effect of stretch from venous pressure on cranial nerve VIII.

Diplopia is a frequent complaint in patients with raised intracranial pressure and papilledema because of stretch on cranial nerve VI. Their vision is horizontally doubled, and the diplopia goes away if one or the other eye is occluded.

Table 3-7. Conditions Associated with Papilledema and Increased Intracranial Pressure—What Are the Possibilities?

- Nutritional/metabolic disorders
  - Enzyme deficiencies
    - Galactokinase
    - Antichymotrypsin
    - 11 β-Hydroxylase galactosemia
    - Cystic fibrosis
    - Deprivational dwarfism
- Endocrine abnormalities
  - Corticosteroid deficiency
  - Corticosteroid excess
  - Thyroid disease: hypothyroidism
  - Pituitary disease: growth hormone tumor
  - Parathyroid disease: hypoparathyroidism
  - Turner's syndrome
  - Adipsic hypernatremia
- Hematologic disease
  - Anemia: iron deficiency
  - Polycythemia vera
- Cerebral venous thrombosis
  - Autoimmune conditions
    - Behçet's
    - Paroxysmal nocturnal hemoglobinuria
    - Idiopathic thrombocytopenic purpura
    - Cryoglobulinemia
    - Cryofibrinogenemia
    - Monoclonal gammopathy
    - Hypocomplementemic urticarial vasculitis
  - Superior vena cava obstruction
  - Tumor (glomus jugulare, cholesteatoma, sarcoid, metastatic, eosinophilic)
  - Otogenic conditions
    - Middle ear infections
    - Chronic mastoiditis
  - Factors in the blood
    - Lupus anticoagulant
    - Anticardiolipin antibody
    - Factor V Leiden (protein C resistance)
    - Prothrombin gene mutation
    - Homocystinemia
    - Paraproteinemia
    - Thrombocythemia
  - Pregnancy
    - Eclampsia
  - Oral contraceptives
  - Androgen therapy (e.g., danazol)
- Circulatory diseases
  - Congestive heart failure
  - Hypertensive encephalopathy
  - Pulmonary emphysema
  - Congenital cardiac disease
- Cerebrovascular malformation
- Subarachnoid hemorrhage
- Head injury
- Renal failure—uremia
- Drugs
  - Antibiotics
    - Tetracycline, minocycline, nalidixic acid, nitrofurantoin
    - Quinolones (Ciprofloxacin)
  - Psychiatric
    - Lithium, chlorpromazine
  - Steroids
  - Oral contraceptives
  - Danazol
  - Leuprolide acetate (Lupron)
  - Levonorgestrel (Norplant)
  - Vitamins A, D
  - 13-*cis* retinoic acid
  - All-*trans* retinoic acid (retinoid used for treating leukemia)
  - Amiodarone
  - Etretinate
  - Perhexiline maleate
  - Indomethacin, ketoprofen
  - Cyclosporine
  - Growth hormone
- Infections
  - Viral meningitis
  - Lyme disease
  - Human immunodeficiency virus
  - Poliomyelitis
  - Acute lymphocytic meningitis
  - Coxsackie B viral encephalitis
  - Guillain-Barré syndrome
  - Infectious mononucleosis
  - Syphilis
  - Cryptococcal meningitis
- Parasitic disease
  - Sandfly fever
  - Trypanosomiasis
  - Torulosis
  - Neurocysticercosis
- Developmental disease
  - Hydrocephalus
  - Aqueductal stenosis
  - Craniostenosis
- Neoplastic disease
  - Leukemia
  - Spinal cord tumors
  - Brain tumors (including gliomatosis cerebri; lymphoma)
  - Lymphoproliferative disorders
    - Sweet's syndrome
    - *P*olyneuropathy, *o*rganomegaly, *e*ndocrinopathy, *m*onoclonal protein abnormality, and *s*kin abnormalities (POEMS syndrome)
    - Castleman's disease
  - Myeloma
- Idiopathic intracranial hypertension (pseudotumor cerebri)
- Other
  - Sarcoid
  - Paget's disease

Source: Adapted from reference 37.

Figure 3-46. Papilledema owing to dural cavernous fistula, an abnormal arterial connection to the dural venous sinus. Dural cavernous fistula occurs infrequently, but papilledema may be its first and only presenting finding. Risk factors include hypercoagulable states and autoimmune conditions. Many investigators suspect that thrombosis may underlie the development of these abnormal connections. Symptoms include pulse synchronous tinnitus. On examination, an audible bruit may be auscultated. The diagnosis can be made by MRI, but frequently angiography is necessary. Treatment is usually ablation of the abnormal channel by way of an interventional radiologic procedure. A. This 60-year-old man complained of pulse synchronous tinnitus and transient visual obscurations. His right disc exhibited grade 3 swelling. The black spot on the temporal margin is a resolving subretinal hemorrhage. B. His left disc also showed grade 3 swelling. Notice the black spot is a resolving subretinal hemorrhage. C. His arteriogram showed that the internal carotid artery had an arterial feeder to the fistula associated with his transverse sinus (*arrow*). Occlusion of the sinus fistula brought improvement of his papilledema, and his symptoms also resolved.

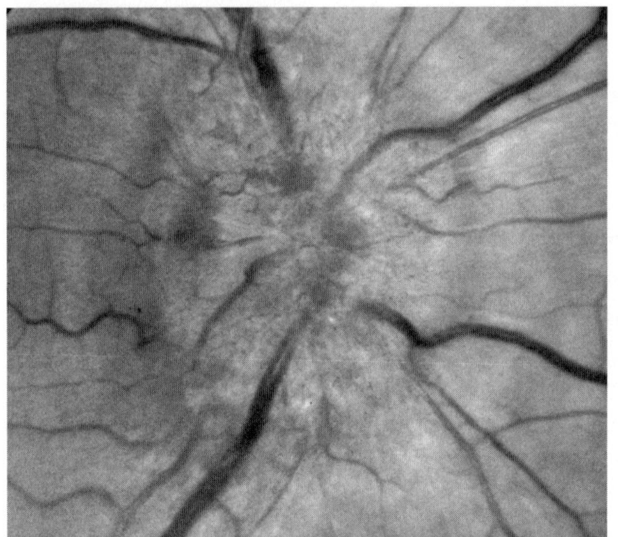

3-46A

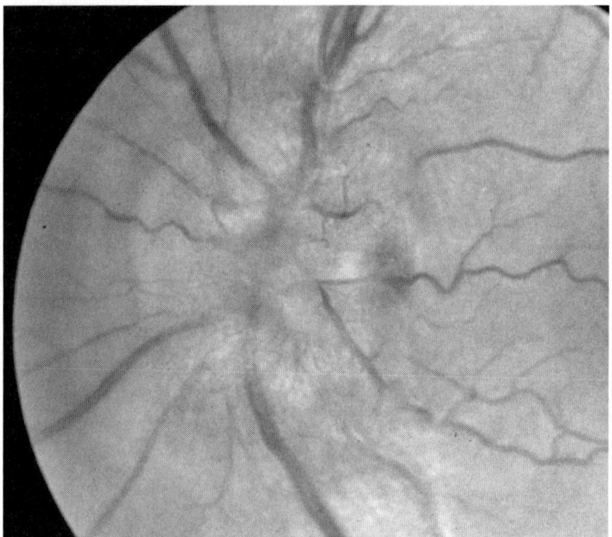

3-46B

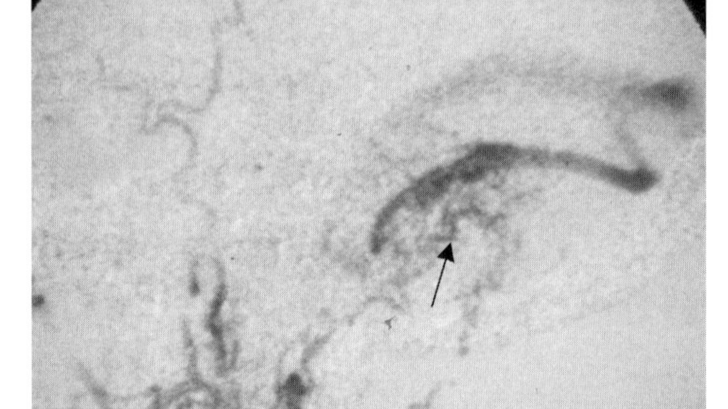

3-46C

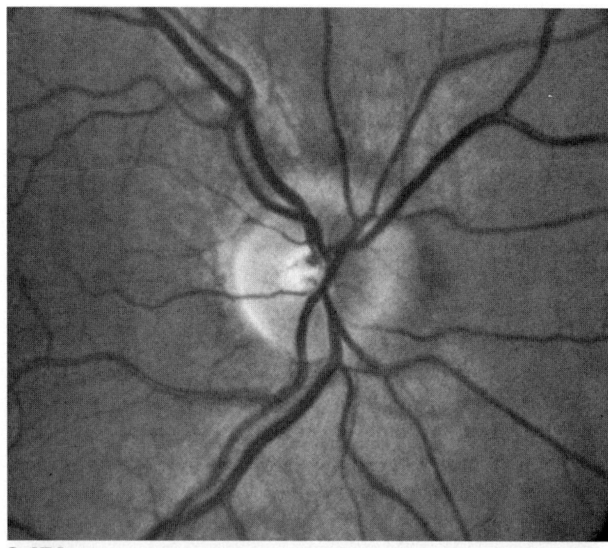
3-47A

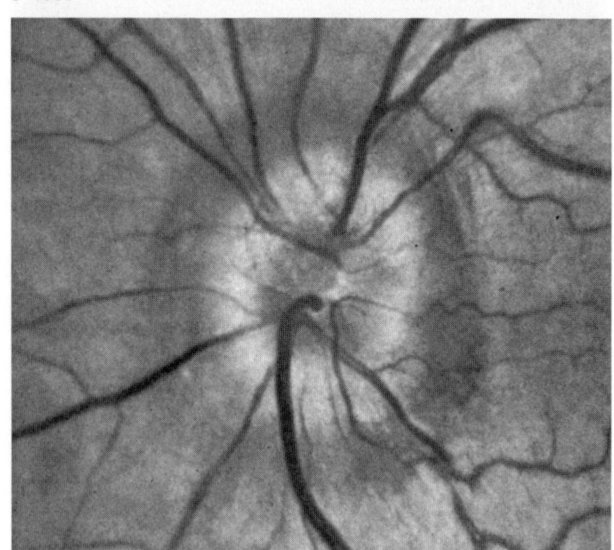
3-47B

Figure 3-47. Papilledema owing to idiopathic intracranial hypertension (IIH) in this woman. IIH is most frequently seen in young women of childbearing age. Although it is present in 1/100,000 people in many countries, it is more common in obese women (10/100,000). The diagnosis is made only after imaging to eliminate other causes of intracranial hypertension, such as venous thrombosis and cerebrospinal fluid examination to eliminate cases of meningitis. Treatment is weight loss and diuretic therapy. Although outcome is generally good for vision, quality of life is severely altered.[37] A. **This 30-year-old woman presented with headaches and transient visual obscurations. She had normal imaging, but an elevated opening pressure on lumbar puncture. A diagnosis of IIH was made. After weight loss and diuretic therapy, her papilledema improved. The right disc shows grade 1 swelling.** B. **The left disc shows grade 3 papilledema.**

SPECIAL PAPILLEDEMA CASES: UNILATERAL SWELLING OF THE OPTIC DISC IN PAPILLEDEMA

A disc can be swollen unilaterally in papilledema. In fact, in some cases disc swelling has been so asymmetric as to mimic Foster Kennedy syndrome (a swollen disc on one side and a pale disc on the opposite side). In idiopathic intracranial hypertension, approximately 10% of cases have asymmetric discs (a difference of at least two grades of papilledema).[40] On occasion, the diagnosis of unilateral papilledema is difficult. Despite a lumbar puncture to measure the pressure, the diagnosis can be unclear, and may require continuous intracranial pressure monitoring.[41] If there is proptosis or limitation of eye movements in the eye with the swollen disc, think of an orbital tumor. If there is pain, redness of the eye, vision loss, and limited motility, think of posterior scleritis (refer back to Table 3-4: Causes of Disc Swelling—Unilateral and Bilateral).

Figure 3-48. Unilateral papilledema owing to IIH in two women who presented with headaches. In IIH, almost 10% of cases have asymmetric discs (a difference of at least two grades of papilledema). A. **Grade 0–1 in one woman with IIH in the right eye, but grade 4–5 swelling in the left eye** (B) **at the same time.** C. **A patient with grade 1 swelling in the right eye and grade 3 swelling in the left eye** (D) **from IIH.**

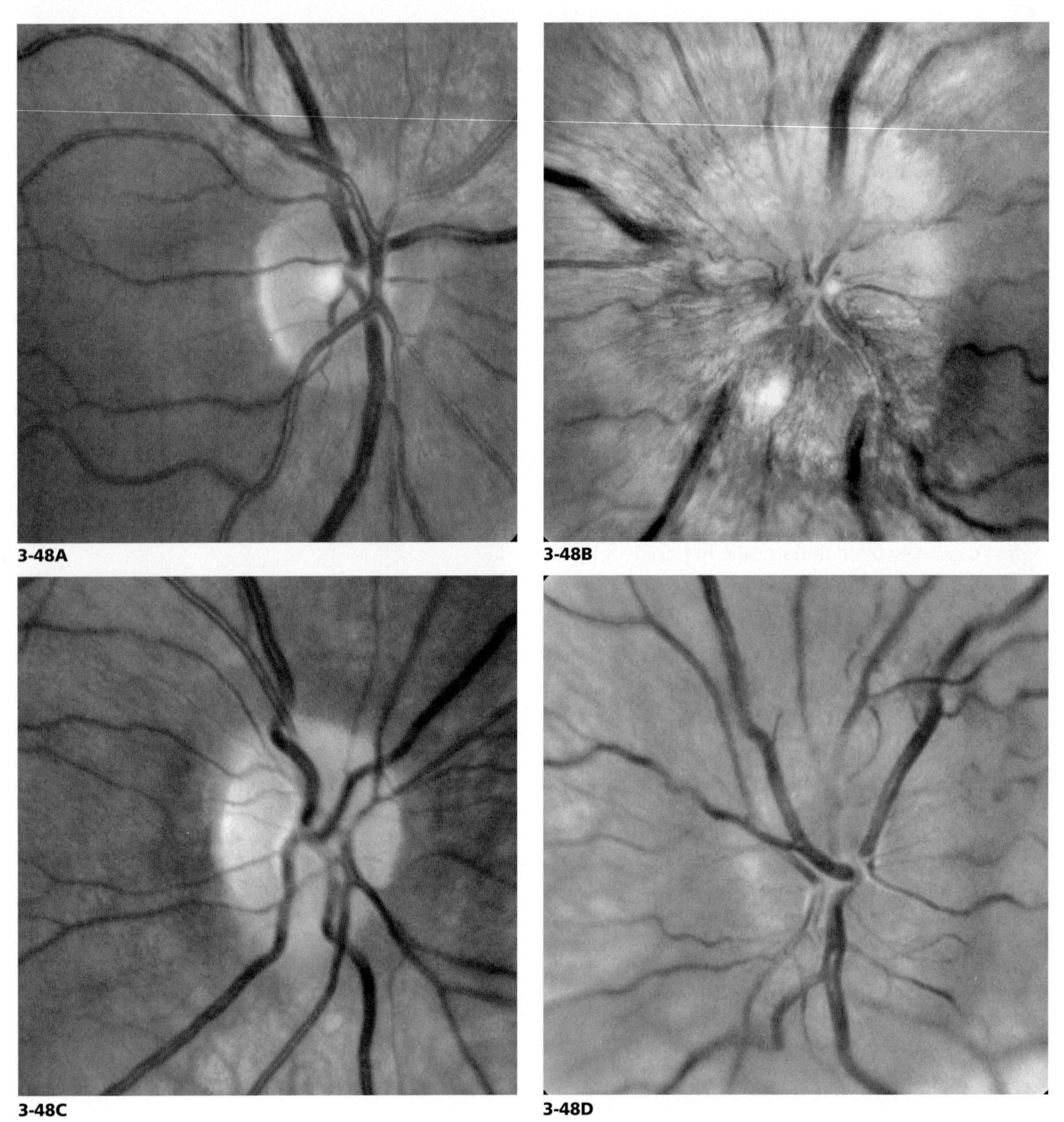

Because of the location of the visual fibers in the optic tract and chiasm, one eye can have a swollen disc and the other may be pale. The classic example of this is the so-called Foster Kennedy syndrome, named for Dr. Foster Kennedy, a New York neurologist who first described the localizing combination.[42] Although the classic description of this combination involves an olfactory groove or frontal lobe meningioma compressing one optic nerve (causing pallor) while increased intracranial pressure causes swelling in the opposite optic nerve, many more cases of this combination of swelling and atrophy are identified as a "pseudo–Foster Kennedy," owing to acute ischemic optic neuropathy in one eye and an old AION in the other.

Figure 3-49. A case of Foster Kennedy syndrome with mild pallor in the right eye (A) **and unilateral papilledema in slightly anomalous, hyperopic discs on the left eye** (B) **owing to a sphenoid ridge/frontal lobe meningioma.** C. **CT shows a large meningioma compressing the chiasm off to the right.** ***Continued***

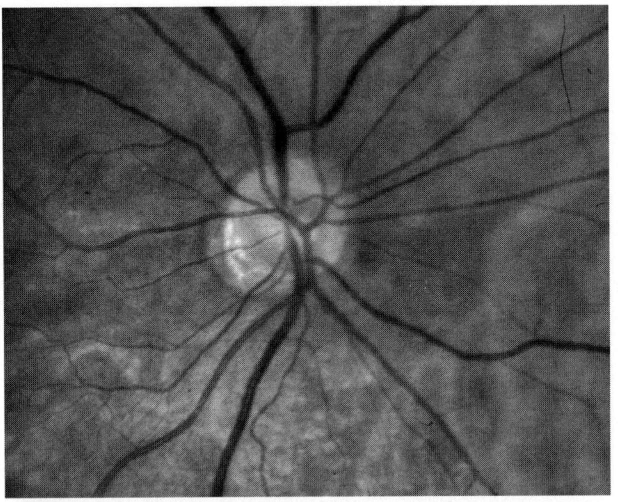

3-49A

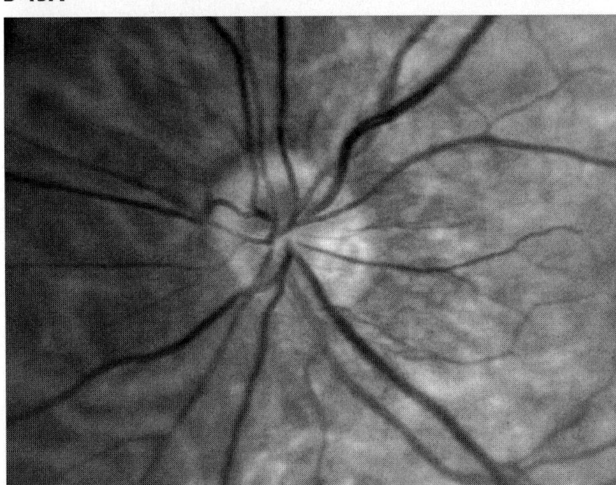

3-49B

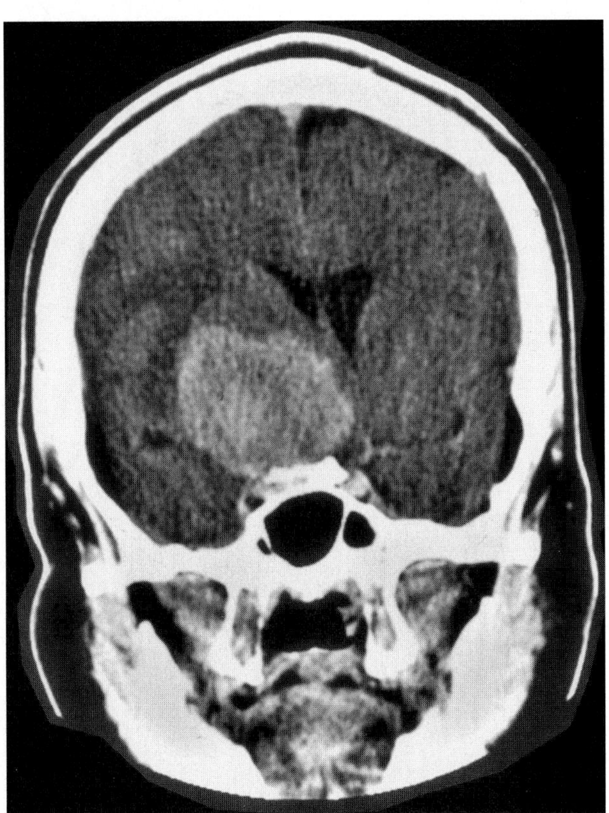

3-49C

Figure 3-49. ***Continued.*** **D. The visual field shows an inferior constriction of the right disc, with a slightly enlarged blind spot on the left disc. E. More commonly, the Foster Kennedy syndrome is pseudo–Foster Kennedy syndrome. This is usually caused by ischemic optic neuropathy. Here you see a pale nerve on the right due to old AION, and an acutely swollen disc on the left (F) owing to a new AION. In this case, loss of visual acuity and visual field in both eyes is a clue that this is not papilledema.**

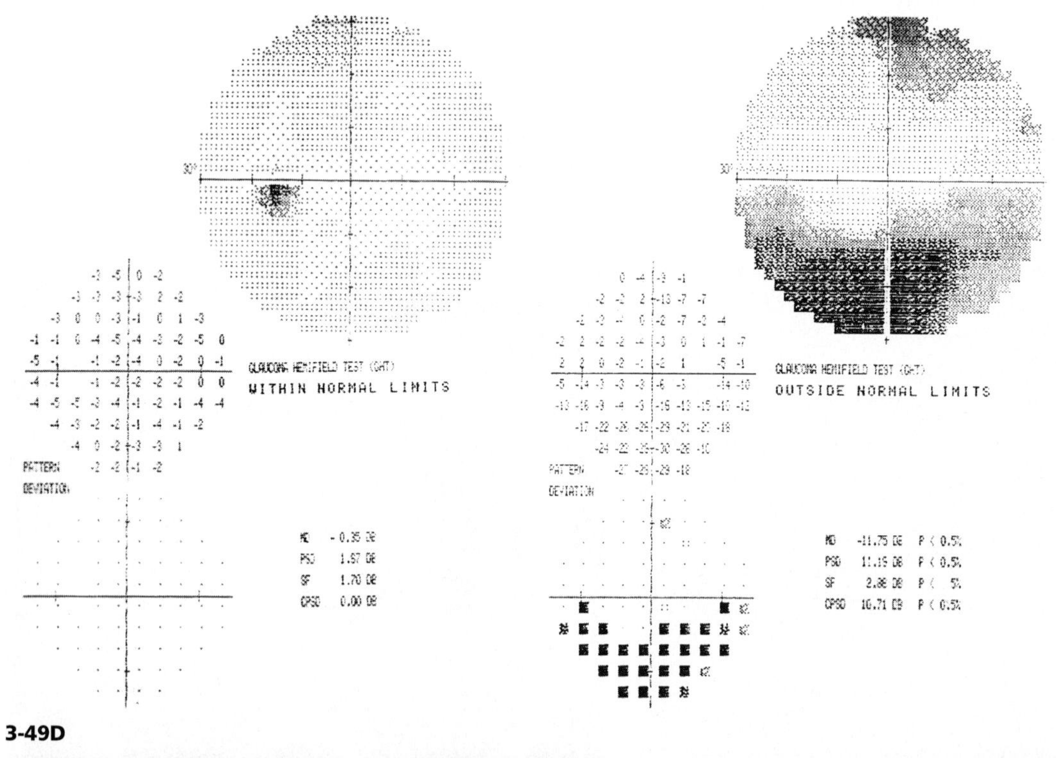

3-49D

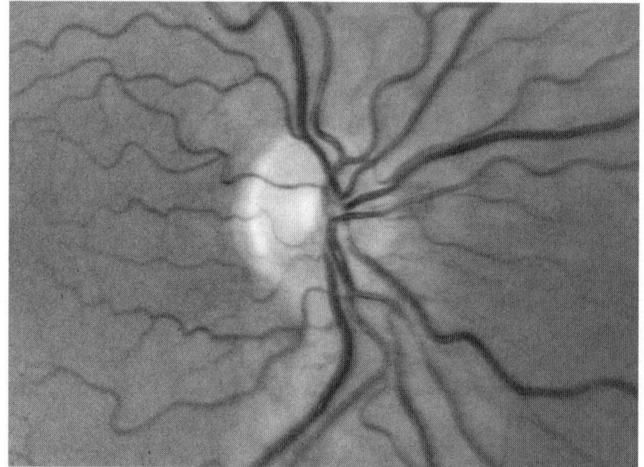

3-49E

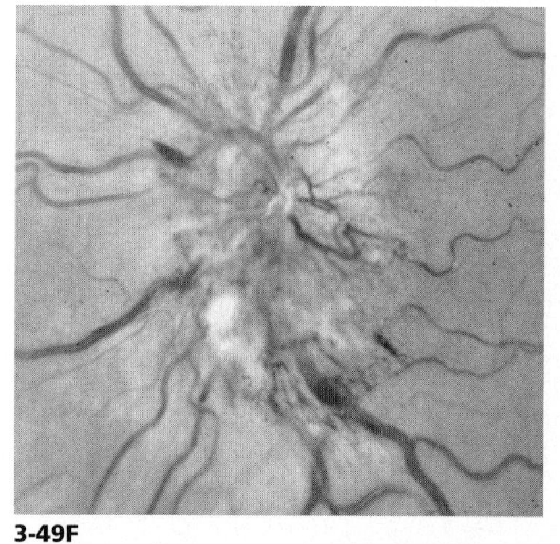

3-49F

A third uncommon disc-swelling papilledema variant is the so-called twin-peaks papilledema. Named for the fact that the swelling is mainly in the superior and inferior pole, this type of papilledema is not only distinctive, but can be localizing of an optic tract lesion (see the discussion on band atrophy in Chapter 4 for a detailed description of the anatomic consideration and causes of this unusual pattern).

Figure 3-50. A. **Twin-peaks papilledema with swelling superiorly and inferiorly and a band of atrophy in between (*arrows*).** B. **Fluorescein angiogram of the disc is even more striking.** C. **Papilledema may be seen superiorly and inferiorly on the disc in the right eye opposite the brain lesion.** D. **On the side of the infiltrating glioma of the thalamus compressing the optic tract, the left disc has slight pallor and little swelling. *Continued.***

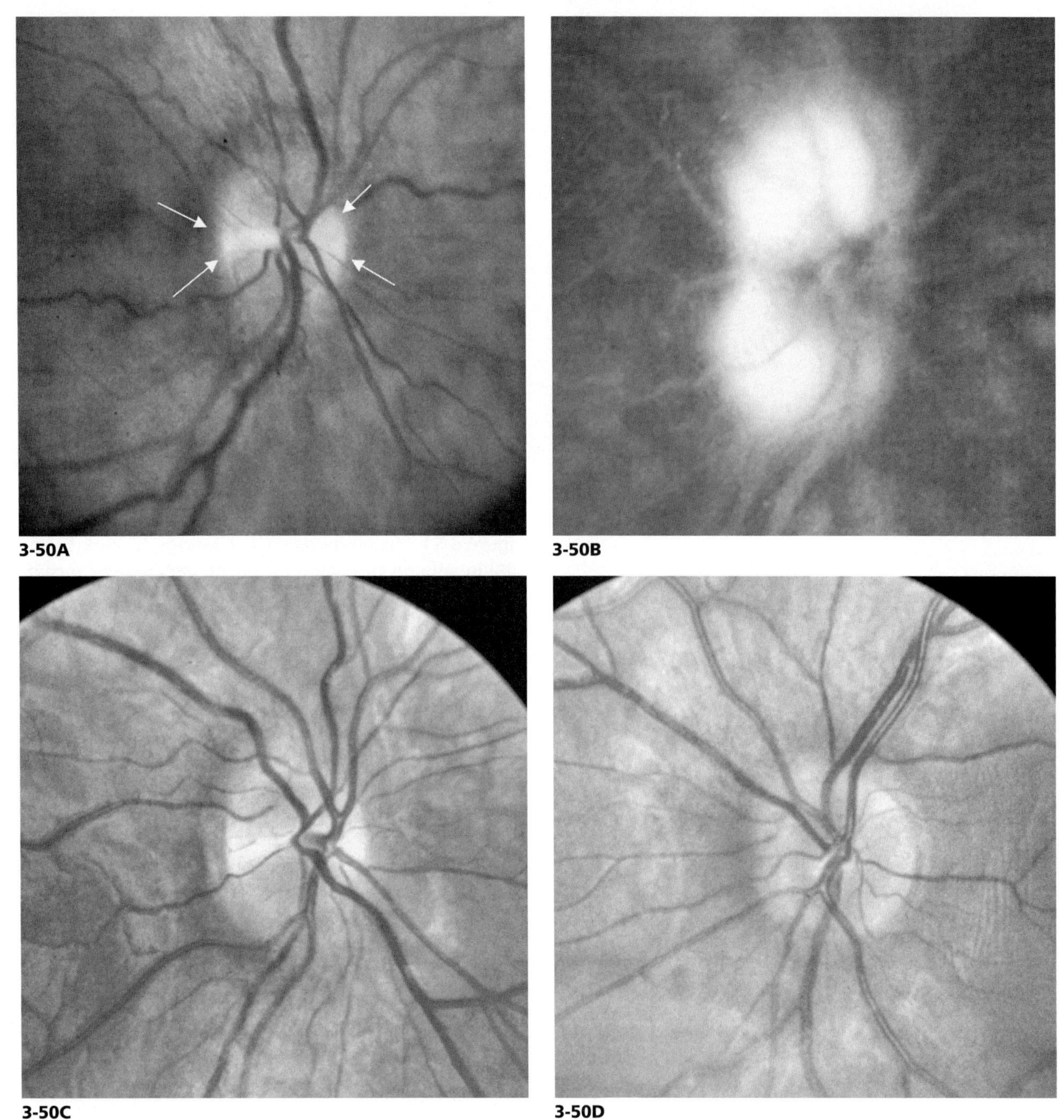

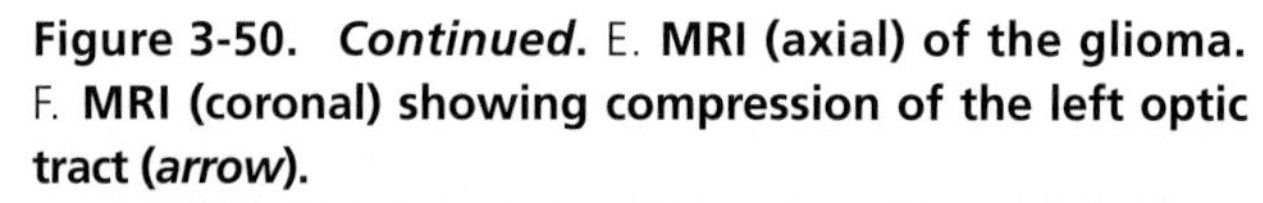

Figure 3-50. ***Continued.*** E. **MRI (axial) of the glioma.** F. **MRI (coronal) showing compression of the left optic tract (*arrow*).**

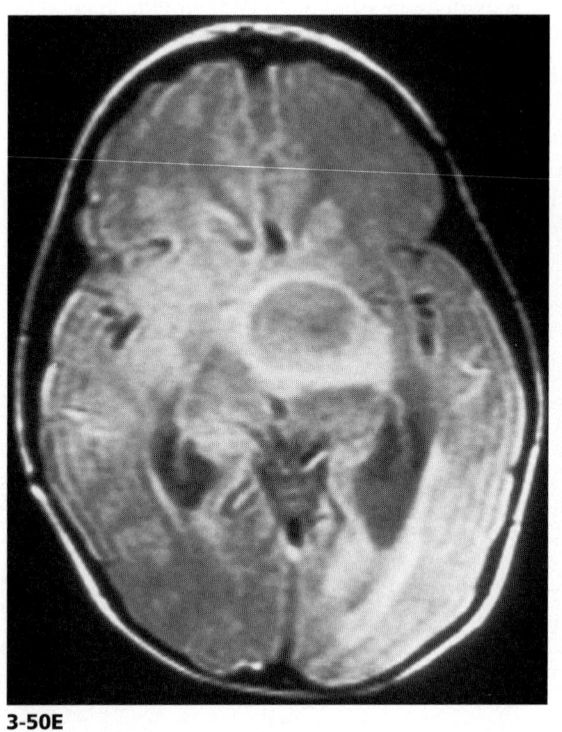

3-50E

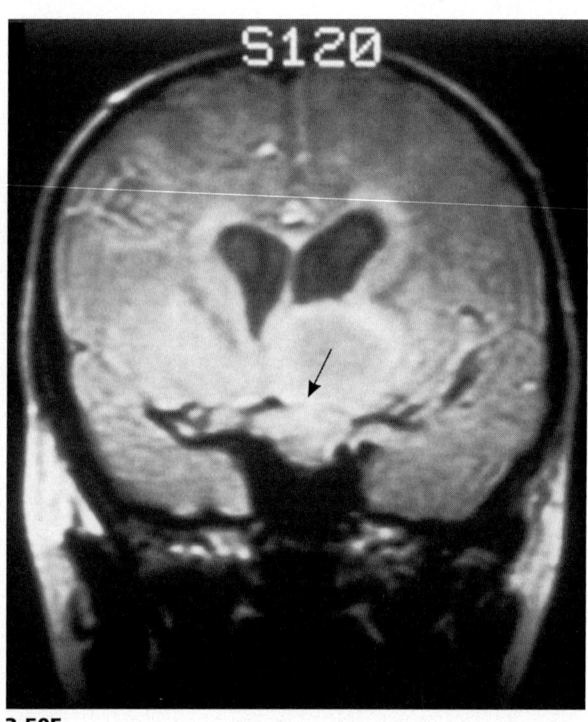

3-50F

Figure 3-51. (opposite page) A. **Findings to look for on MRI in anyone suspected of having papilledema include a dilated optic nerve sheath with a somewhat tortuous or kinked retrobulbar segment of the nerve. MRI with gadolinium may actually show the swollen papilla of the optic nerve in the globe (*arrows*).** B. **On sagittal views on the MRI, look for an empty sella (*arrow*). This may indicate chronicity of swelling. Chronically elevated intracranial pressure frequently causes enlargement of the sella in the vertical direction owing to pulsations of the inferior recess of the third ventricle above it acting as a pile driver. The anterior clinoid can demineralize. A plain skull x-ray could also show the sellar change.** C. **This T2-weighted axial MRI shows dilated nerve sheaths with extra fluid around the nerve. There is so much fluid around the nerve sheath on this MRI that the back of the globe is flattened (*arrow*).** D. **On the coronal view, there is a ring of cerebrospinal fluid surrounding the optic nerve, typical of dilated nerve sheaths associated with papilledema.** E. **This T2-weighted MRI shows extra fluid around the nerve sheath, giving an almost patulous optic nerve directly behind the globe.The usual evaluation of papilledema includes an emergent CT to show any space-**

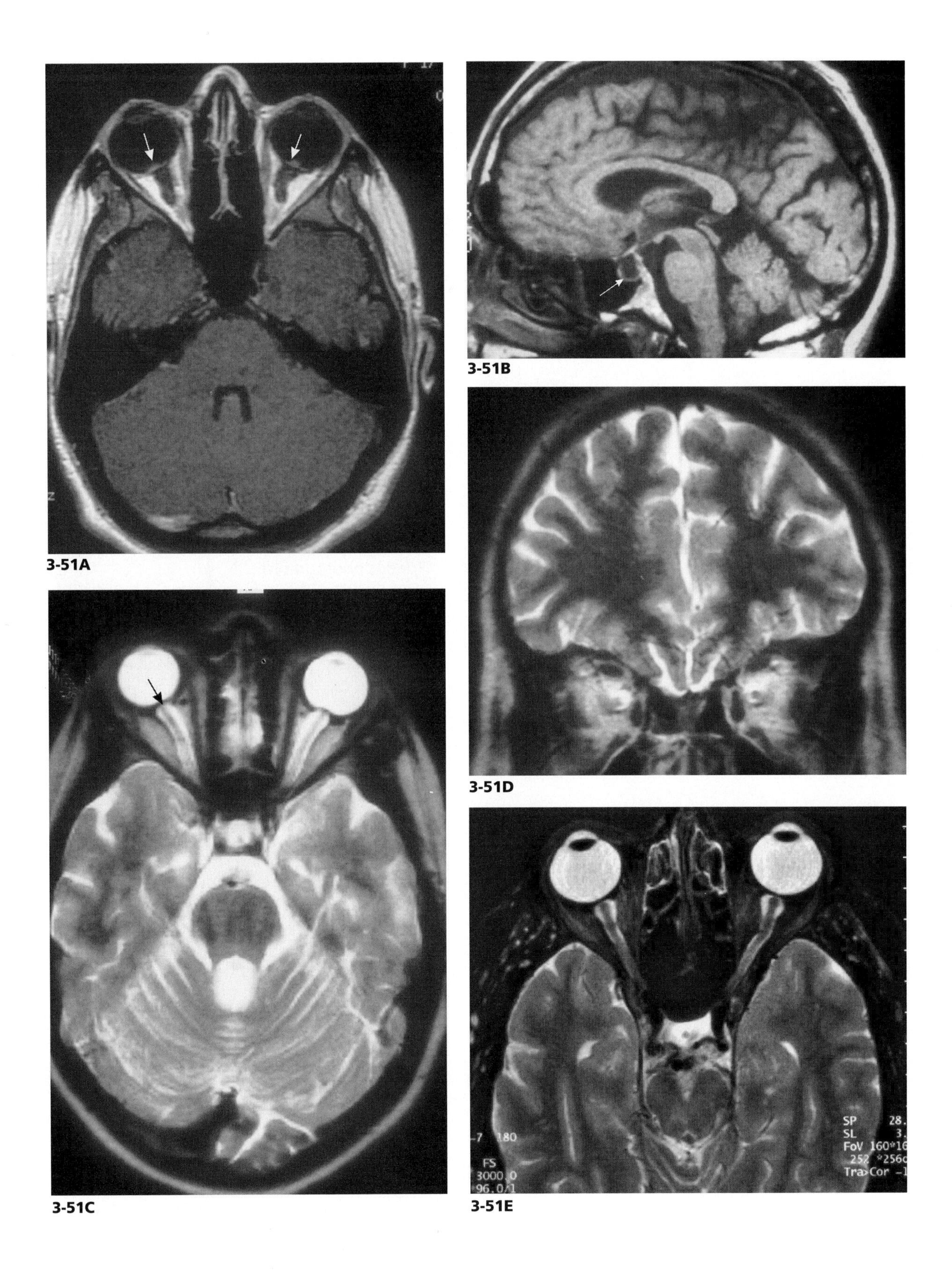

3-51A

3-51B

3-51C

3-51D

3-51E

occupying lesion that would prohibit doing a spinal tap. In some centers, an MRI is readily available and approximately the same price. The information gained from an MRI and magnetic resonance venography (MRV) (looking for venous thrombosis) makes ordering an MRI more cost effective. See Table 3-8 for tests to evaluate papilledema.

Table 3-8. Evaluation of the Patient with Papilledema

Imaging study: MRI or CT; MRV or venography
Cerebrospinal fluid examination: protein, glucose, cells, cytology, culture, opening pressure
Ophthalmic examination:
Visual acuity
Visual field: formal static (e.g., Humphrey visual field) or kinetic (e.g., Goldmann visual field)
Color vision test
Fundus photographs

HOW DOES PAPILLEDEMA CAUSE VISION LOSS?

The vision loss that occurs with papilledema can be thought of as "glaucoma in reverse." Except for enlargement of the blind spot, the forms of vision loss are similar to those seen with glaucoma: visual field constriction and nasal inferior loss. Papilledema can cause vision loss, no matter what the inciting cause.

Figure 3-52. Right (A) and left (B) disc swelling owing to idiopathic intracranial hypertension. The enlarged blind spot is caused by lateral displacement of the rods and cones of the retina by swollen optic nerve fibers, and partially by the hyperopic refractive scotoma from the elevation and swelling of the retinal elements. *Continued.*

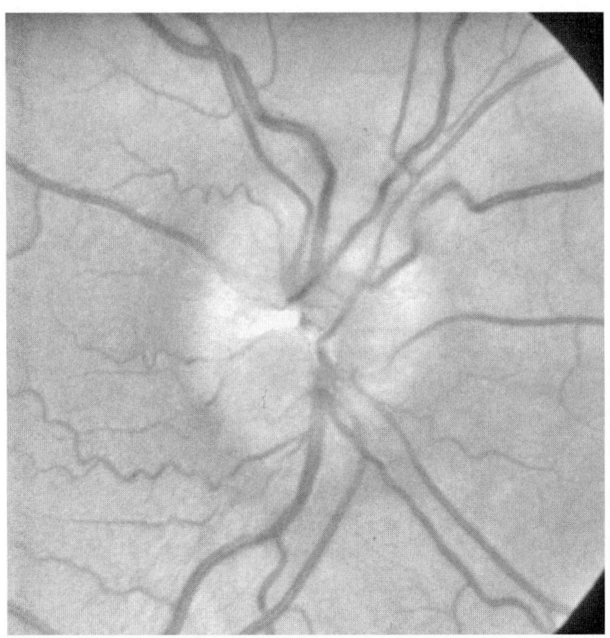

3-52A

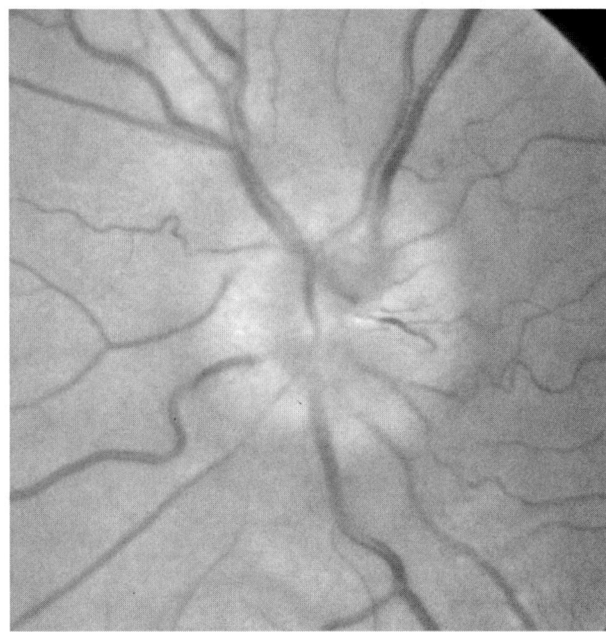

3-52B

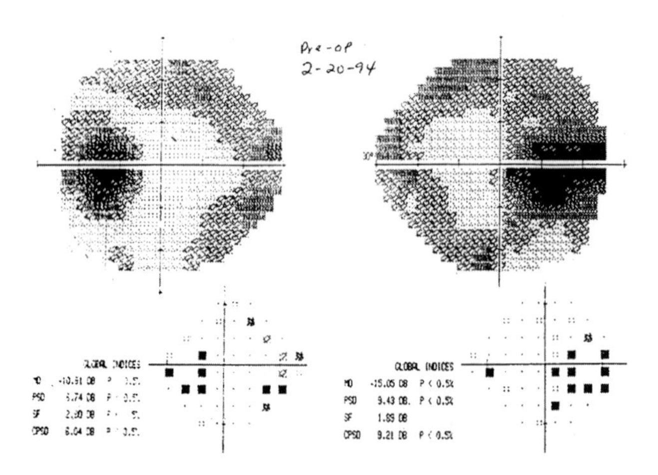

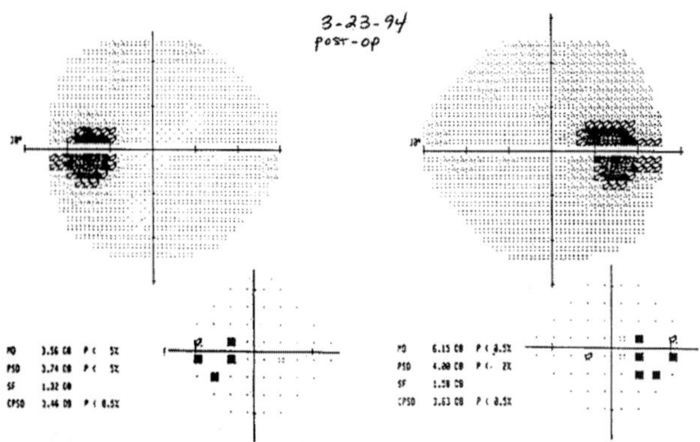

3-52C

Figure 3-52. *Continued.* C. In this case, the visual fields above not only show the enlargement of the blind spot, but also visual constriction. The visual fields below show improvement after an optic nerve sheath fenestration for severe papilledema owing to idiopathic intracranial hypertension, a procedure undertaken after the patient had failed medical treatment with acetazolamide. Her optic disc swelling also improved on the side of decompression (D) and also on the opposite side spontaneously (E).

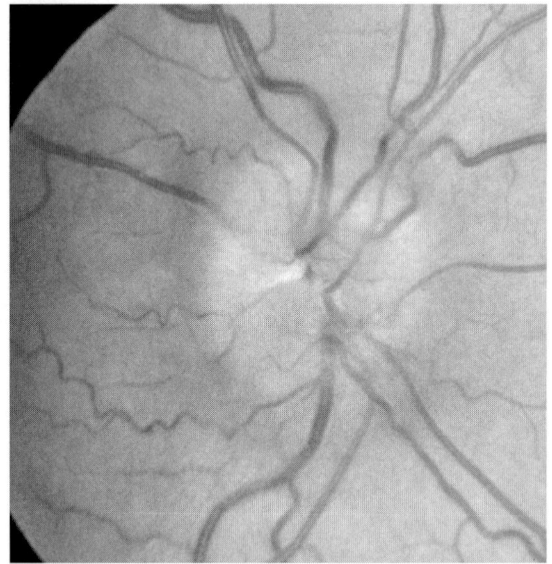

3-52D

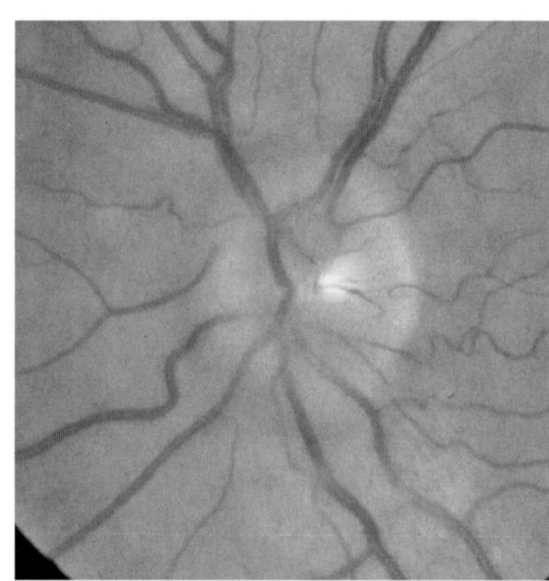

3-52E

Other causes of vision loss in papilledema include further ischemic damage to the optic nerve, axonal loss owing to compression of the swollen fibers against the scleral rim, and acute AION or stroke to the optic disc.

Sudden blindness can occur with papilledema. First, a child with severe papilledema due to a posterior fossa tumor can undergo neurosurgical decompression and awaken blind with no pupillary light reflex. This scenario is thought to be due to an ischemic vascular event owing to altered cerebral and optic disc blood flow, most likely hypotension. A second instance is a sudden failure of a ventriculoperitoneal or lumbar peritoneal shunt, producing a sudden rise in intracranial pressure, which produces papilledema and vision loss.[43]

Treatment of papilledema is usually at first medical, in the form of diuretics aimed at reducing intracranial pressure. When medical treatment fails, surgical treatment with an optic nerve fenestration (or window) in the dural sheath surrounding the optic nerve is helpful in protecting the optic nerve from further damage. A lumbar-peritoneal shunting procedure is sometimes also used.[37]

IS THE SWELLING INFLAMMATORY?

Neuroretinitis is typified by swelling of the optic nerve along with exudates in the retina in a typical pattern (macular star). This pattern is sometimes known as *optic disc edema with macular star* (ODEMS). Neuroretinitis is often seen after a viral illness or cat-scratch disease. Appearance of neuroretinitis is distinctive—totally or segmentally swollen, pale optic disc, linear exudates in the macula and peripapillary region, and, occasionally, vitreous cells. The exudates form deep in the area of the macula, in Henle's layer. The orientation of the nerve fibers in this area leads to the star formation (see Table 3-9 for a list of causes of ODEMS; see also

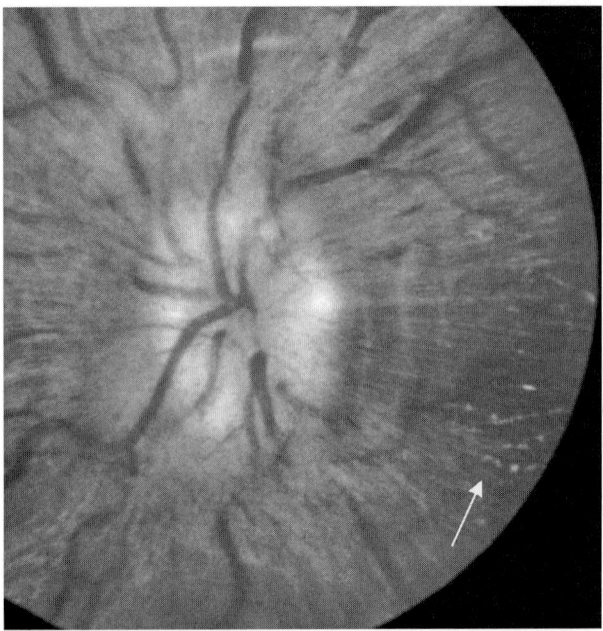
3-53A

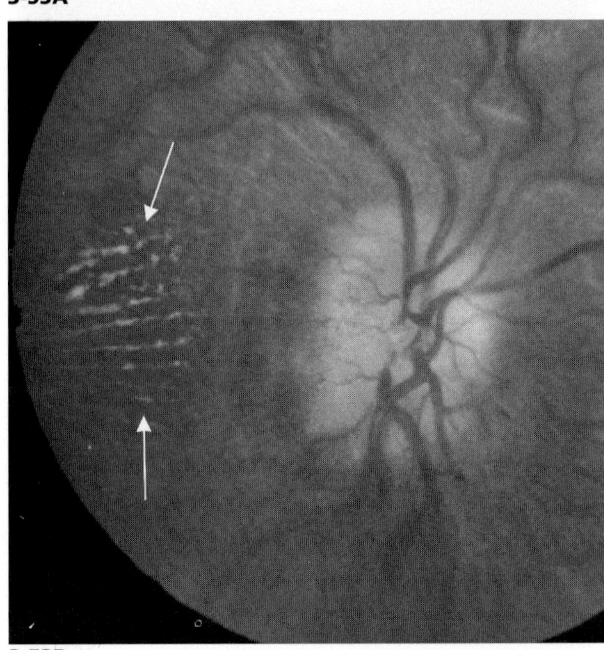
3-53B

anatomic drawing, Figure 10-4B; see also Macular Disorders, Chapter 10, for a discussion of macular stars, see Figures 10-17–10-19). The optic disc edema associated with *Bartonella henselae* (cat-scratch disease) often has an associated peripapillary serous retinal detachment.[44]

Figure 3-53. A,B. **In this case, the woman has idiopathic intracranial hypertension with severe papilledema and a partial macular star (*arrows*).**

Table 3-9. Causes of Optic Disc Swelling and Macular Star

Severe papilledema
AION (with a lot of disc swelling)
Diabetic papillitis, retinopathy
Hypertensive retinopathy with disc swelling
Infections
Mumps
Herpes virus
Influenza virus
Cat-scratch fever (*Bartonella henselae*)
Chickenpox (herpes zoster)
Tuberculous retinopathy
Psittacosis
Mycoses: histoplasma
Syphilis
Lyme disease
Toxoplasmosis
Toxocariasis
Behçet's disease

IS THE SWELLING VASCULAR (HYPERTENSION)?

Severe systemic hypertension can be associated with disc swelling; however, other findings may also be present, including the narrowing of arterioles, artery-vein crossing changes, hemorrhages, cotton-wool spots, and hard exudates (see Chapter 9, Retinopathy—Hypertensive). Although some cases of hypertensive encephalopathy do have disc swelling owing to increased intracranial pressure along with obvious changes on the MRI, some hypertensives may have ischemic optic neuropathy and not true papilledema.[45]

IS THE SWELLING TOXIC?

Methanol

Methanol toxicity is a commonly recognized toxic optic neuropathy most frequently owing to the addition of methanol to ethyl alcohol. Although the disc is swollen acutely, the pathology found at autopsy indicates the lesion is retrobulbar demyelination and later necrosis. After the swelling resolves, optic atrophy occurs, frequently with cupping, and may be indistinguishable from chronic glaucoma.[46,47]

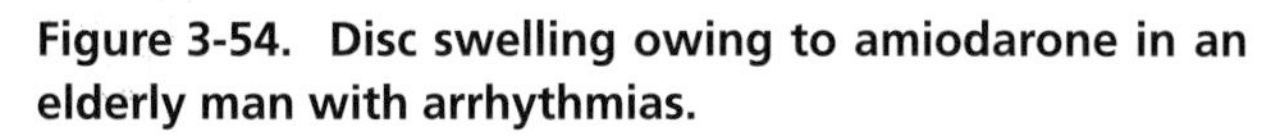

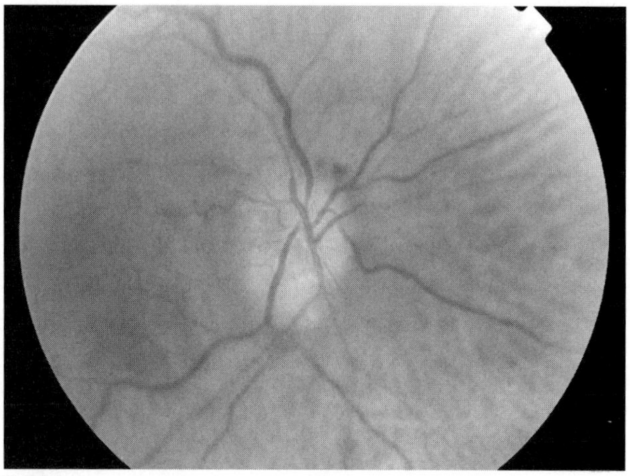

Figure 3-54. Disc swelling owing to amiodarone in an elderly man with arrhythmias.

3-54

Amiodarone

Amiodarone is a drug used for cardiac arrhythmias that causes disc swelling. The swelling is due to axoplasmic stasis, presumably from inhibition of axonal transport related to the drug. There are reports of increased intracranial pressure, as well as ischemic causes of optic disc swelling. Treatment involves stopping the drug. Sometimes the visual fields do not recover. In 1999, Macaluso et al.

reported several characteristics that separate amiodarone toxicity and AION, including insidious onset of vision loss; modest loss of visual acuity (usually 20/20–20/200), resolution of edema taking weeks to months, and bilateral simultaneous involvement.[48]

Table 3-10. Toxins That Produce Disc Swelling

Amiodarone
Methanol
Ethylene glycol
cis-Platinum
Bischloroethylnitrosourea (BCNU or carmustine)
Quinine
Perhexiline maleate

IS THE SWELLING HEREDITARY?—LEBER'S OPTIC NEUROPATHY

Leber's hereditary optic neuropathy (described by Theodor Leber in 1871) is an inherited disorder of the mitochondria. Although women have been described with Leber's optic neuropathy, men are more likely to be symptomatic. The primary Leber's mutations on the mitochondria include the 11778, 14484, and 3460. The typical picture is a painless loss of central vision in one eye, followed by the same in the second eye within weeks to months. The ophthalmoscopic appearance is distinctive, including swelling of the disc owing to swelling of axons and telangiectatic vessels on the disc, and vessel tortuosity. The fluorescein angiogram does not reveal disc leakage. Later, the disc develops diffuse pallor, especially with atrophy of the papillomacular bundle. For an excellent review, see Newman.[49]

Figure 3-55. Typical case of acute Leber's optic neuropathy. A. A 9-year-old boy presented with painless loss of central vision in the right eye. Although his vision in the right eye was decreased to 20/400, the left eye was still 20/20. B. As you can see, however, the left optic disc shows the characteristic findings of telangiectatic disc vessels as well as tortuosity to the arteries and veins. Within 2 weeks, he lost vision in the left eye and developed characteristic bilateral central scotomas. C. Typical Goldmann visual fields associated with Leber's optic neuropathy. Eight months later, he had pallor of the papillomacular bundle. *Continued*

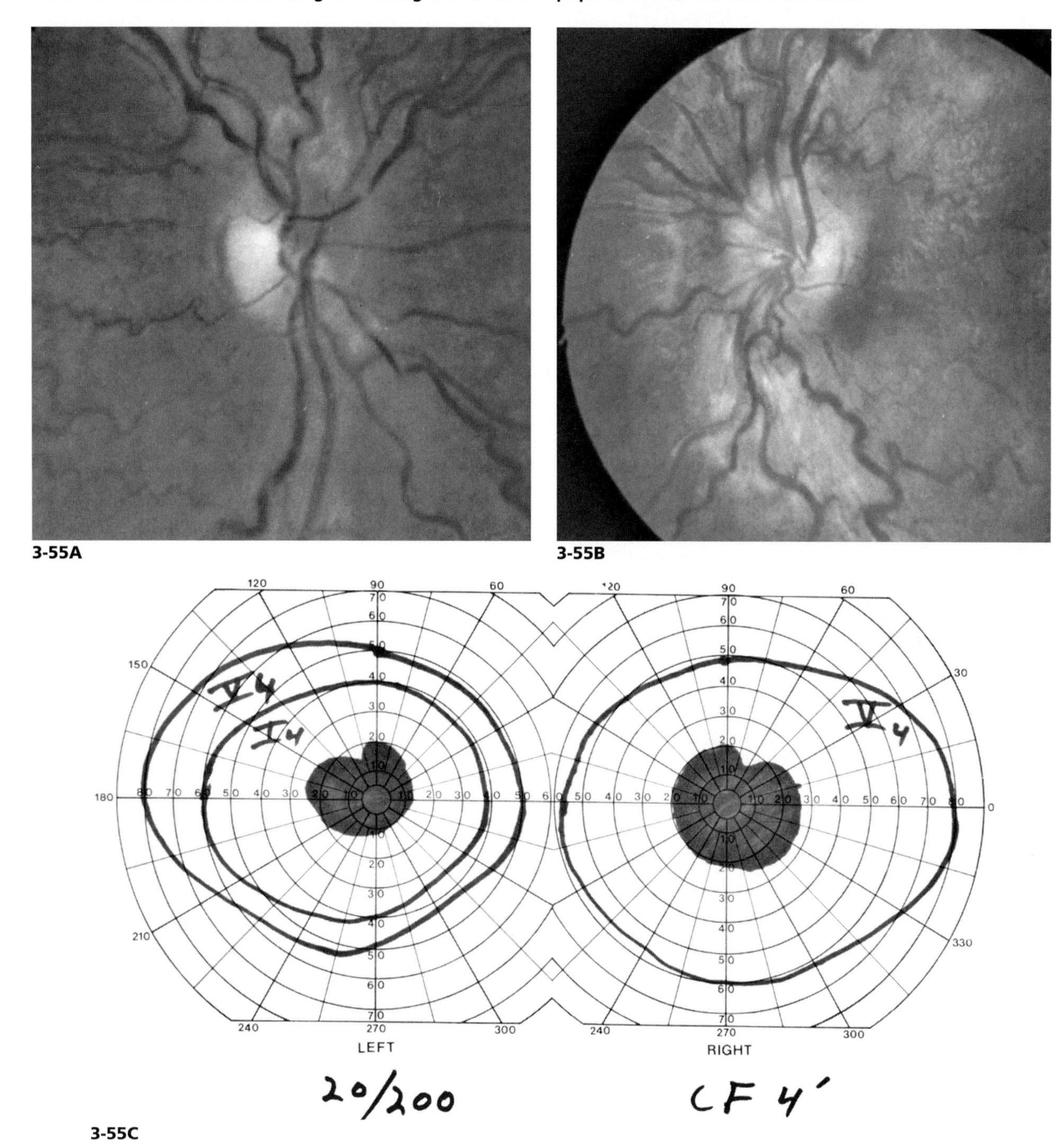

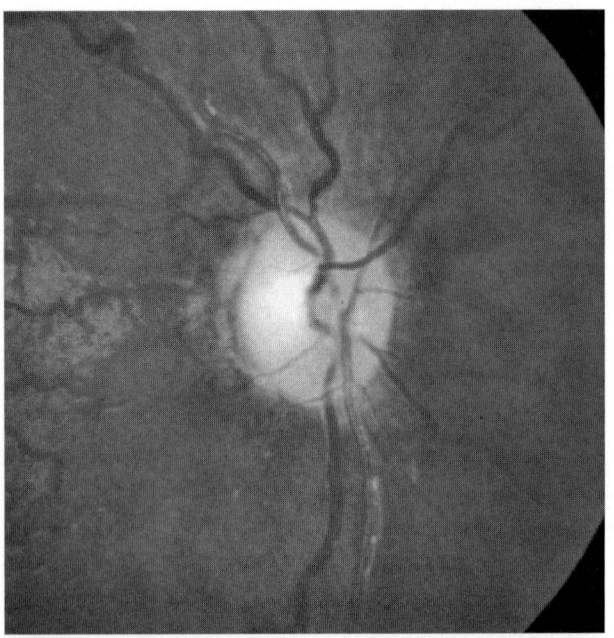
3-55D

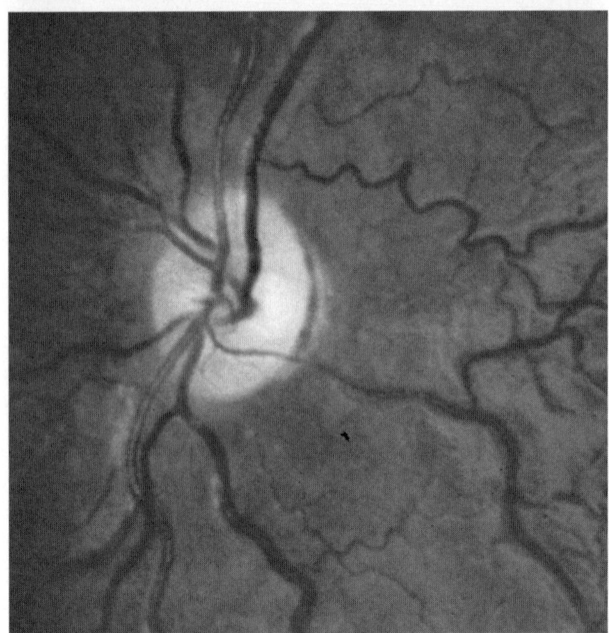
3-55E

Figure 3-55. ***Continued.*** D,E. **At follow-up some time later, there was atrophy.**

UNILATERAL DISC SWELLING

Is the Swelling Inflammatory?—Papillitis or Anterior Optic Neuritis

Papillitis is a general term that describes any swelling of the disc from an ocular process—inflammation, infection, and demyelination. Optic neuritis (from demyelination) with disc swelling is a form of papillitis. Although papillitis can be a unilateral process, bilateral cases are not rare.

Diabetes has been associated with a papillitis as well. In general, this syndrome has been described with younger patients (usually 20–30 years of age, but can be older), type I diabetes (but can be type II) patients, and mild disc swelling without changes in visual function; generally the edema clears without serious sequelae. Diabetic retinopathy, macular edema, and retinal capillary nonperfusion on fluorescein can occur. Differentiation of diabetes papillitis from typical AION or optic neuritis can be problematic, and some believe diabetic papillitis to be a form of AION.[50]

Figure 3-56. A. Diabetic papillitis is fairly common. There may be no loss of visual acuity, and the visual field may not be abnormal. Most think that diabetic papillitis is a form of AION. B,C. Photographs of syphilitic papillitis. The disc is swollen. In addition, there may be a haze over the disc owing to vitreal cells, which obscures the clarity of the disc; on examination, this translates to being unable to focus clearly on the disc. In addition, some papillitis is associated with a macular star formation (see Table 3-9; and Chapter 10, Macular Stars). C. This woman with syphilis had bilateral disc swelling and good visual acuity.

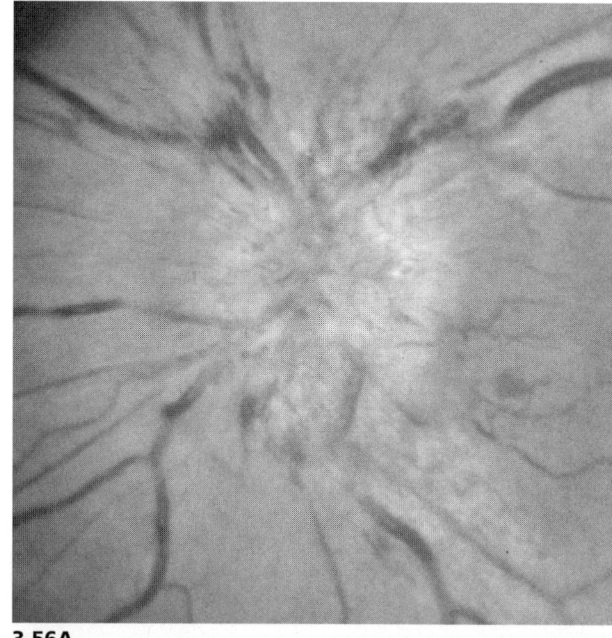

3-56A

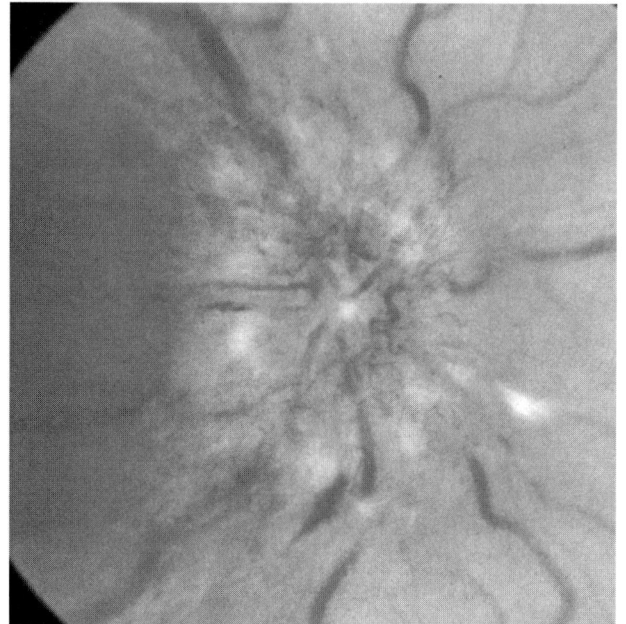

3-56B

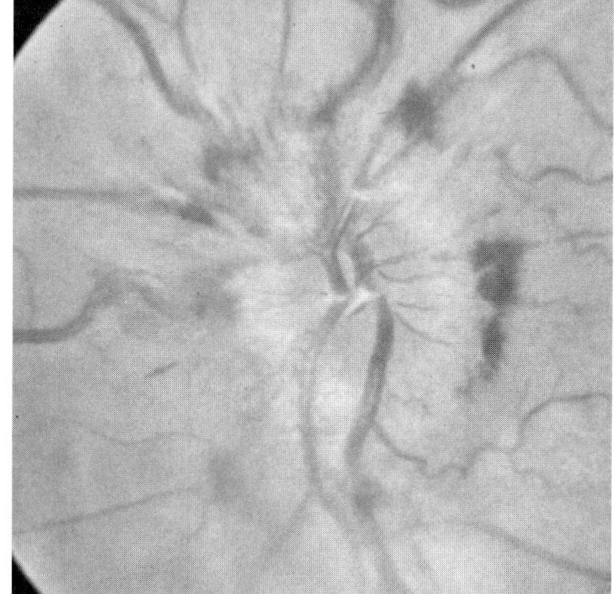

3-56C

Figure 3-57. A,B. **This woman presented with subacute vision loss in the left eye to the level of count fingers and pain on eye movement. Over the next 8 weeks, pallor ensued, but her vision recovered to 20/25. Her cerebrospinal fluid showed normal protein and glucose, but oligoclonal bands were present, and a diagnosis of demyelinating optic neuritis was made. The MRI showed multiple T2 signal periventricular white matter lesions, leading to the diagnosis of multiple sclerosis. Anterior optic neuritis can be associated with a swollen disc. The disc is acutely swollen** (A) **and later shows pallor; notice the "high-water marks" in** B **(*arrows*).**

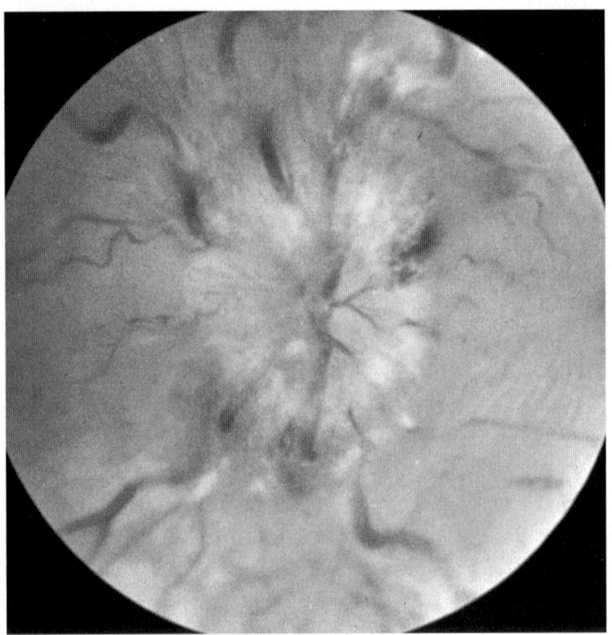

3-57A

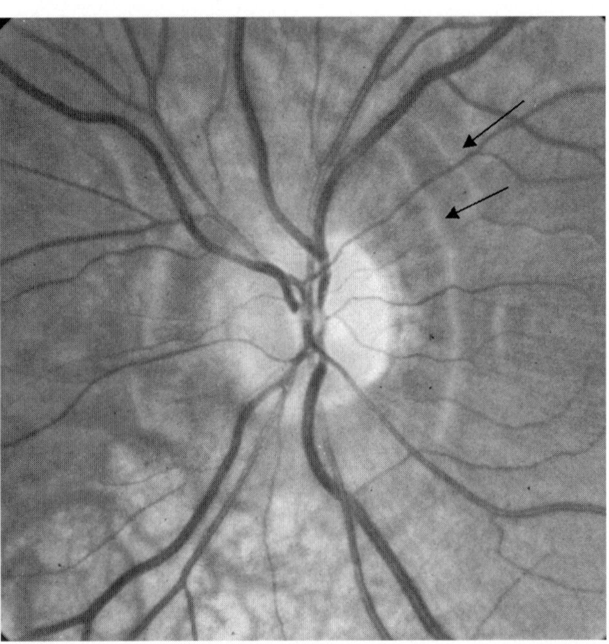

3-57B

Acute anterior optic neuritis is a spectrum of swelling. Whereas most of the cases of retrobulbar optic neuritis have little in the way of swelling associated with profound vision loss, anterior optic neuritis can have more disc swelling. Besides complaining of pain with eye movement, the patient also exhibits loss of visual function and the presence of a relative afferent pupillary defect.

Table 3-11. Differentiation of Papillitis and Papilledema

	Papillitis	Papilledema
History		
Vision loss	Prominent	Usually not prominent
Pain	Present—ocular and with eye movement	Absent (may have headache)
Examination		
Visual acuity	Decreased	Normal
Relative afferent pupil defect	Present	Absent
Visual field	Central scotoma; severe loss	Loss may be nasal; enlarged blind spot; constriction
Appearance of the disc		
Prepapillary haze	Present	Absent
Macular star	Frequent (with neuroretinitis from viral infection)	Rare unless severe swelling—then often hemi-macular star
Optic cup	Obscured by the inflammation	Usually preserved until late
Vessels	Dilated veins, often more than expected for the amount of swelling (especially in papillophlebitis)	Dilated and tortuous; enlargement of the fine capillaries on the disc
Etiology	Infections: virus (herpes), spirochetes (syphilis), human immunodeficiency virus, fungi (cryptococcus); toxoplasmosis	Intracranial mass
	Systemic disease: diabetes	Venous sinus thrombosis
	Demyelination: multiple sclerosis	Cerebrospinal fluid infections—encephalitis, meningitis
	Vasculitis: systemic lupus	Idiopathic (see also Table 3-7)

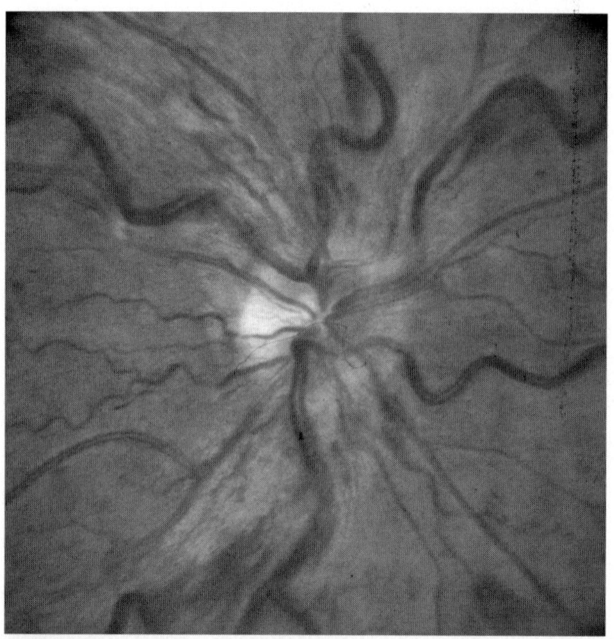
3-58A

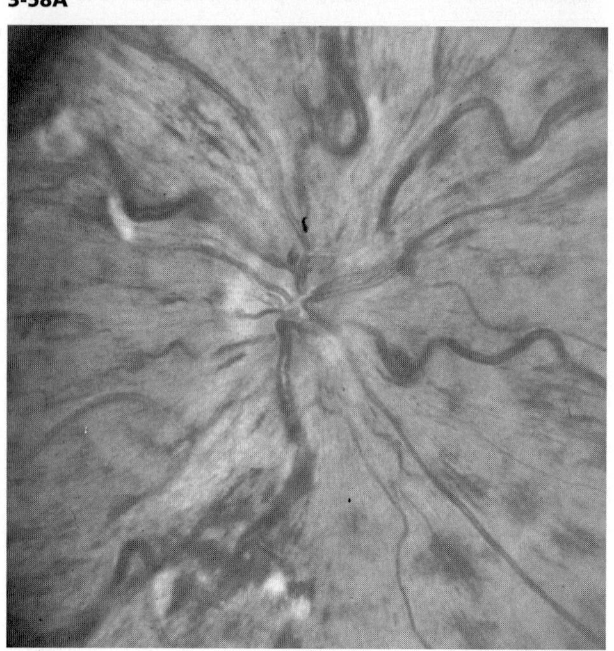
3-58B

VASCULAR CAUSES OF DISC SWELLING

Papillophlebitis can cause central retinal vein occlusion or swelling of the disc owing to a central or branch retinal vein occlusion. The veins are dilated in excess of the swelling of the disc (see Chapter 5 for full details).

Figure 3-58. A,B. **Papillophlebitis causes disc swelling. Papillophlebitis is disc swelling owing to venous congestion and early retinal vein occlusion. Early on, this patient with diabetes mellitus presented with unilateral intermittent visual blurring and 20/20 vision** (A). **The patient has early retinal venous congestion, as shown by the hemorrhages. Later, the venous nature of the swelling becomes more obvious** (B). **The visual acuity was 20/30. Central retinal vein occlusion can be associated with disc swelling (see Chapter 5). (Photographs courtesy of Martin Lubow, M.D.)**

Is the Swelling Ischemic?

Ischemia to the optic disc is fairly common in the older patient, causing unilateral vision loss.

Anterior Ischemic Optic Neuropathy

AION is swelling owing to infarction of the optic disc. Presumably, occlusion of the posterior ciliary arteries causes AION.

There are really two forms of AION: nonarteritic (NA-AION) and arteritic AION owing to giant cell arteritis. The more common form, NA-AION, is associated with hypertension and diabetes. There are clinical features that can differentiate the arteritic and nonarteritic forms of disc swelling. See Chapter 5, Table 5-6 for these features.

Figure 3-59. A. **Ischemia blocks axoplasmic flow by damaging mitochondria in the axoplasm in the prelaminar region. This causes "damming" of axoplasm at the prelaminar region.** B. **Typical NA-AION.** C. **In AION, there may be hemorrhages on the disc.**

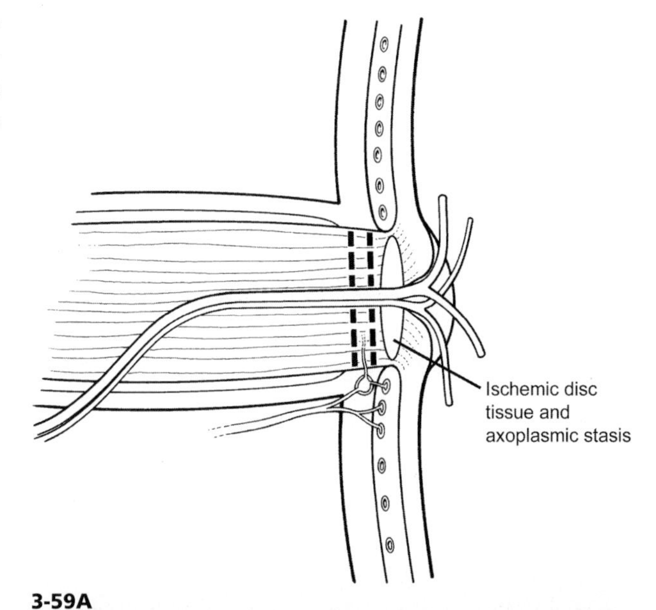

3-59A

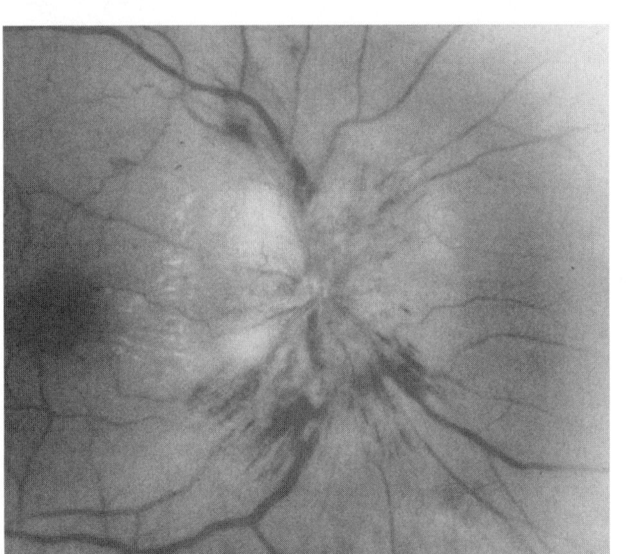

3-59B

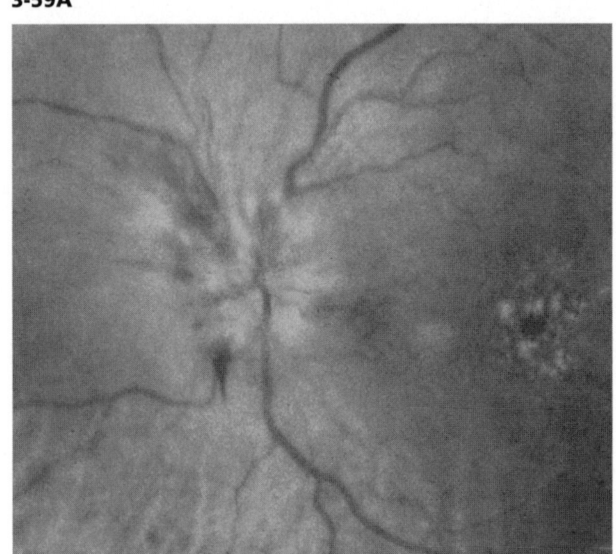

3-59C

Nonarteritic Ischemic Optic Neuropathy

In NA-AION, infarction causes axoplasmic stasis and there is also swelling of the acutely ischemic tissue. Appearance of NA-AION is usually diffuse or sectoral swelling. The swelling appears to have some pallor to it, hence the term *pallid swelling*. There may be hemorrhages and cotton-wool spots nearby. Frequently, the blood vessels are narrowed. The cup is obliterated. Frequently, only part of the disc is affected, with one sector swollen. See Chapter 5 for further discussion of the vascular aspects of AION.

Figure 3-60. A. **AION usually presents with acute, diffuse, unilateral, painless swelling. The feature that helps you make the correct diagnosis is seeing the swelling in the appropriate age group. The opposite disc may have a small cup-to-disc ratio.** B. **Optic atrophy ensues. Notice that the vessels are narrowed and somewhat gliotic.** C. **Another acute AION of the right eye.** D. **Later, optic atrophy occurred. Notice the "high-water mark" (*arrows*).**

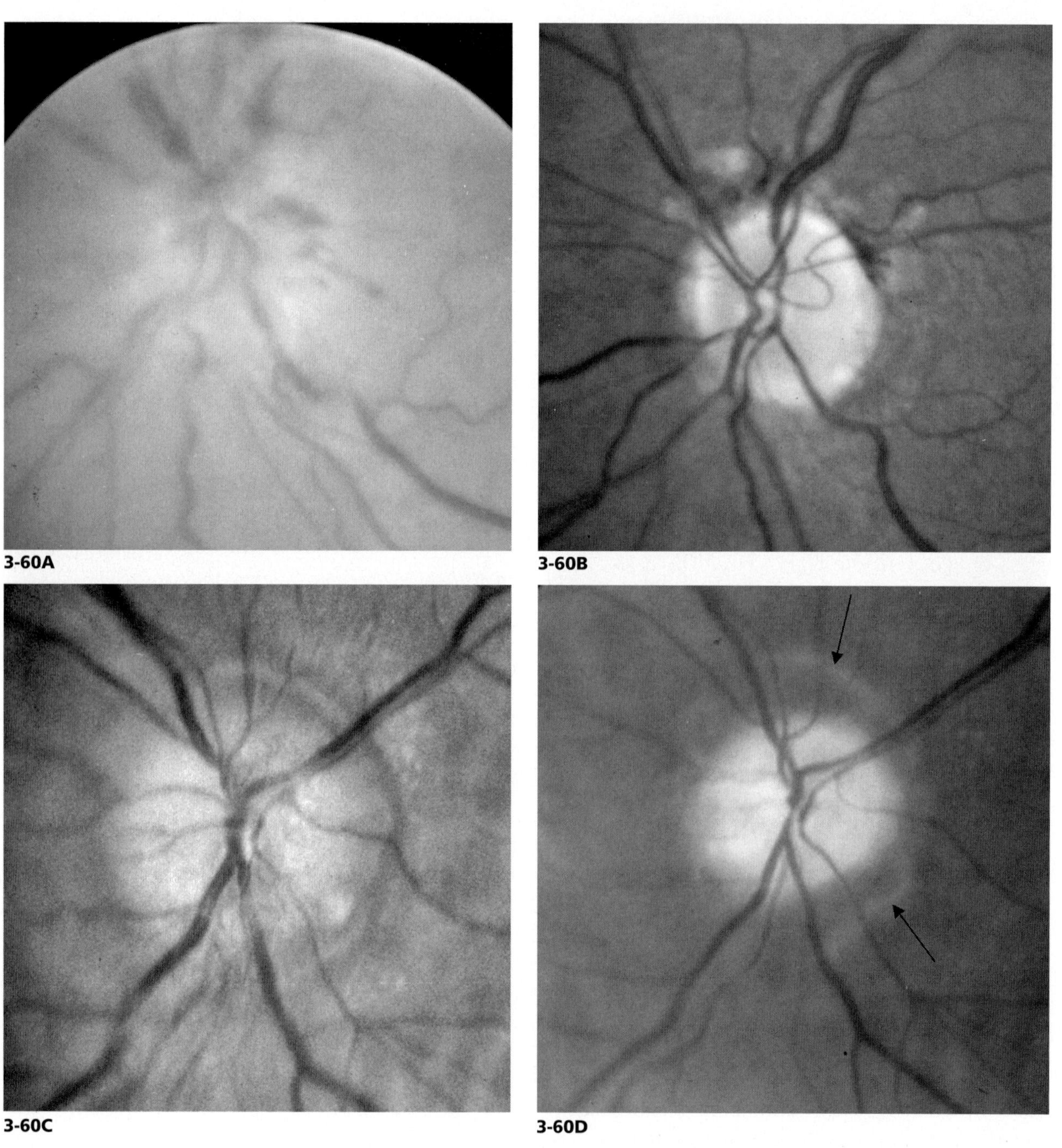

Figure 3-61. A,B. **Sectoral swelling is a distinguishing feature of AION from optic neuritis with swelling.**[51] A. **Inferior disc swelling due to AION.** B. **This disc was sectorially swollen superiorly. In follow-up, the swollen area was pale.**

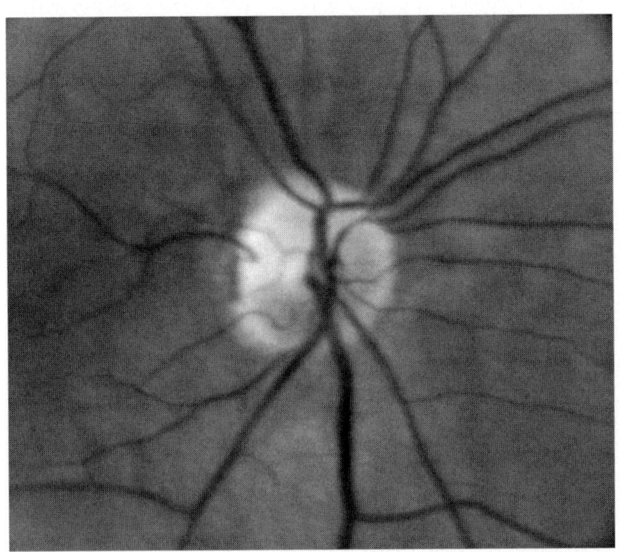

3-61A

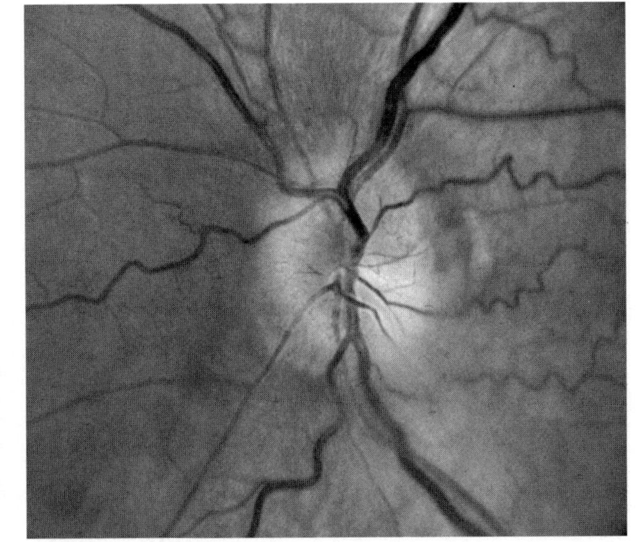

3-61B

Although NA-AION can occur in the young, it occurs usually in older individuals—older than 45 years of age. The etiology of NA-AION is not at all clear, and, although ischemia is a feature of it, ischemia may not be the initial event. There are also definite risk factors for developing NA-AION. First, vascular risk factors such as hypertension and/or diabetes have been associated with the development of AION in most. Another risk factor for the development of AION seems to be "a disc at risk"—that is, a small cup-to-disc ratio. There is an architectural feature of "the disc at risk" for AION; these discs are small, cupless, and crowded. Exactly how this structural factor acts as a risk element is not clear. Furthermore, there is a 40% risk of AION in the second eye within 2 years.[52]

Figure 3-62. The disc at risk. A. **The right disc shows a very small, crowded disc with elevation and no cup. In 2 months the patient had vision loss in the right eye as well.** B. **This diabetic woman presented with acute, painless vision loss in the left eye.** C. **This is a typical disc at risk, without a cup. Part** D **shows the residue from previous AION—note the segmental pallor inferotemporally, indicating a previous attack of AION.**

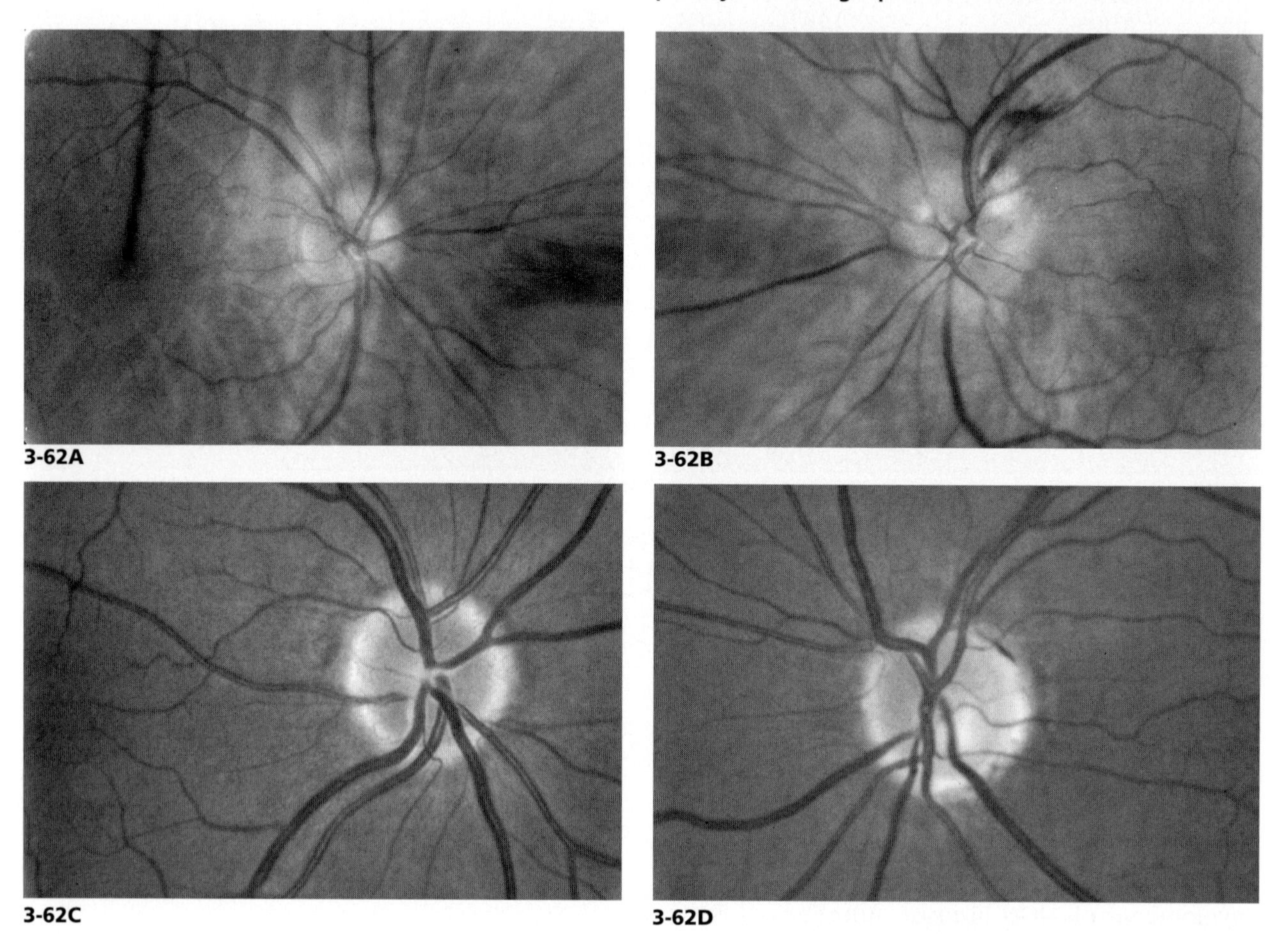

Table 3-12. Risk Factors for Developing Nonarteritic Anterior Ischemic Optic Neuropathy

Hypertension
Diabetes
Small cup-to-disc ratio
Aggressive treatment of blood pressure
Hypotension—spontaneous, associated with dialysis, nocturnal
Smoking
Homocystinemia
Medication: sympathomimetics; amiodarone; sildenafil (Viagra)[53]

Sometimes distinguishing AION from optic neuritis is an issue. There are characteristic disc findings that may be helpful. See Table 3-13.

Table 3-13. Distinguishing AION and Optic Neuritis Swelling

Characteristic	AION	Optic Neuritis
Edema	Diffuse in two-thirds; altitudinal or segmental one-third	Diffuse 90%
Color	Pale swelling 35%	Pale swelling 3%
Hemorrhage on disc	Present 80%	Present 23%
Vessels	Arterial attenuation 33%	Arterial attenuation 5%
	Normal vessels 35%	Normal vessels 68%
Fluorescein angiography	Delay in filling the prelaminar vessels	No delay in filling

Source: Adapted from reference 51.

Symptoms of NA-AION include the painless loss of vision. Many report vision loss on awakening. There may be some pressure sensation around the eye, but only 10–12% report eye pain.[54]

Ophthalmic examination reveals the disc swelling along with decreased visual acuity, a relative afferent pupillary defect in the eye with AION, and visual field abnormalities.

Disc Swelling Owing to Low Intraocular Pressure

Hypotony can cause disc swelling. Markedly *decreased intraocular pressure* or *ocular inflammation* can cause disc swelling owing to axoplasmic stasis. The axoplasm is blocked by normal intracranial pressure which, while normal, is elevated relative to the low intraocular pressure. This causes an obstruction to axoplasmic flow at the level of the lamina cribrosa. Hypotony can also occur with a penetrating wound to the globe, various surgeries to the eye, and anything that damages the ciliary body and reduces the amount of aqueous humor production. Swelling of the disc may not be the most noticeable, whereas retinal edema or macular edema is more common.[55]

DISC SWELLING DUE TO SCLERITIS AND POSTERIOR SCLERITIS

Episcleritis is inflammation of the episclera, which causes redness, pain, and photophobia. The course is benign. *Scleritis*, however, is an inflammation of the sclera caused by vasculitis causing pain, decreased vision, and deep violet–colored sclera. *Posterior scleritis* may have associated pain or redness, but disc swelling, vitriitis, and macular edema can occur. The diagnosis can be made by ultrasonography showing thickening of the sclera, and by CT. There may be hypotony associated with posterior scleritis. Causes of scleritis include autoimmune disease (e.g., rheumatoid arthritis, ankylosing spondylitis, polyarteritis nodosa, Wegener's granulomatosis, systemic lupus erythematosus, ulcerative colitis, psoriatic arthritis), granulomatous disease (e.g., tuberculosis, syphilis, sarcoid), metabolic disease (e.g., thyroid, gout), infectious disease (herpes zoster, herpes simplex, *Pseudomonas*, *Streptococcus*, *Staphylococcus*), external trauma, burns (chemical and thermal), and surgery.[56]

Figure 3-63. Posterior scleritis can cause disc swelling. A. **Notice the very slight redness of the sclera on the right.** B. **There is also a dilated scleral vein on the right.** C. **Posterior scleritis causes disc swelling and sometimes macular edema.** D. **The other eye appears normal.**

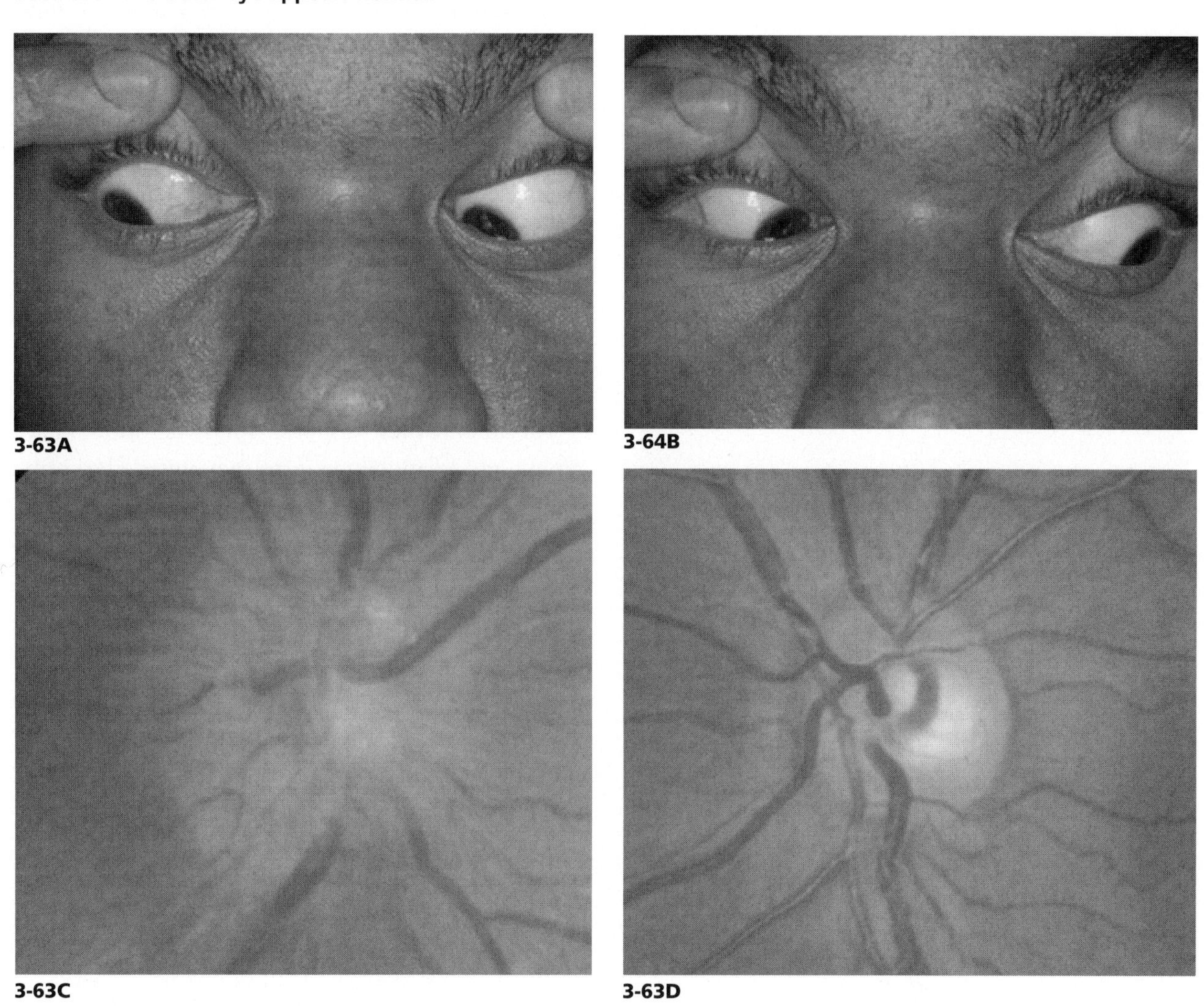

3-63A **3-64B** **3-63C** **3-63D**

SWELLING OWING TO RETINITIS, CHOROIDITIS, OR INFILTRATION

Whenever there is inflammation of the retina or choroid in the eye, the disc is at risk to swell. However, this possibility is made apparent by the changes in the retina and also by the vitreal haze that is present as a result of the inflammation. Look also for hemorrhages and cotton-wool spots (see Chapters 6 and 7).

Infiltrative optic neuropathy may be seen with granulomas such as sarcoid; neoplasms such as lymphoma or leukemia and metastases to the optic nerve head can also cause disc swelling. Cells invade the optic nerve and disc proper; vision loss is variable. Other tumors, such as optic nerve glioma and meningioma, also may invade the optic nerve and cause disc swelling or pallor, or both.

Sarcoidosis, a granulomatous infiltrating condition of unknown etiology, can cause disc swelling in many ways. Direct infiltration of the optic nerve and disc may cause disc swelling. Sometimes a granuloma in or on the disc may be seen. Compression of the vessels at the disc may cause ischemic optic neuropathy. Papilledema owing to increased intracranial pressure can cause bilateral disc swelling. The cause of the increased pressure in some cases is sarcoid compression of intracranial venous sinus structures, and in others it is owing to the sarcoid acting as a mass within the cranium.[57] MRI with contrast helps to sort out the cause of the swelling. The importance of recognizing the disc swelling caused by sarcoid infiltration is that sarcoid optic neuropathy is often treatable with corticosteroids,[58] which may prevent or reverse vision loss.

Figure 3-64. A. Disc swelling owing to sarcoid. This nerve is both compressed and infiltrated. B. This woman had irregular swelling of the disc owing to granulomas of the disc; her swelling was steroid responsive. A biopsy of a hilar node showed sarcoidosis. C. MRI with gadolinium of the orbit shows characteristic optic nerve enhancement (*arrow*). D. This man had severe optic neuropathy to no light perception vision. A mass was seen on imaging studies. A subtotal resection specimen showed infiltrating sarcoid. Sarcoid infiltrates along the Virchow-Robin space. Direct invasion causes swelling or pallor as a result of axonal destruction associated with optic neuropathy. (Reprinted with permission from T Constantino, K Digre, P Zimmerman. Neuro-ophthalmic complications of sarcoidosis. Semin Neurol 2000;20[1]: 123–137.)

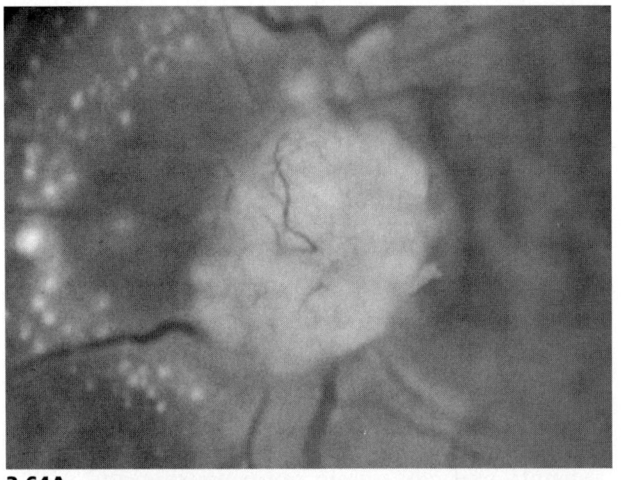

3-64A

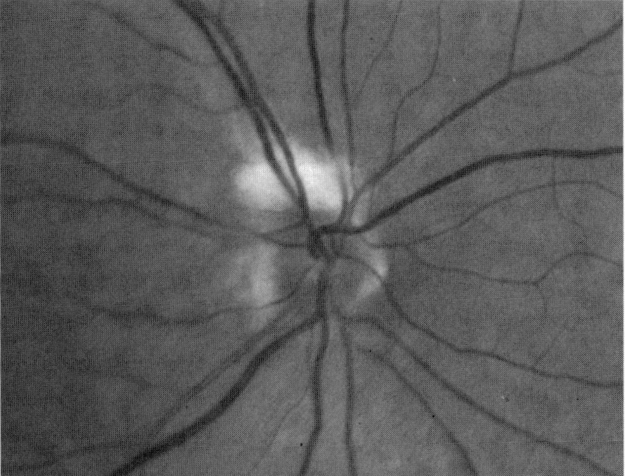

3-64B

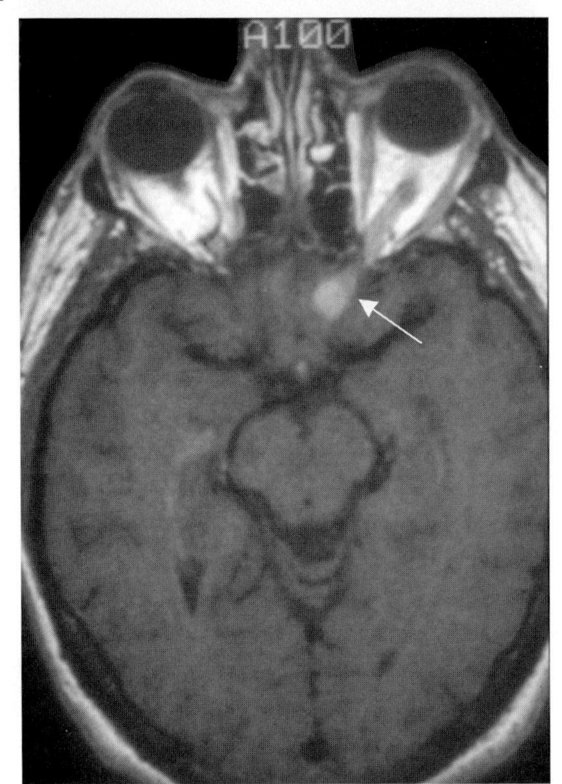

3-64C

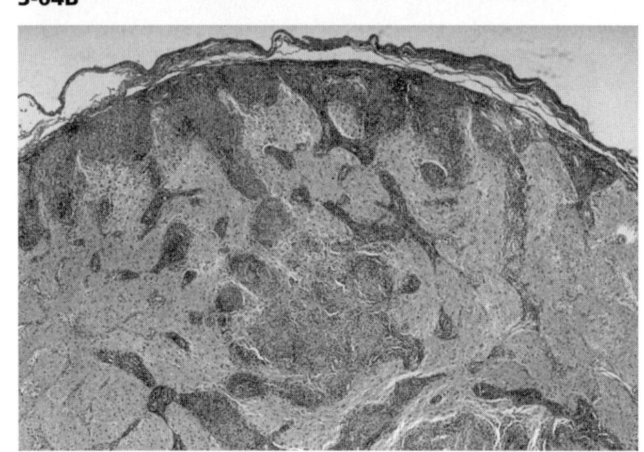

3-64D

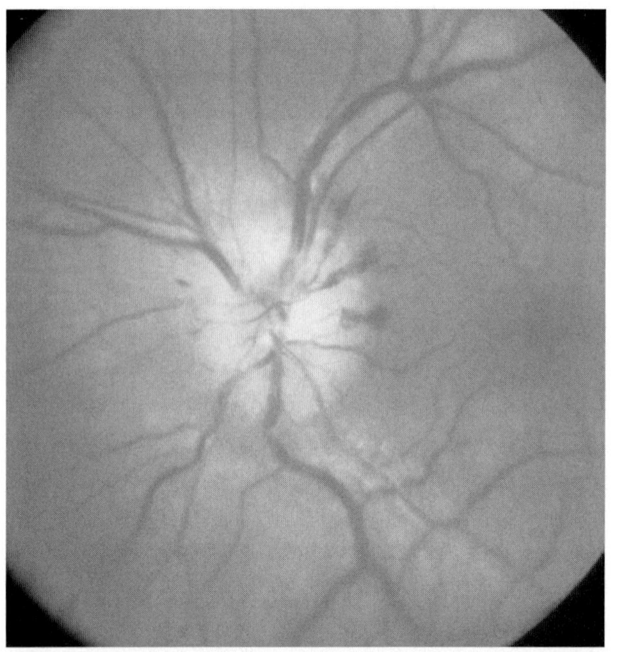

3-65

Leukemia and Lymphoma

Leukemia can cause infiltrative optic neuropathy. Although the patient usually has a history of leukemia at diagnosis, the importance of appearance of disc swelling is that leukemia may affect the central nervous system either by infiltration of the disc or by increased intracranial pressure as a presenting finding. All types of leukemia can affect the optic nerve. Vision loss is variable, and sometimes slight. Chemotherapy with radiation can bring prompt resolution of the swelling. The disc is usually edematous, with a white fluffy infiltrate and peripapillary hemorrhage.

Figure 3-65. Photograph of acute leukemic infiltration. This individual had known leukemia when disc swelling signaled central nervous system leukemia. (Photo courtesy of Paula Morris, CRA.)

Lymphoma can cause disc swelling similar to leukemia and can mimic optic neuritis and AION. Hodgkin's and non-Hodgkin's lymphomas rarely involve the optic nerve.[59]

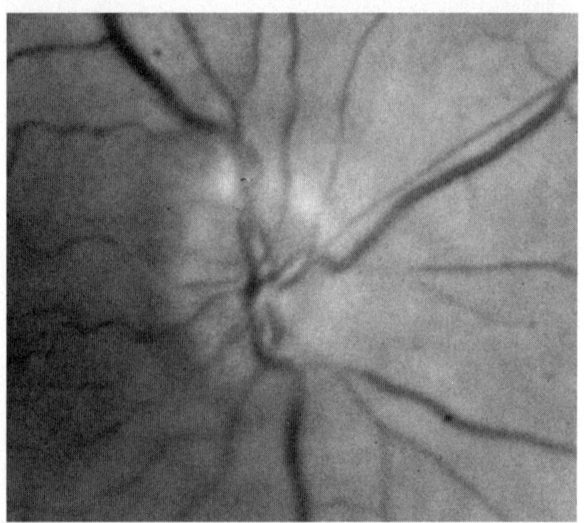

3-66A

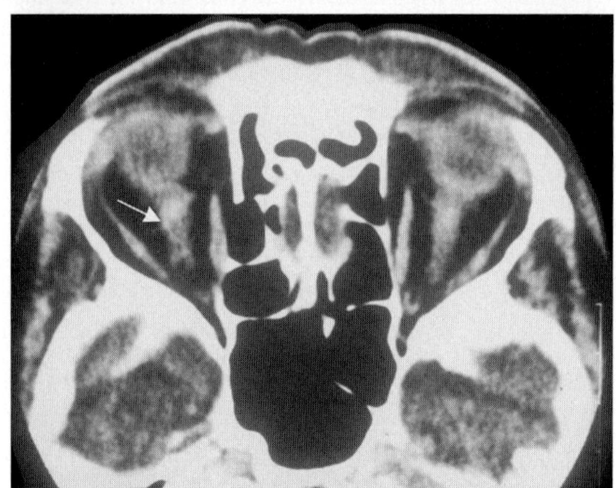

3-66B

Figure 3-66. A. **Infiltrating lymphoma causes disc swelling. This man presented with progressive vision loss in the right eye and disc edema.** B. **A CT scan showed enlarged optic nerves (right more than left). The arrow points to enlargement of the right optic nerve from lymphoma. Biopsy of the right optic nerve sheath revealed non-Hodgkin's lymphoma. (Case courtesy of Roger Harrie, M.D.)**

TUMORS

Although optic nerve glioma in children commonly presents as a pale optic disc (discussed in Chapter 4), *malignant optic nerve gliomas* present in middle age, are more common in men, and vision loss is rapid (within approximately 8 weeks). Outcome is far from benign; death occurs within 1 year of the first symptom.[60] In earlier reports, the presentation was optic atrophy in approximately one-third, with approximately one-half presenting with disc swelling; the rest had normal optic nerves.

Figure 3-67. A. This 45-year-old man presented with vision loss in his right eye; his examination showed severe disc swelling in this eye and vision loss on visual field testing. B. CT showed a markedly enlarged right optic nerve. C. MRI with fat saturation and enhancement and MRI with T2 signals (D) also confirm an enlarged optic nerve. Excisional biopsy of the retrobulbar optic nerve revealed a malignant optic nerve glioma.

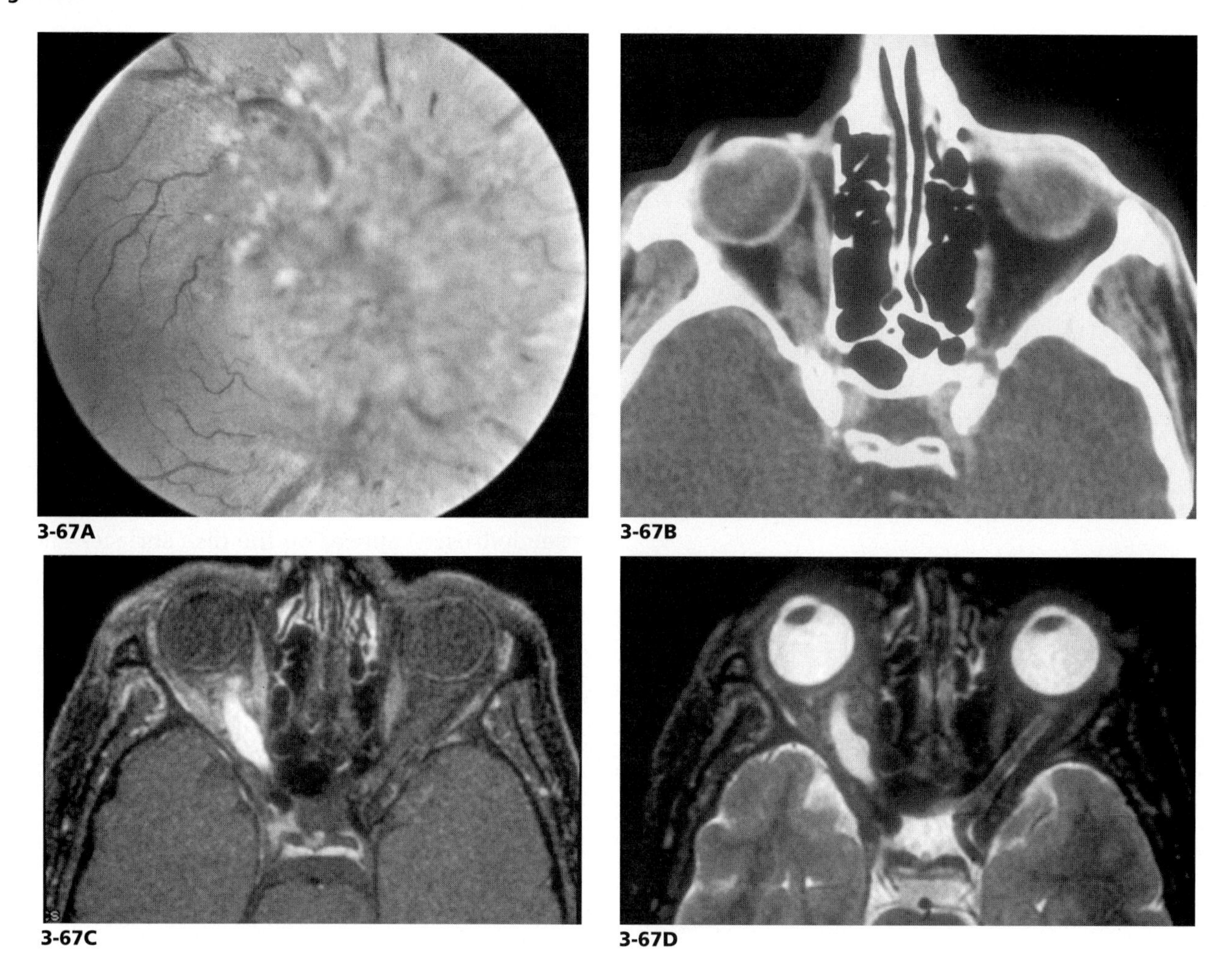

IS THE SWELLING COMPRESSIVE?—TUMORS THAT CAN CAUSE SWELLING

Compressive optic neuropathy from tumors such as meningioma and glioma of the optic nerve can cause disc swelling on one or both sides. Vision loss, often very gradual, is the major complaint even before disc swelling, proptosis, or measurable loss of vision function can be found.

Appearance of the optic nerve in meningioma is that of chronic swelling in approximately one-half of cases; the other one-half has optic atrophy. Venous-venous collaterals or retinochoroidal collaterals appear after compression by tumors has been chronic or may occur with chronic venous stasis, such as after tumorous occlusion of the central retinal vein. This appearance is particularly common in optic nerve meningioma, occurring in approximately one-third of cases (see Chapter 5, Figures 5-34 and 5-35).[61] Furthermore, as with other causes of chronic disc swelling, refractile bodies (pseudodrusen) appear on the disc surface—most commonly seen temporally, and best seen with a red-free filter. Although they may be mistaken for optic nerve drusen, the pseudodrusen disappear when the edema resolves and atrophy ensues.[62]

Figure 3-68. This 35-year-old woman presented with slowly progressive loss of central acuity to 20/30. A. **Her visual field shows progressive constriction over time.** B. **Her disc was chronically swollen, with refractile bodies on the disc surface.** C. **B-scan ultrasonography revealed an enlarged optic nerve (*arrows*), but no optic nerve drusen.** ***Continued***

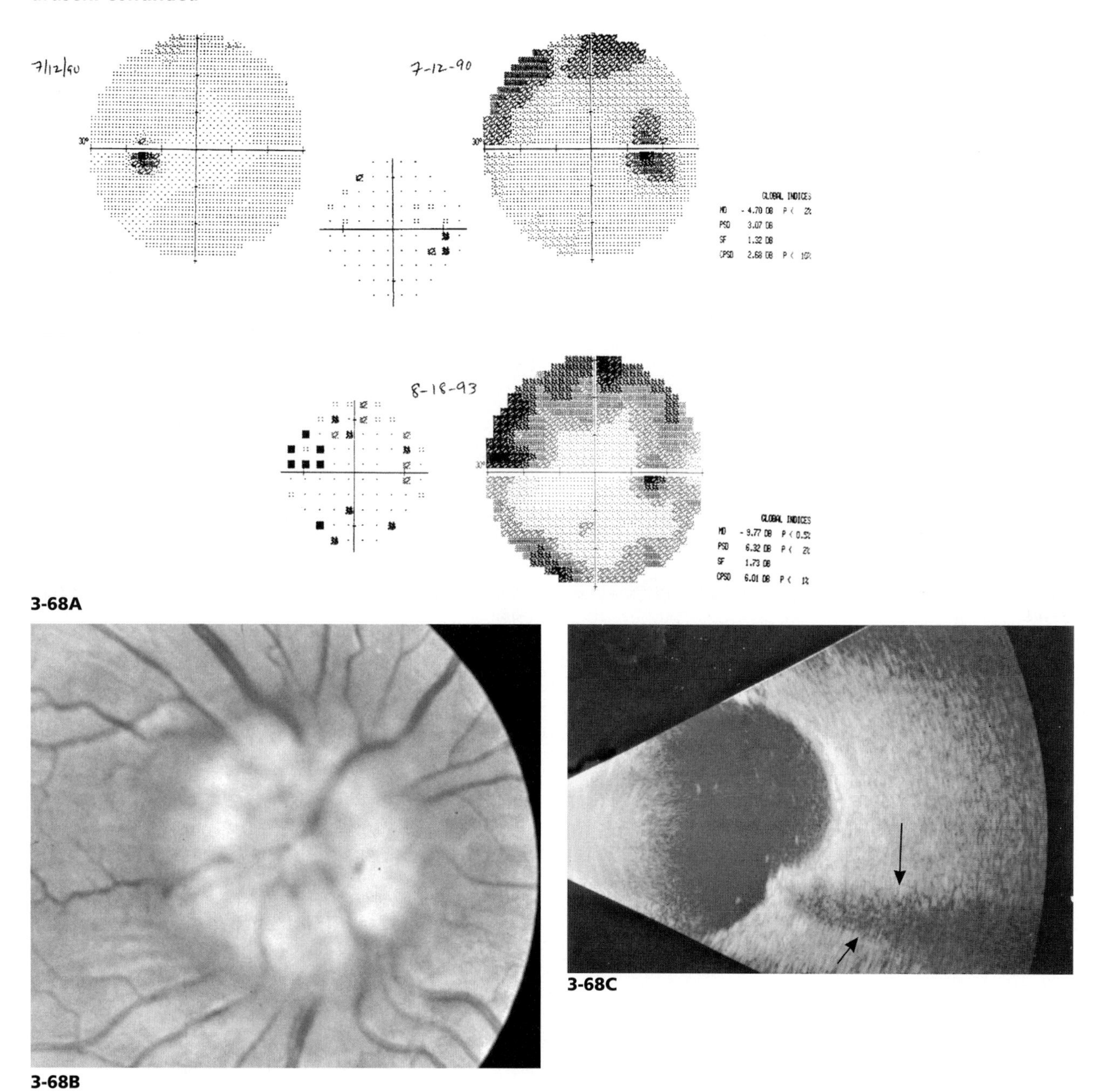

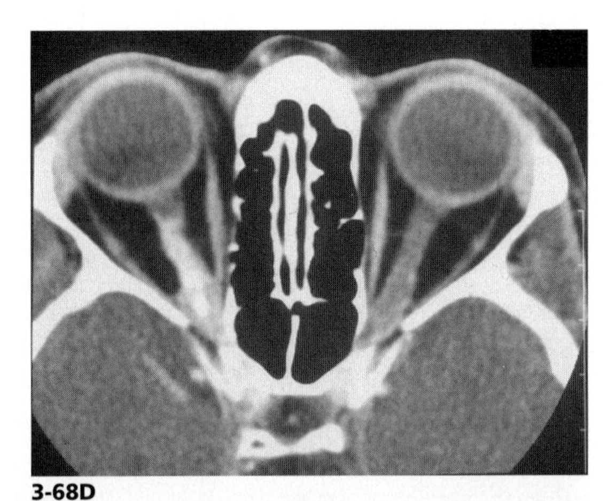

3-68D

Figure 3-68. ***Continued.*** **The CT axial** (D) **and coronal** (E) **scans showed an enlarged calcified optic nerve sheath (*arrow*) considered typical for a sheath meningioma.** F. **The unenhanced MRI showed only a somewhat enlarged optic nerve sheath.**

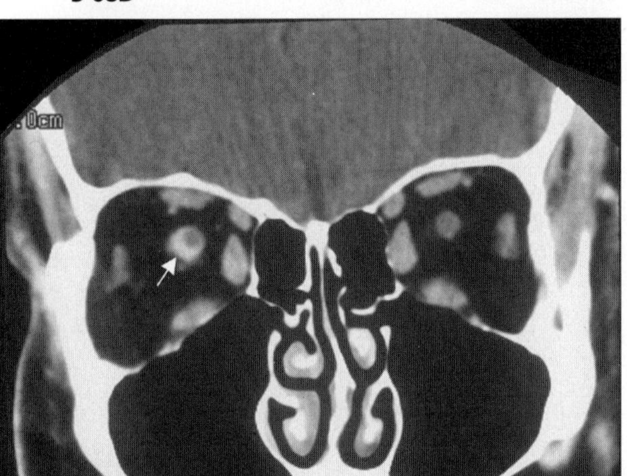

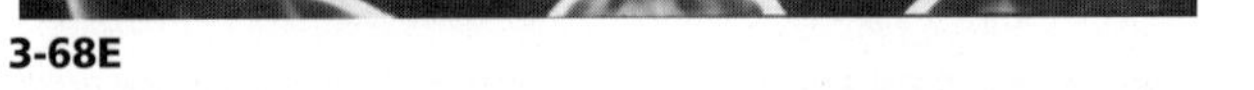

3-68E

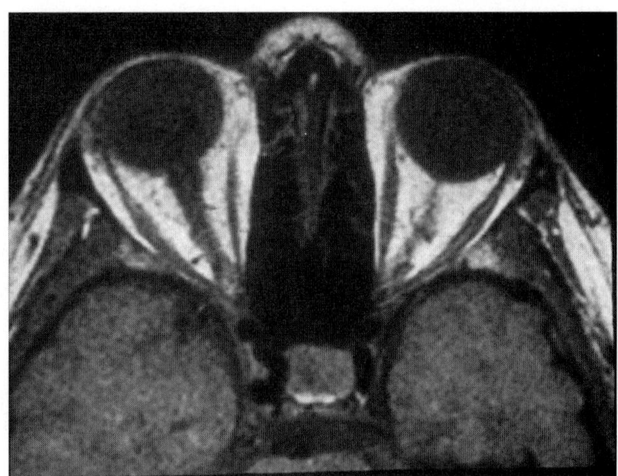

3-68F

METABOLIC CONDITIONS THAT MAY CAUSE OPTIC DISC SWELLING

Although toxic and metabolic conditions have been known to cause optic disc swelling early on, atrophy ensues. Most individuals do not present until there is evidence of vision loss and atrophy has occurred; these conditions are discussed further in Chapter 4.

Practical Viewing Essentials

1. Is the disc truly swollen, or is it an anomalous disc? Look for little red discs, absent cup, and anomalous blood vessels.
2. Look for *all* of the findings of truly swollen discs from papilledema: hyperemia, elevation, blur of the disc margins (especially superiorly and inferiorly), engorged veins, and maintenance of the cup until late.
3. Is the swelling unilateral or bilateral? Recognize bilateral swelling as papilledema and unilateral swelling as usually owing to inflammatory, ischemic, and tumor processes.
4. If there is segmental disc swelling, think ischemia.
5. Correlate a careful history with the examination.
6. If there is visual acuity loss with the disc swelling, think demyelinating, tumor, ischemia, or toxin, not papilledema.
7. Consider all of the broad categories with the potential to cause optic disc swelling.

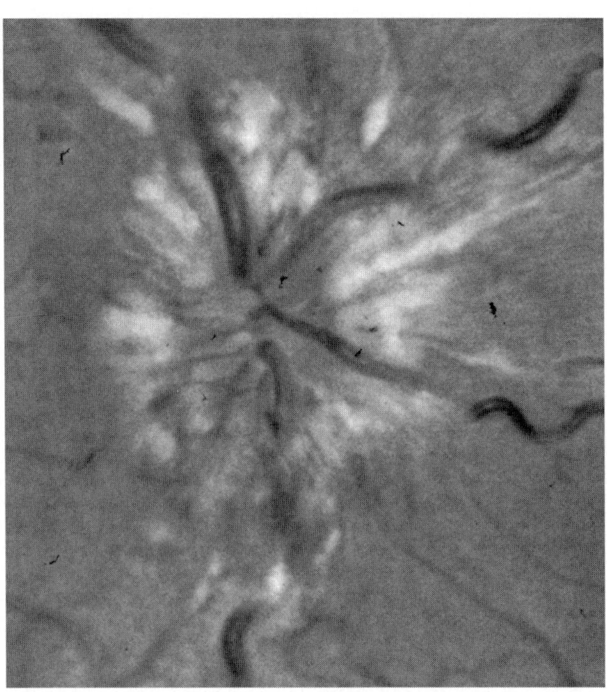

3-69

References

1. Charcot JM. Lectures on the Diseases of the Nervous System. Translated and edited by G Sigerson. New York: Hafner Publishing Company, 1962.
2. Gowers W. A Manual and Atlas of Medical Ophthalmoscopy. London: J & A Churchill, 1879.
3. Brodsky MC. Congenital anomalies of the optic disc. In NR Miller, NJ Newman (eds), Walsh and Hoyt's Clinical Neuro-ophthalmology (5th ed). Baltimore: Williams & Wilkins, 1998;775–823.
4. Lorentzen SE. Drusen of the optic disk, an irregularly dominant hereditary affection. Acta Ophthalmol (Copenh) 1961;39:626–643.
5. Friedman AH, Gartner S, Modi SS. Drusen of the optic disc. A retrospective study in cadaver eyes. Br J Ophthalmol 1975;59(8):413–421.
6. Hoover DL, Robb RM, Petersen RA. Optic disc drusen in children. J Pediatr Ophthalmol Strabismus 1988;25(4):191–195.
7. Mullie MA, Sanders MD. Scleral canal size and optic nerve head drusen. Am J Ophthalmol 1985;99:356–359.
8. Brodsky MC, Baker RS, Hamed LM. Pediatric Neuro-ophthalmology. New York: Springer, 1996.
9. Antcliff RJ, Spalton DJ. Are optic disc drusen inherited? Ophthalmology 1999;106:1278–1281.
10. Sadun AA, Currie JN, Lessell S. Transient visual obscurations with elevated optic discs. Ann Neurol 1984;16:489–494.
11. Kabel I, Otradovec J, Peleska M. Fluorescence angiography in circulatory disturbances in drusen of the optic disk. Ophthalmologica 1972;164(6):449–462.
12. Kurz-Levin MM, Landau K. A comparison of imaging techniques for diagnosing drusen of the optic nerve head. Arch Ophthalmol 1999;117:1045–1049.
13. Boldt HC, Byrne SF, Di Bernardo C. Echographic evaluation of optic disc drusen. J Clin Neuroophthalmol 1991;11:85–91.
14. Rosenberg MA, Savino PJ, Glaser JS. A clinical analysis of pseudopapilledema. I. Population, laterality, acuity, refractive error, ophthalmoscopic characteristics, and coincident disease. Arch Ophthalmol 1979;97:65–70.
15. Coleman K, Ross MH, McCabe M, et al. Disk drusen and angioid streaks in pseudoxanthoma elasticum. Am J Ophthalmol 1991;112:166–170.
16. Cushing H, Bordley J. Observations on experimentally induced choked disc. Bull Johns Hopkins Hosp 1909;20:95–101.
17. Tso MO, Hayreh S. Optic disc edema in raised intracranial pressure. IV. Axoplasmic transport in experimental papilledema. Arch Ophthalmol 1977;95: 1458–1462.
18. Weiss P, Hiscoe HB. Experiments in the mechanism of nerve growth. J Exp Zool 1948;107:315–395.
19. Wirtschafter JD, Rizzo FJ, Smiley C. Optic nerve axoplasm and papilledema. Surv Ophthalmol 1975;20: 157–189.
20. Samuels B. The histopathology of papilloedema. Trans Ophthalmol Soc (UK) 1938;57(2):529–556.
21. Hayreh MS, Hayreh SS. Optic disc edema in raised intracranial pressure. I. Evolution and resolution. Arch Ophthalmol 1977;95:1237–1244.
22. Hoyt WF. Walsh and Hoyt's Neuro-ophthalmology (3rd ed). Baltimore: Williams & Wilkins, 1969.
23. Paton L, Holmes G. The pathology of papilloedema. A histological study of sixty eyes. Brain 1911;33:389–432.
24. Cogan DG. Neurology of the visual system. Springfield, IL: Thomas, 1966;144.
25. Savino P, Glaser JS. Pseudopapilledema versus papilledema. In TM Burde, JS Karp (eds), International Ophthalmology Clinics. Boston: Little, Brown, 1977;115–137.
26. Hayreh SS. Pathogenesis of edema of the optic disc papilledema. Br J Ophthalmol 1964;48:522–543.
27. Hayreh SS. Optic disc edema in raised intracranial pressure. II. Early detection with fluorescein fundus angiography and stereoscopic color photography. Arch Ophthalmol 1977;95:1245–1254.
28. Hedges TR. Papilledema: its recognition and relation to increased intracranial pressure. Surv Ophthalmol 1975;19:210–223.
29. Lindenberg R, Walsh FB, Sacks JG. Neuropathology of Vision: An Atlas. Philadelphia: Lea & Febiger, 1973;4.
30. Selhorst JB, Guderman SK, Butterworth JF, et al. Papilledema after acute head injury. Neurosurgery 1985;16:357–363.
31. Steffen H, Eifert B, Aschoff A, et al. The diagnostic value of optic disc evaluation in acute elevated intracranial pressure. Ophthalmology 1996;103:1229–1232.

32. Hughlings Jackson J. Lecture on optic neuritis from intracranial disease. In J Taylor (ed), Selected Writing of John Hughlings Jackson. London: Hodder and Stoughton, 1932.
33. Cogan DG. Neurology of the Visual System. Springfield, IL: Thomas, 1967;138.
34. Hoyt WF, Beeston D. The Ocular Fundus in Neurologic Disease. St. Louis: Mosby, 1966;6.
35. Sanders MD. The Bowman Lecture: Papilloedema: "The pendulum of progress." Eye 1997;11:267–294.
36. O'Duffy D, James B, Elston J. Idiopathic intracranial hypertension presenting with gaze-evoked amaurosis. Acta Opthalmol Scand 1998;76:119–120.
37. Digre KB, Corbett JJ. IIH: a repraisal. The Neurologist 2001;7:2–67.
38. Corbett JJ, Savino PJ, Thompson HS, et al. Visual loss in pseudotumor cerebri. Follow-up of 57 patients from five to 41 years and a profile of 14 patients with permanent severe visual loss. Arch Neurol 1982;39:461–474.
39. Biousse V, Newman NJ, Lessell S. Audible pulsatile tinnitus in idiopathic intracranial hypertension. Neurology 1998;50(4):1185–1186.
40. Wall M, White WN. Asymmetric papilledema in idiopathic intracranial hypertension: a prospective interocular comparison of sensory visual functions. Invest Opthalmol Vis Sci 1998;39:134–142.
41. Maxner CE, Freeman MI, Corbett JJ. Asymmetric papilledema and visual loss in pseudotumor cerebri. Can J Neurol Sci 1987;14:593–596.
42. Kennedy F. Retrobulbar neuritis as an exact diagnostic sign of certain tumors and abscesses in the frontal lobe. Am J Med Sci 1911;142:355–368.
43. Repka MX, Miller NR, Savino PJ. Pseudotumor cerebri. Am J Ophthalmol 1984;98(6):741–746.
44. Wade NK, Levi L, Jones MR, et al. Optic disc edema associated with peripapillary serous retinal detachment: an early sign of systemic *Bartonella henselae* infection. Am J Ophthalmol 2000;130:327–334.
45. Wall M, Breen L, Winterkorn J. Optic disc edema with cotton-wool spots. Surv Ophthalmol 1995;39: 502–508.
46. Lessell S. Toxic and deficiency optic neuropathies. In N Miller, NJ Newman (eds), Walsh and Hoyt's Clinical Neuro-ophthalmology (5th ed). Baltimore: Williams & Wilkins, 1998;663–679.
47. Sharpe JA, Hostovsky M, Bilbao JM, et al. Methanol optic neuropathy: A histopathological study. Neurology 1982;32:1093–1100.
48. Macaluso DC, Shults WT, Fraunfelder FT. Features of amiodarone-induced optic neuropathy. Am J Ophthalmol 1999;127:610–612.
49. Newman NJ. Hereditary optic neuropathies. In N Miller, NJ Newman (eds), Walsh and Hoyt's Clinical Neuro-ophthalmology (5th ed). Baltimore: Williams & Wilkins, 1998;741–773.
50. Regillo CD, Brown GC, Savino PJ, et al. Diabetic papillopathy. Arch Ophthalmol 1995;113:889–895.
51. Warner JE, Lessell S, Rizzo JF 3rd, Newman NJ. Does optic disc appearance distinguish ischemic optic neuropathy from optic neuritis? Arch Ophthalmol 1997;115:1408–1410.
52. Beri M, Klugman MR, Kohler JA, Hayreh SS. Anterior ischemic optic neuropathy. VII. Incidence of bilaterality and various influencing factors. Ophthalmology 1987;94(8):1020–1028.
53. Egan R, Pomeranz H. Sildenafil (Viagra) associated anterior ischemic optic neuropathy. Arch Ophthalmol 2000;118:291–292.
54. Levin LA, Rizzo JF 3rd, Lessell S. Neural network differentiation of optic neuritis and anterior ischaemic optic neuropathy. Br J Ophthalmol 1996;80(9):835–839.
55. Miller NR, Newman NJ. Topical diagnosis of lesions in the visual sensory pathway. In N Miller, NJ Newman (eds), Walsh and Hoyt's Clinical Neuro-ophthalmology (5th ed). Baltimore: Williams & Wilkins, 1998;265.
56. Sainz de la Maza M, Jabbur NS, Foster CS. Severity of scleritis and episcleritis. Ophthalmology 1994;101 (2):389–396.
57. Constantino T, Digre KB, Zimmerman P. Neuro-ophthalmic manifestations of sarcoidosis. Semin Neurol 2000;20:123–137.
58. Hamilton SR. Sarcoidosis and idiopathic hypertrophic cranial pachymeningitis. In N Miller, NJ Newman (eds), Walsh and Hoyt's Clinical Neuro-ophthalmology (5th ed). Baltimore: Williams & Wilkins, 1998;5465–5538.
59. Kansu T, Orr LS, Savino PJ, et al. Optic neuropathy as an initial manifestation of lymphoreticular diseases. In JL Smith (ed), Neuro-ophthalmology Focus. New York: Masson, 1980;125–136.
60. Hoyt WF, Meshel LG, Lessell S, et al. Malignant optic glioma of adulthood. Brain 1973;96:121–132.
61. Dutton JJ. Optic nerve sheath meningiomas. Surv Ophthalmol 1992;37(3):167–83.
62. Sibony P, Kennerdell JS, Slamovits TL, et al. Intrapapillary refractile bodies in optic nerve sheath meningioma. Arch Ophthalmol 1985;103:383–385.

4 Is the Disc Pale?

[In optic atrophy] the papilla shows no change, neither in its form nor in its dimension; its borders are still well marked. The vessels remain what they were before, . . . the papilla has ceased to be transparent; it strongly reflects the light, on the contrary, and no longer allows us to perceive the vasae propriae in its substance. It follows that it shows no more its normal rosy tint, but, on the contrary, a white, chalky colour, of pearly aspect.

Jean-Martin Charcot[1]

Optic atrophy is not a disease. It is a morphologic sequelae of disease—any disease—which causes shrinkage of cells and fibers and over-all diminution of size of the optic nerve.

R.W. Beck[2]

Terminology describing optic disc pallor can be confusing. *Optic disc pallor* refers to the appearance of the disc—it has a pale color—that appears to be whiter than normal. *Optic neuropathy* refers to impairment of optic nerve function; the disc may or may not be pale. Neuropathy may be due to many entities (e.g., optic neuritis, post-ischemic changes, congenital neuropathy). *Optic atrophy* refers to an irreversibly pale disc in an eye that has reduced visual function (visual acuity and/or visual field); it signifies degeneration of the optic nerve. Before a disc is called *atrophic*, however, visual field and visual function must be tested.

Although pallor is a useful index of atrophy, its value as a criterion is lessened by the wide variation in pinkness of normal discs and by the paradoxic finding of normal visual functions in some cases of extreme pallor. [3]

To diagnose optic atrophy, the history should be consistent with loss or change in vision. For example, the patient notices dimming of vision over the last several days, the vision has been abnormal for a month or a year, or the patient has never really seen very well out of that eye.

One common misinterpretation is the "sudden loss of vision" that turns out to be the sudden *discovery* of previously unappreciated vision loss. Or the history should be consistent with "I have never had good vision in that eye" (in the case of congenital atrophy). Optic neuropathy or atrophy should be associated with visual dysfunction. In addition, the examination of the patient may give clues. Is there an afferent pupillary defect indicating an asymmetric optic neuropathy? Is there a visual field defect? Optic neuropathies/optic atrophy will usually have evidence of visual field abnormalities. Inspection of the disc alone, without history, can lead to misunderstanding and a missed diagnosis.

Is the Disc Really Pale? Mimics of Pallor

Do you have a very bright light source from new batteries? There can be an "illusory impression of whiteness"[4] from a very bright light. After cataract surgery and removal of the lens, the disc frequently appears to be pale because the optical change of the human lens is gone. A darker colored fundus may make the disc look paler than it actually is.

A *large physiologic cup* in a disc is the most common mimic of optic nerve pallor because exposure of the lamina cribrosa, a part of the sclera and, therefore, a "pale" structure, is greater with a large physiologic cup. The whole disc may be considered mistakenly to be pale or atrophic. Myopia can be confused with optic pallor because not only is there often an enlarged optic cup that can be shallow, especially temporally, but, also, there is frequently a scleral temporal crescent that can be mistaken for optic disc pallor. In addition, a white scleral ring or temporal or inferior crescent can mimic optic atrophy.

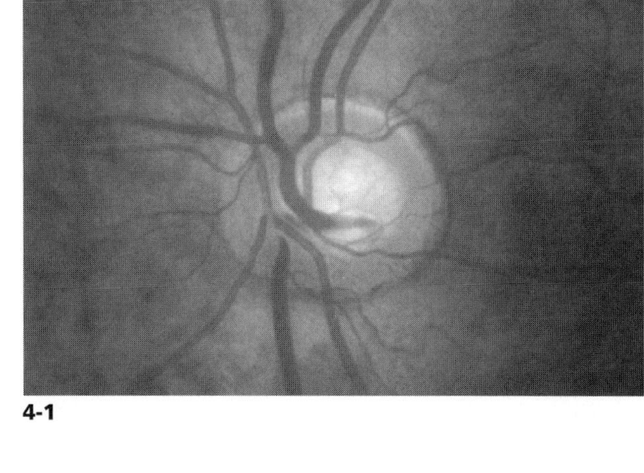

4-1

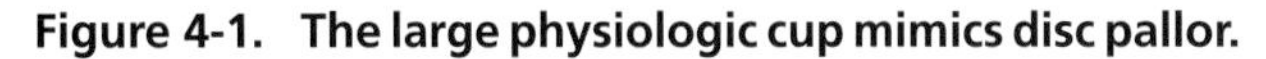

Figure 4-1. The large physiologic cup mimics disc pallor.

Be sure that the pallor is not myelinated nerve fibers.

Figure 4-2. Myelinated nerve fibers may mimic pallor. A. **Myelinated nerve fibers mimicking pallor. Look for the feathery edge typical of myelinated nerve fibers.** B. **Here the entire nerve looks white. However, the whiteness is myelinated nerve fibers.**

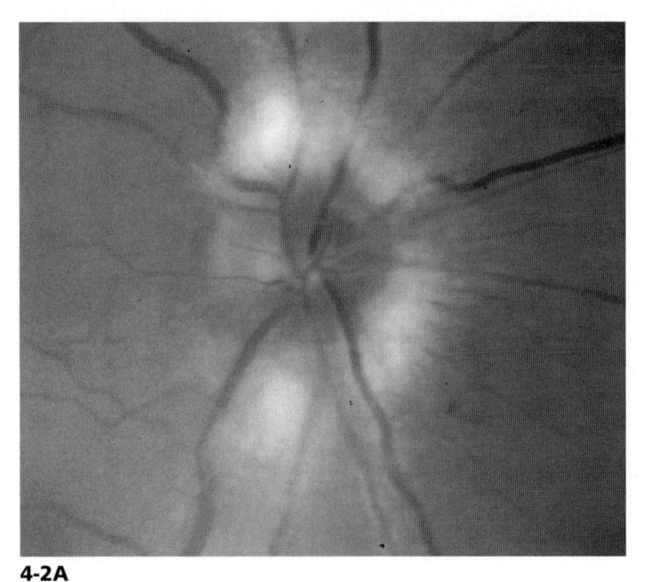

4-2A

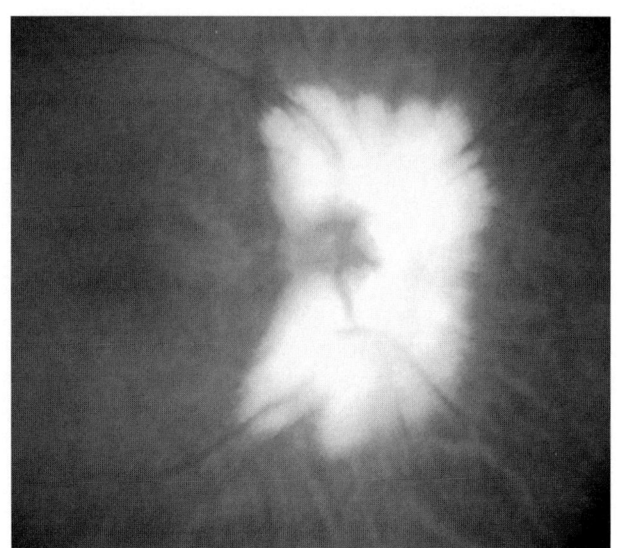

4-2B

In infants, the disc may be slightly gray if myelination of the optic nerve is incomplete, or if the fundus is very blonde. Furthermore, many disc anomalies, like hypoplastic discs or a coloboma of the disc, will give the appearance of disc pallor.

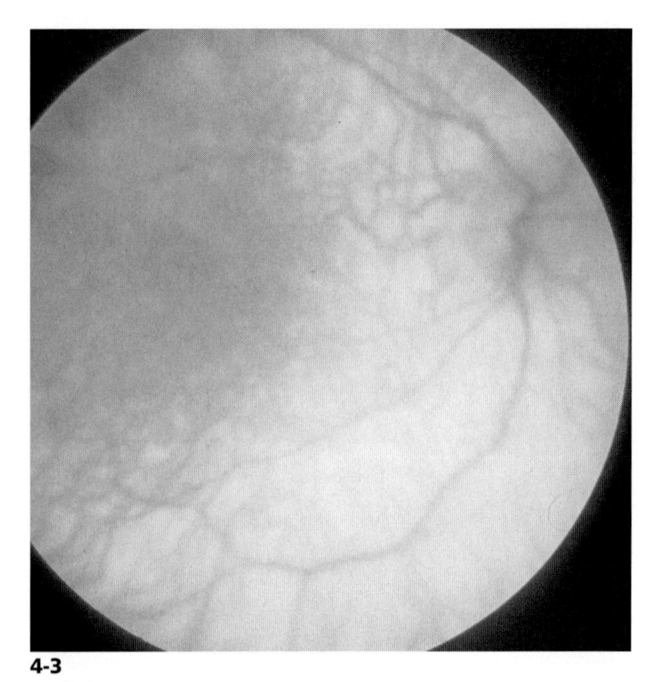

4-3

Figure 4-3. **This blonde fundus makes the slightly gray disc look pale. The color of the surrounding retina can affect the color of the disc. In this case, the almost albinotic fundus makes the color of the disc gray, mimicking optic disc pallor. (Photograph courtesy of Michael Brodsky, M.D.)**

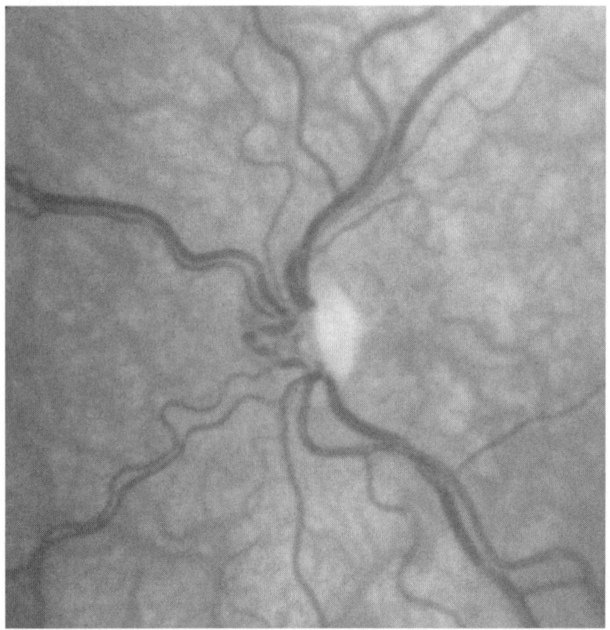

4-4A

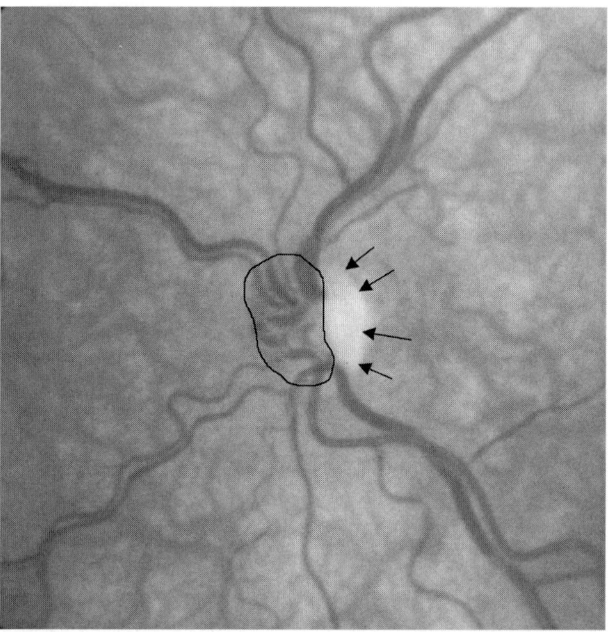

4-4B

Figure 4-4. A. **This hypoplastic disc at first glance looks like a disc with temporal pallor. However, the temporal crescent is not part of the disc. In this case, the fundus is also very blonde, so the disc looks even more pale.** B. **We have outlined the actual disc margin. The arrows are pointing to the scleral edge (a double-ring sign)—that at first glance could be mistaken for part of the disc.**

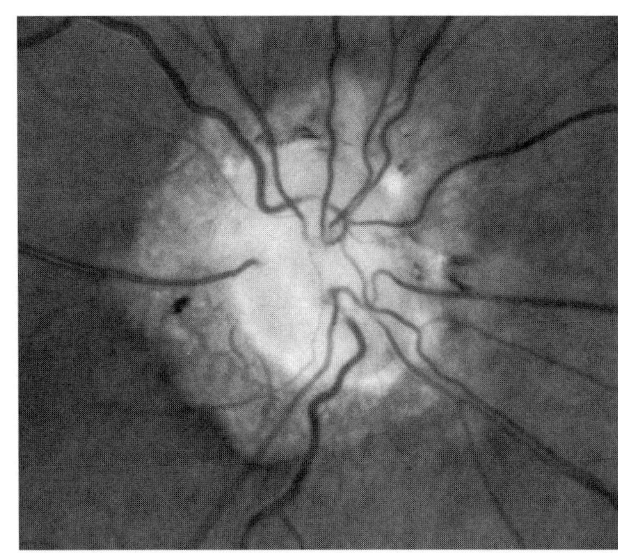
4-5

Figure 4-5. This colobomatous disc has anomalous vasculature and could be mistaken for optic atrophy. Anomalous discs, including optic disc hypoplasia, colobomas, morning glory disc, and optic pits, are probably the next most common mimics of optic disc pallor. See discussion of anomalous discs (see Chapter 11).

Severe anemia transiently can make the disc look pale because of the lack of red blood cells in the small capillaries on the disc.

Table 4-1. Differentiating True Optic Pallor from Pseudopallor

True pallor (see Figure 4-6A)	Pseudopallor (see Figure 4-6B)
Loss of neuroretinal rim	Healthy pink neuroretinal rim with a big cup
Attenuation of blood vessels; vessels may be nasally displaced	Normal blood vessels; may have anomalous branching with anomalous discs
Loss of nerve fiber layer	Normal nerve fiber layer when visible
Progressive cupping	Lamina cribrosa visible
Gliosis of the nerve	Solid color
Segmental pallor (altitudinal pallor, bow-tie, band atrophy)	Post cataract surgery (disc looks pale because lens has been removed)
Pale appearing with any light	Very bright light in ophthalmoscope
Causes: optic neuritis, ischemic optic neuropathy (old); congenital optic atrophy; Leber's optic atrophy; compression by mass (tumor, aneurysm)	Causes: large physiologic cup, myopic disc, anomalous discs; myelinated nerve fibers, anemic disc, optic disc hypoplasia, coloboma

Figure 4-6. A. **True pallor.** B. **Pseudopallor.**

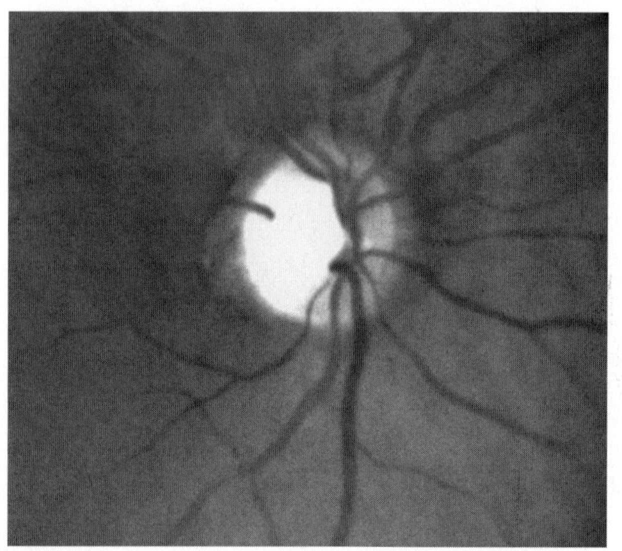

4-6A

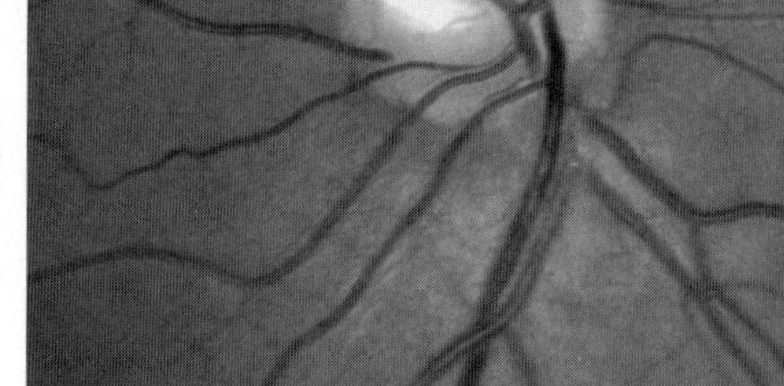

4-6B

Where Does the Disc Get Its Color and What Causes Disc Pallor?

The normal optic nerve gets its color from small vessels on the disc and from the nerve fiber layer. In fact, a histopathologic study showed that the thickness of the optic disc and the small capillaries interdigitating with the nerve fiber layer columns within the disc were most important for the color of the disc. Our ophthalmoscopic light reflecting off of the nerve fiber layer and the capillaries makes the disc look pink. When there is damage to the disc, astrocytes and glial cells cover the capillaries and the light reflects on the surface of those opaque cells and never reaches the capillaries. Furthermore, we also see the lamina, which is also white. Therefore, the disc appears to be white even though there is no vessel dropout. A cupped disc is white because of the scleral lamina cribrosa, which you can easily see. Therefore, the disc appears to be white.[5]

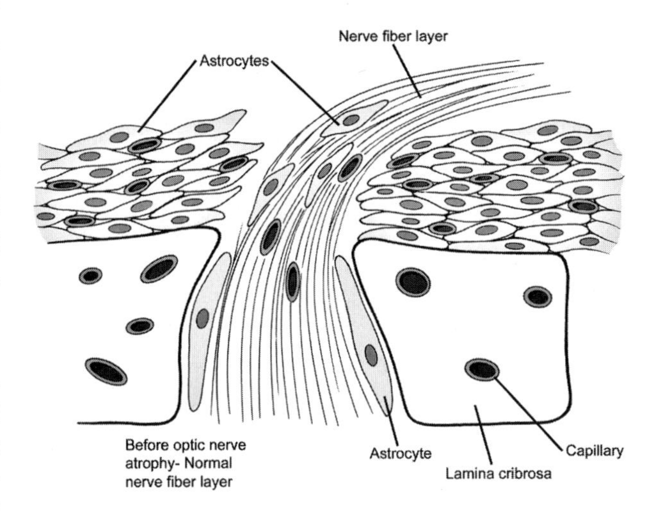

4-7A

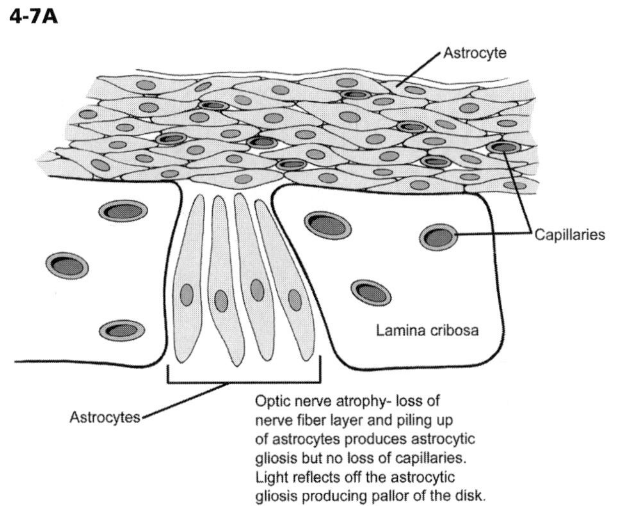

4-7B

Figure 4-7. Review Figure 2-41A. A. **When the ophthalmoscopic light reflects off of the nerve fiber layer and capillaries, the disc looks pink.** B. **Pallor of the disc comes from some capillary dropout and some proliferation of the astrocytes and glial cells. When the the ophthalmoscope light reflects on the surface of opaque glial cells, the visible lamina cribrosa and the disc look white. Furthermore, the loss of the axon bundles, along with changes in the cellular structure, account for the pallor that we see. (Diagrams inspired by Quigley and Anderson.[5])**

When there is damage to the normal optic nerve, the nerve becomes pale. It really is the "tombstone" commerating the causal event. It is what is left behind when the optic nerve is damaged by whatever process.

The entire optic nerve may be atrophic or only sectors may be atrophic. The disc can be *cupped out* in response to the damage—this just means that there is profound loss of disc tissue. The nerve can become *gliotic*—this means that there may have been ischemia or inflammation that caused the loss of tissue replaced by astrocytic glia. This has led some to conclude that there are two forms of optic atrophy: atrophy associated with glial proliferation and fibrotic tissue leading to a more gray disc without cupping and even an irregular disc edge. The second form is a pale disc in which there is cupping, the lamina cribrosa is visible, and the margins of the disc are sharp. This form of pallor is prominent in glaucoma, but can be seen with damage to the optic nerve such as tumor or infarction.[6]

The other concepts that can be useful are the ideas of primary and secondary atrophy. *Primary atrophy* is pallor of the optic disc that occurs as a result of a pathologic process that is not apparent on looking at the disc. There is no defining feature of the pallor—it is just pale (e.g., a completely pale disc from a dominant optic atrophy). Another example would be a totally pale disc, which on imaging is found to be due to compression from a giant carotid aneurysm. Just looking at the disc you could not guess the cause. *Secondary optic atrophy* allows you to make a judgment as to the cause, just from the appearance. For example, if you have pallor of the disc with retinochoroidal collaterals you know that the cause of the pallor is from something compressing the venous structures and/or optic nerve. Altitudinal disc pallor almost invariably is the result of ischemic optic neuropathy—another secondary atrophy. The atrophic nerve after papilledema has a characteristic appearance—hence, another secondary cause of optic atrophy.

Table 4-2. Primary versus Secondary Atrophy

Primary atrophy characteristics	Secondary atrophy characteristics
Primary atrophy due to craniopharyngioma. You can't tell by looking at the disc what the cause of the atrophy is (see Figure 4-8A).	Secondary atrophy: There is a retinochoroidal collateral due to compression from a meningioma. You know just by looking at the disc that the pallor is due to a compressive etiology (see Figure 4-8B).
Retrobulbar optic neuritis.	Sectoral pallor due to anterior ischemic optic neuropathy (AION).
Optic nerve compression.	Post-papilledema atrophy.
Retrobulbar ischemic process.	Band atrophy.
Dominant optic atrophy.	Pale disc with retinochoroidal collateral.
Post-papillitis.	

Figure 4-8. A. **Primary atrophy.** B. **Secondary atrophy. The arrows point to retinochoroidal shunt vessels.**

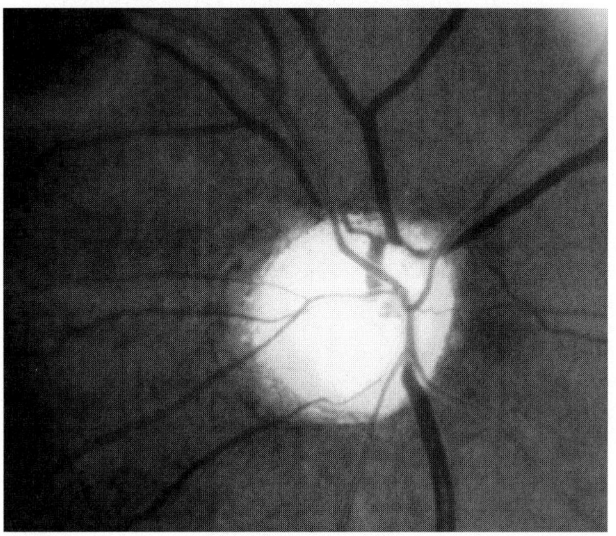

4-8A

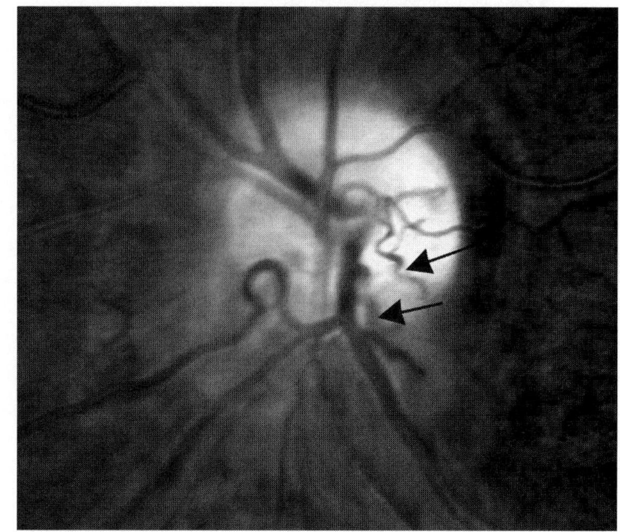

4-8B

Pallor can occur when there is damage to the axons in the retina or optic disc; however, damage to the visual apparatus anywhere along the visual pathway in certain instances can cause the disc to have a specific form of pallor. Sometimes the pattern of atrophy can tell you where the damage is and on occasion can tell you how long the damage has been there. For example, bilateral band atrophy is due to chiasmal disease, but unilateral band atrophy associated with small discs may be the result of geniculocalcarine tract at or before birth (homonymous hemioptic hypoplasia). Just knowing different patterns of pallor may give you a clue as to the cause.

Figure 4-9. Damage to various parts of the afferent visual pathway (optic nerve to occipital lobe) causes the disc to have a distinct appearance—localizing the atrophy to a particular part. If the process is anterior to the chiasm, total pallor or segmental disc pallor (from AION) is the result. If the process is at the chiasm, bilateral band atrophy results. If the process is in the tract, unilateral band atrophy results. If the process is long standing or congenital from the geniculocalcarine tract or occipital lobe, a similar finding of the unilateral band atrophy results, homonymous hemioptic hypoplasia.

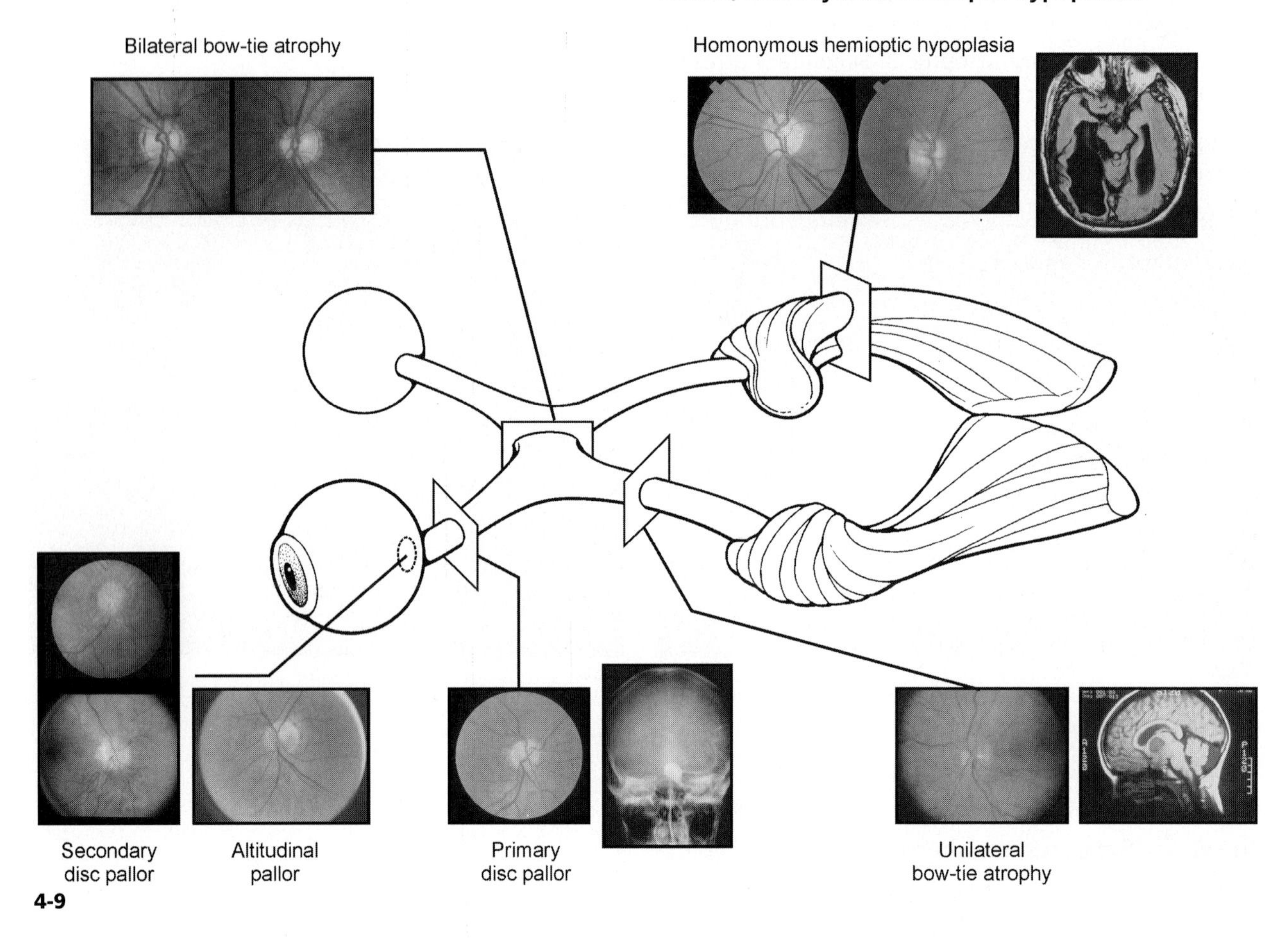

4-9

How Quickly Does Pallor Develop?

Six weeks after a lesion occurs in the optic nerve following transient swelling of the disc, observable loss of the retinal nerve fiber appears. The axon anterior to the lesion will degenerate about the same time. It may take even longer for pallor to be visible.[7] In Leinfelder's study on cats, gliosis of the retina and nerve occurred by 2 months.[8]

The evolution of optic atrophy[9] of a man who suffered a severe gunshot wound, blinding his eye from damage to the optic nerve. The authors followed the man with ophthalmoscopy and photographs:

Immediately: No change in the fundus
Day 12: Very slight disc edema following injury
Day 30: Nerve fiber layer begins to disappear
 Macular light reflex is lost
 Vessels begin to show a kind of sheathing—smaller diameter and straighter
Day 45: Retina begins to mottle
 Reduced vessel diameter; pronounced sheathing of major vessels
 The optic nerve begins to have distinct pallor
Day 60: Loss of the last part of the nerve fiber layer
 Optic pallor is appreciated
 Granularity of the fundus
Day 85: Conspicuous optic pallor
 Retinal granularity increases
No further changes after day 85

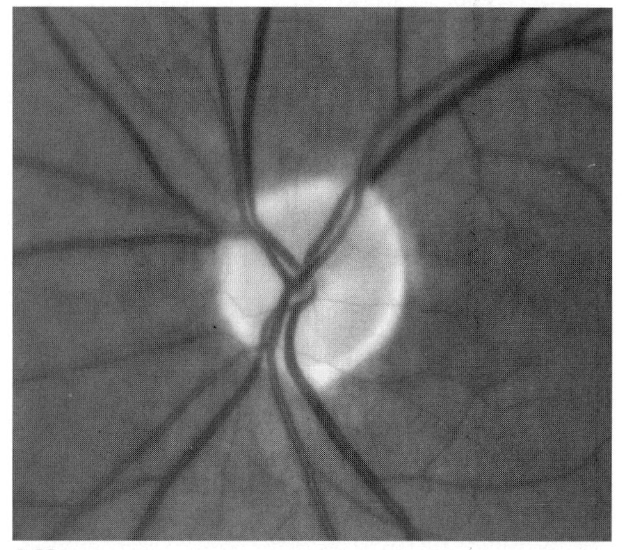

4-10

Figure 4-10. Aside from disc pallor, there are other features of optic atrophy, including cupping, gliosis of the vessels on the disc and of the disc itself, loss of nerve fiber layer (see below), dropout of the vessels on the disc, and decreased capillary blush on the disc.

Are There Other Signs of Optic Nerve Damage?

What does the nerve fiber layer look like? Use the green filter. The nerve fiber layer makes the vessels and retina look just a little fuzzy. In optic neuropathies and optic atrophy, the nerve fibers drop out.

When the nerve fiber begins to disappear, there is a slight decrease in the preretinal opacity, loss of the superficial radial striation, and the choroid shows better and darker. Small vessels previously hidden by the nerve fiber layer are more prominent. The choroidal and retinal pattern is then more prominent.[9]

Nerve Fiber Layer Defects in Optic Neuropathy

Table 4-3. Nerve Fiber Layer Defects in Optic Neuropathy[10]

Defect	Appearance	Cause
No defect (normal nerve fiber layer) (see Figure 4-11A)	Smooth nerve fiber layer—without gaps	—
Slit-like defects (see Figure 4-11B)	See slits in the nerve fiber layer	Glaucoma, nerve fiber layer infarct
Wedge defects (see Figure 4-11C)	Entire wedge of nerve fiber layer loss	Glaucoma, AION
Diffuse atrophy (see Figure 4-11D)	Little visible nerve fiber layer; see RPE and choroid more vividly	Any diffuse process—including glaucoma
Total atrophy (see Figure 4-11E)	No visible nerve fiber; vessels appear more prominent	Diffuse processes—especially vascular

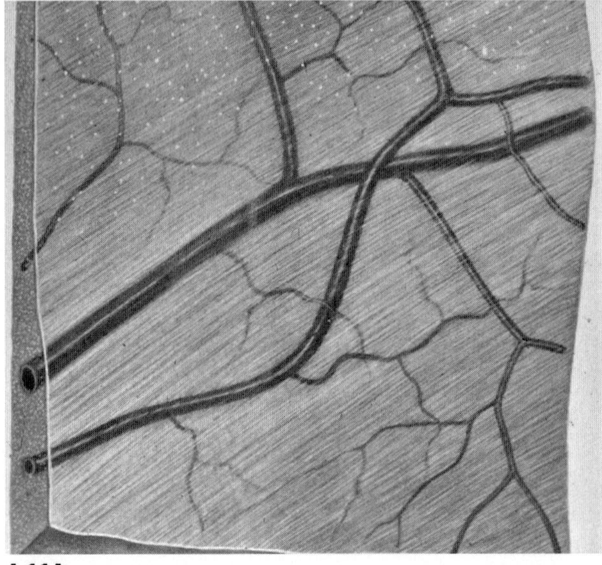

4-11A

Figure 4-11. Nerve fiber layer defects in optic neuropathy. A. **No defect.** ***Continued***

Figure 4-11. ***Continued.*** B. **Slit-like defects,** (C) **wedge defects,** (D) **diffuse atrophy, and** (E) **total atrophy. (Reprinted with permission from reference 10.)**

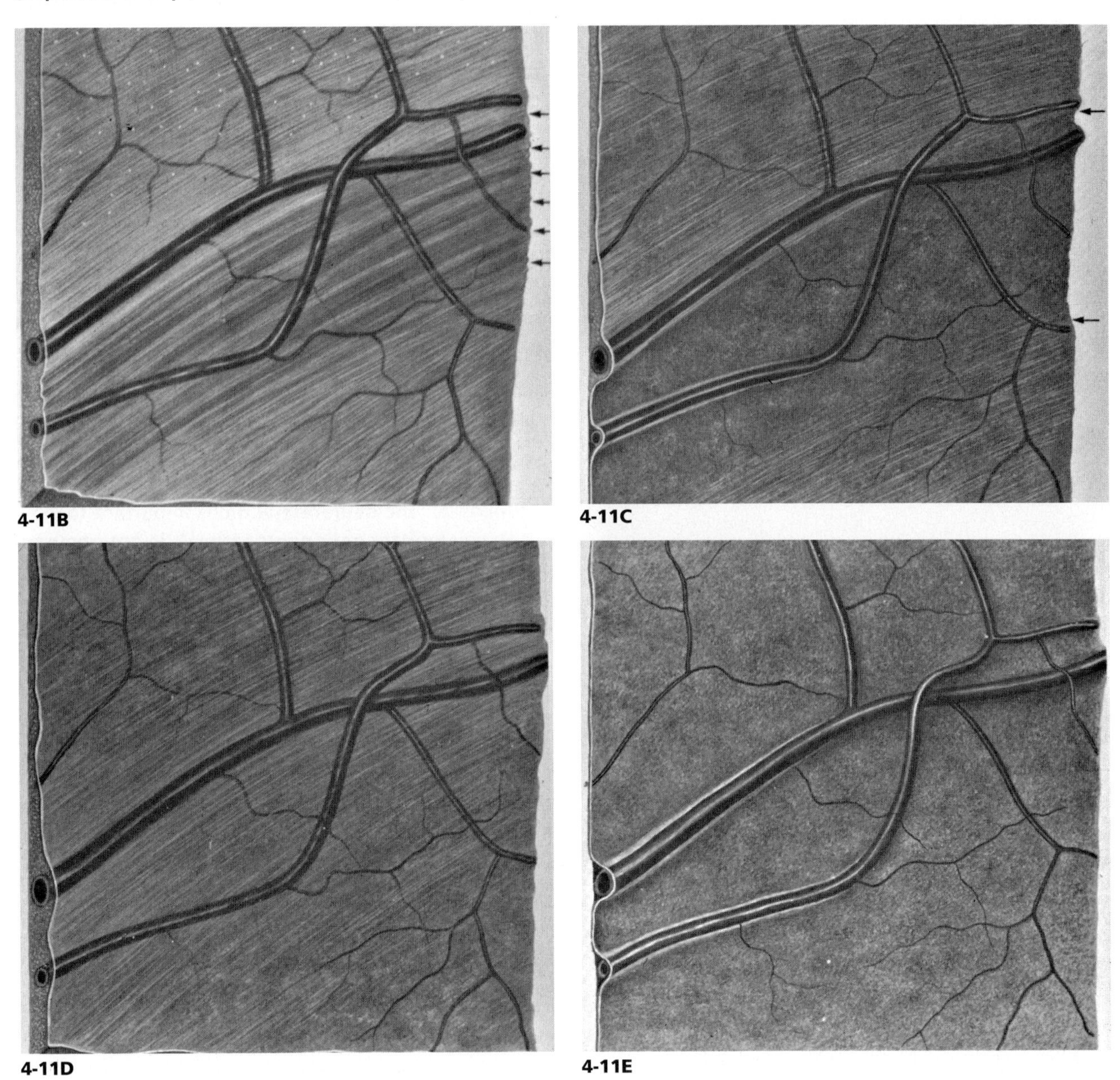

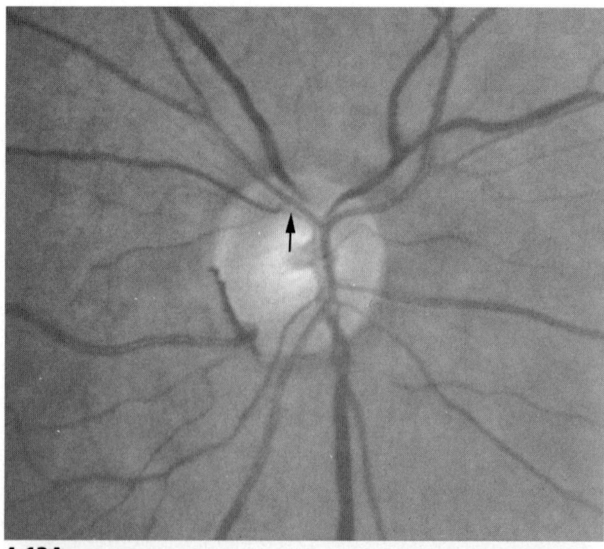

4-12A

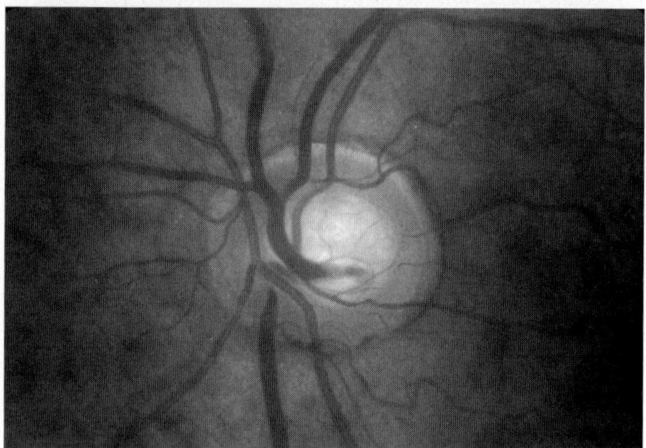

4-12B

Notice the neuroretinal rim when you look for atrophy. The neuroretinal rim is the distance between the scleral canal and the cup. The neuroretinal rim is a reflection of the bulk of the nerve fiber layer and the nerve fiber layer condenses as it approaches the optic disc. The neuroretinal rim is pink to pink-yellow in appearance and has its blood supply delivered in a clock-hour fashion. Should the blood pressure drop or blood supply be interrupted, an ischemic infarct of the disc may occur, making a notch. In glaucoma, the neuroretinal rim may be thinned and notched, as we shall see, but early on the rim will still be present and pink.[11] As a nerve becomes pale due to a process such as compression, the rim may be present, but it pales as axons begin to drop out and gliosis occurs.

Figure 4-12. The neuroretinal rim is important to view when you look for optic neuropathy. A. **In optic neuropathy due to glaucoma, a notch may be present—look superiorly on this disc (*arrow*).** B. **Compare this with a normal neuroretinal rim.**

Is the Pallor Diffuse or Segmental?

Segmental pallor may give a clue as to the type of process occurring. Ischemic optic neuropathy may cause a segmental optic neuropathy. Here you will also see a corresponding visual field defect (e.g., superior pallor will cause an inferior visual field defect).

Figure 4-13. Sectoral pallor (superior or inferior or nasal on the disc) in one eye occurs after a segmental swelling of AION. Ischemic processes frequently cause segmental pallor. A. Notice the temporal segmental atrophy on this disc after AION. B. Superior atrophy occurred after superior disc swelling due to AION. C. The entire superior-temporal aspect of this disc is pale after AION. D. This patient has superior atrophy and also an inferior altitudinal visual field defect. The atrophy is due to AION.

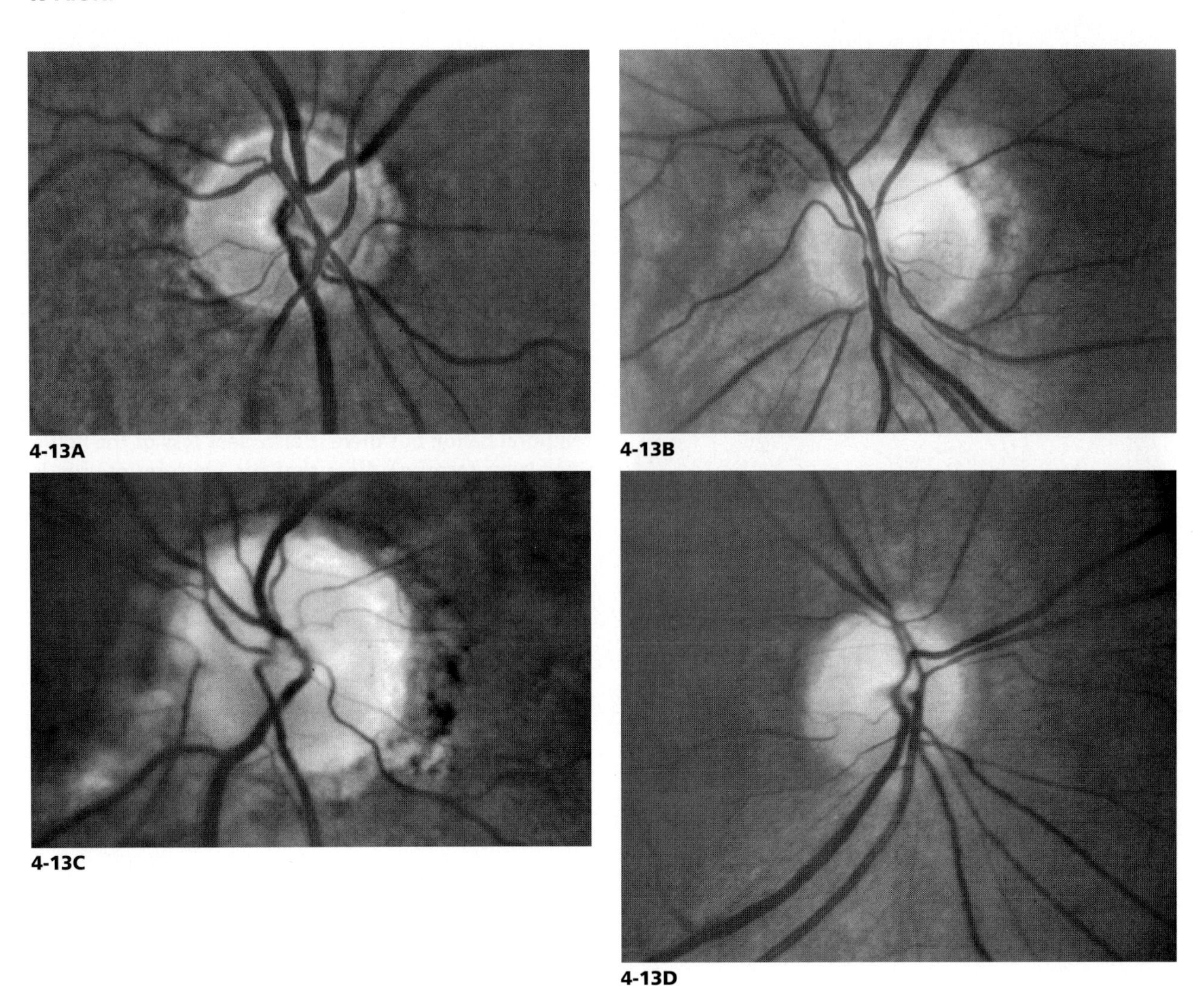

4-13A

4-13B

4-13C

4-13D

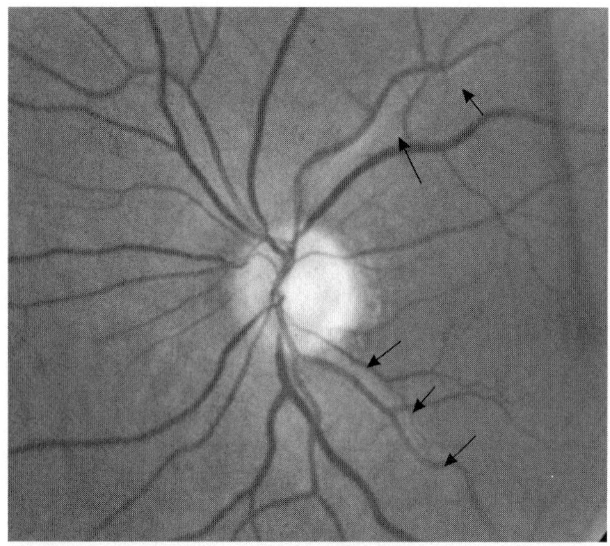

4-14A

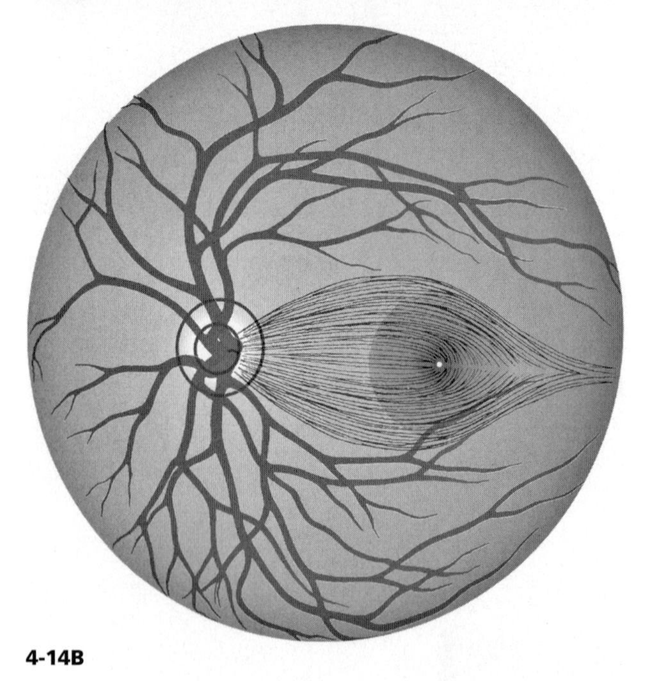

4-14B

THE PROBLEM OF TEMPORAL PALLOR

Temporal pallor is the most common location of segmental optic atrophy, but it is also a much-abused term. Remember not to confuse temporal pallor with an enlarged cup or large myopic discs. Pallor does not equal atrophy. Occasionally, the temporal pallor is so sharply demarcated or asymmetric (worse in one eye than in the other) that it is unmistakable. In that case, a process that has damaged the papillomacular bundle is the usual culprit—and clinically, loss of visual acuity and color vision will be present. Processes that cause temporal pallor include nutritional, toxic, demyelinating, ischemic, and some of the inherited dominant forms of optic atrophy.

Figure 4-14. A. **This woman has had profound loss of her central vision and color vision due to loss of the papillomacular bundle from recurrent bouts of optic neuritis due to multiple sclerosis. Not only can you see the temporal pallor, but there is also clear loss of the nerve fiber layer (*arrows*). Note that the neuroretinal rim is also pale.** B. **Notice the large papillomacular bundle of nerve fiber layer. When this is lost, temporal atrophy ensues.**

Is There Cupping?

We have all been taught that if there is cupping then think of glaucoma. But pathologic cupping is the result of any severe loss of nerve fibers. Hayreh observed that cupping occurs in glaucoma, low-tension glaucoma, and ischemic optic neuropathy—especially the arteritic type.[12] Trobe et al. showed that cupping can also occur following retrobulbar insults such as a tumor or even a posterior ischemic optic neuropathy (PION).[13] Hayreh further showed that cupping was due to a combination of "ischaemic degenerative changes in the neural tissue of the prelaminar region of the optic nerve head, the retrolaminar optic nerve and the lamina cribrosa with retrolaminar fibrosis and bowing backwards of the lamina cribrosa" and that the health of the posterior ciliary arteries that feed this region are of utmost importance to optic neuropathies and cupping.[12] Therefore, many forms of optic nerve damage may be reflected as cupping. So cupping, although a prominent feature in the glaucomas, can be caused by other factors as well—cupping should signal an acquired optic neuropathy if (1) the patient is young, (2) the visual acuity is lower, (3) there is pallor of the neuroretinal rim, (4) there is asymmetry, and (5) there is associated visual field loss (especially if there is involvement of the vertical meridian of the visual field).[14]

Table 4-4. Etiologies of Cupping[14,15]

Glaucoma (most common)
Pituitary tumors (adenomas, apoplexy)
Meningiomas: suprasellar, cavernous sinus, optic nerve sheath, sphenoid wing
Craniopharyngiomas
Epidermoids
Arteriovenous malformation
Aneurysm
Lymphoma
Syphilis

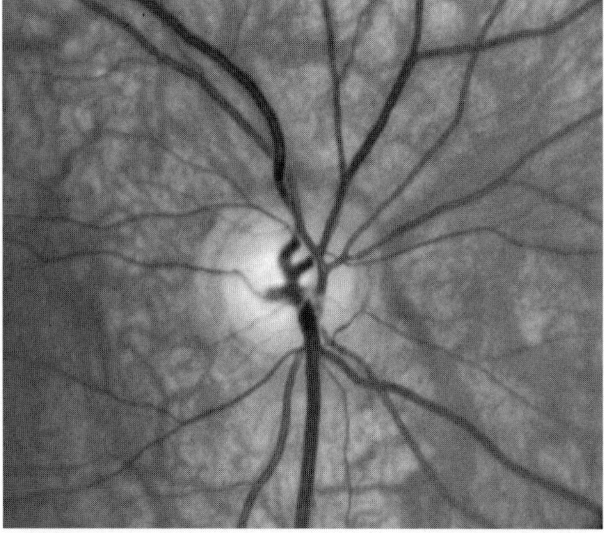

4-15A

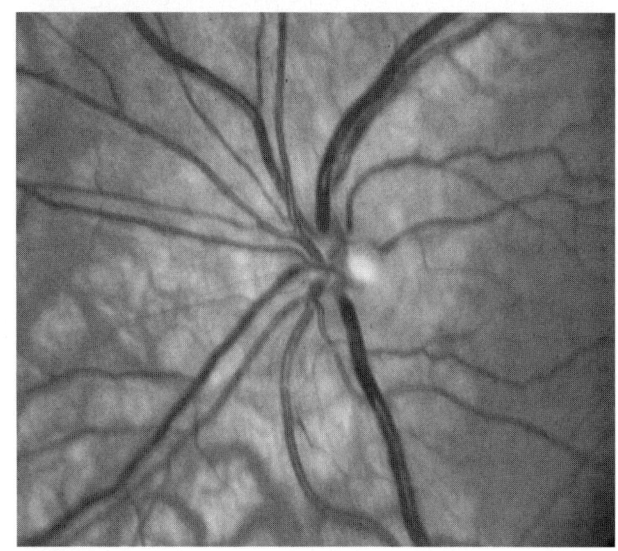

4-15B

Figure 4-15. This young man has a right sphenoid ridge meningioma. He has light perception vision in the right eye (A) and 20/20 vision in the left eye (B). Note that the right disc is cupped (A) compared with the normal left eye (B), and there is pallor of the neuroretinal rim.

What Do the Blood Vessels Look Like?

In most cases of optic atrophy, there is apparent dropout of the very fine blood vessels on the optic disc. There may also be narrowing or attenuation of the larger arterioles.[16]

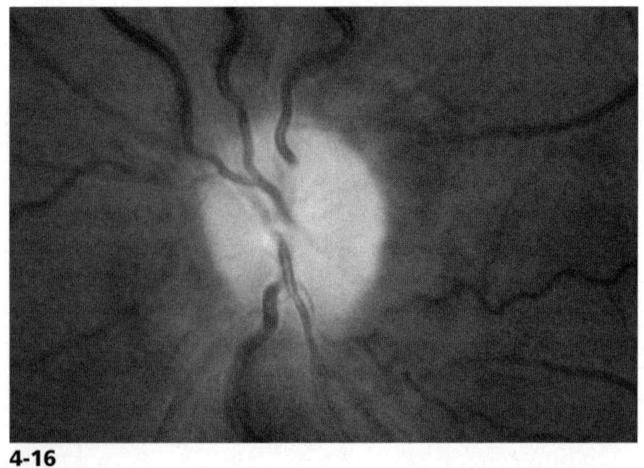

4-16

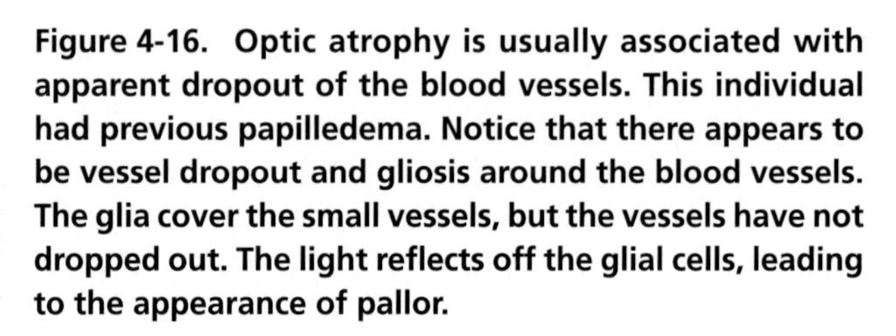

Figure 4-16. Optic atrophy is usually associated with apparent dropout of the blood vessels. This individual had previous papilledema. Notice that there appears to be vessel dropout and gliosis around the blood vessels. The glia cover the small vessels, but the vessels have not dropped out. The light reflects off the glial cells, leading to the appearance of pallor.

Sometimes, the vessels on the disc (large and small) may appear to be attenuated. Attenuation is frequently seen following vascular events such as a prior arterial occlusion or ischemic optic neuropathy. Furthermore, vascular attenuation, on and off the disc, accompanies some of the retinal disorders associated with optic atrophy, such as retinitis pigmentosa. In contrast, sometimes the vessels look enlarged, such as in the retinochoroidal shunt vessels seen in atrophic nerves with underlying optic nerve meningiomas.

Table 4-5. Features to Look for in True Pallor of the Disc[17,18]

Finding	How to use the information
Color of the disc	Not very helpful, unless there is segmental atrophy
Cupping—focal or diffuse loss of the neuroretinal rim	Most useful for identifying glaucoma
Pallor of the neuroretinal rim	Most important for non-glaucomatous atrophy[17]
Nerve fiber layer	Looking for segmental or temporal loss
Vascular attenuation	Helpful in inflammatory, ischemic changes to the nerve (AION, CRA)
Laminar dots (seeing the lamina cribrosa)	Not specific

Can You Tell from the Appearance Alone What the Optic Atrophy Is Owing to?

Although the appearance of the disc in optic atrophy can be helpful (e.g., cupping in glaucoma, altitudinal pallor in AION, attenuation of blood vessels in central retinal artery occlusion), most acquired optic atrophies are not usually diagnosable by the appearance of the disc alone.[17,18]

IS THE DISC PALE UNILATERALLY OR BILATERALLY?

Decide whether there is pallor in one eye or both. What are clues to unilateral pallor? Here again, the history plays an important role in what you should expect. In the history, the patient may be able to tell you that only one eye is affected or that both eyes are affected. If the patient has no idea that something is wrong with his or her vision, the neuropathy could be slowly developing and the patient never covered one eye at a time to test vision. Let the examination work for you. First, go back to the visual acuity—is it the same in both eyes? Is color vision normal in both eyes? The single test that can be helpful in this situation is looking for a relative afferent pupillary defect. Doing the swinging light test and finding a relative afferent defect tells you that at least one eye is worse than the other. If there is no afferent pupillary defect and you think the nerves do look pale, the patient may have bilateral optic neuropathy. Visual field testing by confrontation or formal visual fields also helps you decide whether there is unilateral or bilateral optic neuropathy.

Once you have decided whether the pallor is unilateral or bilateral, you must consider what caused the optic atrophy. Is it congenital or acquired?

Table 4-6. Unilateral or Bilateral Optic Neuropathy?

	Unilateral	Bilateral
History		
Onset	Sudden or gradual	Usually gradual
Pain	Can be present in one eye	Usually absent
Examination		
Visual acuity	Usually affected in one eye	Decreased in both eyes
Color vision	Decreased in one eye	Decreased in both eyes
Relative afferent pupillary defect	Present	Absent; if one eye is worse than the other, may be present
Visual field to confrontation	Unilaterally abnormal	Bilaterally abnormal
Disc pallor	Unilateral pallor	Bilateral pallor
Testing		
Formal visual field	Unilaterally abnormal	Bilateral abnormality
Visual evoked potential	Delayed unilaterally	Bilateral delay

IS THE PALLOR INHERITED/ CONGENITAL OR ACQUIRED?

Congenitally pale optic nerves do occur. Sometimes the optic neuropathy is found on a routine examination and family history may not be available. Checking first-degree relatives (mother, father, sister, brother) may give a clue in this regard.

Table 4-7. Differentiating Acquired from Inherited Optic Neuropathies

Characteristic	Inherited/Congenital	Acquired
Family history	May be present	None
Onset	Often no discrete onset; found on routine examination	Characteristically, onset can be dated to a time or day or week
Symptoms	Decreased vision or none; decreased color vision	Decreasing vision; there may be pain; decreased color vision
Signs	Pale disc—usually diffuse, but can be temporal; disc may be somewhat anomalous	Pale disc—may be altitudinal or sectoral
Evaluation (MR)	Shows small optic nerves and chiasm	May reveal pathology, e.g., T2 signals in white matter; tumor of optic nerve

Table 4-8. Causes of Optic Atrophy: Causes of Acquired Unilateral and Bilateral Optic Neuropathy

Unilateral	Bilateral
Compression: aneurysm (ophthalmic artery or giant), tumor (optic nerve glioma, meningioma, other), Graves' disease (muscle compression)	Compression: suprasellar tumors: pituitary adenoma, craniopharyngioma, parasellar meningioma, chiasmal glioma
Infiltration: sarcoid, lymphoma	Infiltration: sarcoid, lymphoma
Old ischemic optic neuropathy	Long-standing papilledema from brain tumors (cerebellar in children); idiopathic intracranial hypertension; venous sinus thrombosis
	Infectious/postinfectious optic neuritis
Retrobulbar optic neuritis	Arteritic/hypotensive ischemic optic neuropathy
Radiation optic neuropathy	Pallor associated with retinal degeneration
	Unilateral disease presenting bilaterally (optic neuritis, ischemic optic neuropathy, compression, trauma)
Old central retinal artery occlusion	Metabolic disorders
Traumatic optic neuropathy	Diabetes
Disorders that occur bilaterally can seem asymmetric and may appear to be unilateral	Lead
	Vitamin deficiency (B_{12}, thiamine)
	Wernicke's (thiamine)
	Toxins and drugs
	Tobacco, alcohol
	Methyl alcohol
	Isoniazid
	Chloramphenicol
	Inherited disorders
	Glaucoma (usually)
	Congenital structural abnormalities: hydrocephalus
	Disorders that occur unilaterally can occur in both eyes

First, let us consider acquired *unilateral* optic neuropathy/atrophy. You must figure out "What is the optic atrophy due to?"

Table 4-9. How Do You Differentiate among the Unilateral Optic Neuropathies?

Characteristic	Optic neuritis	History of ischemic optic neuropathy	Compressive optic neuropathy	Traumatic optic neuropathy
History				
Age	Younger (younger than 50)	Older (older than 50)	Young (glioma), middle age (meningioma), older (compressive aneurysm)	Any age
Onset	Gradual over 1–10 days	Abrupt: awaken in morning	Very gradual—months to years	After brow trauma
Pain	Yes, often	None	Usually not	Can be painful
Time course	Improves after 2–4 weeks	Improves only slightly	Worsens gradually	Is at its worst from the start; may improve
Examination				
Visual acuity	Often severely affected	Can be affected	Can be spared or affected	Usually affected
Visual field abnormality	Central scotoma, constriction, variable loss	Usually altitudinal defect, constriction, central scotoma	Central scotoma frequent, constriction	Usually constriction
Disc appearance				
Pallor	Usually complete, or early on temporal	May be sectoral pallor	Complete; may see retinochoroidal shunt vessel	Complete or partial
Vessels	Normal	Often narrowed	Retinochoroidal shunt vessel	Vessels may be normal
Testing				
MR/CT scan	May see T2 signals in the white matter; occasional enhancement of the optic nerve or sheath	Usually normal	Will see mass lesion in the orbit or anterior chiasm; CT may show calcification in meningioma	CT may show optic canal or clinoid fracture

Although these distinctions do not always hold because optic neuritis and ischemic optic neuropathy can be bilateral, and tumors can be bilateral, and trauma can be bilateral, this chart is the start of a practical way to make sense of acquired optic atrophy.

OPTIC NEURITIS

The most common cause of unilateral optic pallor in the young (younger than 40 years of age) is *demyelination*. *Optic neuritis* is an inflammatory process of the optic nerve. It can be associated with optic disc swelling, as we have seen in Chapter 3, and papillitis when the optic disc anterior to the lamina cribrosa is involved. The swollen nerve head appearance is seen in one third. As this resolves, optic nerve pallor and perhaps atrophy can develop, depending on the severity of the initial inflammation and the extent of the nerve fiber attrition (see also Figure 3-57).

Figure 4-17. A. **This acutely swollen disc due to optic neuritis became pale later, leading to subsequent pallor** (B). **The MR scan showed typical findings of multiple sclerosis.**

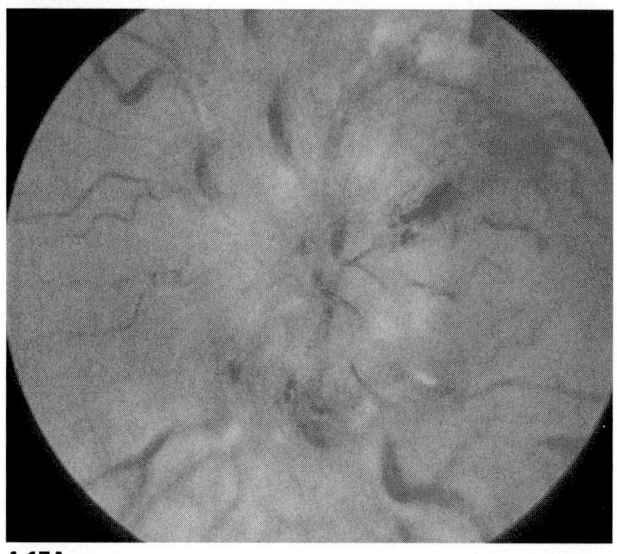

4-17A

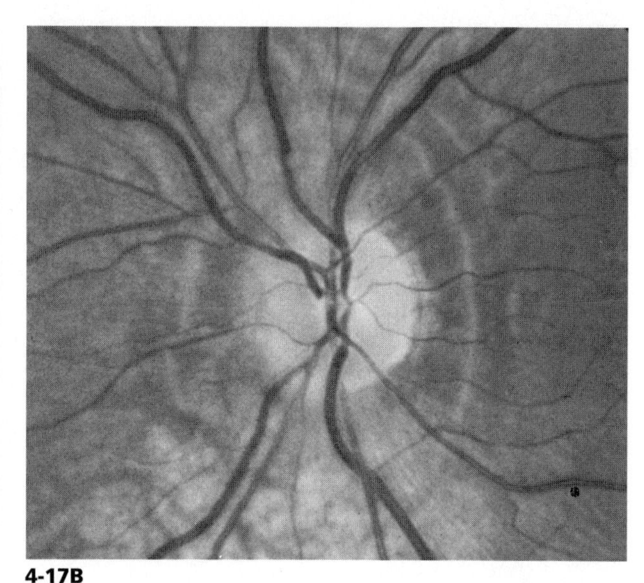

4-17B

Although optic neuritis is most often unilateral, it can be bilateral. Frequently, bilateral optic neuritis occurs after a systemic illness. Children frequently present with bilateral optic neuritis (see Chapter 11).

Figure 4-18. This man had bilateral optic neuritis and vision loss after a flulike illness. His discs were mildly swollen acutely (A, B)**. Although his vision improved, he had residual optic pallor. There is nerve fiber layer drop-out visible in the maculopapillor bundle from 1–6 o'clock in the left eye** (D) **and from 7–10 o'clock in the right eye (*arrows*)** (C) **and left eye (*arrows*)** (D)**. Despite the fact that there was optic neuritis with some disc swelling, there is very little residual pallor as a sign of the previous event. So, you cannot use optic disc pallor alone to tell whether the optic nerve has been insulted.**

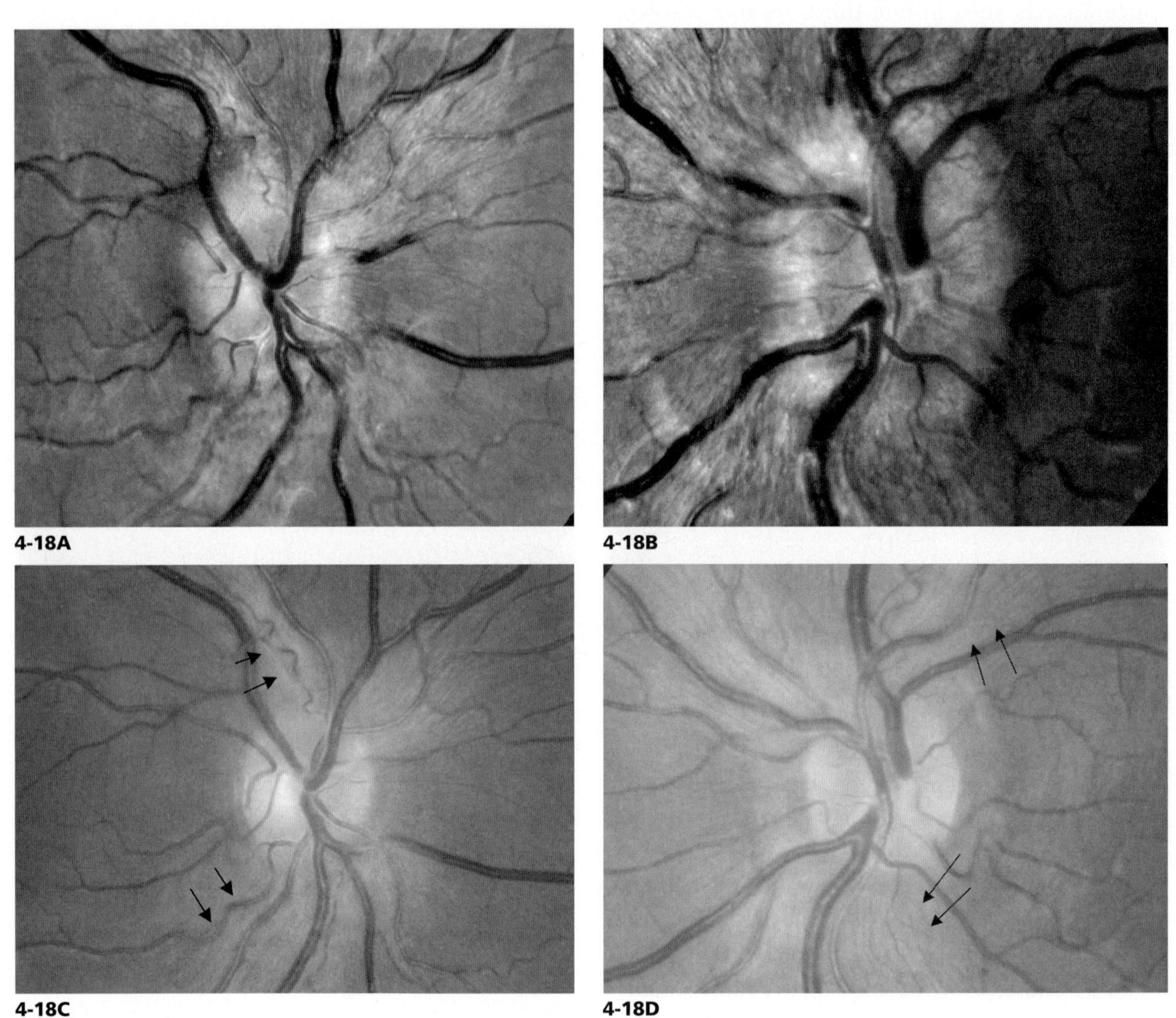

Figure 4-19. **When viewing optic neuropathy, it is very important to look at the nerve fiber layer.** A. **Look for slit and wedge defects (*arrows*) when you are trying to decide if there is an optic neuropathy.** B. **Slit defects seen with red-free photography.** C. **Here you can see the slit defects with red-free better than with colored photography** (D). **If you look closely, you will see the nerve fiber layer. (Photographs are courtesy of William F. Hoyt, M.D.) (Compare with Figure 4-11A–E.)**

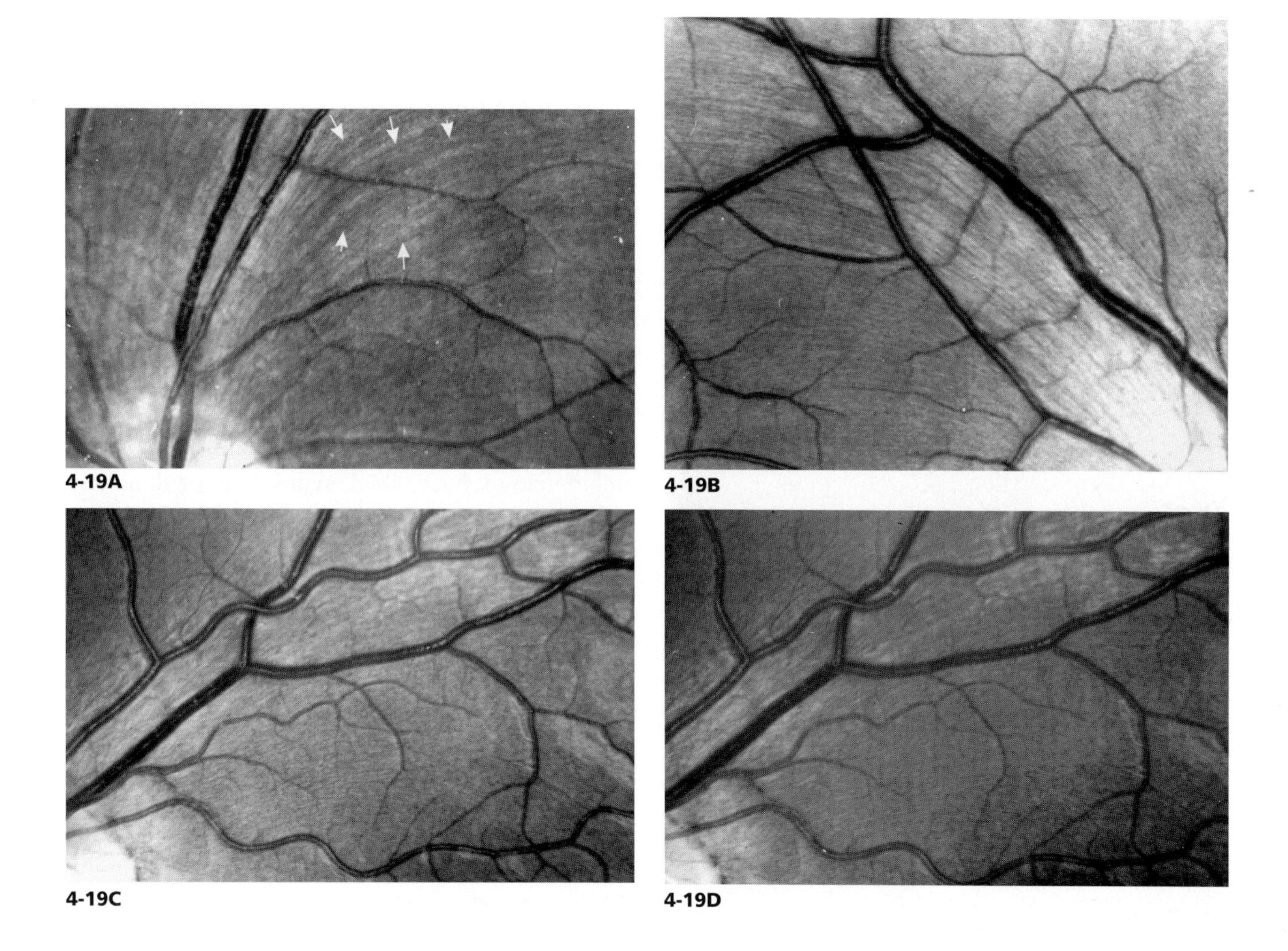

Optic neuritis can also be an inflammation behind the lamina cribrosa, in which case we call it *retrobulbar optic neuritis* . This pattern is seen in about two-thirds of patients with optic neuritis. *Optic neuritis* is a generic term in that it can occur with various inflammations (diabetes, lupus) or infections (syphilis, Lyme disease, meningitis, or encephalitis). The most common cause is demyelination associated with multiple sclerosis. Although optic neuritis can be bilateral, it is most frequently unilateral at the onset when associated with demyelination (multiple sclerosis). Optic neuritis is the presenting symptom (or finding) in multiple sclerosis in about 25% of patients. Furthermore, if one develops optic neuritis without other signs or symptoms of multiple sclerosis, there is a 35–75% chance of acquiring the multiple sclerosis. The disease is more frequent in women aged 20–40 years. There is also a geographic factor, which makes multiple sclerosis more common in cooler climates. In children, optic neuritis is more frequently bilateral and commonly associated with disc swelling.[2] The natural history of a child presenting with optic neuritis subsequently acquiring multiple sclerosis is only 8–26%.[20] In children, there may also be a clear prodromal viral illness.

Symptoms include decreased vision. Complaints include cloud, haze, skim, scum, blur, or dimming. Pain, especially on eye movement, is a strong association with the vision loss in optic neuritis. The time course of the neuritis is usually gradual, worsening over days. Improvement occurs over days to weeks. Ask about previous episodes of diplopia, unsteadiness of gait, truncal numbness, or prior episodes of vision loss, because the optic neuritis may not be the first symptom of multiple sclerosis.

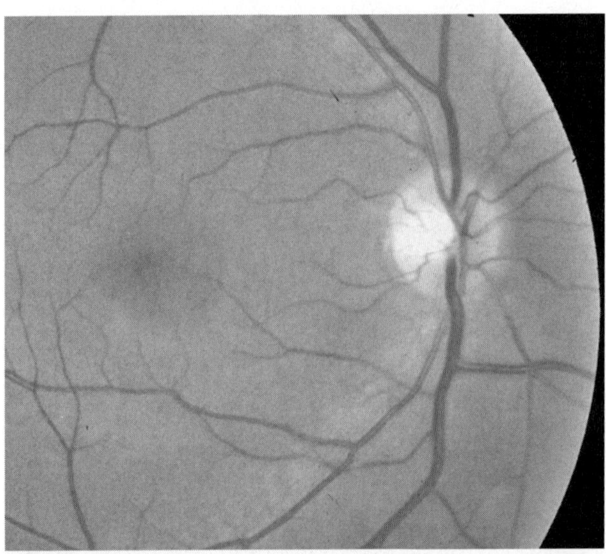

4-20A

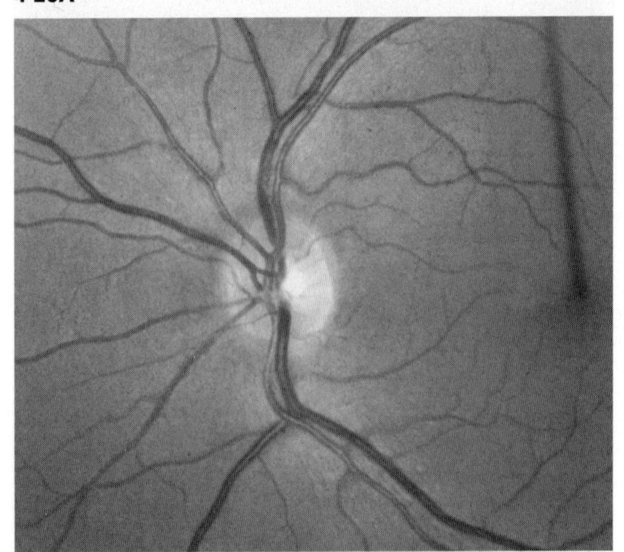

4-20B

Figure 4-20. Most demyelinative optic neuritis is retrobulbar (behind the lamina cribrosa), and early in the event the examiner may not see anything of note in the fundus. This woman presented with acute vision loss in the right eye and pain with eye movement. The MR showed T2 signals in the white matter, and she was diagnosed with optic neuritis due to demyelination. Her right disc showed minor pallor (A) **at onset.** B. **Her left disc showed normal acuity, was not symptomatic, and appeared normal.**

Table 4-10. Other Ocular Findings in Multiple Sclerosis[21]

Optic nerve
Normal (acute retrobulbar optic neuritis in 1/3 of cases)
Swollen (optic neuritis—anterior to lamina cribrosa 1/3 of cases)
Pale (may have had earlier attacks that went unnoticed, 1/3 of cases)
Other patterns: band atrophy from long-standing chiasmal demyelination
Retina
Vitreous cells (rarely)
Venous sheathing
Inflammation (pars planitis)

Devic's optic neuritis is really not a demyelinating neuropathy, but is rather a necrotizing axonopathy including optic neuropathy and spinal cord disease that can be confused with multiple sclerosis, at least initially. The onset is usually unilateral optic neuritis, often without signs of optic disc swelling. However, within months to years, not only is the other eye involved, but the patient also develops a cervical myelopathy. Spinal cord MR is abnormal, but brain MR can be normal. CSF examination does not show oligoclonal bands, but may show elevation in CSF protein and cells. Unlike in multiple sclerosis, the optic neuritis and myelitis rarely improve.

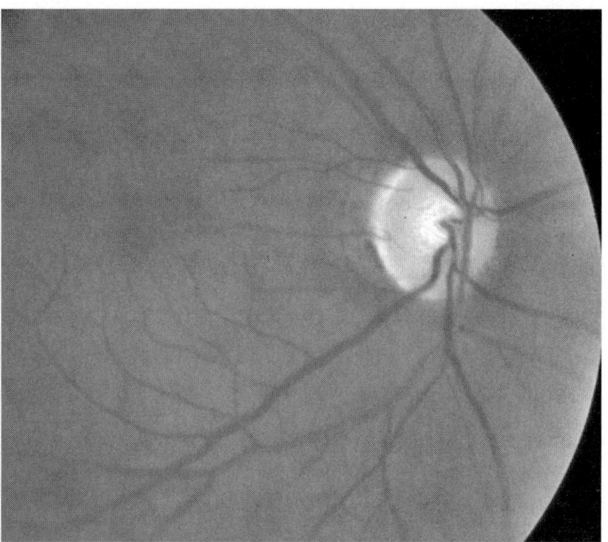

4-21A

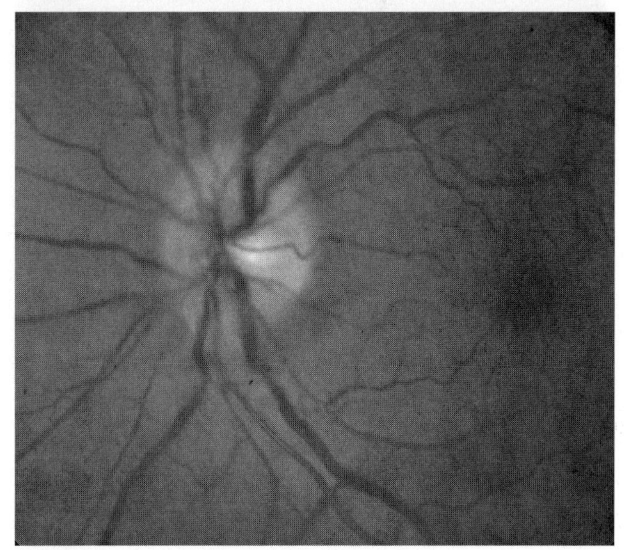

4-21B

Figure 4-21. This 38-year-old woman abruptly lost vision in the right eye (A) **and had mild swelling in the left eye at presentation** (B). ***Continued***

Figure 4-21. ***Continued.*** C,D. **Within 3 months, she lost vision in the left eye, and both of her nerves were pale.** E. **MR axial of her optic nerves revealed thinning of the optic nerve and bilateral demyelination on the T2 signal. Her vision did not recover.** F. **One year later, she developed quadriparesis. Her MR showed extensive demyelination of the cervical cord (*arrow*), and she never recovered her strength.**

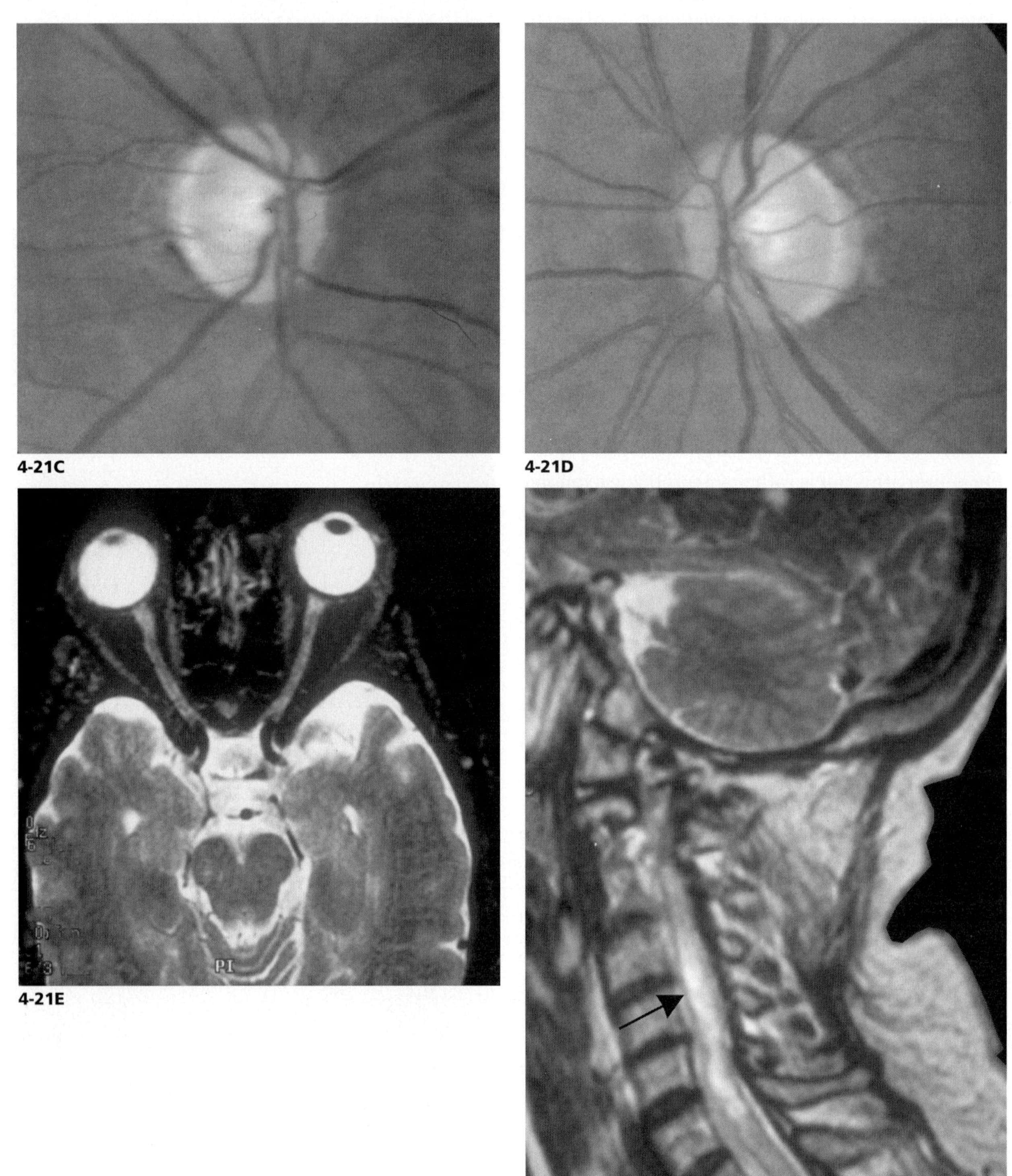

Anterior Ischemic Optic Neuropathy

We have seen that AION usually causes optic disc swelling acutely, followed by optic atrophy. Most patients present with acute or acutely recognized vision loss in one eye. On occasion, a patient may present with unilateral disc pallor due to a previously unrecognized ischemic event. The patient may present with abrupt onset of bilateral vision loss with a swollen disc in one eye and a pale disc in the other eye—also called *pseudo–Foster Kennedy syndrome* (see Figure 3-49E,F).

The cause of ischemic optic neuropathy without disc swelling—PION—is, fortunately, much less common, even rare. Causes of PION include carotid artery disease (often associated with stroke affecting the contralateral side), severe diffuse atherosclerosis, and radical neck dissection.[22] See also the discussion of bilateral PION (see Figure 4-46).

Compressive Causes of Unilateral Pallor

OPTIC NERVE TUMORS

Although some optic nerve gliomas in adults can be associated with disc swelling (see Chapter 3), optic nerve glioma can also be a slow-growing tumor of the optic nerve presenting in childhood, with a mean age of 9 years. Approximately 90% of children present with symptoms by age 20 years. There is no sex predilection. There is a strong association with neurofibromatosis (NF) type I.[23] There are two types of NF.

Type I, the most common of all phakomatoses. The diagnostic criteria include any two of the following: 6 or more café-au-lait spots (>5 mm), Lisch nodules (small fibromas of the iris [see Figure 4-22]), axillary freckling, optic nerve glioma, a first-degree relative with NF-1, or a bone lesion (sphenoid wing dysplasia).

Type II. The diagnostic criteria include a first-degree relative with NF-2 plus an acoustic tumor or any two of the following: schwannoma, neurofibroma, meningioma, glioma, or typical subcapsular cataract.

Appearance of the optic nerve and retina in patients with NF is often normal. However, look for disc pallor or disc swelling indicating an optic nerve tumor. Occasionally, hamartomas can appear in the retina (NF-2 > NF-1).

Table 4-11. Differentiating between NF-1 and NF-2

	NF-1	NF-2
Incidence	1/3000	1/50,000
Cardinal features	Café-au-lait spots; axially freckling; neurofibromas of the peripheral, autonomic, and central nervous system	Acoustic neuroma; juvenile posterior cataract; neurofibroma or other tumor; café-au-lait spots less frequent
Eye findings	Lisch nodule; fibromas of the upper eyelid; optic nerve glioma in 15%	Juvenile posterior cataract; optic nerve meningioma or glioma
Genetics	Chromosome 17	Chromosome 22
Skin features	Café-au-lait spots	Rare
Tumors	Optic nerve glioma	Acoustic neuroma, trigeminal neuroma; cranial nerve neuromas

Ophthalmologic examination is very important when looking for NF-1. First, examine the iris. Lisch nodules are small neurofibromata of the iris.

Figure 4-22. A–C. **NF type I is associated with Lisch nodules, neurofibromas of the eye lids, and optic nerve gliomas producing optic atrophy.** A. **Here you see typical Lisch nodules (*arrow*).** B. **This woman has an optic nerve glioma (*arrow*) of the right optic nerve.** C. **This man has bilateral optic nerve gliomas. He also has prominent neurofibromas of the eyelids (*arrows*).**

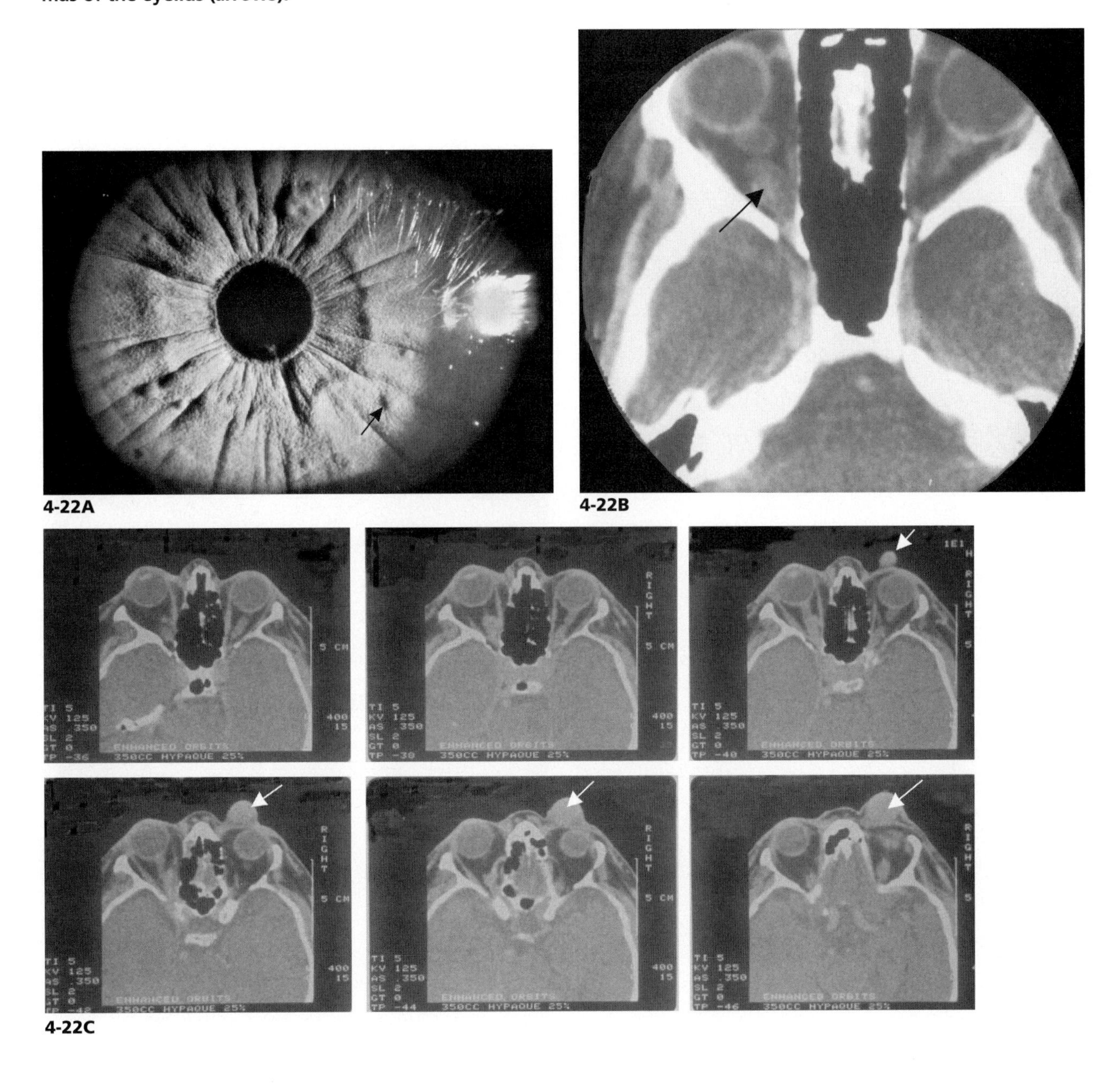

Next, look at the eyelids. Fibromas of the lid are very common. A careful hunt for an optic neuropathy (checking for an afferent pupillary defect, color change, and visual field change) is important because orbital neurofibromas, as well as optic nerve gliomas, can be seen. Further, check for exophthalmos or proptosis that may indicate an orbital tumor.

Skin lesions are another diagnostic criteria for NF. Café-au-lait spots are flat brown discolorations; the presence of 6 or more, larger than 5 mm, is pathognomonic for NF-1. Axillary freckling is another skin lesion.

The disc is usually pale and, because these tumors grow slowly, a child will present with a unilaterally pale optic disc.

Figure 4-23. A. **This 9-year-old girl presented with disfiguring proptosis. An optic nerve glioma was excised in the no-light-perception eye. The disc is diffusely pale.** B. **The MR shows a large globular mass typical of optic nerve glioma behind the globe on the left.**

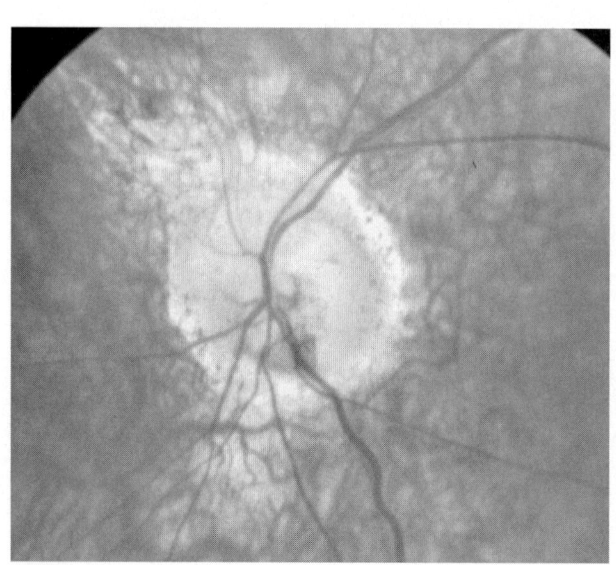

4-23A

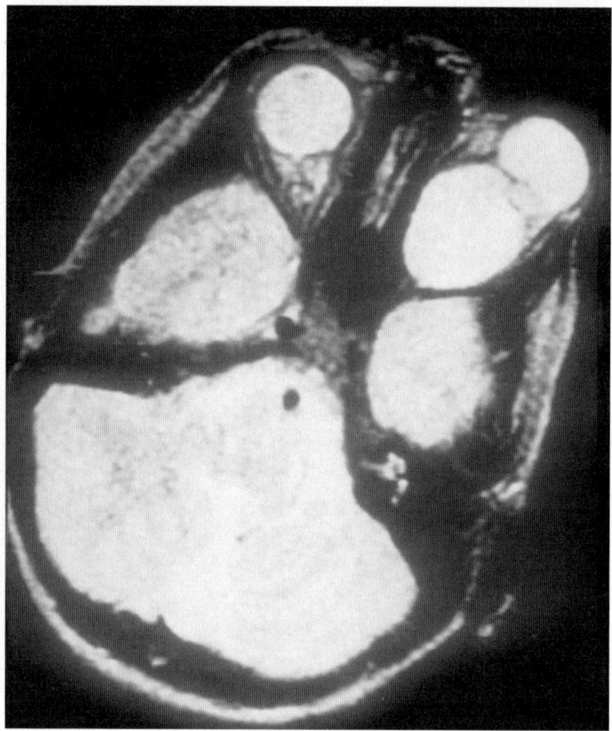

4-23B

Figure 4-24. This 9-year-old girl presented with decreased vision in her left eye. She had known NF-I. A. Her right disc is somewhat small and hypoplastic, and the left disc is pale (B). C. An MR showed an optic nerve glioma on the left. D. The T2 MR shows the enlarged optic nerve with cerebrospinal fluid surrounding the optic nerve. Her vision has been stable, although she does have optic atrophy of the left eye (OS).

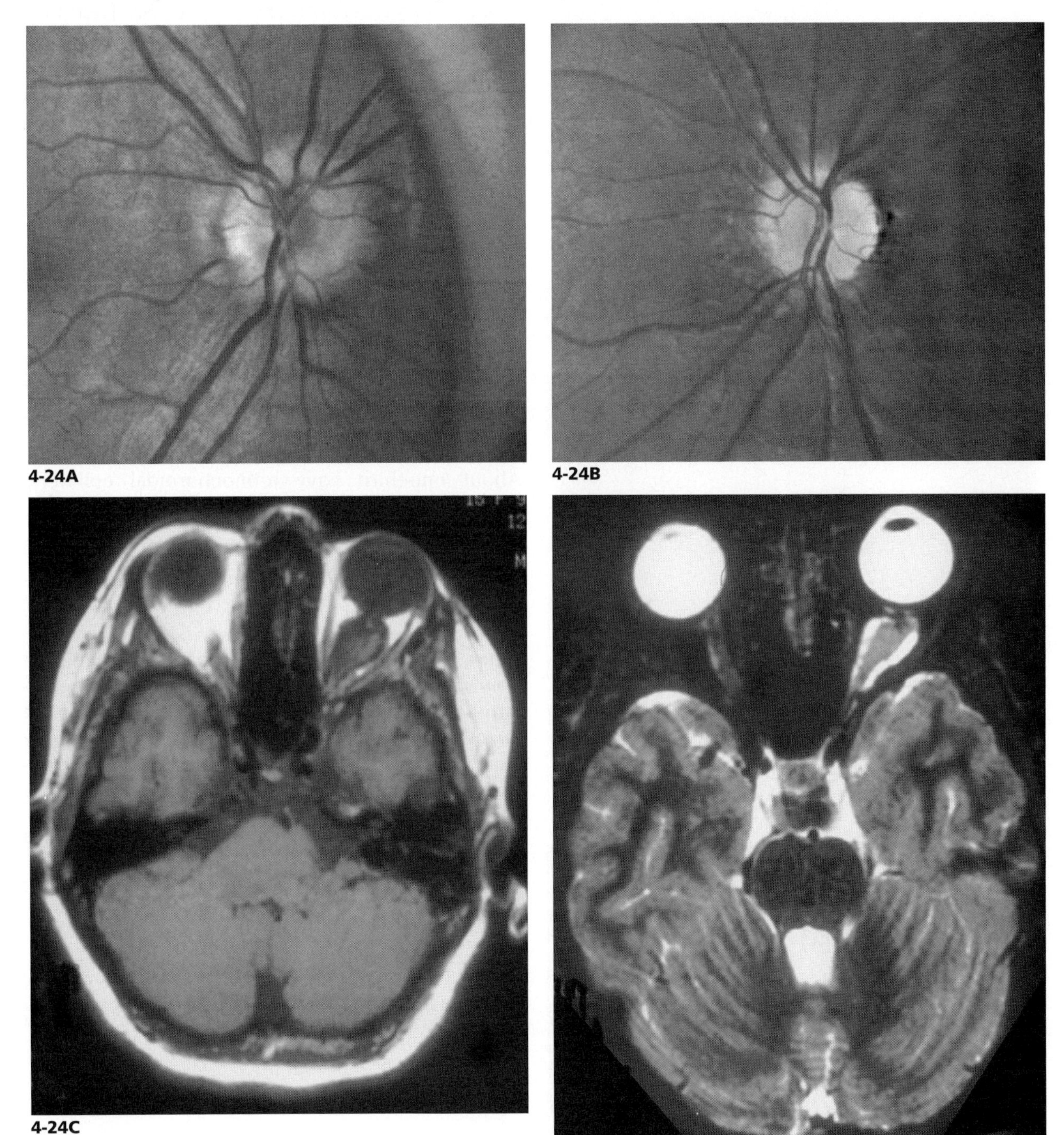

4-24A

4-24B

4-24C

4-24D

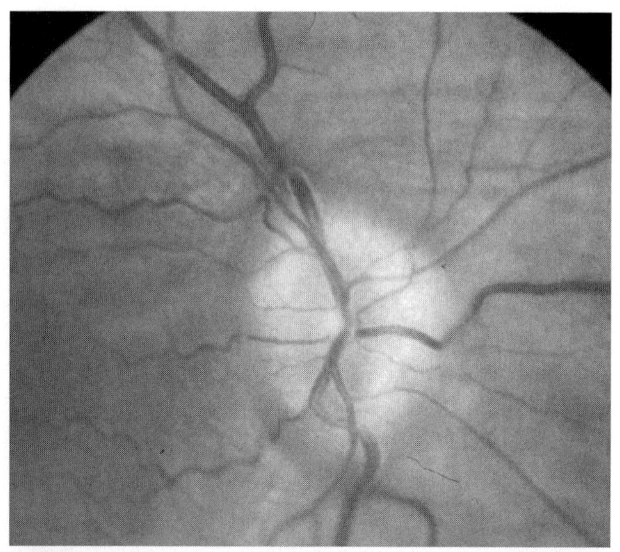

4-25A

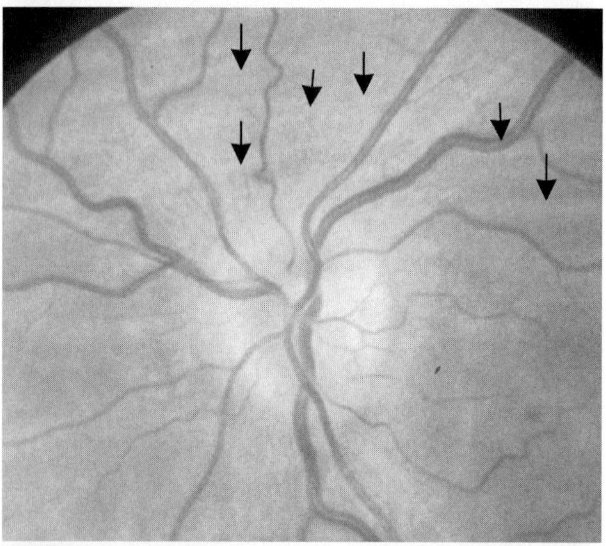

4-25B

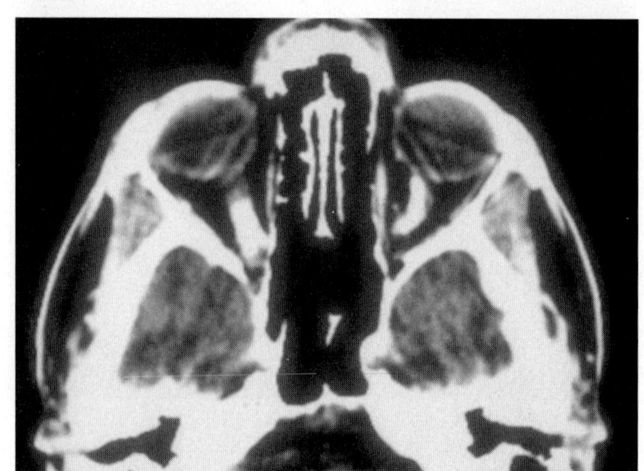

4-25C

Spontaneous improvement has been seen with some optic nerve gliomas (juvenile pilocytic astrocytoma). These were reported in patients (3 months–12 years) with and without NF. Therefore, this fact should be kept in mind when following anyone with optic nerve glioma.[24]

Optic Nerve Tumor: Meningioma

Optic nerve meningiomas are more common in adults (rare in children), and more common in women (61%).[25] Symptoms include slowly developing vision loss, proptosis, and limitation of ocular motility. Almost half have orbital pain and/or headache.

Appearance of the disc in optic nerve meningioma is variable. About half present with optic atrophy and the other half with chronic disc swelling. About one-third have retinochoroidal collateral vessels as a feature of the disc swelling (see the discussion in Chapter 5—retinochoroidal shunts and swelling). Other occasional findings are optic atrophy and choroidal folds.

Figure 4-25. This 40-year-old woman presented with slowly progressive vision loss. A. **She had optic disc pallor of the right disc and** (B) **choroidal folds in the left (*arrows*), which prompted a computed tomography scan.** C. **The computed tomography scan revealed bilateral calcified optic nerve meningiomas.**

Sphenoid ridge meningiomas can also cause a slowly progressive optic atrophy. Look for proptosis and, sometimes, pulsatile exophthalmos.

Optic Neuropathy from Radiation

See Radiation Retinopathy, Chapter 9.

OPTIC NERVE COMPRESSION: VASCULAR—OPHTHALMIC ARTERY ANEURYSM

Carotid-ophthalmic artery aneurysms compress the optic nerve from below, usually at the optic foramen. The location, therefore, makes it very likely that these aneurysms will produce a slowly progressive optic neuropathy. Giant ophthalmic artery aneurysms are more common in middle-aged women and are frequently bilateral.

Appearance of the disc is usually diffuse pallor. Because these slowly develop, and can even compress the chiasm or optic tract, look for band atrophy in the opposite eye. Remember that there is only 3–5 mm between the optic nerve and the optic tract. Think of optic tract compression, especially if visual acuity is preserved.

Figure 4-26. A. **This individual had slowly progressive vision loss of the right eye (notice the diffuse pallor).** B. **The left disc shows early band atrophy from optic tract compression by the huge intracranial aneurysm. To appreciate the band atrophy, look at the color of the disc at 12, 3, 6, and 9 o'clock. 12 and 6 are pink and 3 and 9 are pale in comparison.** ***Continued***

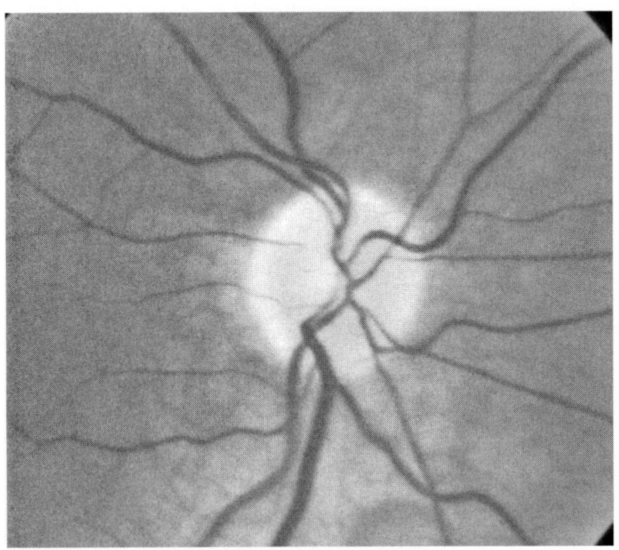

4-26A

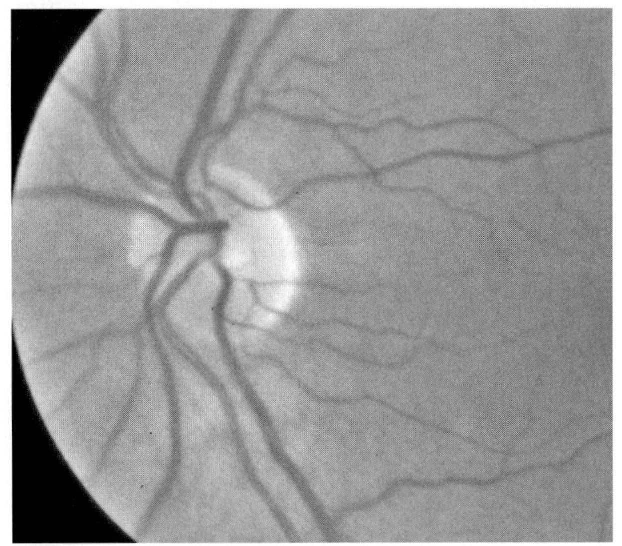

4-26B

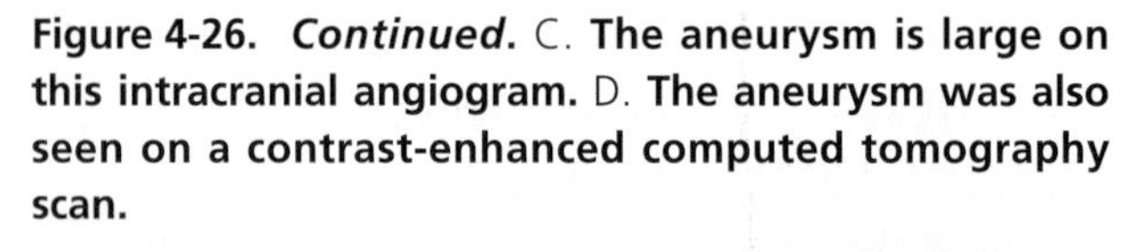

Figure 4-26. ***Continued.*** **C. The aneurysm is large on this intracranial angiogram. D. The aneurysm was also seen on a contrast-enhanced computed tomography scan.**

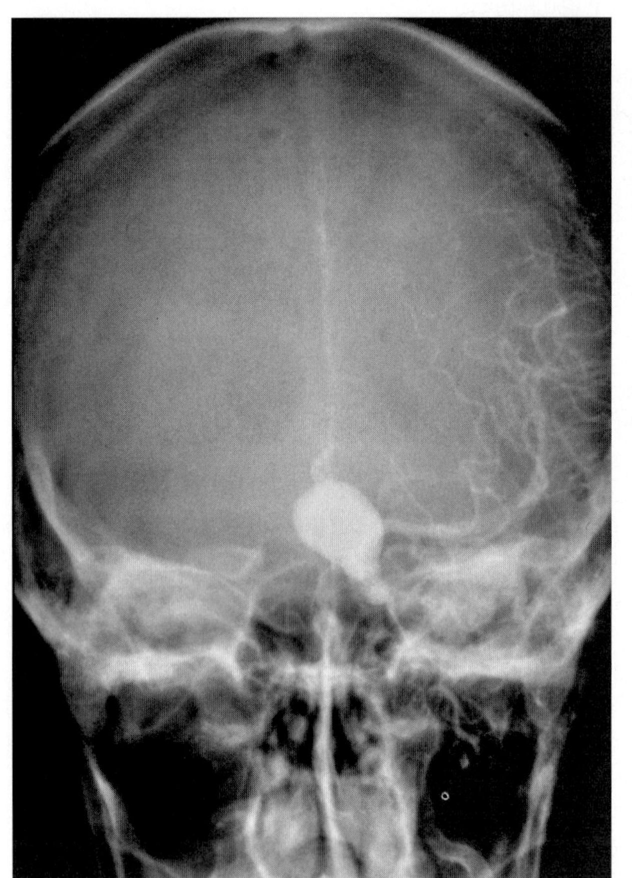

4-26C

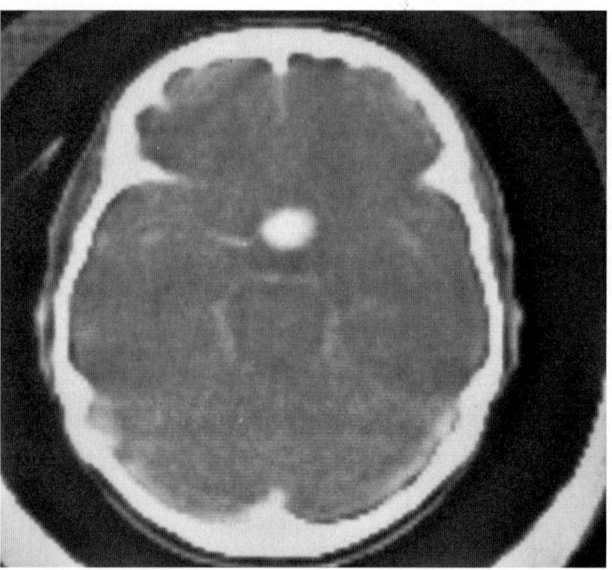

4-26D

Bilateral Optic Atrophy

Just as we found that the history and examination were integrally involved in making the correct diagnosis in unilateral optic atrophy, bilateral optic atrophy requires your best history and examination because there are so many possibilities.

Table 4-12. Differentiating Forms of Bilateral Optic Neuropathy

	Glaucoma	Compression	Ischemic	Postpapilledema	Toxic-metabolic	Congenital	Hereditary	Neurodegenerative
Examples	Open-angle, closed-angle, low-tension	Mass, tumor, aneurysm at chiasm or tract	Hypotensive/blood loss AION, bilateral PION	After any cause of papilledema (tumor, IIH, venous thrombosis)	Vitamin deficiency (B_1, B_{12}); chloramphenicol; ethambutol	Hydrocephalus, intrauterine insult	Leber's optic atrophy, Kjer dominant optic atrophy	Childhood metabolic disorders, spinocerebellar ataxia with optic atrophy
History	May have family history	Gradual vision loss, possible increasing eye prominence	Following blood loss, hypotension; lumbar surgery	History of tumor, IIH, venous sinus thrombosis	Exposure history; drug history; hobbies, diet, vomiting; smoking, alcohol intake	Usually see signs of vision loss early on in children	Vision loss usually in childhood or young adulthood	Some abnormal at birth, whereas others see normally and then develop the abnormality
Age	Usually older	Any age	Any age—usually older	Any age	Usually older age group; any age	Childhood/infant	Child/infant/young adult	Infant/child/adult
Onset	Slow, gradual, over years	Usually slow and gradual	Abrupt after surgery	Gradual loss with papilledema	Gradual vision loss	Can be present at birth and stable, or slowly progressive, as in hydrocephalus	Variable, and insidious; Leber's optic neuropathy often abrupt onset	Variable—most progressive and gradual
Course	Progressive	Progressive	Not progressive	Can be progressive if the inciting cause still exists (pressure is still elevated)	Progressive	Stable or progressive	Progressive	Progressive

Continued

Table 4-12. *Continued*

	Glaucoma	Compression	Ischemic	Postpapilledema	Toxic-metabolic	Congenital	Hereditary	Neurodegenerative
Examination								
Visual acuity	Normal until late	Can be affected early on if macular fibers (central vision) affected	Severely affected—often no light perception	Visual acuity affected late	Visual acuity affected	Visual acuity is variable	Variable acuity	Variable acuity
Other features	Increased intraocular pressure	Loss of smell; endocrinologic dysfunction (amenorrhea, galactorrhea)	May have swelling acutely, or none	History of headache; neurologic examination	Poorly reactive pupils	Check head size; other dysmorphic features; retinal examination for congenital infection	Hearing loss with some; check for diabetes or other metabolic disorders	Hearing loss, peripheral neuropathy, dementia, ataxia, retinal degenerative disease
Visual field	Arcuate bundle defects typical—nasal inferior loss	Central scotoma; bitemporal defect; homonymous hemianopia	Severely affected; sometimes unrecordable	Severely constricted visual fields	Central scotoma; visual field constriction	Central scotoma, visual field constriction	Central scotoma	Variable

Disc appearance	Increased cupping, decrease in neuroretinal rim; commonly asymmetric; pallor usually late finding	If chiasmal compression—band atrophy common; if tract—band atrophy in the contralateral eye	Initially normal; later, severe atrophy	See fibrous tissue on the disc, high water marks	Hyperemia of the disc early on—may see hemorrhage in Wernicke's; later atrophy—especially see dropout of the papillomacular bundle	Diffuse pallor; anomalous disc	Pallor may be sectoral or diffuse	Diffuse pallor
Vessels	Normal	Usually normal	Attenuated	Sheathing on the disc	Normal	Normal	Normal; Leber's optic neuropathy; tortuous vessels	Variable
Testing								
MR/CT	Sometimes required to rule out compressive abnormality; MR/CT is normal	Shows mass lesion compressing chiasm and optic nerve tract	MR/CT is normal	MR may reveal cause for increased intracranial pressure; look for empty sella	MR/CT normal; in Wernicke's see changes in mamillary bodies and lentiform nucleus; other tests: B_{12}, B_1, lead, complete blood cell count, chemistry	MR or CT important to evaluate for structural abnormality like hydrocephalus	MR/CT normal	MR/CT may be abnormal—gray matter or white matter abnormal; atrophy

GLAUCOMA

Glaucoma is the most common optic neuropathy; progressive cupping of the optic disc due to increased intraocular pressure together with visual field abnormalities and local disc susceptibility factors characterize this neuropathy. We can think of it as papilledema in reverse. That is, the pressure of the eye in a sense causes compression on the disc from within the eye. Traditionally, glaucoma is divided into primary or secondary forms. Primary forms are considered to be closed-angle, chronic simple (open-angle), low-tension–open-angle, juvenile, and congenital.

Table 4-13. Defining the Glaucomas

Type	Characteristic features	Who gets it
Primary glaucoma		
Closed-angle	Prodrome ocular pain usually unilateral with closure along with blurred vision; pupil dilates, conjunctival edema. The disc does not acutely cup.	Shorter eyes (hyperopia) with smaller cornea, shallow anterior chamber, thicker lens that is more anterior. Inherited. Age—older. Eskimos (40 times more likely than in those with white European ancestry)
Open-angle (chronic simple)	Bilateral, but can affect eyes asymmetrically; insidious onset with no symptoms until visual field defects.	Increased intraocular pressure; hereditary; age (older)
Low-tension, normal pressure	Very insidious onset, with normal pressures; bilateral	Inheritance; myopia, age (older), black race, hypertension, vascular disease, migraine[19]
Congenital[20,28,29]	Classically, epiphora, photophobia, blepharospasm; older children may be asymptomatic	Associated with congenital anomalies (e.g., microcornea, neurofibromatosis); buphthalmos
Secondary glaucoma	Variable presentation depending on the condition causing it; open angle may present with progressive cupping; closed angle may be more acute	Eye formation abnormalities; inflammatory (uveitis), vascular (neovascularization), inherited developmental disorders, trauma and tumor; drugs; surgery (cataract)

Adapted from references 26–29.

Secondary forms of glaucoma are due to inflammatory, vascular, trauma, or tumor etiology in the eye. The most common form of glaucoma is chronic simple. Most primary care physicians and neurologists see patients with open-angle glaucoma and low-tension glaucoma. Knowing when to refer the patient for further evaluation and work-up by an ophthalmologist is the primary goal.

Primary glaucomatous optic neuropathy affects at least 2 million people in the United States. Over half of these have increased intraocular pressure, but a significant portion do not.[30] Prevalence of open-angle glaucoma is 1.2–2.1% of people and prevalence increases with age (0.9% ages 43–54, but 4.7% of people >75).[31]

Look for evidence of glaucoma, including cupping, nerve fiber layer defects, notching of the neuroretinal rim, nasalization of blood vessels, elongation of the vertical cup, and peripapillary atrophy.

Table 4-14. Features to Look for on the Disc for Evidence of Glaucoma

Features
Cupping
Nerve fiber layer defects (slits, especially temporally off the disc)
Notching of the neuroretinal rim
Nasalization of the blood vessels
Elongation of the vertical diameter of the cup
Asymmetry of cup-to-disc ratio from eye to eye
Hemorrhages at the disc margin and in the peripapillary disc region
Peripapillary disc atrophy
Atrophy of the optic disc

Adapted in part from reference 32.

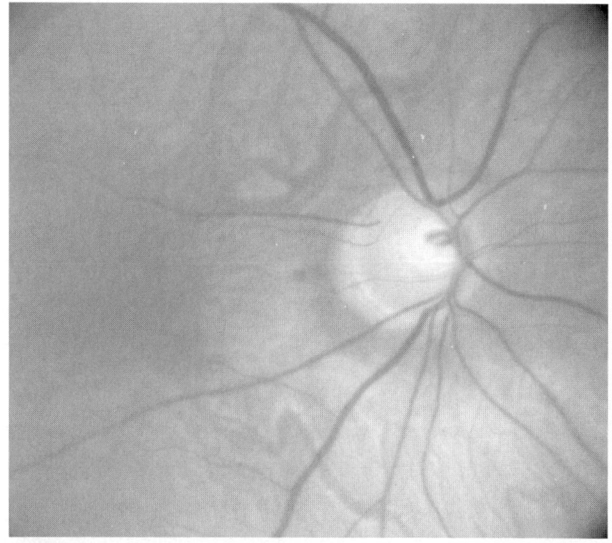

4-27A

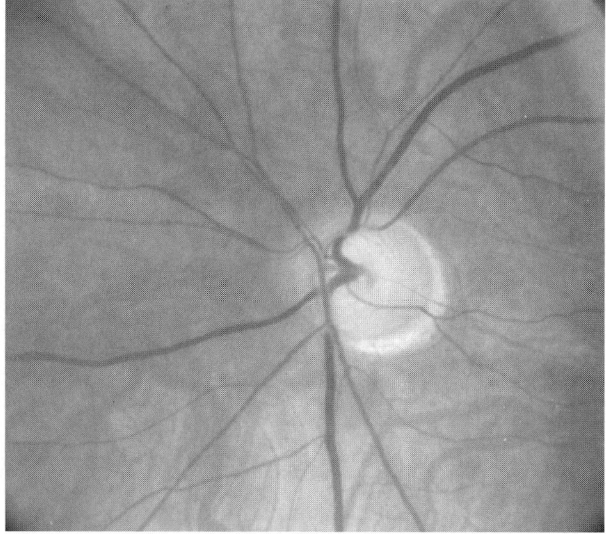

4-27B

Figure 4-27. A, B. **Appearance of the disc in glaucoma is determined first by an enlarged cup as the number of nerve fibers decrease. Notice how the vessels dive into the excavated cup at the neuroretinal rim. (Photographs courtesy of F. Jane Durcan, M.D.)**

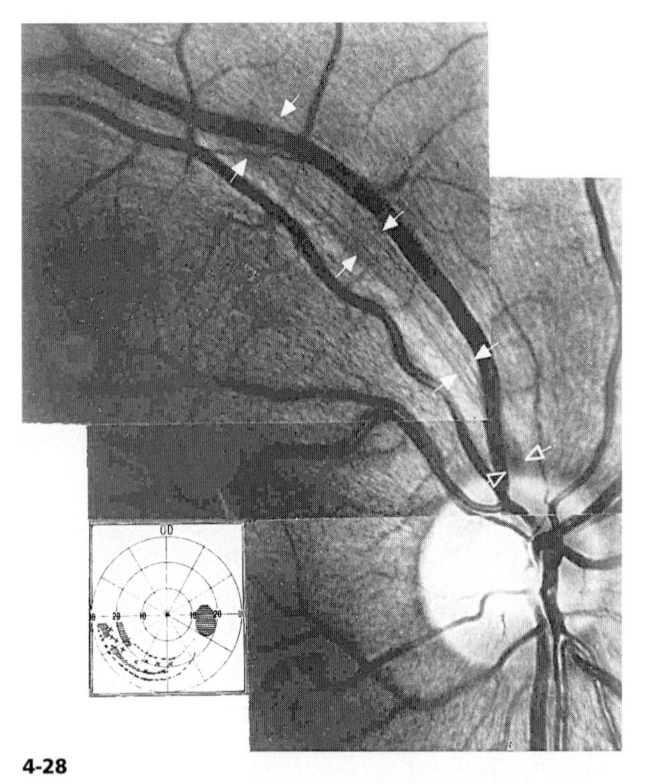

4-28

Figure 4-28. **The nerve fiber layer can show bundle defects. Use the green light (red-free) to view the nerve fiber in any one in whom you suspect glaucoma.[13] If you see a defect, frequently the visual field will be abnormal and show an arcuate or altitudinal defect even to confrontation testing. Here is an inferior arcuate (because it arcs from the disc) visual field defect. The open arrows show an almost wedge defect right at the disc. The other arrows outline the nerve fiber layer defect as it courses superiorly in the retina. (Photograph courtesy of William F. Hoyt, M.D.)**

Figure 4-29. A. **The neuroretinal rim becomes thinner; in particular the rim superotemporally and inferotemporally may develop a notch, which is usually superior or inferior and rarely nasal or temporal.[32]** B. **We have outlined the cup with the superior notch (*arrow*) so that the notching of the cup is accentuated. (Photograph courtesy of F. Jane Durcan, M.D.)**

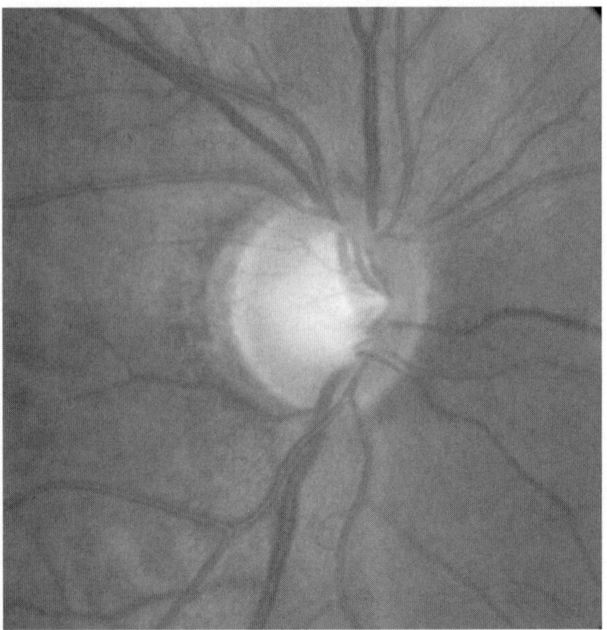

4-29A

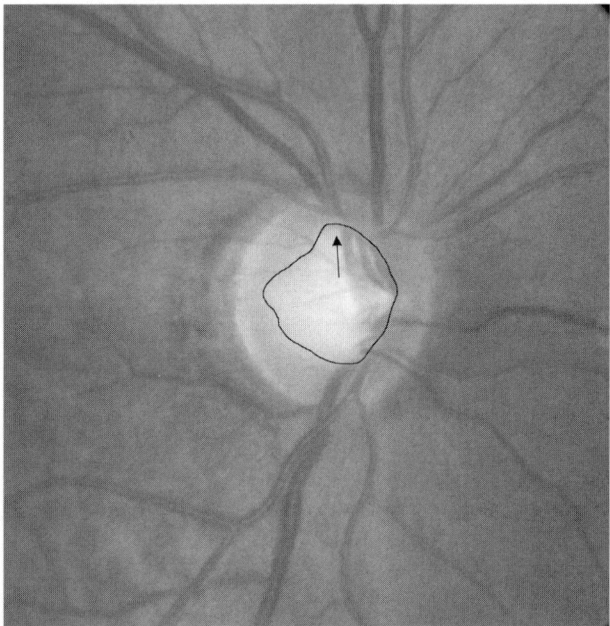

4-29B

Figure 4-30. A. The central retinal vessels become nasally displaced on the disc. Although vessel displacement is not specific to glaucoma, it is one way to recognize a large cup. Notice that this patient's fundus is tessellated, and you can easily see the choroidal vessels. B. Typical nasal displacement of vessels in glaucoma. Note also the extreme narrowing of the neuroretinal rim at 6 o'clock. (Photographs courtesy of F. Jane Durcan, M.D.)

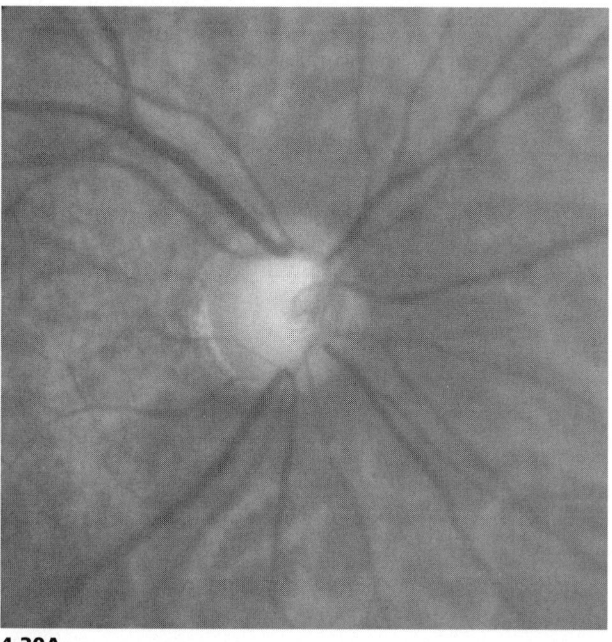

4-30A

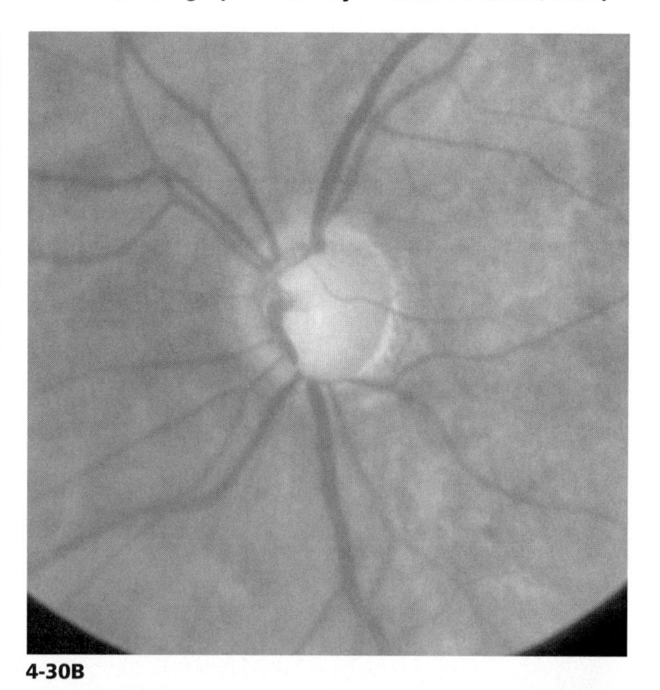

4-30B

Figure 4-31. A. Notching may increase to the edge of the neuroretinal rim—almost like an acquired pit. This patient has a superior arcuate defect. B. The neuroretinal rim is notched and elongated. We have outlined the area of the cup where it extends inferiorly.

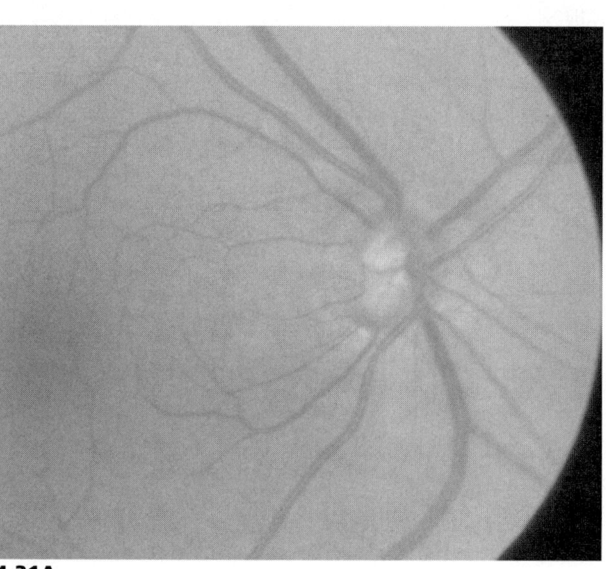

4-31A

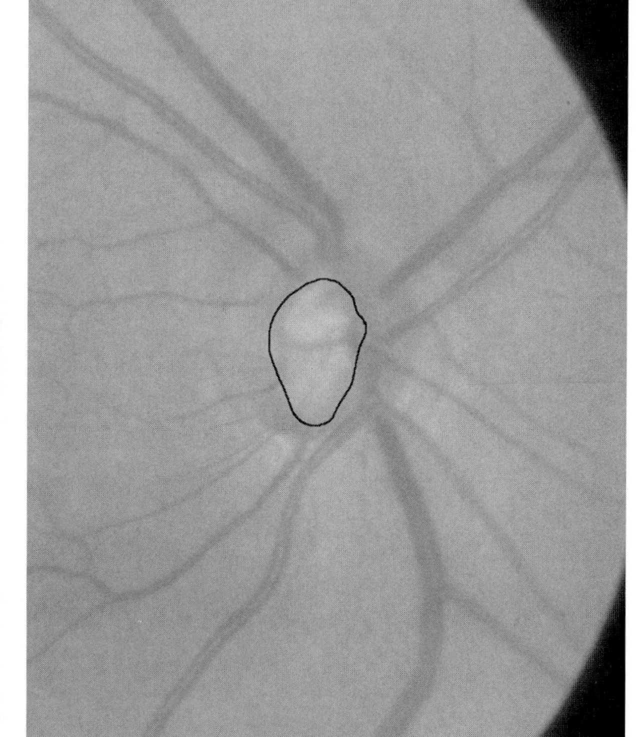

4-31B

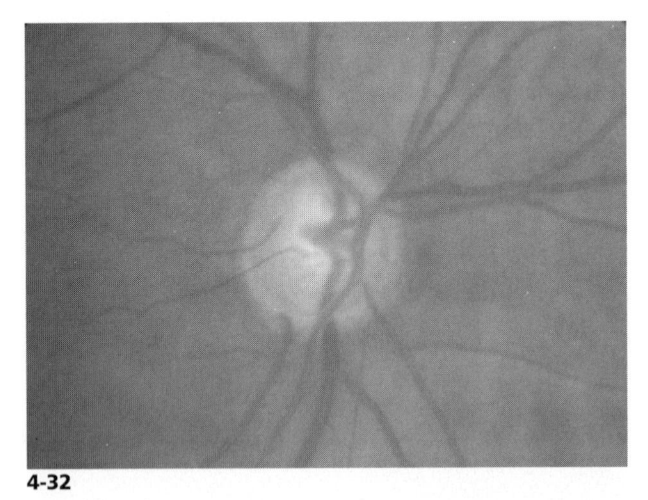

4-32

Figure 4-32. The cup may elongate. The vertical diameter of the cup may be greater than the horizontal diameter. As glaucoma progresses, the cup enlarges, the lamina cribrosa is pushed back, and vessels dive into the cup while the neuroretinal rim closes in. In fact, a vertical cup-to-disc ratio of greater than 0.6 is associated with a high probability of glaucoma. (Photograph courtesy of F. Jane Durcan, M.D.)

Figure 4-33. There is usually a difference between the cup size in each eye in glaucoma. The cup-to-disc ratio is about 0.6 on the right disc (A) **and 0.4 on the left disc** (B)**. Normally, cups are symmetric. When you see asymmetric cupping, think of glaucoma. (Photographs courtesy of F. Jane Durcan, M.D.)**

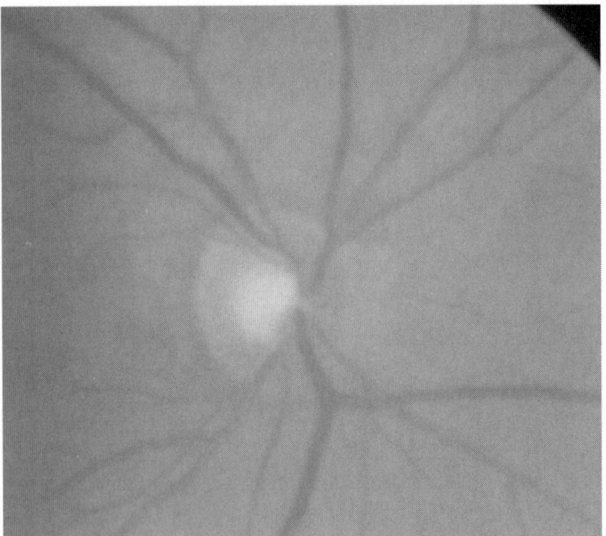

4-33A

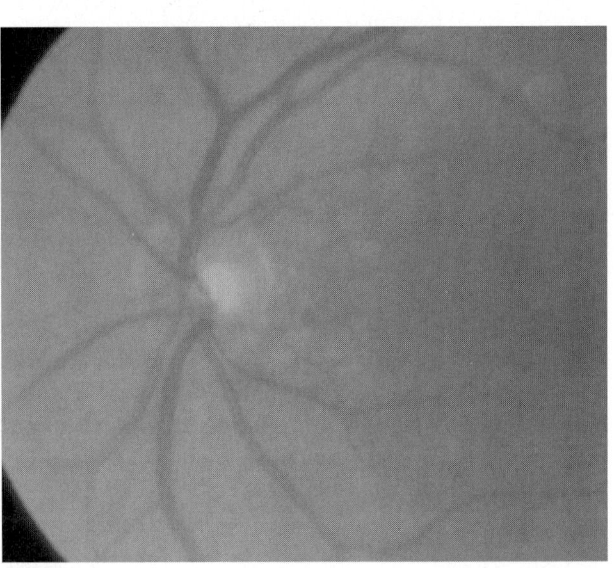

4-33B

Figure 4-34. Look for small hemorrhages at the disc margin in glaucoma. A. **Here you see a hemorrhage along the inferior margin of the disc (*arrow*). There is also a notch at about 3:30 on the disc.** B. **See the small splinter hemorrhage at approximately 7 o'clock at the disc margin (*arrow*).** C. **Peripapillary hemorrhages deep along the disc margin can also occur, such as in this case (*arrows*). (Photographs courtesy of F. Jane Durcan, M.D.)**

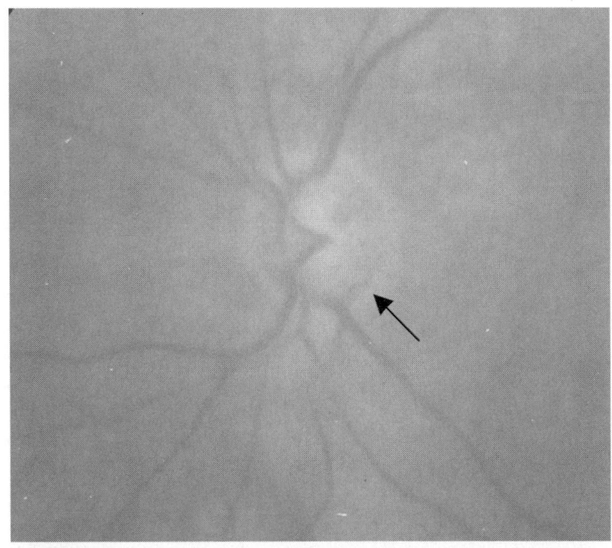

4-34A

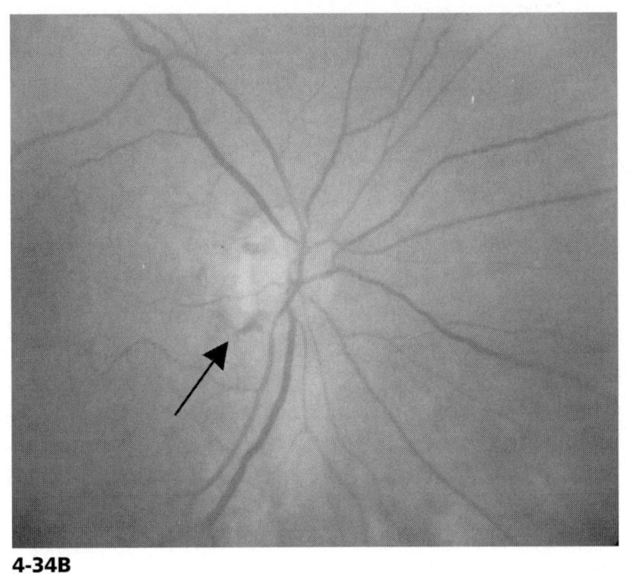

4-34B

4-34C

There may be small splinter hemorrhages at the disc margin (7–30% have such a hemorrhage). Although splinter hemorrhages are not specific for glaucoma, they are present with higher frequency in glaucoma.[33] Look for peripapillary atrophy—a partial or complete halo of choroidal or pigment epithelial atrophy. Interestingly, low tension glaucoma changes cannot be differentiated from high pressure glaucoma changes—they appear the same.

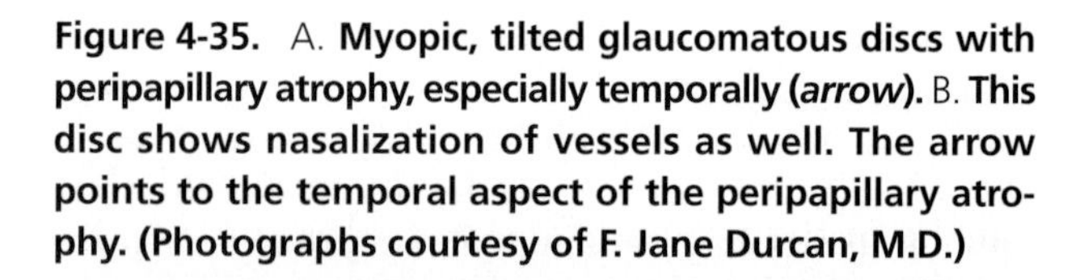
Figure 4-35. A. **Myopic, tilted glaucomatous discs with peripapillary atrophy, especially temporally (*arrow*).** B. **This disc shows nasalization of vessels as well. The arrow points to the temporal aspect of the peripapillary atrophy. (Photographs courtesy of F. Jane Durcan, M.D.)**

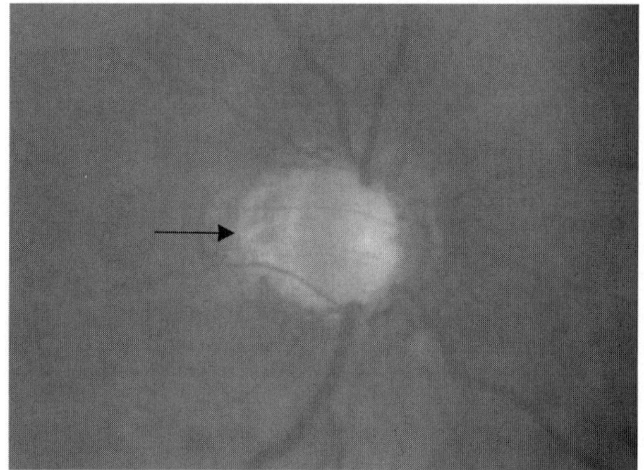
4-35A

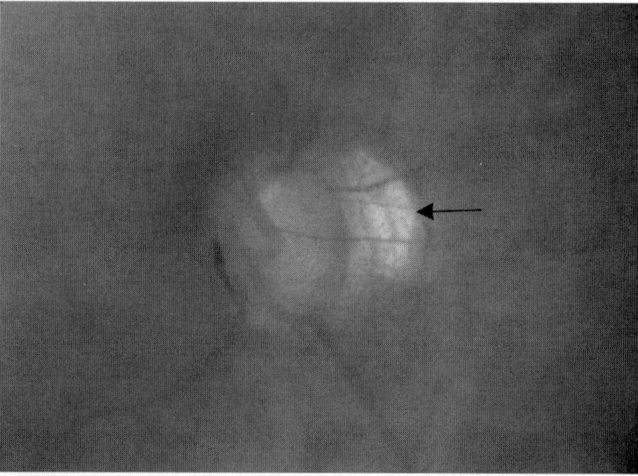
4-35B

Many patients with myopia and glaucoma have tilted discs with a scleral crescent, enlarged cups and shallow discs with thinning of the neuroretinal rim superiorly and inferiorly. Peripapillary atrophy occurs with aging, myopia, and glaucoma. Therefore, observing the peripapillary area is important.[32]

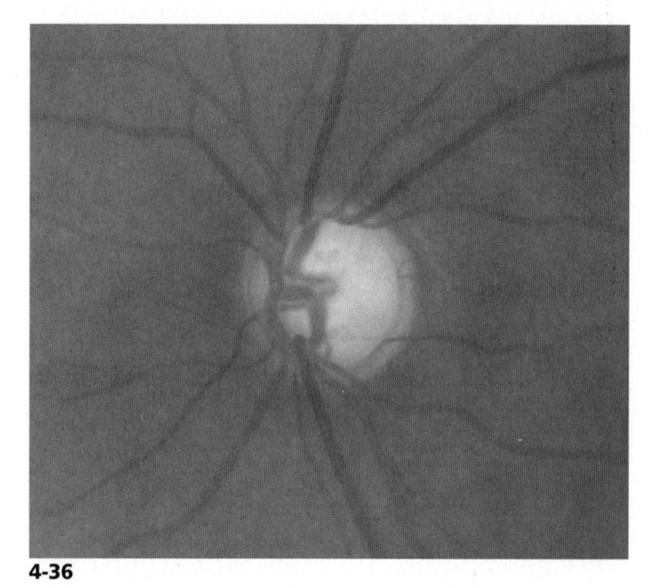
4-36

Figure 4-36. Atrophic glaucomatous discs show thinning of the neuroretinal rim, "saucerization" (i.e., shallow cupping), evidence of peripapillary atrophy, and pallor of the neuroretinal rim.[32] Some of these will also have retinochoroidal collateral vessels. (See Chapter 5, Retinochoroidal Collaterals with Glaucoma, Figure 5-36.) (Photograph courtesy of F. Jane Durcan, M.D.)

If there are any "angle closure attacks," symptoms are more dramatic. Although angle closure may affect both eyes, symptoms are in one eye. There may be prodromal attacks, which are similar to acute attacks, but much milder. Acute angle closure with very high intraocular pressure causes blurred vision, even markedly decreased to light perception; halos may be observed, especially around lights; pain—sometimes intense—around the eye radiating to the temple; eyelid edema; tearing; congestion of the conjunctiva (red eye); and the pupil may be mid-position and fixed to light. The pain with glaucoma attacks may be in the eye or in the brow, and is usually a steady ache but may have the features of migraine, including nausea, vomiting, fatigue, and anxiety.

Table 4-15. Causes of Cupping That Mimic Glaucoma

AION (especially arteritic form)
Congenital disc anomalies (coloboma and optic nerve pits)
Optic nerve compression (Graves', tumors)
Chiasmal compression
Toxic neuropathies

In many of these cases of cupping due to conditions that mimic glaucoma (Table 4-15), the residual neuroretinal rim is paler than in glaucoma.[13] However, MR will be needed for definitive diagnosis in some of these situations.

The main thinking about the etiology of glaucoma has always centered around the pressure within the eye as a mechanical force producing cupping and vision loss. These forces alter the lamina cribrosa itself and alter axonal transport. However, vascular factors are rising in importance as the increased recognition of low pressure or normal pressure glaucoma demands that alternative explanations be considered. Furthermore, individual genetic susceptibility to these factors is now known to play an important role.[34]

COMPRESSION AS A CAUSE OF BILATERAL OPTIC ATROPHY

When a mass in the suprasellar space or frontal lobe compresses the intracranial portion of the optic nerve and chiasm, optic atrophy and optic nerve pallor bilaterally ensue.

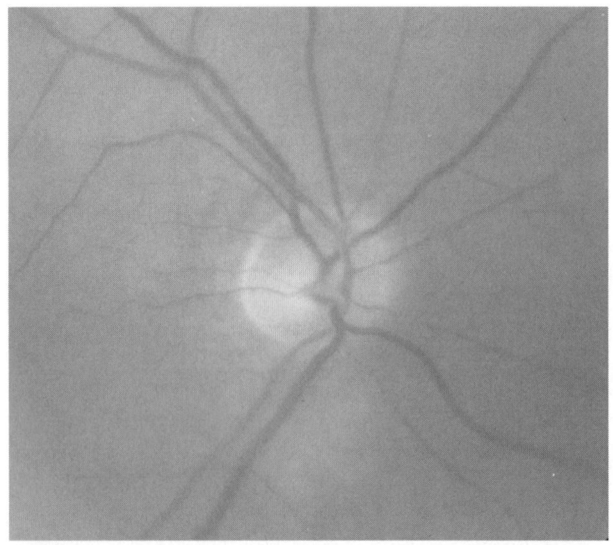

4-37A

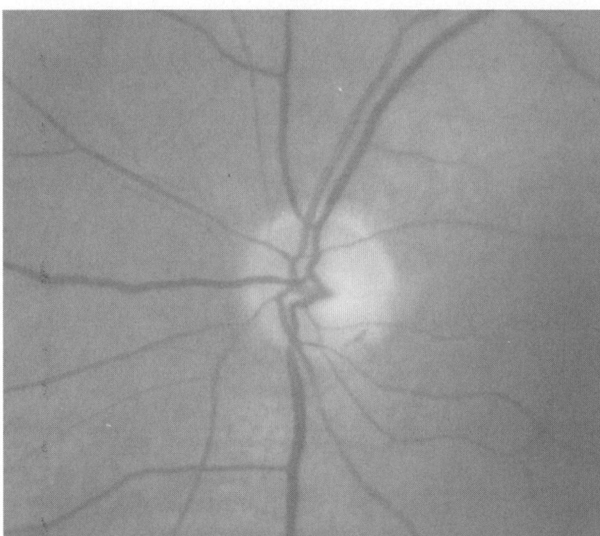

4-37B

Frontal lobe tumors, especially those arising from the olfactory groove, such as meningiomas, can go undetected for some time. A presentation of disc swelling in one eye and atrophy in the other eye, Foster Kennedy syndrome, was discussed in Chapter 3 on disc swelling. However, if the compression is gradual and severe, frontal lobe tumors can also present with bilateral optic atrophy.

Even very large pituitary tumors rarely cause papilledema. They also very rarely cause visual field defects and optic atrophy until they are very large. Microadenomas cause no vision loss. Small and medium-sized tumors, unless located strategically under the optic nerve, do not cause vision loss. Large tumors cause remarkably small visual field defects, and only huge tumors cause major field loss in the majority of patients.

Craniopharyngiomas compressing the chiasm cause swelling of the optic discs and subsequent profound atrophy out of proportion to the size of the tumor. These tumors are very destructive of nerve tissue, which may be related to chemical meningitis, secondary to leakage from the cystic components of the tumor as well as the mass effect.

Figure 4-37. This elderly man presented with progressive vision loss and pale optic discs. A pituitary adenoma was found. A. **Right eye,** (B) **left eye.** C. **The MR shows a large pituitary adenoma with extension toward the left, giving a slightly more atrophic nerve on the left.**

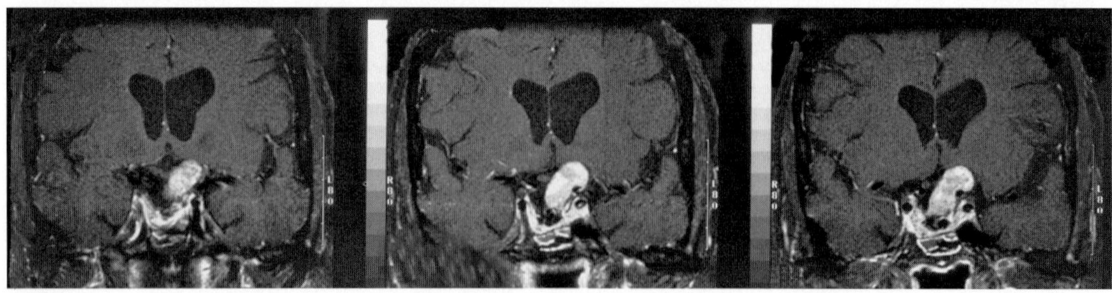

4-37C

Figure 4-38. These discs are severely pale due to a craniopharyngioma. The atrophy was profound even though the tumor was not excessively large.

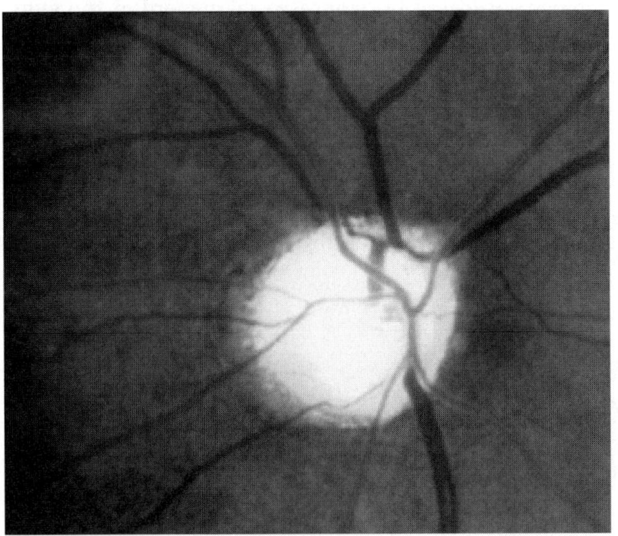

4-38A

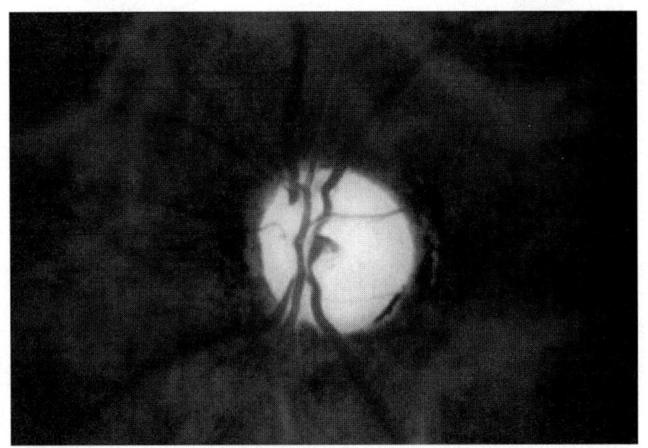

4-38B

Chiasmal compression has several symptoms that are worth remembering. Besides the complaint of slowly progressive vision loss and dimming of the temporal visual field in each eye, patients complain of loss of depth perception (such as used in threading a needle) and diplopia, not only due to a cranial nerve (III, IV, or VI paresis) but also due to a phenomenon called *hemifield slide* .

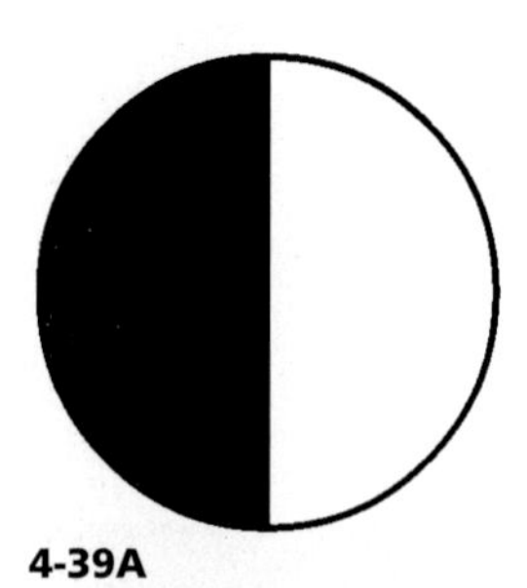

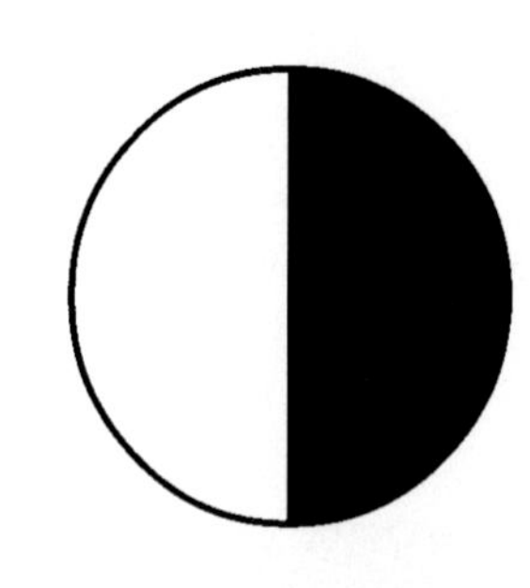

Figure 4-39. A. **The typical visual field of chiasmal compression is a bitemporal hemianopia.** B. **Hemifield slide occurs due to the loss of the temporal visual fields when the nasal fields of each eye may not fuse because there is a minor vertical or horizontal misalignment of the eyes. The result is a kind of diplopia. Below is a copy of the printed phrase that a woman with bitemporal hemianopia made to show us what this looked like to her.**

4-39A

How to apply
People who think they or someone they know may be eligible for SSI can apply, or get more information, by contacting any social security office.

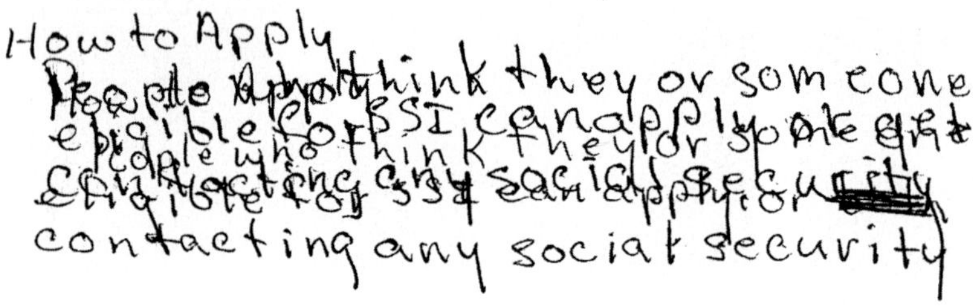

4-39B

BAND ATROPHY

Learn also to recognize the pattern of pallor in this chiasmal compression. It is one of the few "localizing" forms of bilateral segmental pallor, called *band atrophy.* To understand the appearance, you must understand the anatomy. First, the crossing nerve fibers, which are compressed in chiasmal lesions, have their cell bodies in the *nasal* hemi-retina; this gives the bitemporal visual field defect. When thinking about the pattern of atrophy associated with chiasmal compression, make the fovea the center of the retina as the dividing portion between the nasal and temporal half of the fovea.

Figure 4-40. (opposite page) A. **The diagram shows the temporal fibers from the retina, which course through the chiasm uncrossed and are usually not the first to be compressed, whereas the nasal fibers, which are the crossing fibers, become atrophic. This area will be pale.** B. **This disc displays band optic atrophy. Because the nasal hemifield fibers are lost, a band of fibers on both sides of the disc serving the nasal retina and nasal macula will be atrophic, giving the "band" or "bow-tie" appearance. This disc shows band atrophy due to a suprasular meningioma compressing the chiasm.**

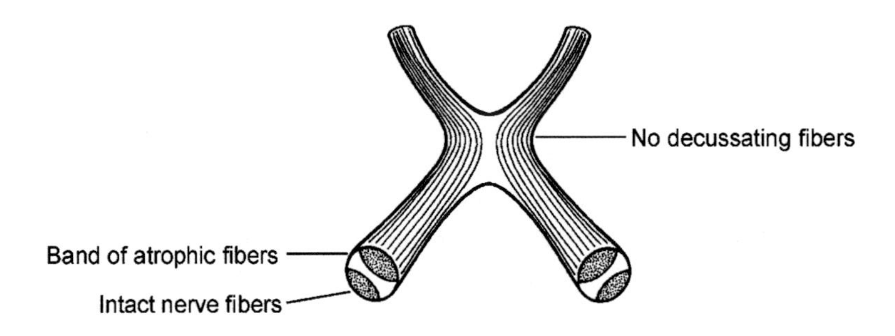

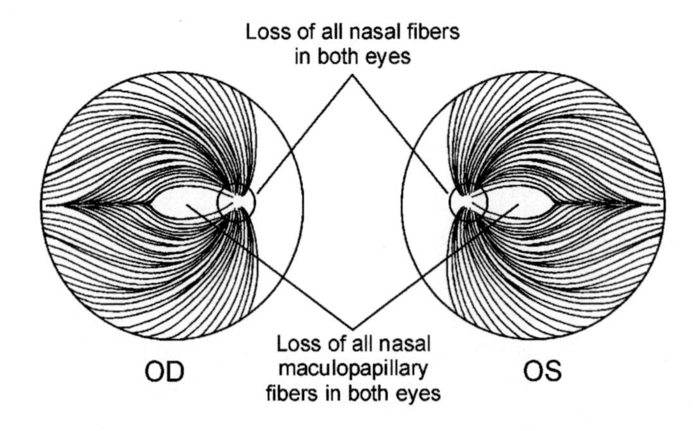

Failure of development or traumatic disruption of chiasmal crossing fibers produces bilateral "band atrophy"

4-40A

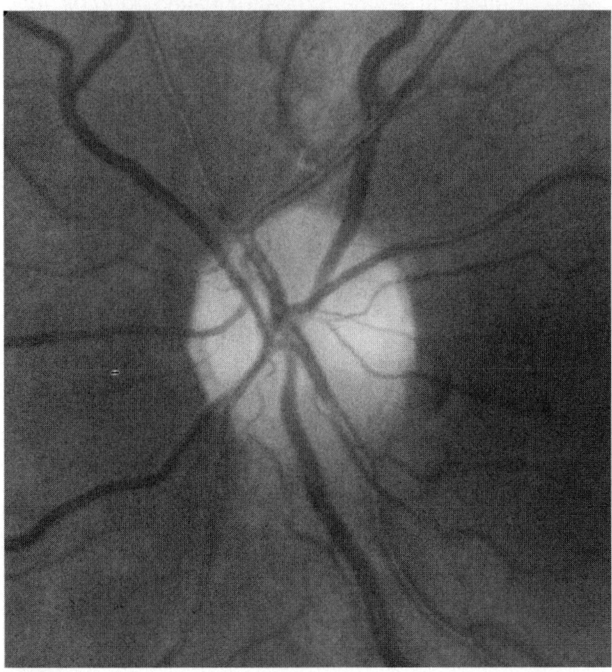

4-40B

Gowers described band atrophy of tract origin early on in his monograph:

In the case of longest duration, in which the hemiopia was persistently complete, in the course of years the whole of the disc of the eye in which the area lost was on the temporal (and therefore greatest), became perceptibly paler than the other, the tint of the two being at first equal. A similar slight pallor of the disc opposite to the cerebral lesion has been noted by others in cases of hemiopia of long duration.[36]

Figure 4-41. This young girl developed hydrocephalus after a motor vehicle accident and closed head injury. Notice the band atrophy in both discs (*arrows*) (A and B)**; The MR axial** (C) **and coronal** (D) **scans show splaying of the chiasm.**

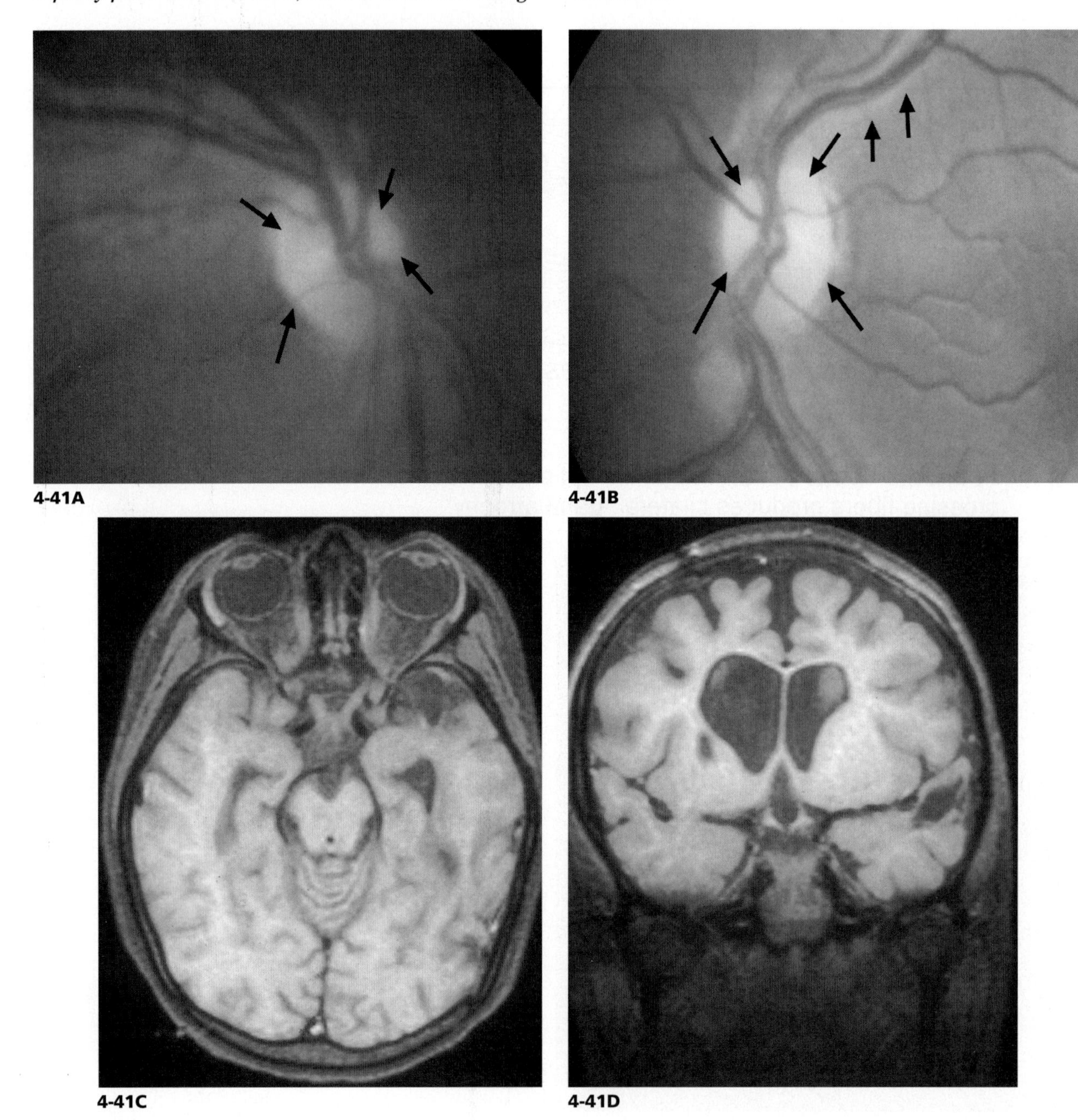

Figure 4-42. A. This young man had chiasmal neuritis as part of his global picture of multiple sclerosis. He, too, shows a form of band atrophy. B. The arrows outline the dropout of the nerve fiber layer. C. Axial contrast-enhanced MR showing enhancement of the left optic nerve into the chiasm (*arrow*). D. Coronal contrast-enhanced MR showing enhancement of the left optic nerve and chiasm (*arrow*). *Continued*

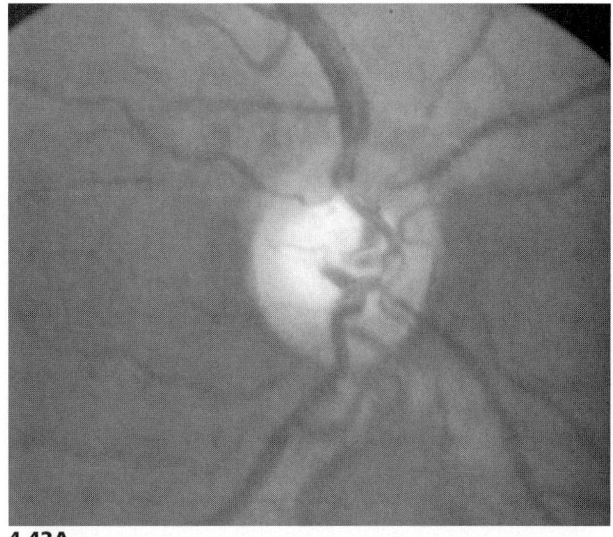

4-42A

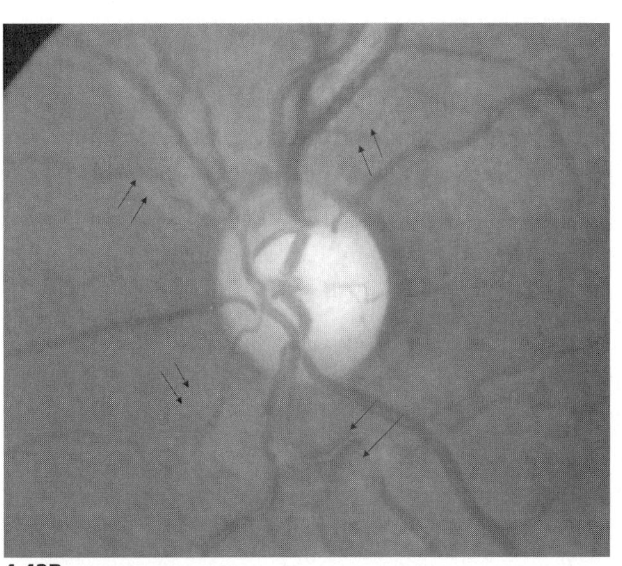

4-42B

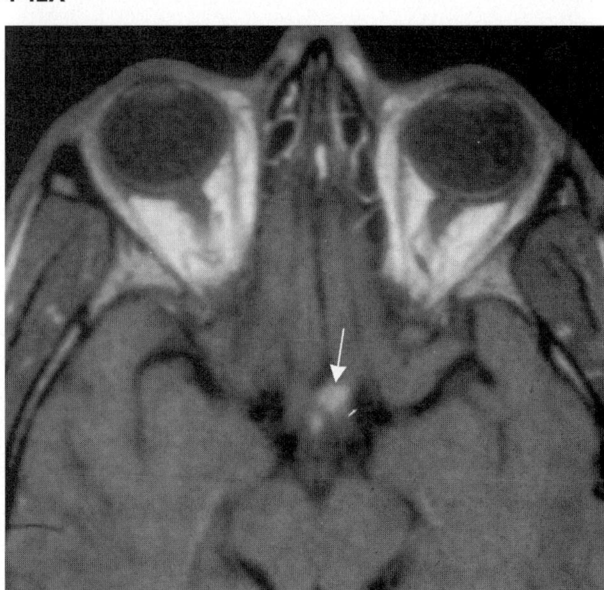

4-42C

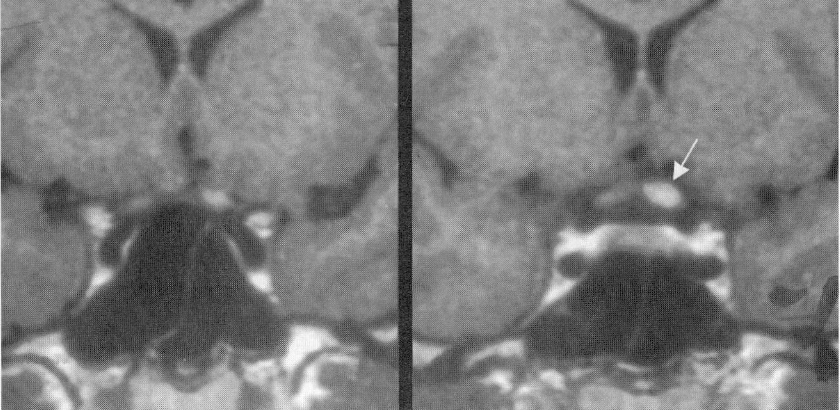

4-42D

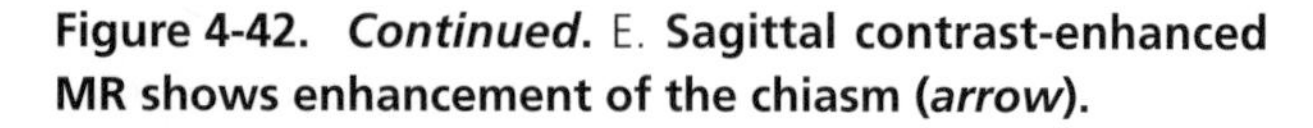

Figure 4-42. ***Continued.*** E. **Sagittal contrast-enhanced MR shows enhancement of the chiasm (*arrow*).**

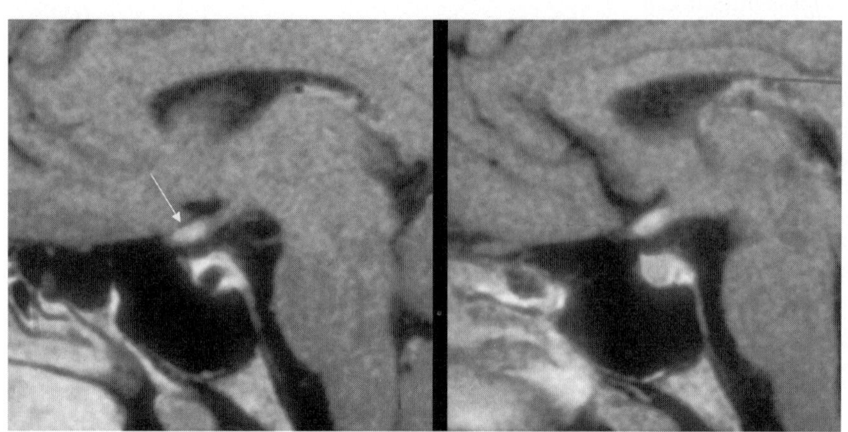

4-42E

OPTIC ATROPHY OWING TO OPTIC TRACT DISEASE

Parasellar lesions may also compress the optic tract with a variably complete homonymous hemianopia. A tract lesion can also cause a distinct bilateral segmental atrophy that is recognizable. In the eye that is contralateral to the lesion—the temporal field eye—the nasal retinal ganglion axons are compressed. Therefore, in the optic tract damage, only the contralateral disc has the band atrophy appearance and the ipsilateral disc may look normal or slightly atrophic with temporal pallor, as opposed to the chiasmal lesion, with loss of the nasal hemi-retinal nerve fiber layer in both eyes. Another clinical clue to a tract lesion, aside from the appearance of the optic disc, is a relative afferent pupillary defect in the contralateral (band atrophy) eye in which 30% more of nasal fibers are lost.

Figure 4-43. A. **This individual had a left tract lesion with acquired band atrophy in the contralateral eye (right eye) and only slight pallor in the ipsilateral eye (left eye). Pathology of tract homonymous is quite distinct.[35] (See also Figure 4-40B.)** ***Continued***

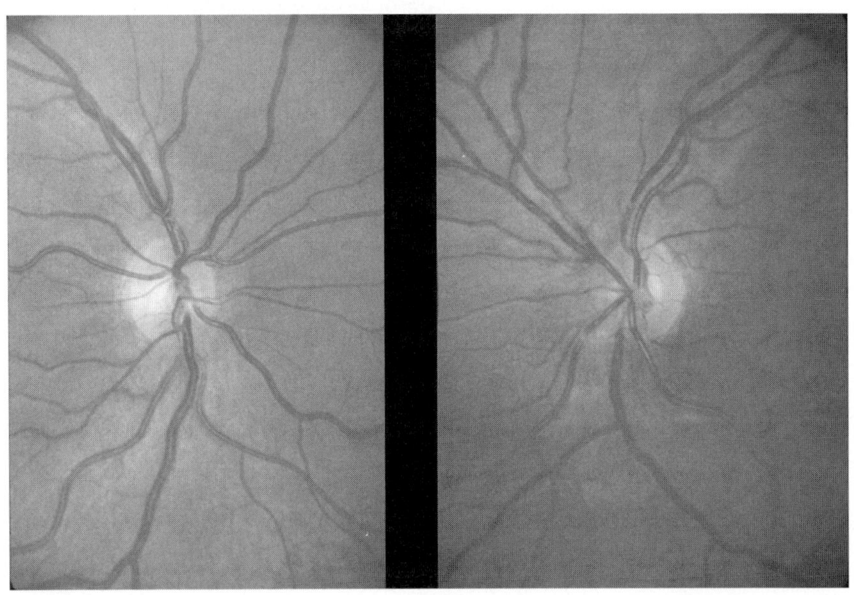

4-43A

Figure 4-43. ***Continued.*** B. **The nasal crossing fibers and the temporal fibers from the same side in the optic tract give a distinct band atrophy in the contralateral eye to the compression. The ipsilateral disc may look diffusely pale or normal (see the caption of Figure 11-9). (Reprinted with permission from reference 39.)**

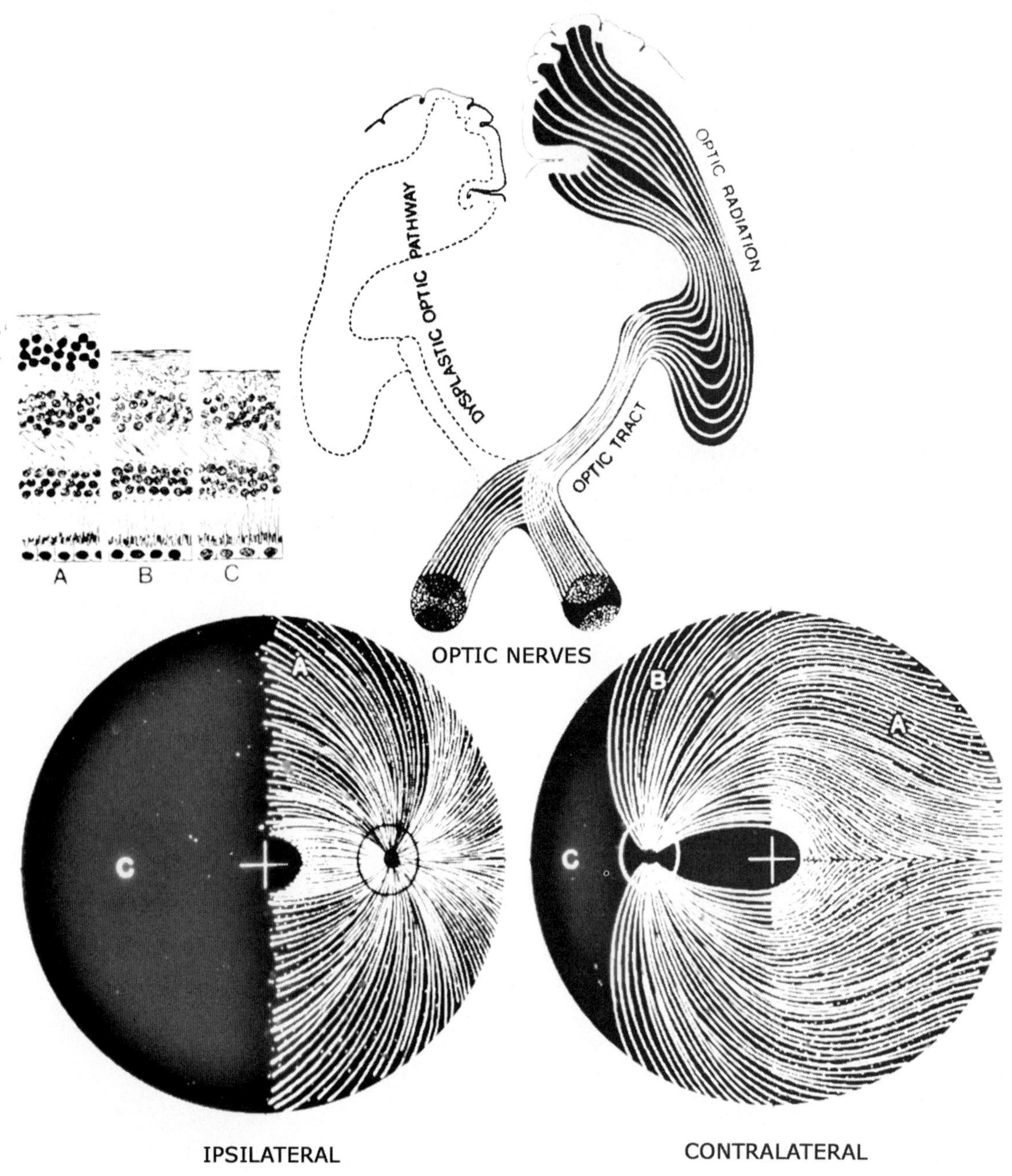

4-43B

Figure 4-44. This young woman suffered a stroke affecting her right occipital lobe at a young age. A. **She had a left homonymous hemianopia and typical findings of a tract lesion: mild diffuse pallor in her right eye (ipsilateral to the lesion) and contralateral band atrophy** (B) **contralateral to the lesion.** C. **MR showing atrophy of the right tract and occipital lobe.**

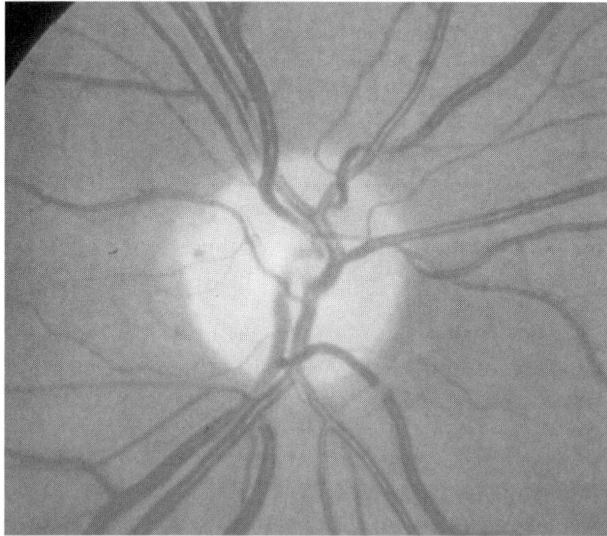

4-44A

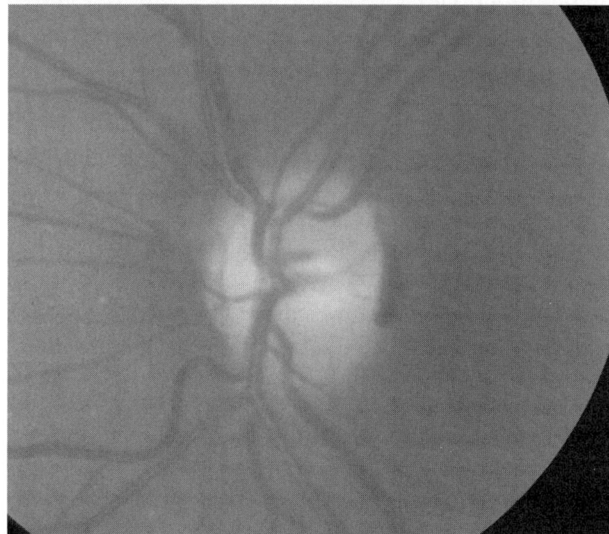

4-44B

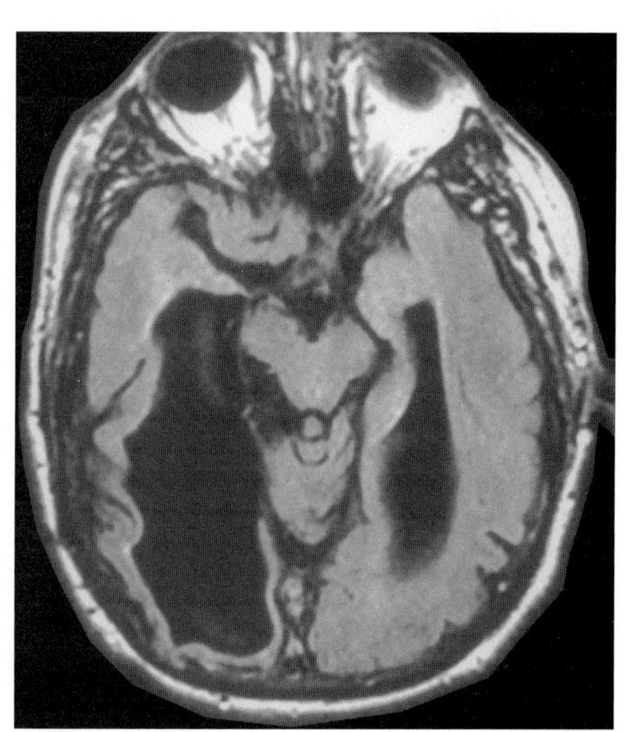

4-44C

Lesions of the lateral geniculate give typical visual field defects depending on what part of the geniculate is damaged, but the optic atrophy appears similar to the atrophy seen in a tract lesion. The usual cause of such a defect is infarction of the lateral (sometimes called *posterior choroidal*) choroidal artery, usually a branch off of the posterior cerebral artery,[37] or the anterior choroidal artery, a branch off of the internal carotid artery.

Related to tract lesions, *congenital homonymous hemioptic hypoplasia* —caused by a lesion (not typically compression, but because the disc defect is again segmental, it is included here) acquired at an early age (usually before or at birth)—has a characteristic disc pattern as well. First, these lesions are usually from congenital or early in utero occipital damage, although optic tract lesions can also occur; therefore, the characteristic disc appearance with this lesion is the result of transsynaptic degeneration. Second, the cause of congenital hemianopia can be variable—cerebral hemiatrophy, vascular malformation, porencephalic cysts, or in utero strokes. Third, and typically, patients are really unaware of their visual field defect.[38] The disc in the contralateral eye shows the band or bow-tie atrophy due to loss of the nasal retinal hemifield fibers. The ipsilateral eye shows atrophy and loss of nerve fibers superior and inferior on the disc. The other characteristic described by Hoyt is the slightly small optic discs bilaterally (hence, *hypoplasia* was added to the name).[39]

Table 4-16. Ophthalmoscopic Features of Hemioptic Defect

Feature	Ipsilateral to hemispheric defect	Contralateral to hemispheric defect
Disc size	Small	Small
Disc shape	Round	Vertically slightly oval
Disc color	Pallor temporally	Band atrophy
Vessels on the disc	Reduced number temporally	Reduced number nasal and temporal
Nerve fiber layer	Slight decrease temporally	See arcuate fiber loss temporal and nasally
Foveal reflex	Distinct nasal; less distinct temporal	Indistinct nasal; normal temporal

Adapted from reference 39.

Table 4-17. Other Causes of Compressive Bilateral Optic Atrophy

- Tumors
  - Meningioma—frontal, sphenoidal, bilateral nerve sheath
  - Craniopharyngioma
  - Pituitary adenoma (prolactinoma, growth hormone secreting)
  - Dysgerminomas (parasellar)
  - Gliomas
  - Metastatic disease
- Aneurysms
- Cysts (arachnoidal)
- Sphenoidal mucocele
- Fibrous dysplasia
- Craniosynostosis
- Osteopetrosis

Figure 4-45. A young man with a right optic neuropathy—notice the difference in the two discs (right eye, A; left eye, B)—from compression of the right optic canal due to fibrous dysplasia, shown here with computed tomography axial (C) and coronal (D) scans. The arrows show the dysplastic bone of the optic canal. Fibrous dysplasia can cause a slowly progressive unilateral or bilateral optic neuropathy. Acute vision loss is also due to hemorrhage from dysplastic bone. The radiographic findings are usually diagnostic.[40]

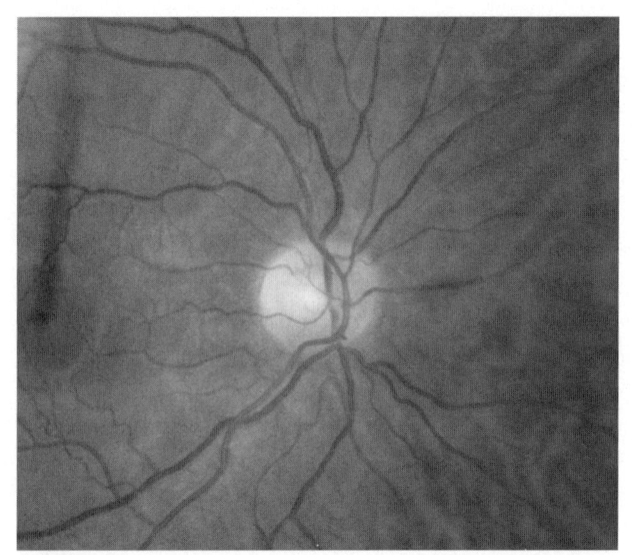

4-45A

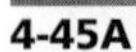

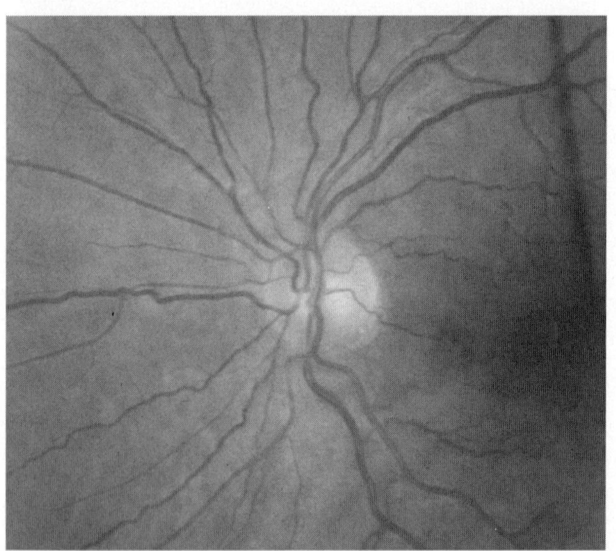

4-45B

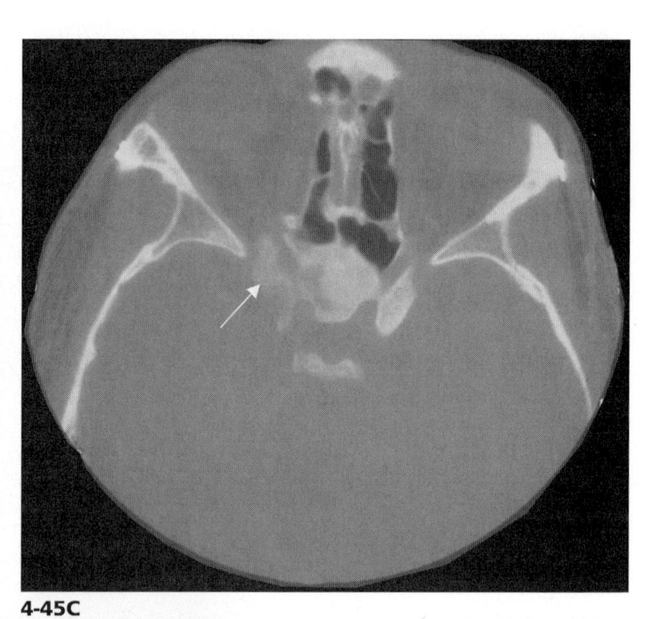

4-45C

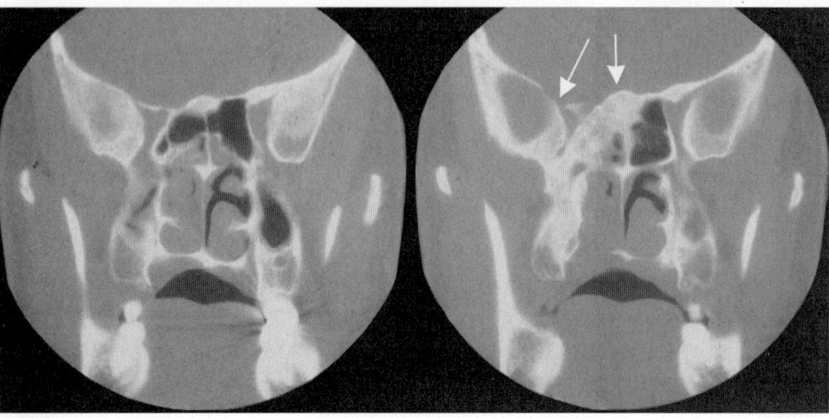

4-45D

OPTIC ATROPHY—ISCHEMIA

Ischemic causes of bilateral optic atrophy include bilateral AION (after the swelling is gone), bilateral PION from arteritis or after systemic hypotension due to spontaneous or iatrogenic hemorrhage, or lumbar disc surgery. Because we have already discussed AION in the chapter on optic disc swelling (Chapter 3), here we discuss the syndrome of bilateral PION.[41]The associations with this type of ischemic damage include severe blood loss after any type of surgical procedure, without documented hypotension; with prolonged hypotension, especially in individuals with anemia; lumbosacral back surgery—thought to be partially due to improper positioning with the face down causing globe compression, and the use of hypotension to reduce bleeding,[42] but also reported in those with proper positioning[43,44]; and coronary bypass surgery.[22]

Table 4-18. Reported Causes of Unilateral or Bilateral AION or PION following Surgical or Medical Procedures

Cardiopulmonary bypass surgery (most frequently reported)
Lumbar disc surgery
Large amount of blood loss
Bilateral radical neck dissection
Coronary catheterization
Cardiac arrest
Cardiomyoplasty
Hip surgery
Mitral valve surgery
Cholecystectomy
Parathyroidectomy
Hemodialysis
Pneumonectomy

Adapted from reference 44.

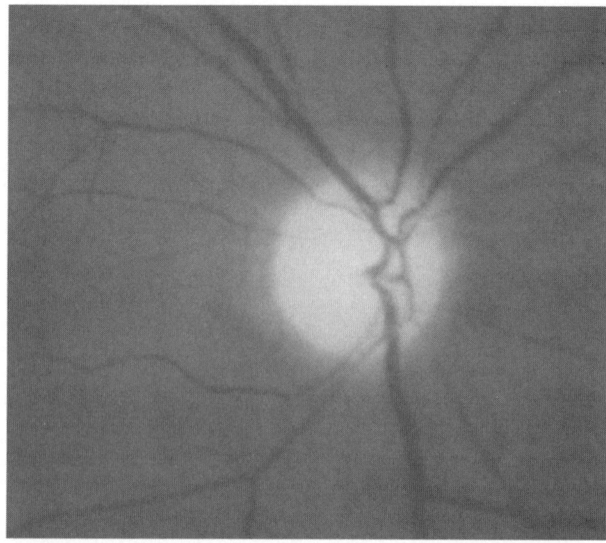

4-46A

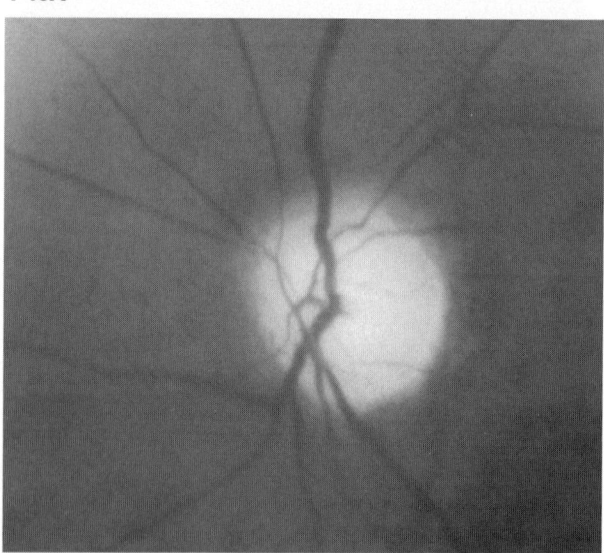

4-46B

The exact etiology of bilateral blindness after blood loss and surgery is not known, but the vision loss is thought to be caused by release of vasopressin and catecholamines, causing a vasospasm and infarction of the posterior optic nerve.[44] Presurgical anemia, blood loss at the time of surgery, and hypotension may be other important factors. The disc with a small cup may be at risk for ischemic damage. When the patient awakens from surgery or is examined after an injury with the complaint, "I can't see," vision loss is severe. The appearance of the optic nerve immediately after the insult may show only slight swelling of the disc, but more often there is no distinctive feature. The key to the diagnosis of the cause of the vision loss is a poor or absent pupillary light reflex. When the bilateral disc atrophy ensues in 6–8 weeks, the diagnosis of PION is made.

Occasionally, when the pupil reflexes are normal, the bilateral vision loss is secondary to occipital ischemia causing cerebral blindness. This may partially resolve, leaving unilateral or bilateral homonymous hemianopia. Rarely, acute chiasmal apoplexy can present as bilateral vision loss. These and other potential conditions can be sorted out clinically and radiographically.

Figure 4-46. This older woman had cardiac bypass surgery and minor hypotension. She awoke blind with normal optic nerves. Within 6–8 weeks, severe optic atrophy became apparent. A. **Right disc pallor, severe and diffuse.** B. **Left disc pallor, severe and diffuse.**

Post-papilledema optic atrophy occurs after papilledema has resolved. See discussion of papilledema and its formation.

The appearance of optic atrophy following papilledema is distinctive. The disc is generally pale and the surface is gliotic. There may also be intraretinal "high water marks," which are lipoproteinaceous exudates and pigment in the peripapillary area. Finally, the vessels may be sheathed with glia. Post-papilledema atrophy does not occur in all eyes that have had papilledema, but in patients who had swollen discs years before and were unaware of it, the appearance of post-papilledema atrophy may be confusing in the analysis of their fundus.

Figure 4-47. After the acute swelling diminished (A), **this man was left with bilaterally pale optic discs from increased intracranial pressure.** B. **Note the "high water marks" (*arrowheads*) as well as the pigmentary changes around the disc. There is also some gliosis (*arrows*).**

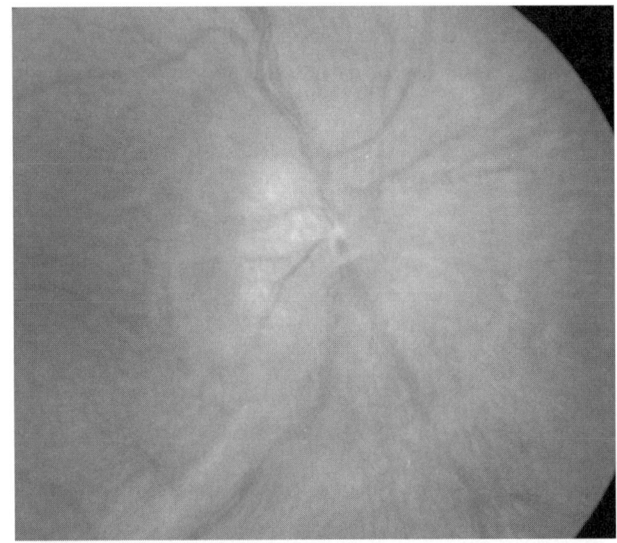

4-47A

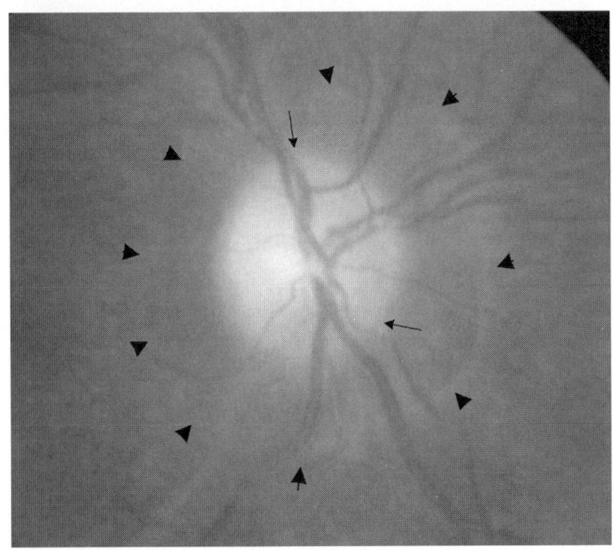

4-47B

TOXIC OPTIC NEUROPATHY

Toxic/nutritional abnormalities cause bilateral optic neuropathy and retinopathy. Bilateral vision loss can be the toxic manifestation of certain drugs that damage the retinal elements (rods and cones), the support cells (amacrine cells) in the retina, the ganglion cells, or the axons that make up the optic nerve. Toxins can be multifactorial and may affect the system at more than one location. Sometimes it is difficult to distinguish toxic retinopathy from optic neuropathy, especially if the damage is in the central visual pathway (like the macula or maculopapular bundle). In general, peripheral retinal damage causes constriction of the visual pathway (constriction of the visual fields) with normal visual acuity. Damage to the retinal pigment epithelium causes a pigmentary change in the retinal appearance (see Retina). If the toxic effect is on the ganglion cells or axons, axoplasmic flow leads to bilateral disc swelling, changes in the retinal nerve fiber layer, and residual gliosis. Optic nerve and ganglion cell damage may depress the central visual acuity. Most toxins or medications produce symmetric changes in the optic nerve or retina unless the toxin is injected into the blood supply of the optic nerve. Although many of the agents listed below also cause an initial disc swelling or hyperemia, eventually these toxins or deficiencies cause atrophy. Toxic optic neuropathy and nutritional deficiency optic neuropathy should be included in the differential diagnosis for retrobulbar optic neuritis, optic atrophy, amblyopia, and central scotoma.[45–60]

Bedside evaluation should include Snellen visual acuity, color vision testing, Amsler grid testing, and, occasionally, visual evoked potentials and focal electroretinogram (see Table 4-19, Chapter 9 [retinal toxins, Table 9-16], and Chapter 10 [macular toxins, Table 10-10]).

For a complete list of drugs reported to cause optic neuropathy, see Lessel.[45]

Anti-tuberculous drugs have been associated with optic nerve damage. The drugs involved include ethambutol and isoniazide. Ethambutol appears to have dose-related toxicity such that the incidence increases with higher doses: 15% incidence at 50 mg/kg per day; 5% incidence at 25 mg/kg per day; 1% incidence at 15 mg/kg per day. Visual acuity can be monitored monthly with periodic visual field analysis.[60]

There are common themes in toxic optic neuropathies. Can you recognize toxic optic neuropathy by appearance of the optic disc?

Appearance, in general, is one of three things: (1) swelling—slight and diffuse, bilateral and symmetric, (2) hyperemia followed by atrophy—usually temporally because the papillomacular bundle seems to be most often affected, (3) slowly developing temporal atrophy (1–5 clock hours on the disc), and (4) loss of visual acuity and color vision.

Table 4-19. Toxic/Nutritional Agents Associated with Neuropathy

Agent	Toxic sequelae and symptoms	Optic nerve	Diagnosis/special treatment
Nutritional deficiencies			
Thiamine (? Folate)	Ophthalmoplegia, ptosis; altered mental state; loss of memory; Wernicke's encephalopathy	Optic neuropathy—slight disc swelling; cecocentral scotoma; hemorrhages can be seen early on	Thiamine and folic acid
B_{12}	Caused usually by pernicious anemia; myelopathy due to posterior column dysfunction; dementia	Bilateral central and cecocentral scotoma; may see sub-clinical abnormalities on visual evoked potential (VEP)	B_{12} level; complete blood cell count, bone marrow evaluation; treat with IM hydroxycobalamin
Starvation	Vision loss, peripheral neuropathy	Cecocentral scotoma	Replace vitamins; feed
Drugs			
Ethambutaol[47,48]	Used for tuberculosis (TB) treatment; dose related; usually after 7 mos	Color loss: blue-yellow first; central scotoma; rare disc swelling	Stop the drug—follow color, visual acuity; usually improves
Isoniazid[49]	Used for TB treatment; causes peripheral neuropathy; dose related	0.6–6.0% optic neuropathy and increases with dosage; hyperemia first sign, then temporal atrophy; cecocentral scotoma	Follow with color vision, contrast sensitivity; treat with pyridoxine
Rifampin	Tx TB; causes peripheral neuropathy, seizure, encephalopathy	Cecocentral scotomas; disc swelling; dyschromatopsia	Stop drug and take pyridoxine
Chloramphenicol[50]	Tx certain infections; causes anemia	Optic neuritis with loss of central visual acuity; dyschromatopsia, swollen discs; causes ganglion cell loss	Stop the drug; occasionally reversible
Amiodarone[51]	Tx arrhythmias; decreases thyroid hormone, causes tremor; peripheral neuropathy; corneal keratopathy	Disc swelling both from axoplasmic stasis (ischemia) and increased intracranial pressure	Follow color vision and fundus photographs 2 times each yr
Perhexiline maleate[52]	Anti-anginal medication; can see a keratopathy associated with use	Disc swelling with increased intracranial pressure; thought to have a similar mechanism to amiodarone	Usually resolves
Deferoxamine	Tx iron poisoning	Central scotoma; pigmentary retinopathy and optic neuropathy	Abnormal electroretinogram, VEP, electrooculography

Continued

Table 4-19. *Continued*

Agent	Toxic sequelae and symptoms	Optic nerve	Diagnosis/special treatment
Chloroquine	Tx malaria; tinnitus and deafness	Optic neuropathy; retinal pigment epithelium toxicity with macula "bull's eye appearance" (see Chapter 10)	Amsler grid, visual field every 6 mos (central 10°)
Hydroxyquinolones: Iodochlorhydroxquin[53]	Had been promoted falsely as a treatment for diarrhea; causes optic neuropathy, myelopathy, peripheral neuropathy subacute myelopticoneuropathy (SMON) in Japan	Optic neuropathy; decreased color vision; blindness (5%)	Stop the drug
Quinine	Tx leg cramps	Disc swelling; pan retinopathy	Discontinue drug—may have residual permanent vision loss
Disulfiram (Antabuse)	Tx alcoholism	Retrobulbar neuritis	Discontinue the drug
Dapsone	Tx leprosy; other	Optic neuropathy at high doses	Discontinue
Methotrexate	Tx malignancy, autoimmune conditions; bone marrow suppressant, hepatitis, renal	Optic neuropathy	Reduce dose; discontinue
Chlorambucil	Tx malignancy, Behçet's syndrome	Disc edema	Stop drug
BCNU[54]	Tx malignancy	Optic neuropathy; intraretinal vasculitis with nerve fiber layer infarcts; especially prominent unilaterally after intra-arterial injections	Stop drug; may be permanent
Vincristine[55]	Tx malignancy; GI, leukopenia; rare often secondary to IV or intravitreal injection	Optic neuropathy due to ganglion cell loss and axonal loss	No recovery
Cisplatin[56]	Tx malignancy; intra-arterial injections	Retrobulbar optic neuropathy and disc swelling	May not improve
Tamoxifen[57]	Tx breast malignancy	Dose-related retinopathy with refractile retinal changes in the optic nerve and macula (inner plexiform layer—Henle's layer)	Can be reversible
Tobacco	Tobacco products, especially cigar and pipe; also cigarettes; not clear that alcohol is associated	Progressive color vision loss; centrocecal scotoma	Stop smoking; treat with IM hydroxocobalamin

Methanol[58,59]	Wood alcohol metabolized to formic acid; blindness is the main result; metabolic acidosis (from formic acid); meningismus; agitated encephalitis; GI symptoms (pancreatitis); liver disease; lung disease; putaminal necrosis reported[33]	Retrobulbar nerve is "fixed" in formic acid; focal demyelination of the optic nerve behind the lamina; early disc swelling from axoplasmic stasis followed by cecocentral scotoma and optic neuropathy and atrophy	Consider treatment with B_{12}; stop smoking; ethanol, folic acid, leucovorin
Formaldehyde	Used to treat bladder tumors; used to treat bladder inflammation	Similar to methanol	Treatment the same as methanol
Lead	From batteries burned and lead paint; headache, tremor; peripheral neuropathy; look for lead lines on x-rays	Papilledema from increased intracranial pressure; in adults, lead may cause optic atrophy and stippling of the retina	Tx: chelating agent
Ethylene glycol	Antifreeze; causes nausea, vomiting, coma; headache peripheral neuropathy	Can cause increased intracranial pressure and papilledema; also causes optic neuropathy	Diagnosis: oxalate crystals in urine; acidosis; Tx: bicarbonate, ethanol, hemodialysis
Methyl bromide	Neurotoxin: altered mental status; peripheral neuropathy	Central scotomas; axonopathy of optic nerve; hyperemia, optic neuritis	Stop exposure
Thallium	GI, alopecia, headache, rash, peripheral neuropathy	Optic neuropathy-cecocentral scotoma	Vitamin treatment; stop exposure

BCNU = bischloroethylnitrosourea (carmustine); Tx = treatment of.
Adapted from references 46,60.

Figure 4-48. This man presented with decreased central acuity bilaterally. He smoked, drank alcohol, and had a poor diet. A. **The disc was hyperemic initially, and** (B) **mild temporal pallor ensued. His vision recovered somewhat after he quit smoking.**

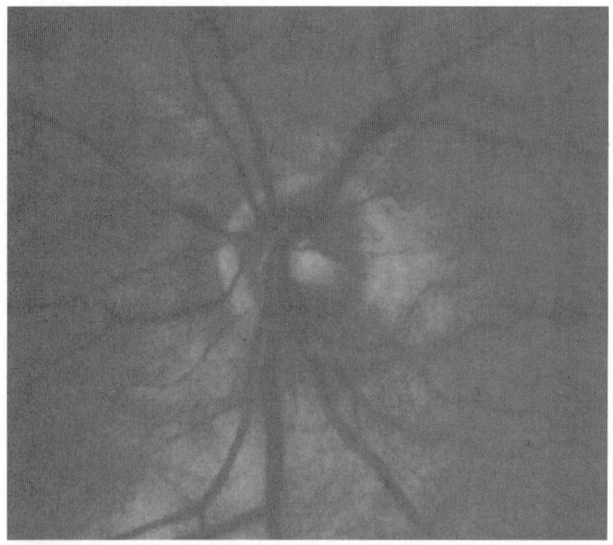

4-48A

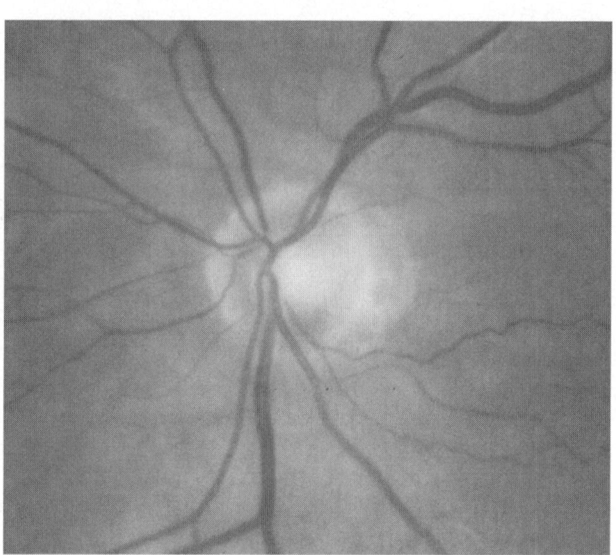

4-48B

Figure 4-49. This gentleman presented with decreasing vision. He was found to have bilateral temporal pallor (A, right eye B, left eye) and (C) partial central scotomas on his visual field. Workup for other causes of optic neuropathy, including a scan, was negative. He smoked and drank alcohol.

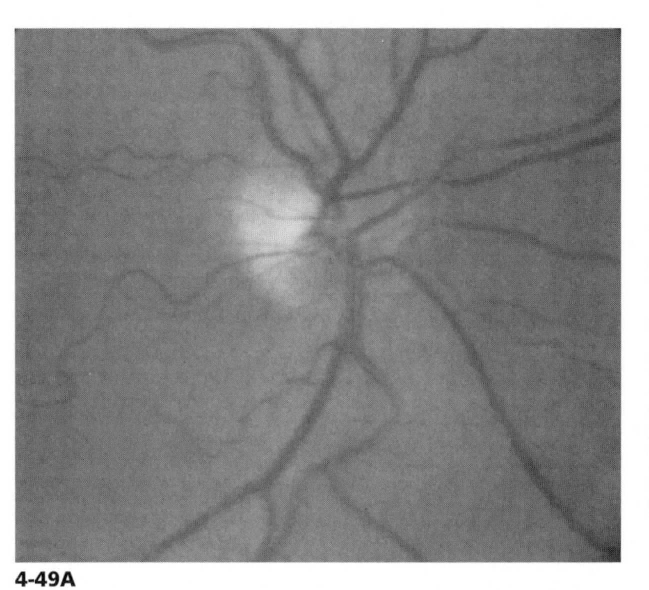

4-49A

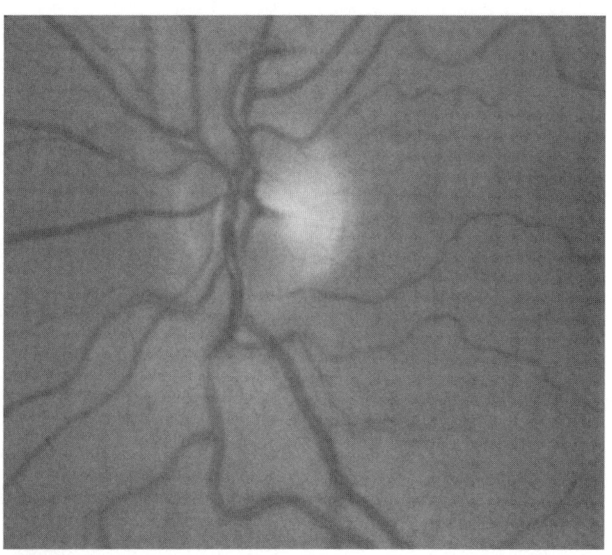

4-49B

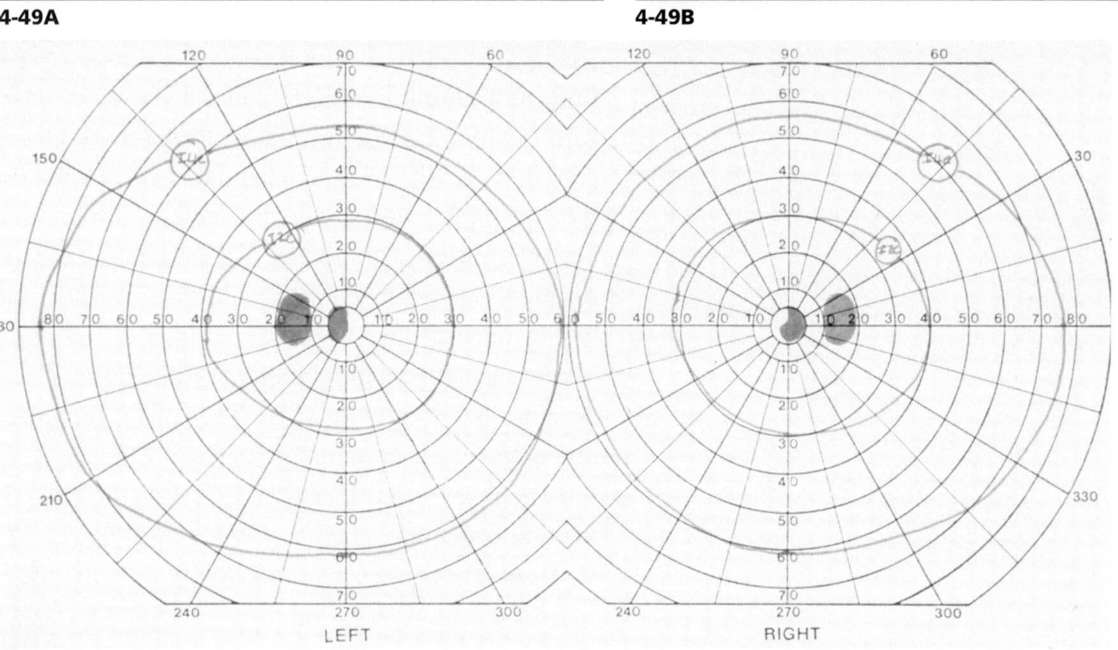

4-49C

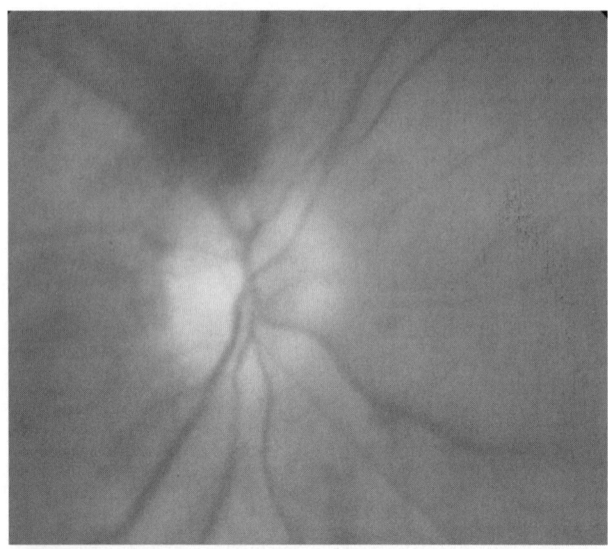

4-50A

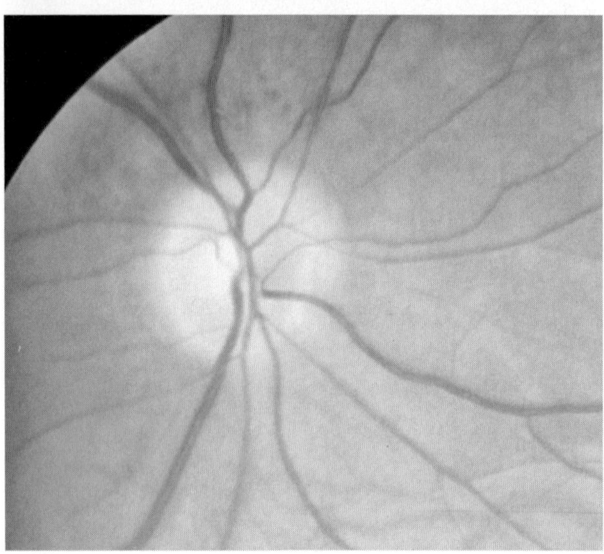

4-50B

Although toxic/nutritional neuropathies are fairly rare, you *must* be able to recognize them; in many cases stopping the offending agent results in resolution of symptoms. Also, be aware that some of these patients may have Leber's optic neuropathy that has been unmasked during treatment or in association with these agents.

Figure 4-50. A,B. **This 35-year-old woman underwent a gastric bypass for weight loss. She developed nausea and vomiting and had significant weight loss. She had no alcohol consumption. She presented with extraocular muscle abnormalities, ptosis, and confusion, and responded to intravenous thiamine. On examination, however, disc pallor was noted. She also had bilateral hemorrhages. Interestingly, Wernicke's initial case reports also included a woman with hyperemesis gravidarum associated with optic disc pallor and hemorrhages. (See M Victor, RD Adams, GH Collins. The Wernicke-Korsakoff syndrome. Philadelphia: FA Davis, 1989.)**

HYDROCEPHALUS OPTIC NEUROPATHY

Congenital brain disorders can also be associated with bilateral optic neuropathy. Probably the most common disorder is congenital hydrocephalus. Hydrocephalus can occur congenitally for a number of reasons, including aqueductal stenosis, Arnold-Chiari malformation, and after intracranial hemorrhage or infection. Appearance of the optic nerve is usually bilateral pallor. Although there may be acute swelling with hydrocephalus, optic atrophy is the more common presentation. Because the third ventricle compresses and spreads the chiasm, band atrophy may also be present (see Figure 4-41 for band atrophy associated with hydrocephalus).[61]

Figure 4-51. This woman had long-standing chronic hydrocephalus that was only found after she was evaluated for bilateral diffuse optic atrophy. A,B. Her right and left discs show chronic bilateral optic atrophy. C. Her MR shows bowing and stretching of the chiasm by the third ventricle.

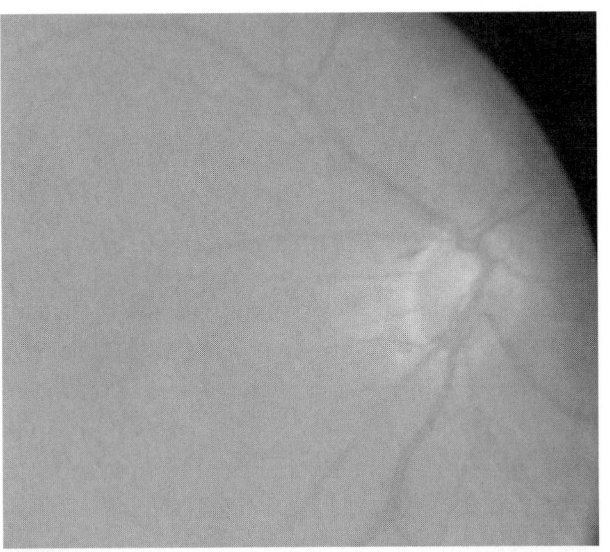

4-51A

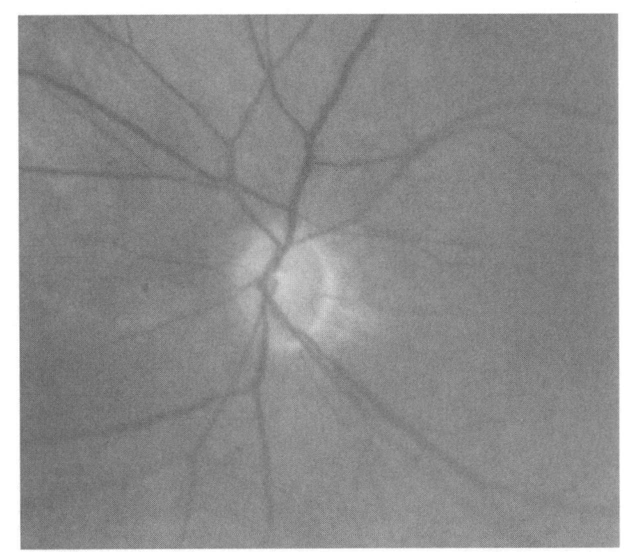

4-51B

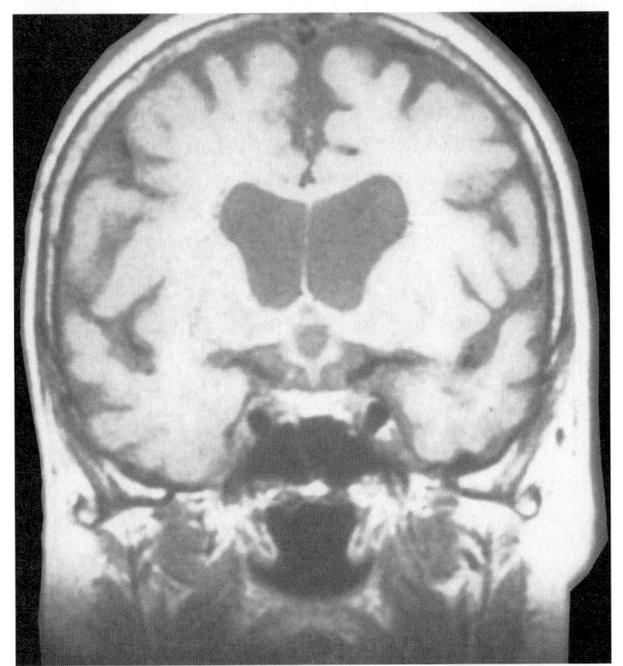

4-51C

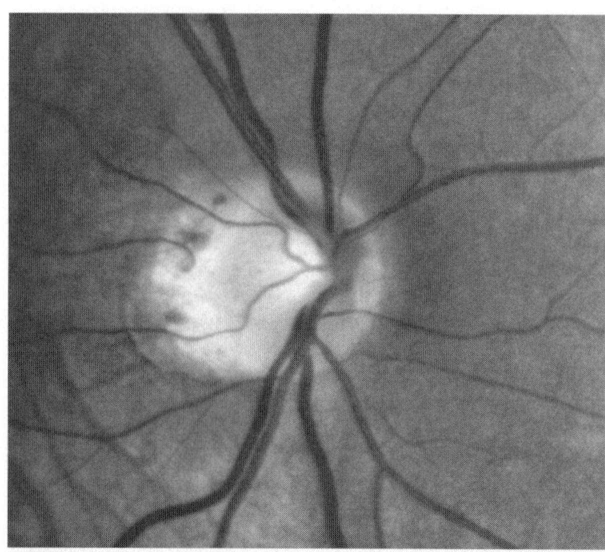

4-52A

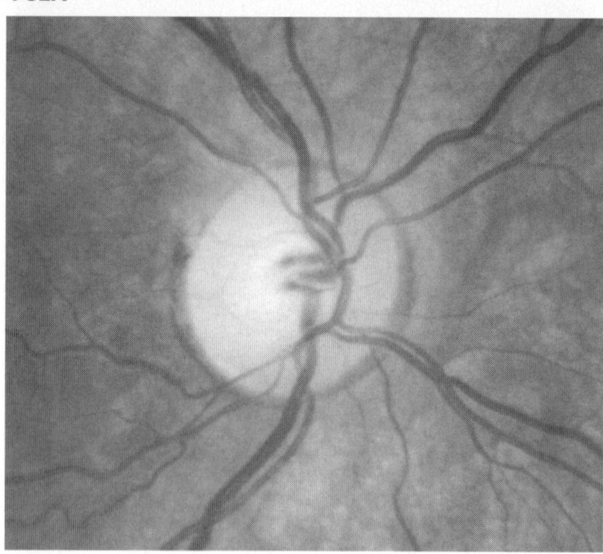

4-52B

The causes of optic pallor related to hydrocephalus are: (1) *long-standing papilledema* from increased intracranial pressure and subsequent atrophy, (2) *chiasmal stretching* by a dilated third ventricle from the deformation of the brain or skull, (3) *chiasmal stretching* from the third ventricle, (4) *transsynaptic degeneration* because many of these cases occur in utero, and (5) *iatrogenic complications* of shunt placement in the optic nerve, tract, and radiations.[20,61,62]

HEREDITARY OPTIC NEUROPATHY

Hereditary optic neuropathies can be dominant (present at age 4–8 with mild vision loss), or recessive (present at age 1–9 with moderate to severe vision loss), and may occur with associated conditions, including spinocerebellar degeneration (Friedreich's ataxia; mental retardation), diabetes, and deafness (Friedreich's ataxia, diabetes insipidus, Usher's syndrome, Refsum's syndrome, and Laurence-Moon-Biedl syndrome) (see Chapter 11).

Figure 4-52. The son presented with bilateral optic atrophy of unknown etiology after he failed a school visual examination. When looking for dominant optic atrophy, look at the parents. When we examined his mother, we found a similar kind of atrophy. A, **mother;** B, **son.**

Leber's hereditary optic neuropathy initially presents with unilateral central vision loss, usually associated with variable disc swelling (slight or none) and tortuous small vessels, after which optic atrophy gradually develops. Second eye involvement may be immediate or follow by months or years (see the description in Chapter 3).

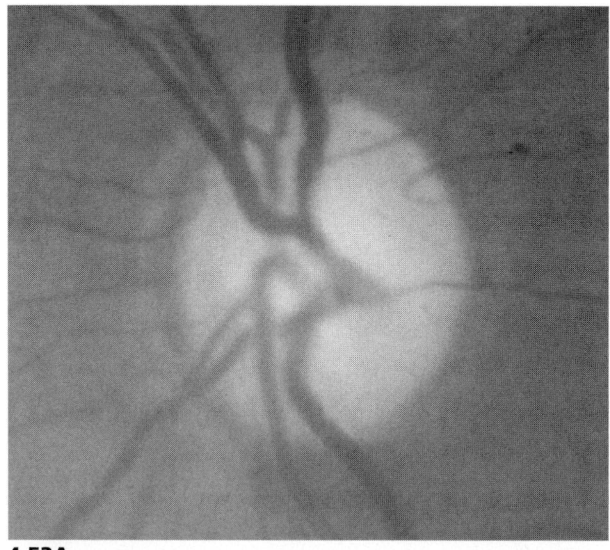
4-53A

Figure 4-53. A. A mother was legally blind due to known Leber's optic neuropathy. B. Son's right disc. Her son lost vision at age 25. His vision has been reduced, but he is able to work (not drive). C. Son's left disc. Notice the dropout of the nerve fiber layer just temporal to the disc (*arrows*).

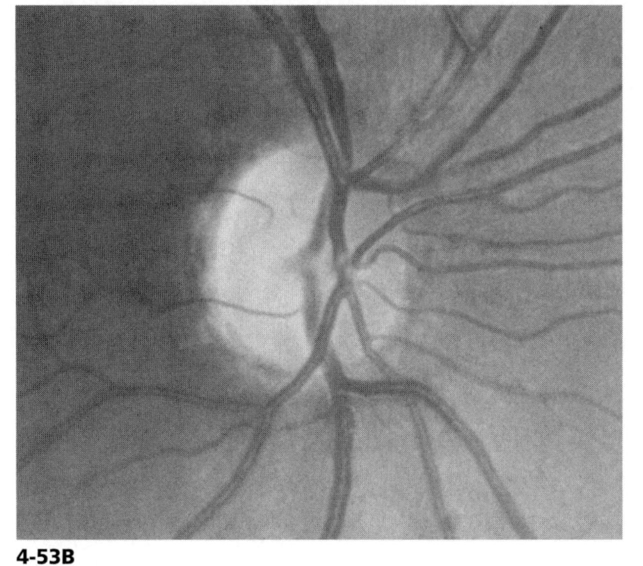
4-53B

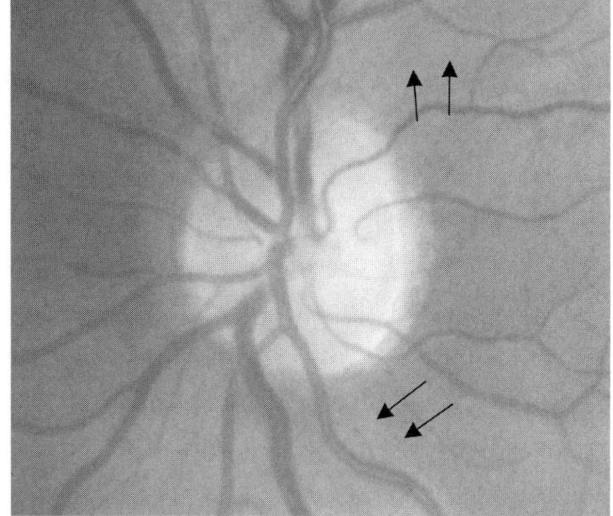
4-53C

Some neurodegenerative conditions, which affect the nervous system, have been associated with optic atrophy. Because most of these are also genetically acquired, they can be found presenting in children as well. The reason for separating neurodegenerative from hereditary optic atrophies is that the hereditary optic neuropathies tend to be isolated to optic neuropathy, whereas the neurodegenerative conditions affect other parts of the nervous system. Although Kjer's dominant optic atrophy can progress, many of the hereditary optic atrophies are fairly stable. Neurodegenerative conditions progress and visual elements may worsen over time; that's why they are called *degenerative*. Degenerative conditions in the nervous system caused by gray matter disease present with dementia, seizures, or movement disorders, whereas white matter disease presents more with peripheral neuropathy and gait disorder. For more information about neurodegenerative conditions associated with optic atrophy see Chapter 11.[20]

Practical Viewing Essentials

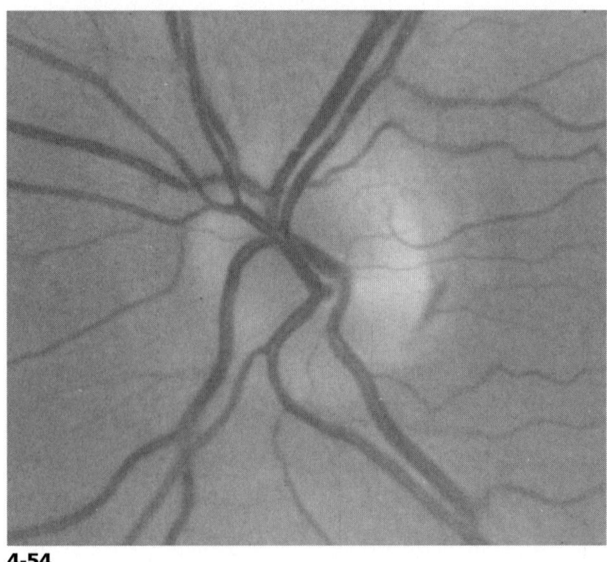

4-54

1. Do not just look at the color of the disc.
2. Using the red-free filter, is there nerve fiber dropout?
3. Is there enlargement of the cup?
4. What is the appearance of the neuroretinal rim?
5. What is happening with the small arterioles on the disc?
6. Decide whether the pallor is unilateral or bilateral.
7. Use characteristics of the history and examination to guide your evaluation and diagnosis.
8. Learn to recognize localizing atrophies: band atrophy, segmental atrophy, temporal atrophy.
9. Watch for toxic optic neuropathies because they are treatable.
10. If a child has optic atrophy, examine the parents.

References

1. Charcot JM. Lectures on the Diseases of the Nervous System. Translated and edited by G. Sigerson. New York: Hafner Publishing, 1962.
2. Beck RW. Optic neuritis. In NR Miller, NJ Newman (eds), Walsh and Hoyt's Clinical Neuroophthalmology. Baltimore: Williams & Wilkins, 1998;599–647.
3. Cogan D. Neurology of the Visual System. Springfield, IL: Charles C Thomas, 1980;133.
4. Hoyt WF, Beeston D. The Ocular Fundus in Neurologic Disease. St. Louis: Mosby, 1966.
5. Quigley HA, Anderson DR. The histologic basis of optic disk pallor in experimental optic atrophy. Am J Ophthalmol 1977;83:709–717.
6. Ballantyne AJ, Michaelson IC. Textbook of the Fundus of the Eye. Baltimore: Williams & Wilkins, 1970.
7. Frisén L. Ophthalmoscopic evaluation of the retinal nerve fiber layer in neuro-ophthalmologic disease. In JL Smith (ed), Neuro-ophthalmology Focus. New York: Massey, 1979.
8. Leinfelder PJ. Retrograde degeneration in the optic nerves and retinal ganglion cells. Trans Am Ophthalmol Soc 1938;36:307–315.
9. Lundström M, Frisén L. Evolution of descending optic atrophy. A case report. Acta Ophthalmol (Copenh) 1975;53:738–746.
10. Hoyt WF, Frisén L, Newman NM. Fundoscopy of nerve fiber layer defects in glaucoma. Invest Ophthalmol Vis Sci 1973;12:814–829.
11. Miller NR, Newman NJ. Topical diagnosis of lesions in the visual sensory pathway. In NR Miller, NJ Newman (eds), Walsh and Hoyt's Clinical Neuroophthalmology. Baltimore: Williams & Wilkins, 1998;286–289.
12. Hayreh SS. Pathogenesis of cupping of the optic disc. Br J Ophthalmol 1974;58:863–876.
13. Trobe JD, Glaser JS, Cassady J, et al. Nonglaucomatous excavation of the optic disc. Arch Ophthalmol 1980;98:1046–1050.
14. Greenfield DS, Siatkowski RM, Glaser JS, et al. The cupped disc. Who needs neuroimaging? Ophthalmology 1998;105:1866–1874.
15. Bianchi-Marzoli S, Rizzo JF, Brancato R, Lessell S. Quantitative analysis of optic disc cupping in compressive optic neuropathy. Ophthalmology 1995; 102:436–440.
16. Papastathopoulos KI, Jonas JB. Focal narrowing of retinal arterioles in optic nerve atrophy. Ophthalmology 1995;102:1706–1711.
17. Trobe JD, Glaser JS, Cassady JC. Optic atrophy. Differential diagnosis by fundus observation alone. Arch Ophthalmol 1980;98:1040–1045.
18. Warner JE, Lessell S, Rizzo JF, Newman NJ. Does optic disc appearance distinguish ischemic optic neuropathy from optic neuritis? Arch Ophthalmol 1997;115:1408–1410.
19. Trobe JD, Glaser JS, Cassady JC. Optic atrophy. Differential diagnosis by fundus examination alone. Arch Ophthalmol 1980;98:1040–1045.
20. Brodsky, MC, Baker RS, Hamed LM. Pediatric Neuro-ophthalmology. New York: Springer, 1996.
21. Davis EA, Rizzo JF. Ocular manifestations of multiple sclerosis. Int Ophthalmol Clin 1998;39:49–57.
22. Kelman SE. Ischemic optic neuropathies. In NR Miller, NJ Newman (eds), Walsh and Hoyt's Clinical Neuro-ophthalmology. Baltimore: Williams & Wilkins, 1998;549–598.
23. To KW, Rabinowitz SM, Friedman AH. Neurofibromatosis and neural crest neoplasms: primary acquired melanosis and malignant melanoma of the conjunctiva. Surv Ophthalmol 1989;22:373–379.
24. Parsa CF, Hoyt CS, Lesser RL, et al. Spontaneous regression of optic gliomas: thirteen cases documented by serial neuroimaging. Arch Ophthalmol 2001;119:516–529.
25. Dutton, JJ. Optic nerve sheath meningiomas. Surv Ophthalmol 1992;37:167–185.
26. Lowe RF, Ritch R. Angle closure glaucoma. In R Ritch, MB Shields, T Krupin (eds), The Glaucomas. St. Louis: Mosby, 1989;825–837.
27. Werner EB. Low-tension glaucoma. In R Ritch, MB Shields, T Krupin (eds), The Glaucomas. St. Louis: Mosby, 1989;797–812.
28. Dickens, CJ, Hoskins H. Diagnosis and treatment of congenital glaucoma. In R Ritch, MB Shields, T Krupin (eds), The Glaucomas. St. Louis: Mosby, 1989;773–785.
29. Dickens CJ, Hoskins HD. Epidemiology and pathophysiology of congenital glaucoma. In R Ritch, MB Shields, T Krupin (eds), The Glaucomas. St. Louis: Mosby, 1989;761–772.

30. VanBuskirk EM, Cioffi GA. Glaucomatous optic neuropathy. Am J Ophthalmol 1992;113(4):447–452.
31. Klein BE, Klein R, Sponsel WE, et al. Prevalence of glaucoma. The Beaver Dam Eye Study. Ophthalmology 1992;99:1499–1504.
32. Broadway DC, Nicolela T, Drance SM. Optic disk appearances in primary open-angle glaucoma. Surv Ophthalmol 1999;43(Suppl):S223–S243.
33. Diehl DL, Quigley HA, Miller NR, et al. Prevalence and significance of optic disc hemorrhage in a longitudinal study of glaucoma. Arch Ophthalmol 1990;108:545–550.
34. Fechtner RD, Weinreb RN. Mechanisms of optic nerve damage in primary open angle glaucoma. Surv Ophthalmol 1994;39:23–42.
35. Savino PJ, Paris M, Schatz NJ, et al. Optic tract syndrome. A review of 21 patients. Arch Ophthalmol 1978;96(4):656–663.
36. Gowers W. A Manual and Atlas of Medical Ophthalmology. London: J & A Churchill, 1879.
37. Frisén L, Holmegaard L, Rosencrantz M. Sectorial optic atrophy and homonymous, horizontal sectoranopia: a lateral choroidal artery syndrome? J Neurol Neurosurg Psychiatry 1978;41:374–380.
38. Brodsky MC, Baker RS, Hamed LM. Pediatric Neuro-ophthalmology. New York: Springer, 1996; 26–27.
39. Hoyt WF, Rios-Montenegro EN, Behrens MM, Eckelhoff RJ. Homonymous hemioptic hypoplasia. Fundoscopic features in standard and red-free illumination in three patients with congenital hemiplegia. Br J Ophthalmol 1972;56(7):537–545.
40. Katz BJ, Nerad JA. Ophthalmic manifestations of fibrous dysplasia. A disease of children and adults. Ophthalmology 1998;105:2207–2215.
41. Hayreh SS. Posterior ischemic optic neuropathy. Ophthalmologica 1981;182:29–41.
42. Katz DM, Trobe JD, Cornblath WT, Kline LB. Ischemic optic neuropathy after lumbar spine surgery. Arch Ophthalmol 1994;112:925–931.
43. Alexandrakis G, Lam BL. Bilateral posterior ischemic optic neuropathy after spinal surgery. Am J Ophthalmol 1999;127;354–355.
44. Remigio D, Wertenbaker C, Katz DM. Post-operative bilateral vision loss. Surv Ophthalmol 2000;44:426–432.
45. Lessell S. Toxic and deficiency optic neuropathies. In NR Miller, NJ Newman (eds), Walsh and Hoyt's Clinical Neuro-ophthalmology. Baltimore: Williams & Wilkins, 1998;663–679.
46. Walsh F, Hoyt WF. Clinical Neuro-ophthalmology (3rd ed). Baltimore: Williams & Wilkins, 1969;2540–2745.
47. Woung LC, Jou JR, Liaw SL. Visual function in recovered ethambutol optic neuropathy. J Ocul Pharmacol Ther 1995;11:411–419.
48. DeVita EG, Miao M, Sadun AA. Optic neuropathy in ethambutol-treated renal tuberculosis. J Clin Neuroophthalmol 1987;7:77–86.
49. Jimenez-Lucho VE, del Busto R, Odel J. Isoniazid and ethambutol as a cause of optic neuropathy. Eur J Respir Dis 1987;71:42–45.
50. Godel V, Nemet P, Lazar M. Chloramphenicol optic neuropathy. Arch Ophthalmol 1980;98:1417–1421.
51. Macaluso D, Shults WT, Fraunfelder FT. Features of amiodarone-induced optic neuropathy. Am J Ophthalmol 1999;127:610–612.
52. Gibson JM, Fielder AR, Garner A, Millac P. Severe ocular side effects of perhexilene maleate: case report. Br J Ophthalmol 1984;58:553–560.
53. Nelson E. Subacute myelo-optico-neuropathy (SMON). Ann Intern Med 1972;77:468–470.
54. Kupersmith MJ, Frohman LP, Choi IS, et al. Visual system toxicity following intra-arterial chemotherapy. Neurology 1988;38:284–289.
55. Sanderson PA, Kuwabara T, Cogan DG. Optic neuropathy presumably caused by vincristine therapy. Am J Ophthalmol 1976;81:146–150.
56. Maiese K, Walker RW, Gargan R, Victor JD. Intra-arterial cisplatin-associated optic and otic toxicity. Arch Neurol 1992;49:83–86.
57. Ashford AR, Donev I, Tiwari RP, Garrett TJ. Reversible ocular toxicity related to tamoxifen therapy. Cancer 1988;61(1):33–35.
58. Sharpe JA, Hostovsky M, Bilbao JM, Newcastle NB. Methanol optic neuropathy: a histopathological study. Neurology 1982;32:1093–1100.
59. Onader F, Ilker S, Kansu T, et al. Acute blindness and putaminal necrosis in methanol intoxication. Int Ophthalmol 1998–99;22(2):81–84.
60. Grant WM. Toxicology of the Eye. Springfield, IL: Thomas, 1974.
61. Chou S, Digre KB. Neuro-ophthalmic findings in hydrocephalus and shunt malfunctions. Clin Neurosurg 1999;10:587–608.
62. Corbett JJ. N-O complications of hydrocephalus and shunting procedures. Semin Neurol 1986;6:111–123.

5 Amaurosis Fugax and Not So Fugax—Vascular Disorders of the Eye

In no other structure of the body are the termination of an artery and the commencement of a vein presented to view and information regarding the general state of the vascular system is often to be gained from an inspection of their size, texture, and conditions of the circulation within them.

William Gowers[1]

Transient and long-lasting monocular vision loss related to arteriolar occlusive and venous occlusive disease is part of what makes looking at the retina and the disc such an immediately gratifying diagnostic tool. Nowhere else in the body can one so clearly see blood vessels to the capillary level.

Because the eye is such a vascular structure, disorders of the blood vessels frequently affect vision. As we have seen in viewing the disc for swelling or pallor, knowing the history helps us to know what to expect when we look at the disc and retina. The historical features to consider in evaluating anyone with transient vision loss thought to be related to vascular changes include the age and general health of the patient; family history of stroke, myocardial infarction, and migraine; and the types of drugs taken (e.g., vasoconstricting agents, cocaine use, cigarette smoking). Specific historical questions should include whether one or both eyes are affected, the sequence of loss (e.g., abrupt, slow, stepwise), the duration of loss, the mode of return of vision (if any), and associated symptoms (e.g., weakness, numbness, pain). By knowing the vascular anatomy and historical features, the examiner knows what to be looking for in the examination of the disc and ocular fundus.

Introduction to the Vascular Supply of the Eye

The blood supply to the globe derives from the ophthalmic artery which, in turn, derives from the internal carotid artery, with greater or lesser contribution from the middle meningeal artery.[2] The ophthalmic artery passes through the optic canal, inferior to the optic nerve, and branches within the orbit to form muscular, lacrimal, posterior ciliary, and central retinal artery segments. These ophthalmic artery branch vessels anastomose with the middle meningeal, supratrochlear, anterior, and posterior ethmoidal arteries, all of which derive from the external carotid system. Thus, if the internal carotid artery is occluded, the blood supply to the retina may derive exclusively from the external carotid system. Furthermore, embolic material from the stump of the occluded internal carotid artery can embolize to the retina in a retrograde fashion through the external carotid collateral vessels.

Figure 5-1. A. Diagram of the overall blood supply to the eye; the most important source of blood is from the internal carotid artery via the ophthalmic artery and central retinal artery. However, the external carotid communications are potential collaterals to the eye. Look at the numerous opportunities for the external carotid artery branches to communicate with the globe and the internal carotid circulation. The lighter gray is from the internal carotid artery, and the darker gray is from the external carotid artery. See the corresponding color figure on the accompanying CD-Rom. B. Here you see a person with an occluded internal carotid artery. The person had episodic vision loss (amaurosis fugax). How could this be, with the occluded internal carotid artery? The person's amaurotic events were coming from the external carotid via collaterals. The arrow points to the occluded stump of the internal carotid artery.

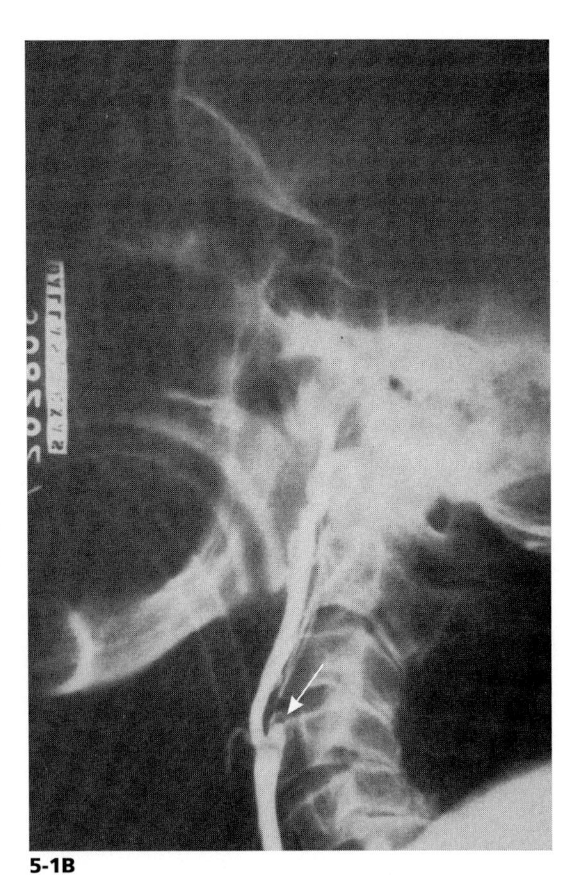

5-1B

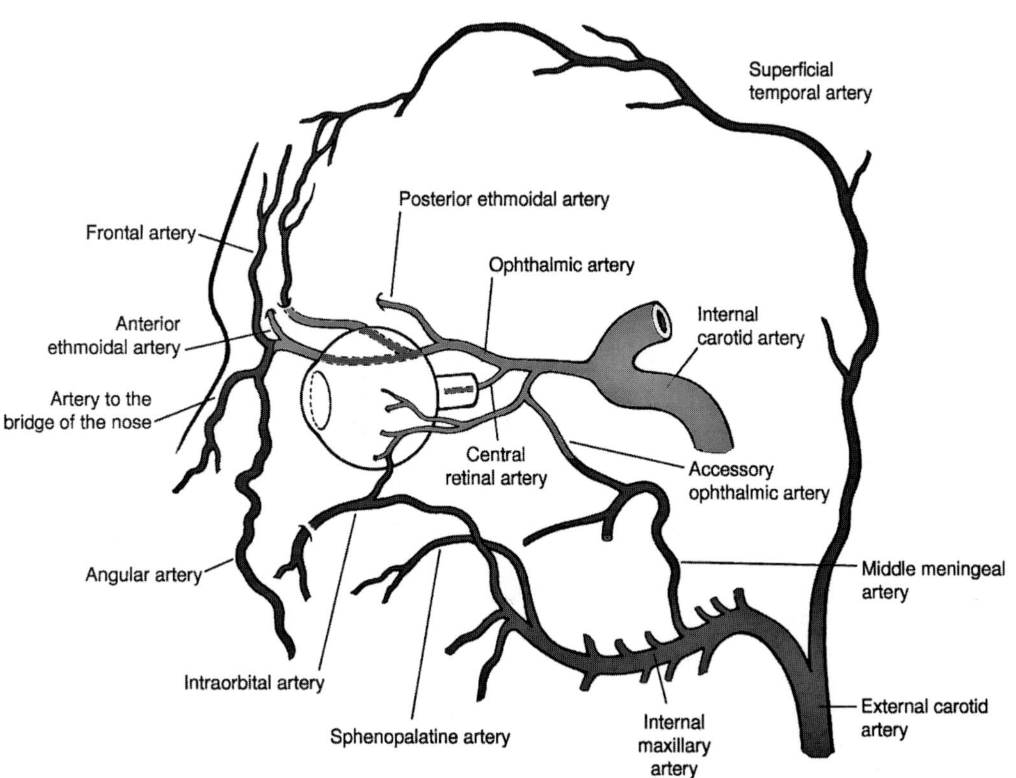

5-1A

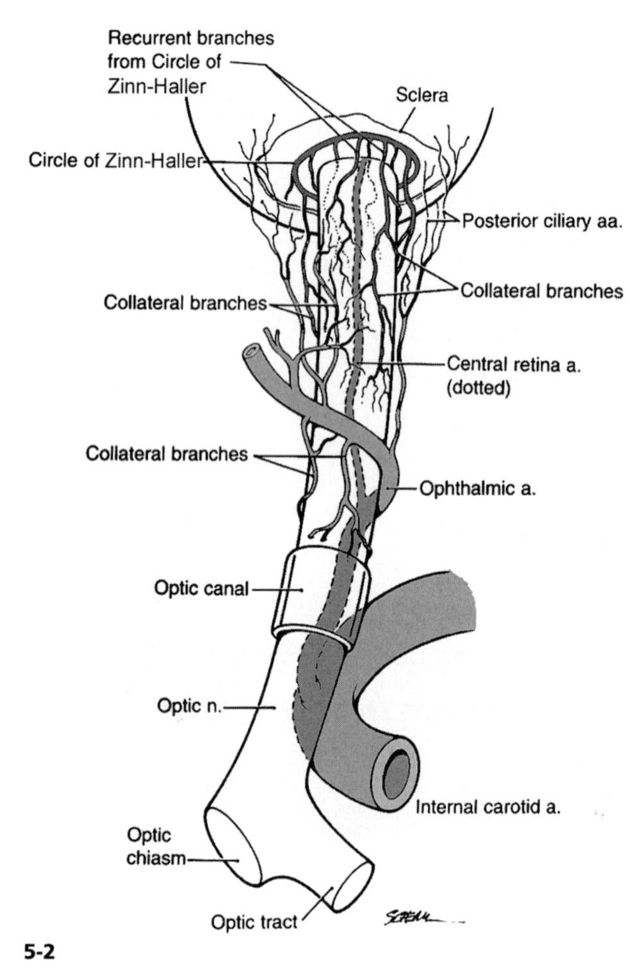

5-2

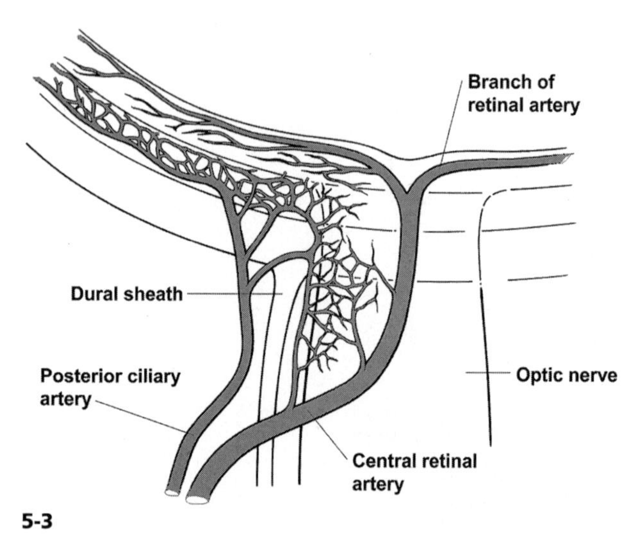

5-3

The external carotid artery circulation has important potential collaterals that connect the external and internal carotid artery blood supply. The external carotid can also serve as a source of embolism to the eye.

Figure 5-2. The internal carotid artery supplies the globe by way of the ophthalmic artery, through two major branches: The central retinal artery and the posterior ciliary arteries. The central retinal artery penetrates the dural sheath with the central retinal vein and enters the optic nerve, providing the blood supply to the internal surface of the retina. The ciliary arteries supply the choroid and the optic disc via a circumferential set of connecting arterioles (the circle of Zinn-Haller) that penetrate the sclera around the optic nerve.

Figure 5-3. The posterior ciliary arteries supply the choroid and the retrolaminar area of the disc. The central retinal artery supplies the retina.

The ciliary arteries provide blood supply to the choroid and the retrolaminar area of the optic nerve. In approximately one-third of persons, one or more ciliary arterioles penetrate the retina at the disc margin, and provide a variable amount of blood supply to the retinal ganglion cell and nerve fiber layer. In even fewer instances, a large segment of the retina is supplied by a major blood vessel (superior or inferior branch to the retina) that appears to be a branch of the central retinal artery, but is actually a ciliary artery. Rarely, the retina has a totally ciliary blood supply.[3]

Despite the fact that ciliary and central retinal arteries are both branches of the ophthalmic artery, occlusion of ciliary arteries appears rarely as a manifestation of embolic disease, whereas ciliary artery occlusion is common with arteritis. Embolic occlusion of the central retinal artery is common, but is much less commonly the result of arteritis.

Figure 5-4. A. The cilioretinal artery provides ciliary circulation blood supply to the retina. Here you see the artery entering at the lateral aspect of the disc. B. Remember to look for the cilioretinal artery leaving the disc. In this case, the cilioretinal artery is shown temporally; it has a hook-like appearance. C,D. This woman has bilateral cilioretinal artery vessels (*arrows*) that extend toward the macula. Notice that she also has "little red discs" (cupless, hyperemic "discs-at-risk"). In the event of a complete central retinal artery occlusion (CRAO), these cilioretinal arterial branches may provide the only blood available to the retina. The location of these vessels determines whether significant vision is preserved. Furthermore, occlusion of the cilioretinal arterioles, especially in the papillomacular bundle, may cause serious vision loss. E. This man has a large cilioretinal artery that supplies the superior temporal portion of his retina. The left arrow points the origin of the cilioretinal artery, and the right arrow points to its course.

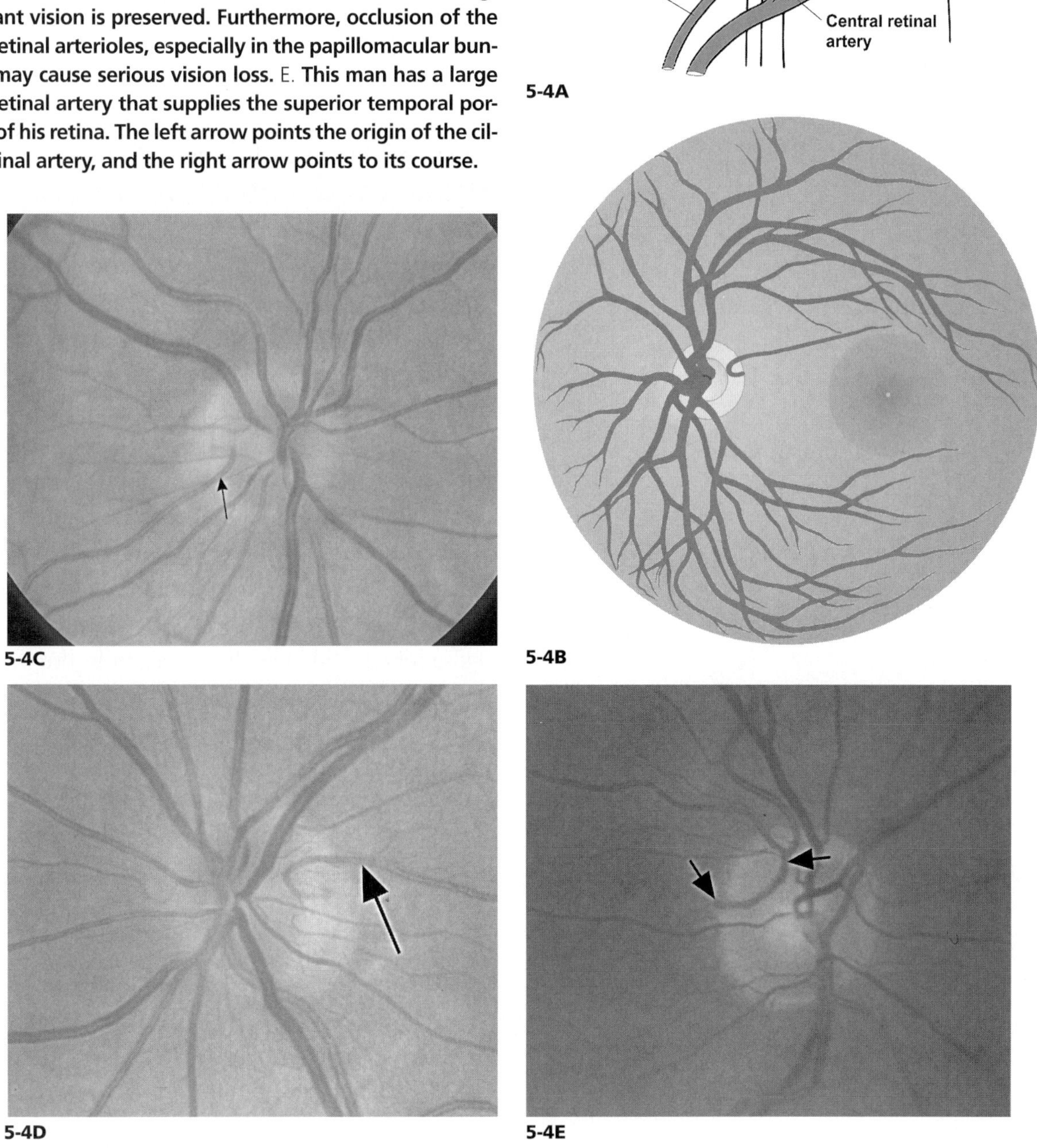

Blood Supply to the Optic Disc

The deep optic disc has a choroidally derived (posterior ciliary) blood supply in the laminar and retrolaminar area, whereas the visible surface of the disc derives its blood supply from small branches of the central retinal artery (see Chapter 2, Table 2-2). Axons converging on the margin of the disc derive their blood supply from superficial radial peripapillary capillaries.

Evaluating a Patient for Suspected Vascular Disease

Evaluation of a patient with vascular disease affecting the eyes should always start with blood pressure in both arms; unequal blood pressures can signal central vascular disease such as aortic atherosclerosis or inflammation. Evaluation of the heart, including heart rate, regularity of heart rate, and auscultation of the heart for murmurs and extra sounds (such as an S3) is equally important.

Where should you listen for bruits? Bruits can be auscultated at the supraclavicular region as well as all along the carotid artery. The bruit is usually high-pitched and may be focal over the carotid bifurcation. Occasionally, a bruit can be heard over the eye. To do this, use the diaphragm, because the lid tissue may plug the hole in the bell. Always have the patient close both eyes and then open the one *not* being auscultated to eliminate the noise produced by muscle contraction.

Viewing the Fundus for Vascular Disease—General Principles

What should you notice about the disc and retinal vasculature in those patients in whom you suspect vascular disorders? First, view the disc itself: Is it normal, swollen, or pale? Next, view the blood vessels: Are the arteries and veins of normal caliber? Follow each individual artery out from the disc to at least the first branch. Is there evidence of vascular occlusion? Are the veins of normal caliber? Is there evidence of embolic material? Are there crossing changes? Is there perivascular nerve fiber layer swelling? Do you observe a hemorrhage? Are there arterial pulsations or venous pulsations (see Chapter 2)?

WAYS TO STUDY BLOOD FLOW AT THE BEDSIDE—FINGER OCULAR PLETHYSMOGRAPHY

One way to test blood flow at the bedside is to do a crude assessment of blood flow to the eye. Look at the disc through the ophthalmoscope, and get the central retinal artery and vein into view. Apply the slight pressure of your finger through the lid on the lateral sclera. Very slight pressure causes the retinal vein to collapse. Normally, a moderate pressure on the sclera causes the central retinal artery to pulse, or "wink." The first collapse of the artery is the diastolic pressure. In patients with underlying occlusive atherosclerotic disease, a very slight pressure occludes or causes the central retinal artery to pulse or occlude. If the central retinal artery is occluded, there is no pulse, no matter how hard you press on the sclera through the eyelid.[4]

View the collapse of the central retinal vein (see Video 5-V-1A on the accompanying CD-Rom) and the winking of the central retinal artery (see Video 5-V-1B on the accompanying CD-Rom).

Ophthalmodynamometry is rarely performed these days: It measures the pressure exerted on the globe by a piston depressed into the sclera (like finger ocular plethysmography) and gives a numerical pressure. This technique can be helpful when looking for carotid artery disease. The procedure is most easily performed by two people. One person holds the ophthalmodynamometer plunger against the lateral sclera, depressing the plunger gradually and continuously increasing the amount of pressure. The other person views the central retinal artery through a dilated iris with the ophthalmoscope. First, the vein collapses, and then the artery begins to "wink" or pulse at the examiner. The point at which the artery begins to wink is the diastolic reading. The plunger is pulled back until the winking stops, and then the person who is doing the observation says "under." The plunger is again pushed down until the winking starts and the observer says "over." When more pressure is applied to the globe and systolic blood pressure is exceeded, the arteriole blanches and stops pulsating. By gradually reducing the pressure, the arteriole fills again, and this point is the systolic reading. The observer again gives the signal of "over" or "under" while the other person exerts pressure using the plunger and notes the numerical reading.

Although it is possible to measure pressures in millimeters of mercury while simultaneously looking at intraocular pressure, most readings are done to compare one side with the other. Variation between the two sides is usually less than 15%[5]; however, 5% of patients have an ophthalmic artery which is a direct branch of the middle meningeal artery. Thus, this test is invalid in 1 patient in 20, because the middle meningeal artery is a branch of the external carotid system.

These techniques have been rarely used to study the blood flow to the eye since the advent of magnetic resonance angiography, ultrasonography (color ocular blood flow Doppler and transcranial Doppler), and, particularly, fluorescein angiography.

OTHER WAYS TO VIEW THE VASCULATURE AND BLOOD FLOW TO THE EYE

Originally described by David et al.,[6] as well as Hollenhorst and Kearns,[7] the arm-to-retina time in fluorescein angiography was determined by two observers watching with the direct ophthalmoscope or indirect ophthalmoscope as fluorescein was injected. Normal arm-to-retina time is between 10 and 16 seconds, and a delay of more than 1–2 seconds between sides was a possible indication of carotid artery disease.[7] David et al. determined that the difference between the two eyes is not more than 1 second, with a mean difference of 0.5 seconds.[6] Presently, high-speed photography has replaced this simple viewing technique. Today, the photographers note the time of injection as time 0, with each photograph seconds or minutes from the time of injection. The arm-to-retina time gives the physician an indication of the speed of circulation to the eye, and is prolonged in congestive heart failure as well as when there is atherosclerotic or inflammatory disease producing a significant block of the carotid or other vessels.

Of course, there are more sophisticated ways to assess the blood flow to the eye. First, imaging techniques such as magnetic resonance imaging and magnetic resonance angiography show anatomic detail of the internal carotid artery without angiocatheterization; this technique does not usually show the anatomic detail of the ophthalmic artery, let alone the blood flow to the disc. Ultrasonography, including orbital colored Doppler and transcranial Doppler, assesses the ophthalmic artery blood flow and often the posterior ciliary arteries behind the disc. Fluorescein angiography probably remains the gold standard for assessing blood flow to the nerve and retina.

Transient Monocular Vision Loss or Amaurosis Fugax

Amaurosis derives from the Greek word αμαυρωοσζ, meaning blindness. Fugax is the Latin form of the Greek word φυγαχ, for fleeting—which together means: "fleeting blindness." Transient monocular blindness is commonly, but not invariably, due to recurrent embolization. The phrase *amaurosis fugax* has been so attached to embolic causes of vision loss that the term *transient monocular blindness* or *transient monocular vision loss* is preferable.

The source of emboli may be directly arterial or venous. Arterial emboli arise from a cardiac ventricular, atrial, or valvular source; from a "shagbark" atherosclerotic aorta; or from more distal vessels, classically the internal carotid artery. Embolic presentation of transient monocular blindness is usually quite abrupt, and frequently there are repetitive incidences. Because atherosclerotic major arterial occlusion is more gradual, there is a greater likelihood of collateral arterial supply and no visual symptoms.[5] Vasospastic disease may cause episodic amaurosis, but embolic causes need to be sought assiduously. Nonetheless, migraine can, on rare occasions, cause monocular amaurotic events. If the source is from the venous side, it occurs via the right heart and a patent foramen ovale. The clinical circumstance is repeated Valsalva maneuvers, causing a venous to arterial right-to-left shunt through a patent foramen ovale.

Caveat: The use of the term *amaurosis fugax* carries a lot of diagnostic emotional baggage; it implies

Table 5-1. Causes of Transient Monocular Blindness

- Ocular
  - Tear film abnormality
  - Transient elevation of intraocular pressure
  - Cells or blood in the anterior chamber
- Optic disc disease (transient, seconds-long vision obscuration)
  - Papilledema from whatever cause of increased intracranial pressure
  - Optic nerve drusen
  - Optic disc congenital anomalies (coloboma)
  - Myopia
- Optic nerve disease
  - Compressive optic neuropathies—occasionally gaze-evoked blindness
  - Orbital hemangioma or osteoma
  - Papilledema
  - Thyroid eye disease
- Vascular
  - Carotid artery atheromatous emboli
  - Anastomotic (external carotid) arterial emboli (stump syndrome)
  - Venous and right-to-left shunts (watch for relationship of events to Valsalva maneuver)
  - Retinochoroidal collaterals
  - Cardiac sources (account for the majority of emboli)
    - Valvular—including post-rheumatic valvular disease; mitral valve prolapse; bicuspid aortic valve
    - Tumor—(atrial myxoma)
  - Patent foramen ovale
  - Atrial septal aneurysms >1 cm
  - Aortic arch "shag-bark" atherosclerosis
  - Vasculitis—temporal arteritis; Takayasu arteritis
  - Hypotension from arrhythmia, drugs, postural changes, or blood loss
    - Frank Yatsu's rule of forties: mean BP <40 mm Hg; heart rate <40/min or >160/min
  - Vasospasm (including migraine)
- Hematologic abnormalities
  - Hypercoagulable states
    - Antithrombin III
    - Factor V Leiden deficiency
    - Protein C and S deficiency
    - Polycythemia
    - Sickle cell disease
    - Hyperhomocystinemia
    - Thrombocytopenia purpura
  - Antiphospholipid antibodies
    - Anticardiolipin antibodies
    - Lupus anticoagulant
  - Thrombocytosis
- Metabolic causes
  - Diabetes
  - Hypertension
- Iatrogenic
  - After cardiac catheterization, cardiac bypass
  - Carotid angiography, carotid endarterectomy

Note: Although some of these events do not truly cause blindness, the patient may overdo his or her alarm and describe visual changes as vision loss.

an embolic cause. Because emboli have been attributed largely to an atherosclerotic carotid artery, there tends to be an arrest of differential diagnostic thought if nothing is found in the carotid artery. The table of causes of transient monocular vision loss emphasizes that there are *many* pathophysiologic events that have the potential to cause transient loss of vision in one eye.

As embolic material passes through a vessel or vessels in the retina, it triggers retinal depolarization, producing spots or flashes described as looking like sparklers, shooting stars, or, as one patient said, "looking like minnows flashing away from the edge of a pond when one steps near." If the emboli stick, they cause monocular altitudinal, quadrantic, or other segmental losses of vision. The "shadelike" vision loss (like a curtain coming up or down or, rarely, from the side) is a staple complaint, but an embolic source is not always found.

Dr. Shirley Wray systematically reviewed more than 850 cases of transient monocular blindness and made several observations about these cases, as well as developed a classification system that allows us to think about transient monocular blindness caused by vascular occlusion.

Table 5-2. Types of Transient Monocular Blindness (Wray's Classification)

Features	Type 1: transient retinal ischemia	Type 2: retinal vascular insufficiency	Type 3: vasospasm	Type 4: unclassifiable multiple etiologies
Age group	Any age	Older age	Younger and older ages	Any age
Cause	Embolus (thrombus) from carotid artery, heart, or aorta; antiphospholipid antibodies	Extracranial arterial occlusive disease or internal and external carotid artery	An intermittent retinal vascular insufficiency without permanent impairment of retinal perfusion	Heart defects, underlying systemic lupus erythematosus
Onset	Abrupt	Gradual	Abrupt to gradual	Abrupt
Provoking features	None	Systemic hypotension; venous hypertension; steal phenomenon	Migraine	None known
Vision loss	Complete or partial—curtain ascending or descending; sideways moving blind	Complete or partial; acuity normal, but contrast changed; bright objects brighter; flickering edge to objects; glare of white paper; colored lights	Complete or progressive visual field narrowing	Partial
Duration of event	Secs–mins	Mins–hrs	Mins	Variable—secs, mins
Recovery	Complete	Complete	Complete/some loss	Complete

Features	Type 1: transient retinal ischemia	Type 2: retinal vascular insufficiency	Type 3: vasospasm	Type 4: unclassifiable multiple etiologies
Pain	No	Yes—aching over orbit, face worse upright	Frequently—before, during, or after	No
Mechanism	Embolus	Hypoperfusion	Vasospasm of optic artery or central retinal artery	Multiple
Other features	Total vision blackout	Visual aberrations	Peripheral loss sparing central visual field	—
Risk of vision loss/death	Permanent vision loss <3%/annum	Higher risk of stroke and myocardial death	Variable	—
Risk factors	Generalized arteriosclerotic vascular disease; fibromuscular hyperplasia; angiitis, systemic lupus, Behçet's syndrome, moya moya syndrome; hypercoagulable state	Severe atherosclerosis; Takayasu's arteritis; giant cell arteritis	Migraine; giant cell arteritis; periarteritis nodosa, eosinophilic vasculitis	Systemic lupus
General examination	Auscultation of neck, eye	Blood pressure, palpation of arteries	Livedo reticularis	Splinter hemorrhages of fingernails
Other ocular findings	Look for signs of embolism in conjunctiva	Rubeosis of iris, poor pupillary light reflex, ischemic uveitis (not steroid responsive)	Anterior ischemic optic neuropathy, retinal infarction	None
Fundus examination	Retinal emboli; central retinal artery occlusion, branch retinal artery occlusion, anterior ischemic optic neuropathy (AION)	Low pressure retinopathy—dot/blot hemorrhage, microaneurysms, segmental narrowing of veins, pulsating retinal artery, anterior ischemic optic neuropathy; cupping, choroidal infarct	During attack look for narrowing of the arteries first, with subsequent narrowing of venous circulation (see Video 5-V-2 on the accompanying CD-Rom)	No defects appreciated
Fluorescein angiogram	May reveal emboli, normal	Marked prolongation of arm-to-retina time, slowed arteriovenous time	Narrowing of arteries during attack, normal in between	Normal

Source: Adapted from SH Wray. Amaurosis fugax. In RJ Tusa, SA Newman (eds), Neuro-ophthalmological disorders. New York: Marcel Dekker, 1995; SH Wray. Visual aspects of extracranial disease. In EF Bernstin (ed), Amaurosis Fugax. New York: Springer 1988;72–89; SH Wray. Transient monocular blindness. In J Bogousslavsky, L Caplan (eds), Visual Symptoms (Eye) in Stroke Syndromes. Cambridge: Cambridge University Press 1995;68–79.

Arterial Occlusion

CENTRAL RETINAL ARTERY OCCLUSION

Occlusion of the central retinal artery produces abrupt loss of vision and a characteristic fundus appearance. The nerve fiber layer becomes opaque and obscures the vessels to some extent. This opacification is owing to cloudy swelling of the ganglion cells and axons, and is not interstitial edema. In those individuals who have cilioretinal arteries that supply the retina surrounding the optic disc, there may be patches of pink, healthy-appearing retina. The arterial vessels are narrowed, and the blood forms blocklike segments that resemble boxcars or cattle trucks. Finally, the macula takes on a bright red appearance, as contrasted with the surrounding pale ischemic retina. The "cherry-red" macula is owing to the preservation of the normal choroidal blood supply and the contrast of the healthy oxygenated tissue with the infarcted pallid tissue. A cherry-red macula of different cause can be seen with other genetic conditions (see Chapter 10, What Is That in the Macula?, and Chapter 11, Practical Viewing in Children).

Figure 5-5. (opposite page) A. **An embolus usually occludes the central retinal artery, often at the lamina cribrosa.** B. **When the central retinal artery is occluded, the entire retina is pale. The intact choroidal circulation (perfused by branches off of the short posterior ciliary arteries) beneath the macula maintains the normal macular color. Most of the time, embolic material is not seen in the central retinal artery because it is just behind where you are viewing on the disc.** C. **In CRAO, the macula is red (hence, "cherry-red spot") because the choroidal circulation beneath the macula is intact. The surrounding retina is pale because of swelling of the infarcted retinal ganglion cells and axons.** D. **Close-up of the cherry-red macula.** E. **Another CRAO with a cherry-red macula. (Photograph courtesy of Paula Morris, CRA.)**

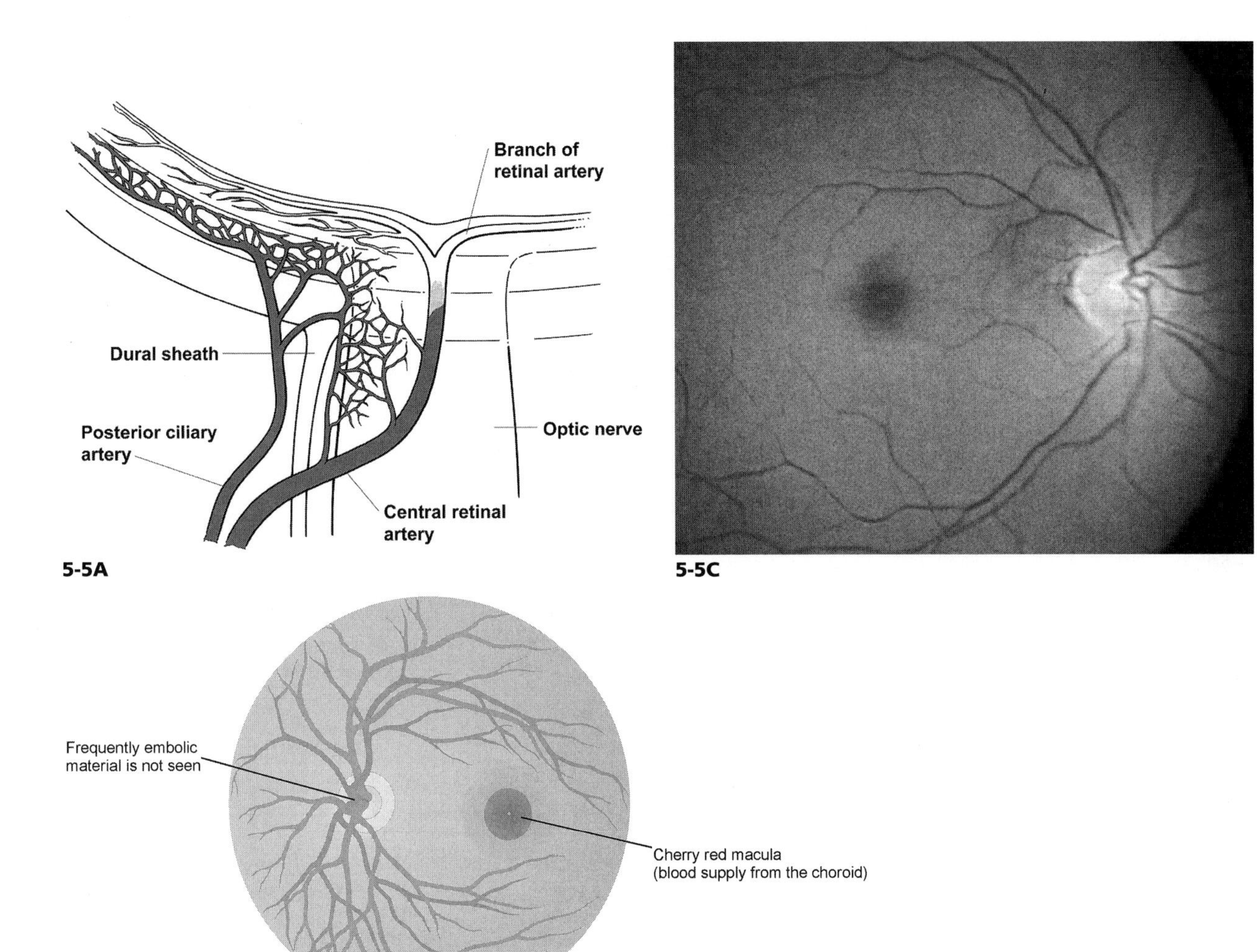

5-5A

5-5C

5-5B

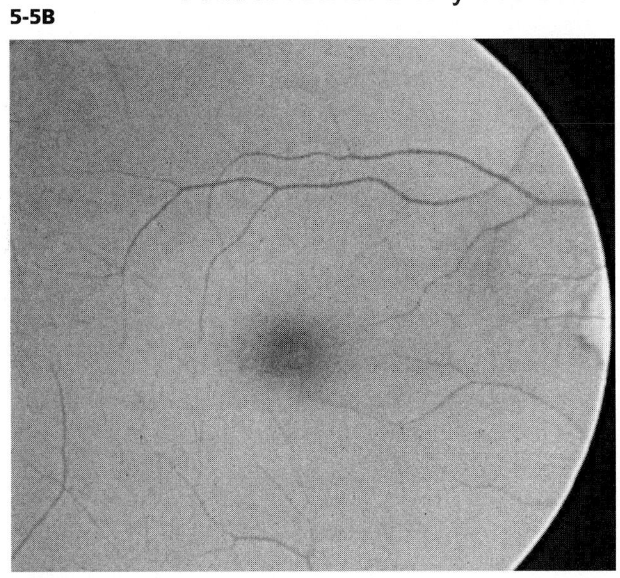

5-5D

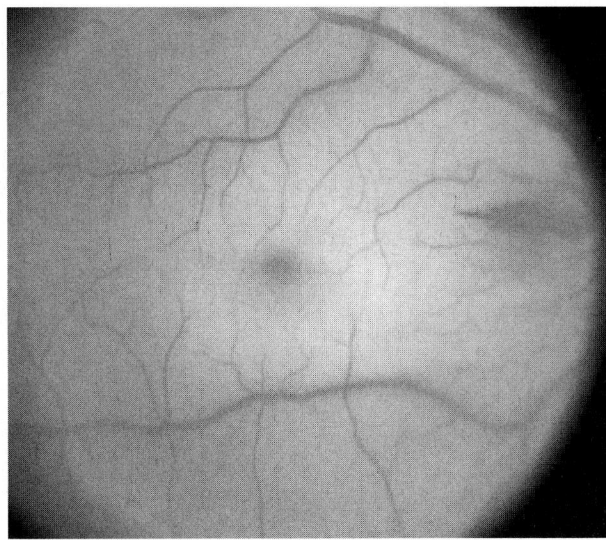

5-5E

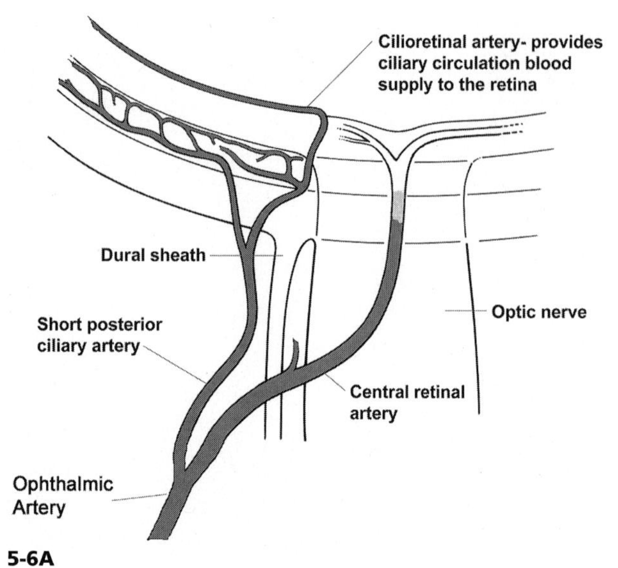

5-6A

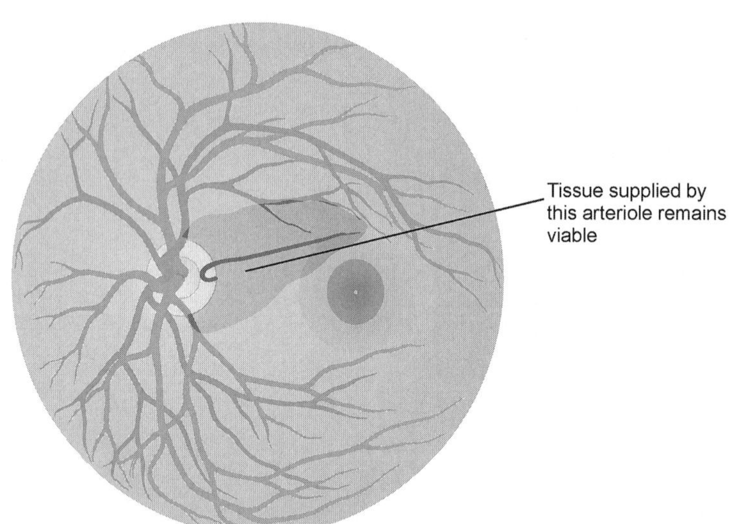

CRAO with cilioretinal artery sparing

5-6B

Figure 5-6. A. **During a CRAO, the presence of a cilioretinal artery allows for preservation of some retinal tissue.** B. **The retina is pale in a CRAO, but when a cilioretinal artery is present, there is a tongue of normally perfused tissue along the cilioretinal artery.** ***Continued***

Figure 5-6. ***Continued.*** C. **If there is a cilioretinal artery, the entire retina is pale, except for those retinal elements supplied by the cilioretinal artery, which remain normal in color. In these cases, visual acuity may be maintained despite a striking loss of visual field. This is the optic fundus of an artist who was able to continue working with central vision preserved by the cilioretinal artery (*arrow*).** D. **Another CRAO with cilioretinal artery sparing.** E. **The visual field from the patient in** (D) **would have been completely obliterated by a CRAO. However, because the cilioretinal artery was there and was not occluded, a small central visual field remained, leaving the patient with excellent central vision.**

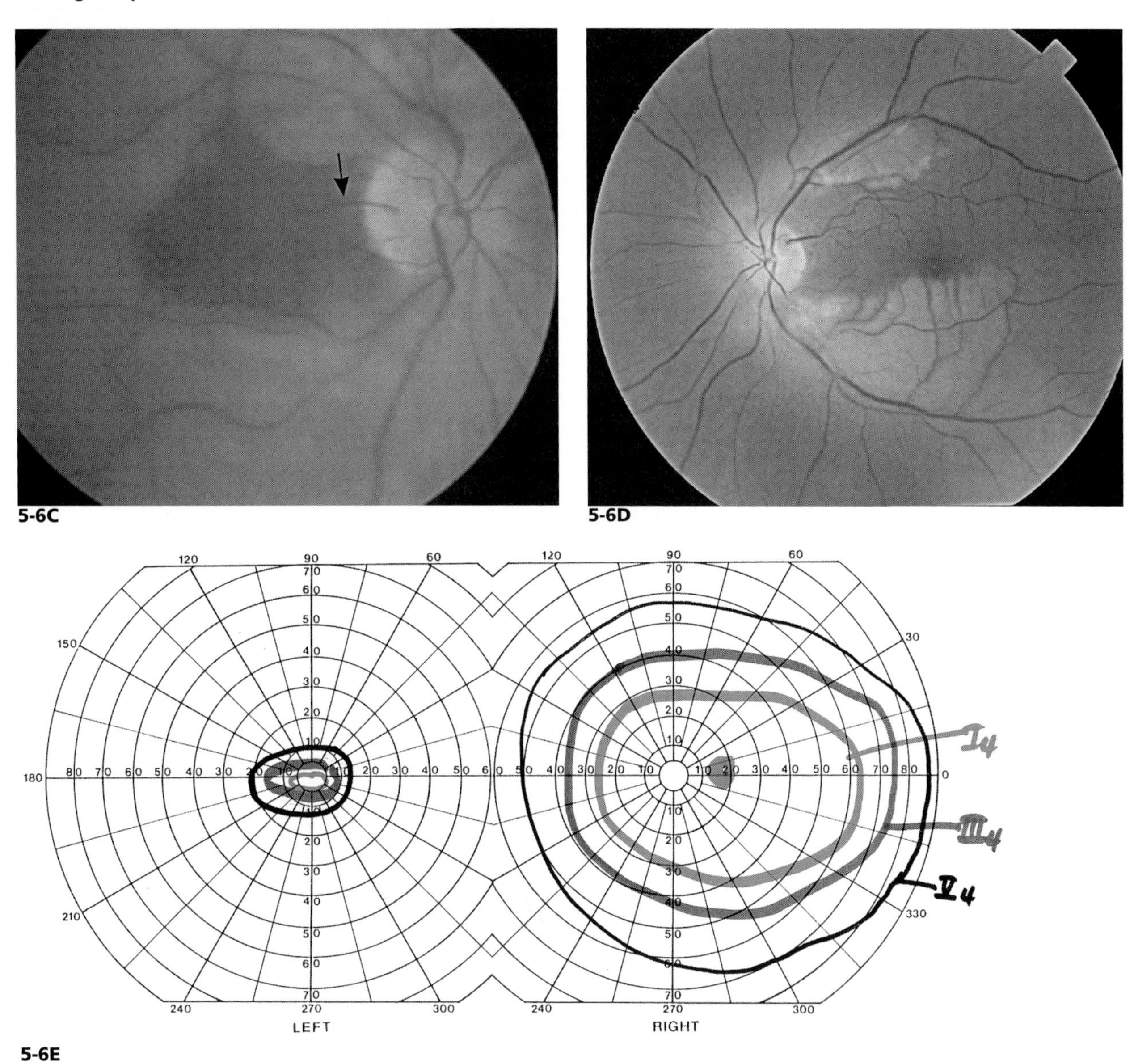

The retinal tolerance time for total ischemia of monkey retina is 96–120 minutes after complete occlusion of the central retinal artery, followed by reperfusion.[2] If a patient has a full-blown picture of CRAO by the time you first see the eye, it is highly unlikely that any intervention will succeed in returning vision.

Table 5-3. Treatment of Acute Central Retinal Artery Occlusion

Treatment
Carbogen 15% CO_2 and 100% oxygen
IV Acetazolamide 1 g followed by:
Anterior chamber paracentesis
Possible tissue plasminogen–activating factor (t-PA)
Hyperbaric oxygen (experimental)

Rarely, the treatment sequence shown in Table 5-3 restores vision. The duration of vision loss is critical, of course.

Days after the occlusion, pallor of the disc ensues with arterial narrowing and variable vascular sheathing. Hemorrhages are uncommon. Aside from optic disc pallor, what might you expect to see months after a CRAO? Optic disc pallor and atrophy are invariably present, along with arteriolar narrowing. Experimental CRAO does not cause peripapillary atrophy or reduction in the size (width) of the neuroretinal rim; this fact may help to determine the cause of undiagnosed optic atrophy, because glaucomatous changes in the disc are associated with peripapillary atrophy and reduction of the neuroretinal rim.[8]

CRAO always should be considered embolic until proven otherwise. Clues to the source of an embolus are discussed with branch retinal artery occlusion (BRAO), in which, with rare exception, embolic occlusion is the cause. Other causes of

CRAO to consider are atheromatous occlusion of the central retinal artery, inflammatory vascular occlusion such as temporal arteritis or polyarteritis nodosa, central retinal artery vasospasm, and poor flow to the eye as the result of high intraocular pressure or decreased perfusion pressure by extracranial disease or hypotension.

Emboli caught at the level of the optic disc or those that migrate more peripherally may have characteristics that allow one to identify a probable source. Many more emboli occur and pass through the vessels without "sticking" than are ever appreciated. Ultrasonography can give one appreciation of an upstream "chirping" of continuing spontaneous embolic events from downstream atherosclerotic plaques. This embolic noise may be worsened with carotid palpation or massage, rough carotid auscultation, and during arteriography or even shaving the neck with an electric razor.

BRANCH RETINAL ARTERY OCCLUSION

When a branch of the central retinal artery is occluded, the arcuate nature of the distribution of the nerve fiber layer is clearly demonstrated, as is the horizontal separation of the superior and inferior arterial blood supply to the retina. Instead of a cherry-red macula, there can be a hemi–cherry-red macula. It is likely you will see the cause of the vascular occlusion at the point of obstruction or broken up in multiple smaller downstream vessels. Many emboli migrate through the capillaries and leave only small hemorrhages, a nerve fiber infarct, or nothing in their wake. As opposed to CRAO, which may not always represent embolic occlusion, BRAO is virtually always the result of embolic events until an exhaustive source for embolic sources has proven negative. Intravascular coagulopathy (anticardiolipin antibodies) may rarely produce branch artery obstruction. Rarely, BRAO is associated with a viral infection.[9]

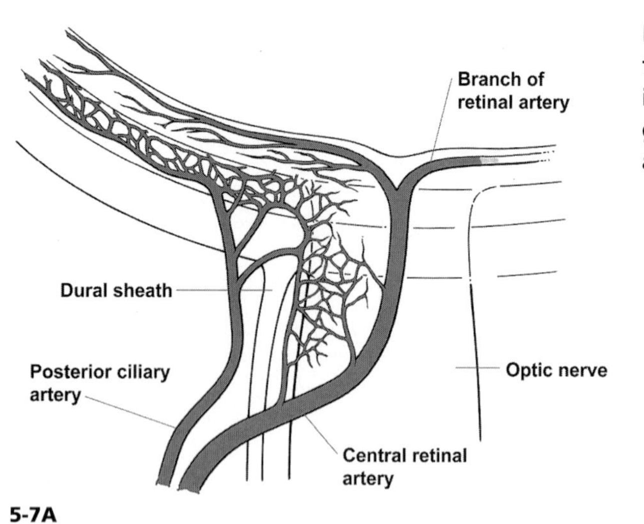

5-7A

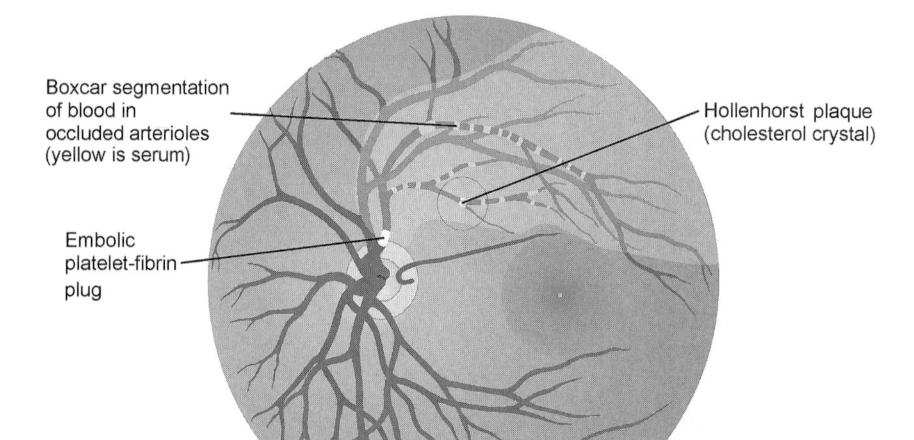

5-7B

Figure 5-7. A. **A BRAO is literally an occlusion of one of the branches from the central retinal artery.** B. **The retina is pale where the branch retinal artery is occluded, giving a demarcation line between the healthy retina and the infarcted pale retina.** ***Continued***

Figure 5-7. *Continued*. C. Here is a superior temporal BRAO causing pallor of the retina and a "hemi-macular cherry-red spot." D. The patient had an inferior nasal visual field defect corresponding with the superior temporal occlusion. E. This patient had an inferior temporal BRAO owing to an embolism. F. The corresponding fluorescein angiogram shows a cut-off of the retinal artery and disc staining, indicating ischemia to the disc as well.

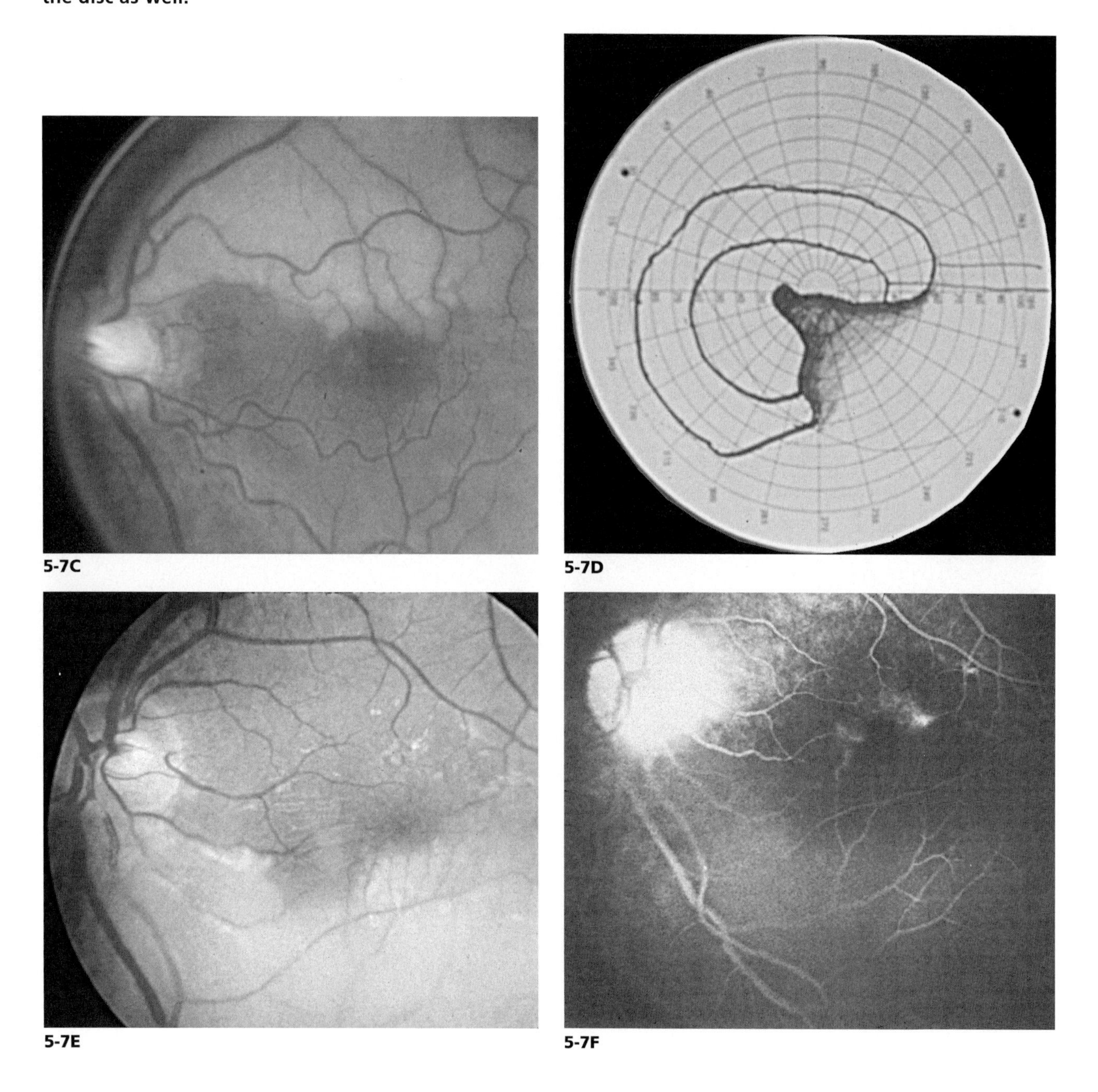

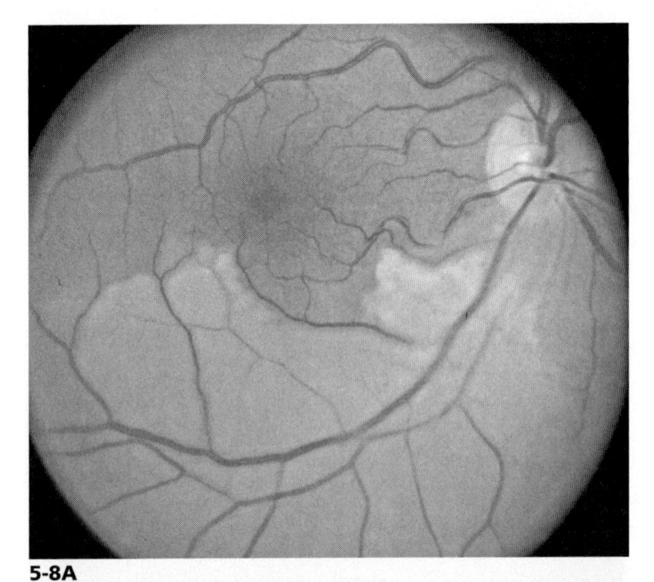

5-8A

Figure 5-8. A. **This woman had a BRAO caused by vasculitis. The retina is pale, but the disc appears almost normal.** B. **One month later, the pallor of the retina is resolving, and the disc is starting to pale slightly.** C. **Three months later, one cannot detect any retinal pallor; however, the disc is pale inferiorly and somewhat cupped.**

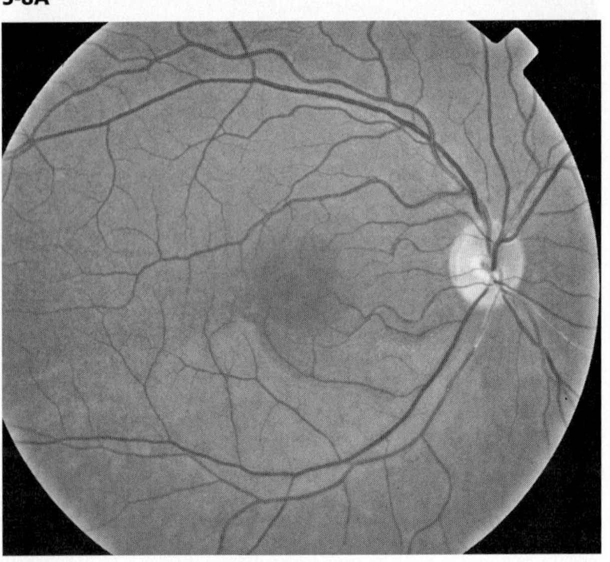

5-8B

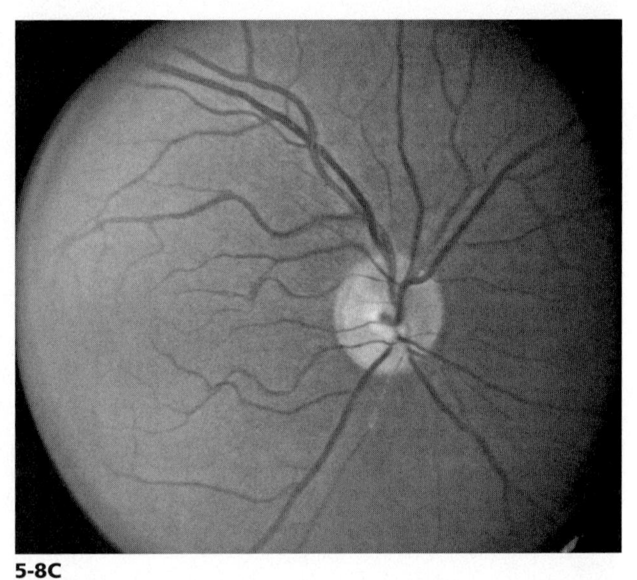

5-8C

Figure 5-9. A woman with sarcoid in her lacrimal gland underwent steroid injections into her lacrimal gland. She suffered acute visual blurring when the steroid entered her central retinal artery through an arterial anastomosis in the orbit, between the external carotid circulation and the central retinal artery. A. The retina is pale from multiple small BRAOs; there is a blot hemorrhage off of the right. B. The red-free photograph accentuates the pallor with multiple small occlusions. C,D. An early fluorescein angiogram shows cut-offs of multiple retinal arterioles. E. Late in the angiogram (10 minutes elapsed), some of the vessels have stained but there is still poor filling of other vessels.

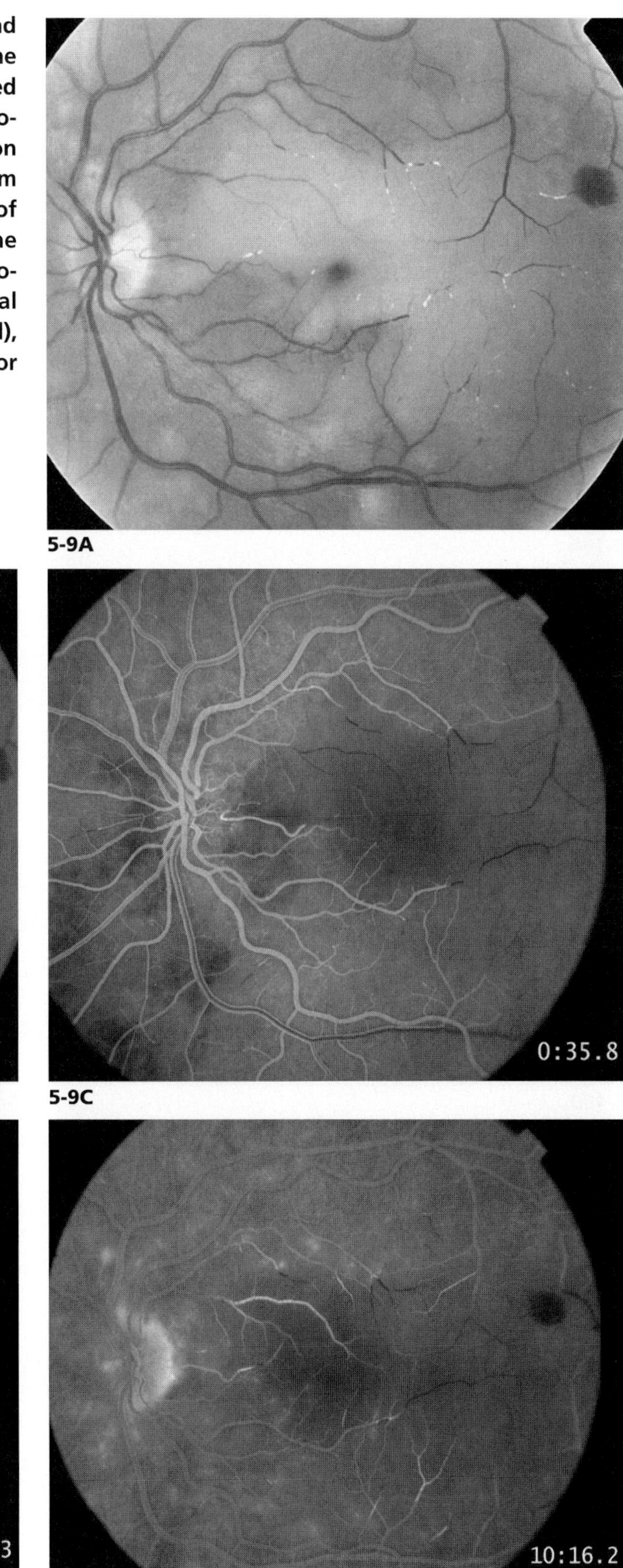

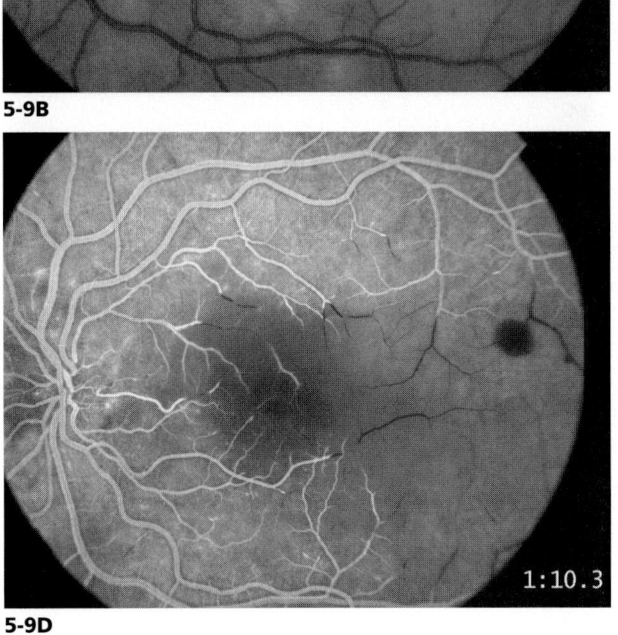

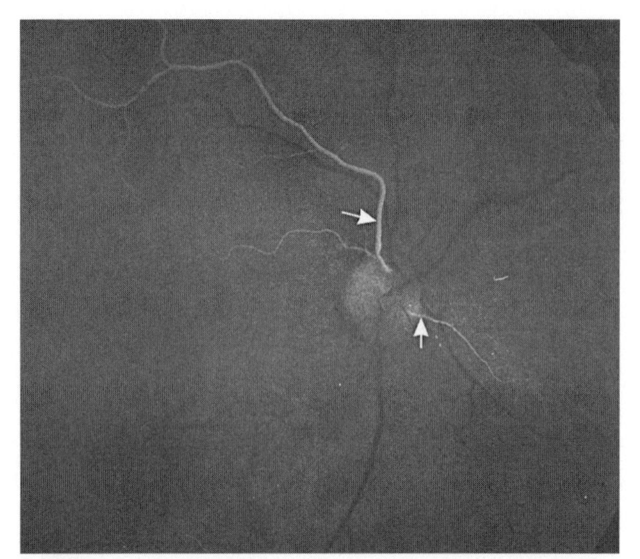

5-10A

Figure 5-10. A. **In this inferior branch retinal artery occlusion, you see the superior branch retinal artery and the cilioretinal artery filling first (*arrows*) on this fluorescein angiogram.** B. **The rest of the retinal arteries fill afterward.** C. **The flow is slow in the inferior branch circulation related to the arterial occlusion; note that the veins are still in the phase of "laminar flow" (the stripe down each side of the vein) (*arrow*).**

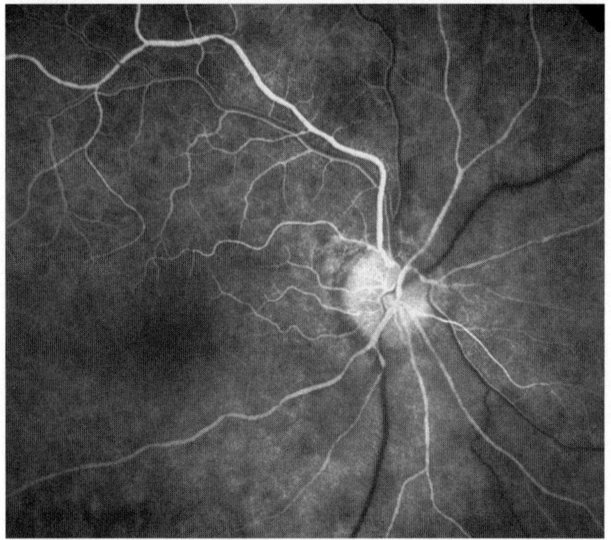

5-10B

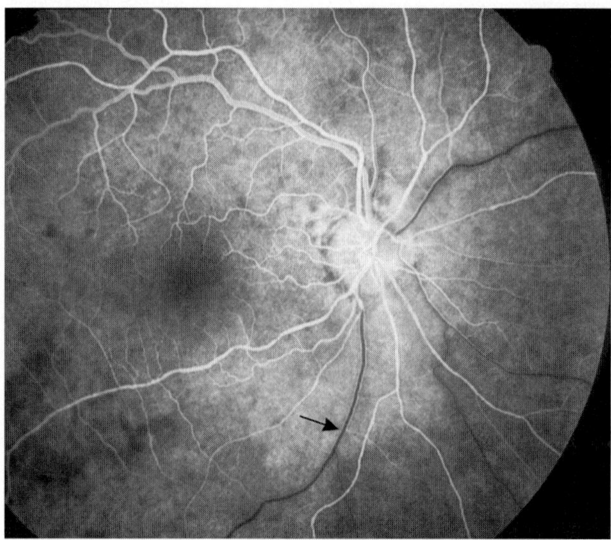

5-10C

Venous stasis retinopathy can occur as a complication of an embolic BRAO.[10]

CILIORETINAL ARTERY OCCLUSION

On occasion, the cilioretinal artery alone is occluded. The posterior ciliary vessels that penetrate the lamina cribrosa to supply the retina (cilioretinal artery) become affected in giant cell arteritis, resulting in a characteristic tonguelike retinal infarct that proceeds from the edge of the disc out onto the retina and meanders usually along the papillomacular bundle. Although in older individuals the most important cause to look for is giant cell arteritis, other causes can be present as well, including embolic occlusion or trauma to the posterior ciliary arteries. The visual field defect is commonly a paracentral scotoma when the occlusion is temporal off of the disc toward the macular area.

Figure 5-11. A. **Although embolic occlusion is possible, occlusion of the cilioretinal artery in an individual older than 65 years of age is evidence of giant cell arteritis until proven otherwise. The central retinal artery, once it has pierced the sclera, loses its elastic lamina, whereas the ciliary artery has an internal elastica, which is a major point of inflammation in giant cell arteritis.** B. **A drawing of an occlusion of the cilioretinal artery shows a pale peninsula of infarction jutting in toward the macula.** C. **This woman had papilledema with progressive visual field loss. She underwent an optic nerve sheath decompression, but suffered a cilioretinal artery occlusion during the surgical procedure. You can see the pale retina just temporal to the swollen disc (*arrows*).** ***Continued***

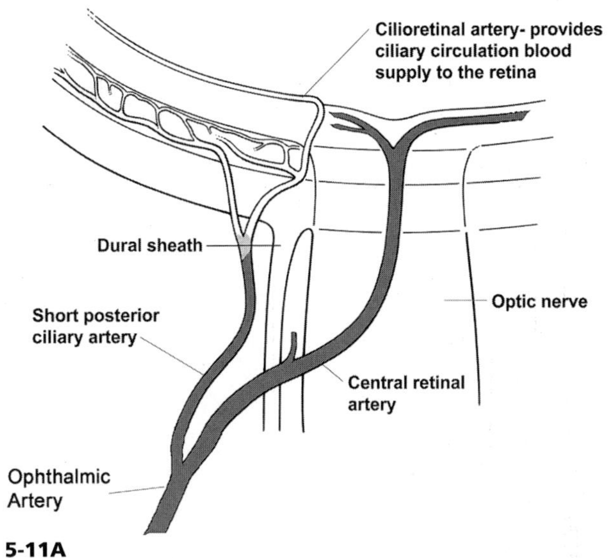

5-11A

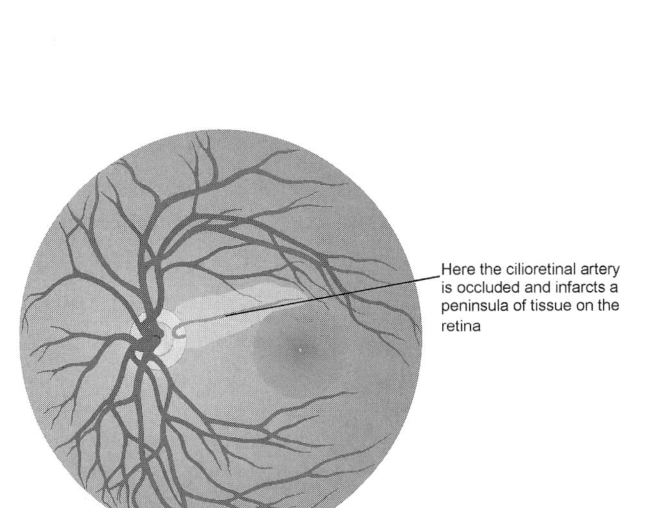

5-11B

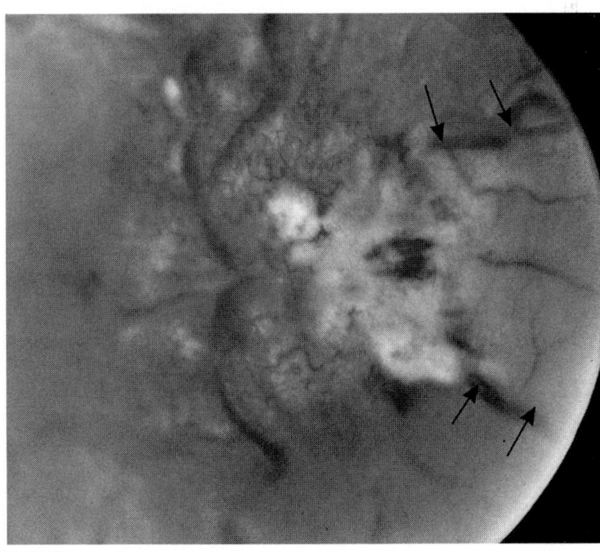

5-11C

Figure 5-11. *Continued.* D. **This man presented with acute central vision loss and an isolated cilioretinal artery occlusion. An extensive evaluation for temporal arteritis and an embolic source was unrevealing. The arrowheads outline the infarcted tissue; the arrow points to the cilioretinal artery.** E. **This man had biopsy-proven giant cell arteritis and presented with an isolated cilioretinal artery occlusion. Notice that there are also cotton-wool spots on the disc and that the disc is slightly swollen. The arrows point to the cilioretinal artery occlusion.**

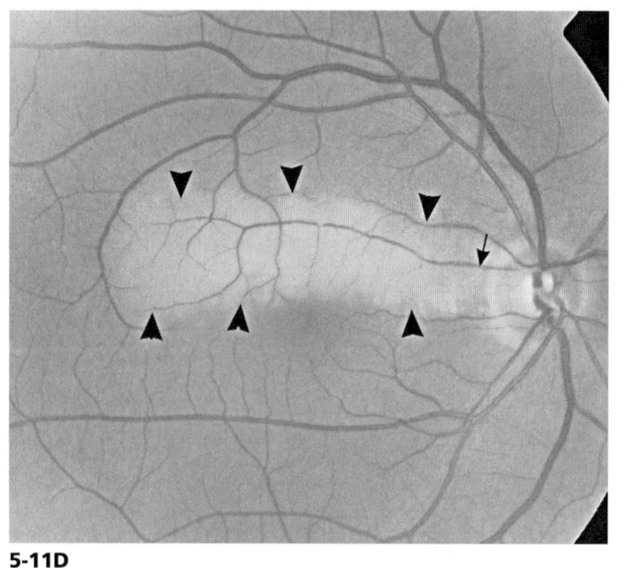

5-11D

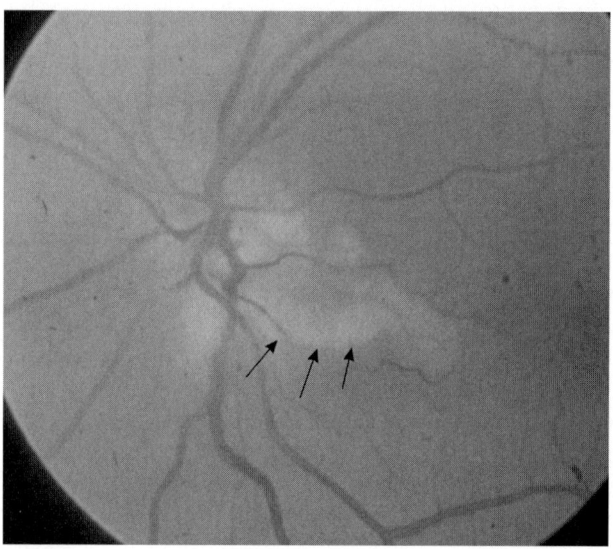

5-11E

The result of occlusions of the branch retinal artery or cilioretinal artery is ischemia to the retina at retinal arteriolar bifurcations, in which emboli lodge for various periods of time, leading to nerve fiber layer infarcts of varied ages, dot and blot hemorrhages, and white-centered hemorrhages known as *Roth's spots* . Roth's spot hemorrhages probably occur most commonly today in the setting of artery-to-artery embolization and in shaken baby syndrome, but have acquired a mythical status as being characteristic of subacute bacterial endocarditis. Any time these hemorrhages are seen, one should give some thought to subacute bacterial endocarditis, but recall that they are seen in a multitude of settings (see discussion of Roth's spots in Chapter 7).

OTHER SIGNS OF ARTERIAL OCCLUSION

Boxcar Appearance

A boxcar appearance of a segmented column of blood indicates slow flow or abnormal flow in a vessel. Segmentation of cells occurs most commonly in the veins, but can also be seen in the arteries. Other causes of a boxcar appearance include hyperviscosity syndromes and cardiac failure. In fact, at the time of cardiac arrest, one can ophthalmoscopically look for segmentation of the blood columns in the retina to evaluate the effectiveness of the resuscitation.[5]

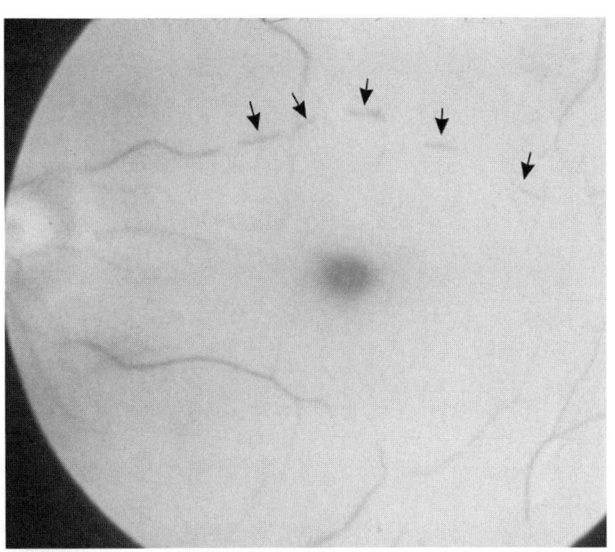
5-12A

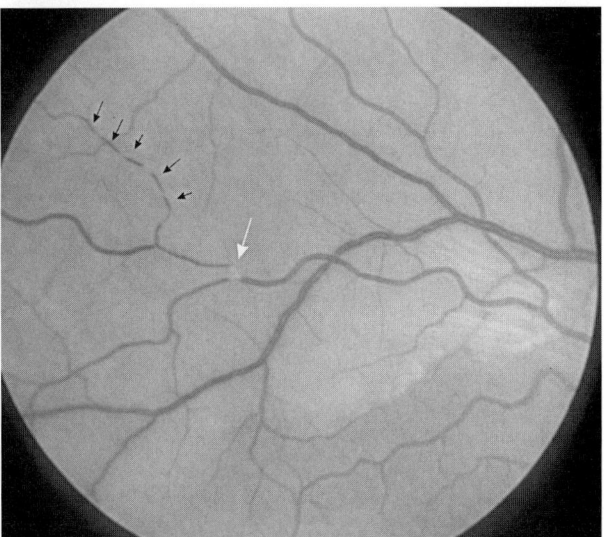
5-12B

Figure 5-12. A. **Here is a cherry-red macula from a CRAO—notice also the boxcar formations within the retinal arteries (*arrows*).** B. **This woman had a BRAO. You can appreciate the embolus in a branching retinal artery (*white arrow*). Boxcar formation is visible here, also (*black arrows*).**

Cholesterol Emboli

Cholesterol emboli, crystals known as *Hollenhorst plaques*, are parts of the grumous material found on the surface and within the cavity of ulcerated atherosclerotic plaques. These crystals within an arteriole glisten and have a refractile quality as the light is played over them. Colors are bright yellow-white to coppery, depending on the amount of blood passing in front of them.

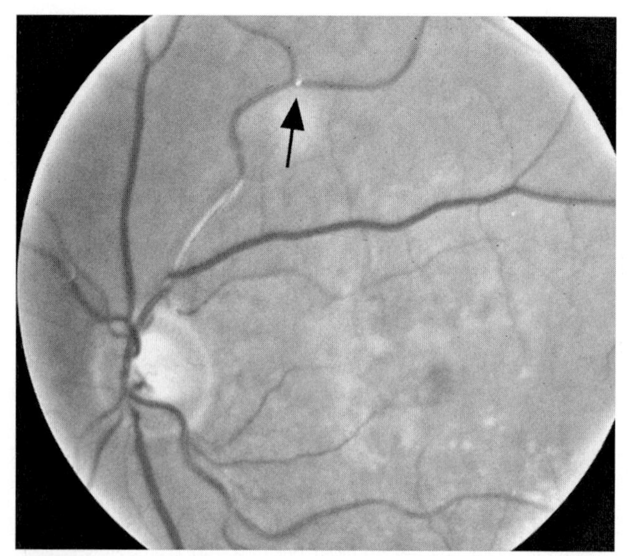

5-13A

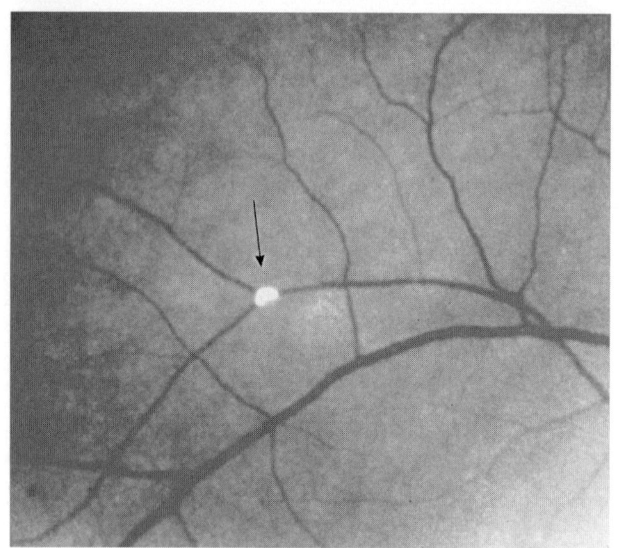

5-13B

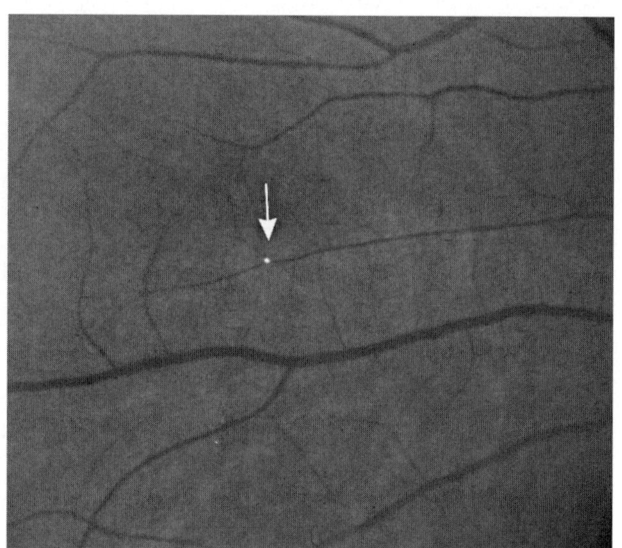

5-13C

Figure 5-13. A. **A Hollenhorst plaque is a yellow-orange plaque often seen at branch points of arteries. This patient had a BRAO due to a Hollenhorst plaque related to carotid vascular disease (*arrow*).** B. **This plaque is shiny. There was no associated BRAO, and it was found incidentally. Evaluation showed carotid vascular disease.** C. **This plaque (*arrow*) is hard to see—you would need to rotate the light back and forth to pick up a flicker of reflection.**

Dr. Robert W. Hollenhorst was an ophthalmologist who practiced at the Mayo Clinic. He had an abiding interest in vascular disease. In 1961, Hollenhorst stated the following:

Among 235 patients who had occlusive disease within the carotid arterial system and 93 patients with clinical symptoms and signs of involvement of the vertebral-basilar system, 31 (9.4%) had from a single plaque to several dozen bright plaques that were orange, yellow, or copper in color and situated at various bifurcations in some of the retinal arterioles . . . these plaques had a characteristically bright orange-color and reflected the light of the ophthalmoscope often in a heliographic position and tended to lodge simultaneously at several bifurcations of the same arteriole as though they were fragments of a larger plaque. [11]

Hollenhorst also offered the following advice for viewing the plaques with the ophthalmoscope[7]:

1. The plaque reflects the light brightly in one direction more than the other—so if the light is turned to different angles, the plaque will shine brighter (therefore, turn your ophthalmoscope in different directions as you are viewing the retinal arterioles in order to see some of the smallest plaques).
2. If you compress the globe and view the plaque within the vessel you will see a bright reflection flashing on and off with each pulsation.
3. Occlusion of an entire arteriole by a large plaque is infrequent (therefore, most of these do not occlude the artery).
4. If you see a plaque at one proximal bifurcation, look downstream because they tend to break off and lodge in smaller and more distal bifurcations.
5. The plaque may look larger than the vessel. Although the cholesterol plaque is wider than the blood column, it is not wider than the arteriole.

The importance of recognizing a Hollenhorst (cholesterol) plaque is that at least 90% of patients with visible embolic plaques have vascular disease, and 15% die within the first year of this finding and 55% are dead within 7 years. The cause of death is most frequently heart disease.[12]

Fibrin-Platelet Emboli

Fibrin-platelet emboli are common and simply reflect other collections of embolic material, long in clotting material and short in refractile cholesterol crystals.

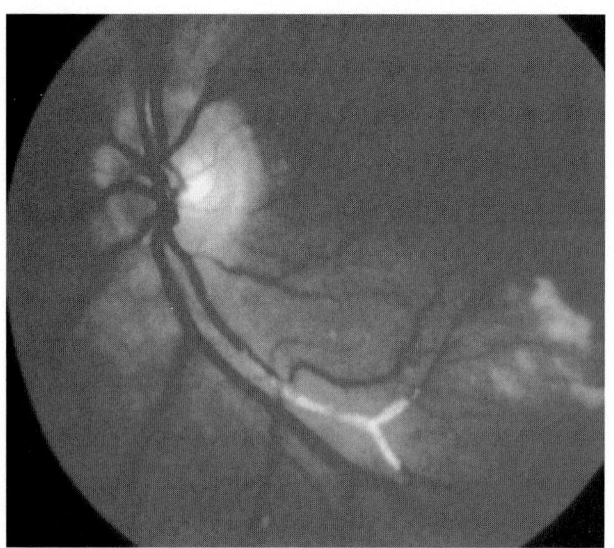

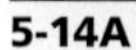

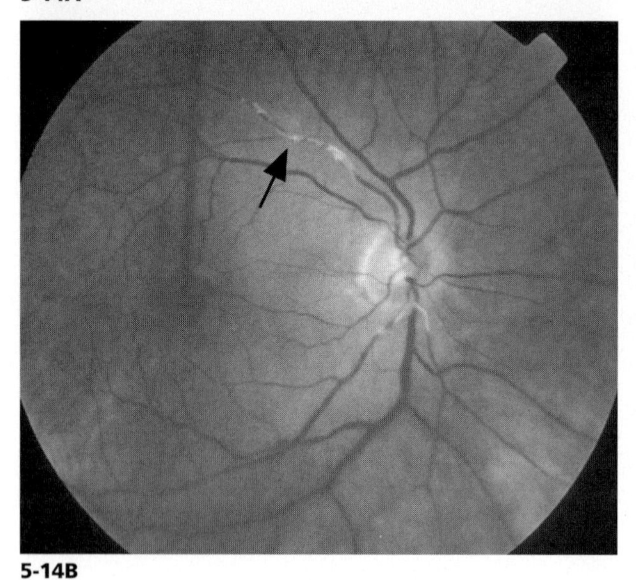

5-14B

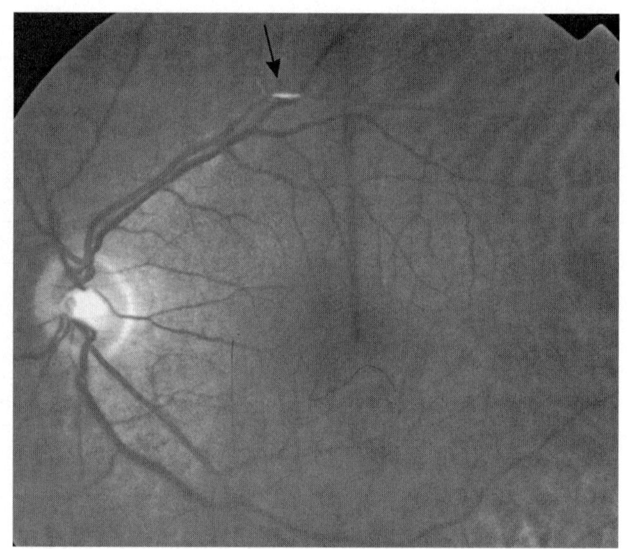

5-14C

Figure 5-14. These patients all had platelet fibrin emboli causing BRAO. Although the retinal pallor subsided, the emboli remain. A. **This clot outlines an entire arteriole to a branch. There are also cotton-wool spots distally.** B. **The occlusion is along an arteriole (*arrow*).** C. **This occlusion is just past a branch point (*arrow*).**

Evaluation of patients with fibrin-platelet emboli should include a full evaluation of the heart valves (e.g., floppy mitral valve, rheumatic disease, systemic lupus), carotid artery disease (including carotid artery plaque), and hypercoagulable workup. Look for a patent foramen ovale.

Calcific Emboli

Calcific emboli are fragments from a damaged valve. These are uncommon, or at least are recognized uncommonly. In contrast to the yellow- or copper-colored refractile emboli of Hollenhorst, these particles tend to be irregular and flat white. Calcific plaques tend to occlude the blood vessel right on the disc. The occlusion usually presents as arterial occlusion and less commonly as transient monocular vision loss.

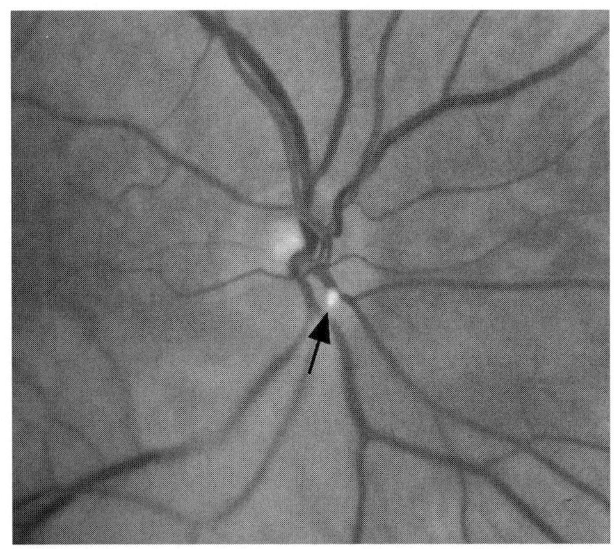

5-15

Figure 5-15. Look at the inferior branch of the central retinal artery on the disc and you will see a calcific embolus (*arrow*). (Photograph courtesy of Shelly Cross, M.D.)

Talc Emboli

Talc emboli in drug addicts are not common, despite the common use of talc to cut heroin. The distribution suggests that talc emboli are the result of passage of talc through a patent foramen ovale to both retinas after intravenous injection. Cough or other Valsalva maneuvers cause increased right heart pressure and a right-to-left shunt.

Tumor Emboli

Tumor emboli come from the surface of an atrial myxoma. Although rare, the diagnosis of atrial myxoma is urgent because of the extreme friability of the tumor and inexorable embolization until it is removed.

Fat Emboli

Fat emboli in the retina occur basically in two clinical settings. The first, but by no means a common occurrence, is with flat bone and long bone fractures. Even when fat emboli were looked for by indirect ophthalmoscopy in a group of orthopedic vehicular accident patients, only 4% of the group had evidence of retinal fat embolism.[13] Chest, neck,

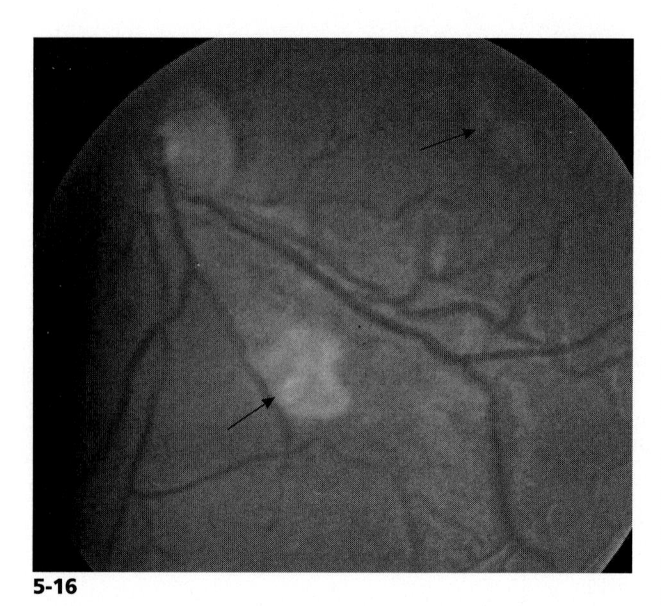

5-16

throat, and conjunctival petechiae are also seen. Fat emboli also occur with pancreatitis, in which large quantities of serum lipids occur with lipase in the blood stream. Patients with fat emboli to the brain frequently have an episode of what looks like a confusional state owing to a metabolic encephalopathy; showers of fat emboli to the brain may produce multiple focal neurologic signs and even reversible decorticate posturing or asterixis (see Chapter 14).

Figure 5-16. Fat emboli are rare. Here you see the occlusion of a vessel along with a large, ameboid cotton-wool spot (*arrow*). This fat embolus was seen in a 29-year-old man with hemorrhagic pancreatitis who presented with an acute confusional state. His confusion cleared, but he was left with petechiae on his chest and fat emboli in the retina without vision loss.

Table 5-4. Assessing Embolic Type

	Type of Embolus					
	Cholesterol	**Calcific**	**Platelet/fibrin**	**Fat**	**Myxoma***	**Talc**
History	TMB	TMB and/or vision loss	TMB and/or vision loss	Confusion, usually incidental	TMB + neurological events; subacute bacterial endocarditis without rheumatic history	No symptoms
Risk factors	Hypertension, smoking; older age	Rheumatic heart disease	Heart disease or carotid disease; systemic lupus erythematosus; fibromuscular dysplasia	Pancreatitis, surgery on long bones	—	Intravenous drug abuse
Appearance	Shiny, bright yellow; bifurcations	Dull white; usually larger vessel—on disc	Long, smooth segments with ends	Multiple infarcts	White material in the central retinal artery	Fine speckles of white in vessels
Source	Carotid artery	Heart—aortic or mitral valve	Valve or carotid artery	Long bone fracture, pancreatitis	Myxoma of left atrium	Drug use and patent foramen ovale
Evaluation	Auscultate carotid, carotid duplex, angiogram	Auscultate heart, echocardiogram, electrocardiogram	Carotid artery and heart evaluation	Serum amylase, urine for fat globules	Heart evaluation, echocardiogram	Echocardiogram
Treatment	Carotid endarterectomy or aspirin	Anticoagulation	Aspirin, carotid endarterectomy, anticoagulation	Self-limited	Anticoagulation, open-heart surgery	Avoid IV drug abuse

TMB = transient monocular blindness.
*Data in this column from DG Cogan, SH Wray. Vascular occlusions in the eye from cardiac myxomas. Am J Ophthalmol 1979;80:396–403.

POSTERIOR CILIARY ARTERY OCCLUSION

When the posterior ciliary artery is occluded two things may happen: If a branch of a person's posterior ciliary artery extends into a cilioretinal artery, you may see a typical cilioretinal artery occlusion. More frequently, when the posterior ciliary artery is occluded, an infarction of the disc ensues. Review the discussion of disc swelling associated with anterior ischemic optic neuropathy (see Chapter 3).

Figure 5-17. A. **Notice that when the posterior ciliary artery is occluded there is loss of blood flow to the optic disc, the choroid, or both. The ciliary artery has its elastic lamina (unlike the central retinal artery), and therefore is susceptible to giant cell arteritis.** B. **When the disc loses its blood supply, swelling takes place and a stroke to the optic nerve occurs called *anterior ischemic optic neuropathy.***

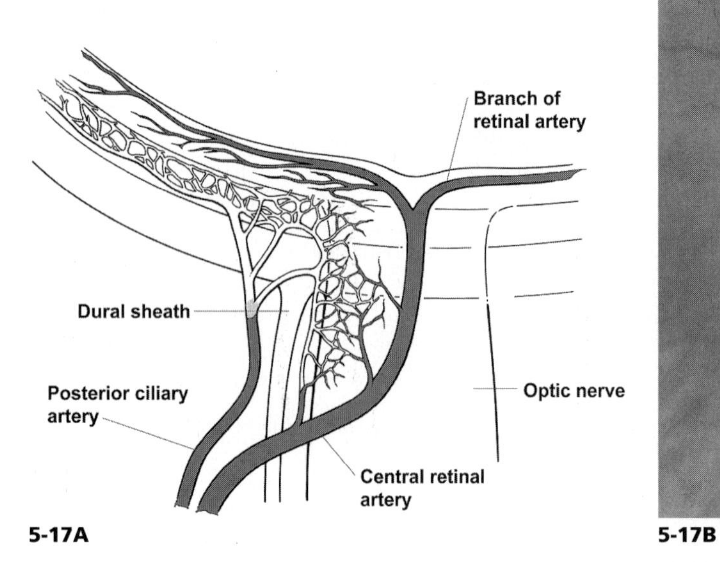

5-17A

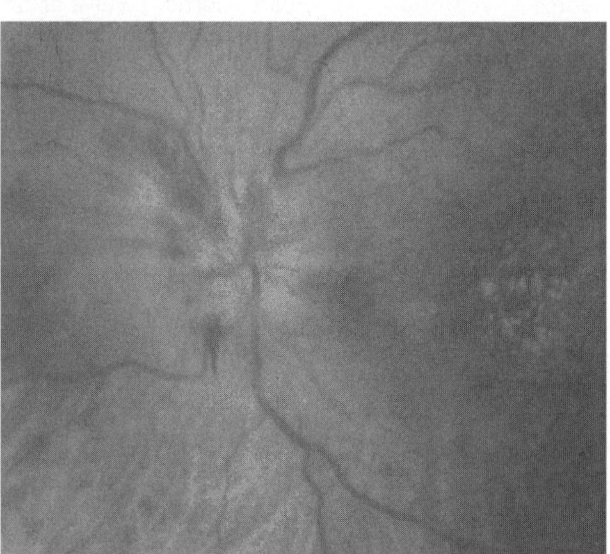

5-17B

Figure 5-18. Fluorescein angiography is sometimes helpful and shows changes of the small vessels on the disc and late staining. A. The clinical appearance of NA-AION is a swollen disc. B. Typical fluorescein angiogram of NA-AION early on shows lack of filling of the posterior ciliary arteries (*arrowheads* outline the nonfilling choroid) and early disc staining. C. Later, the disc stains and leaks owing to the breakdown of the blood retinal barrier.

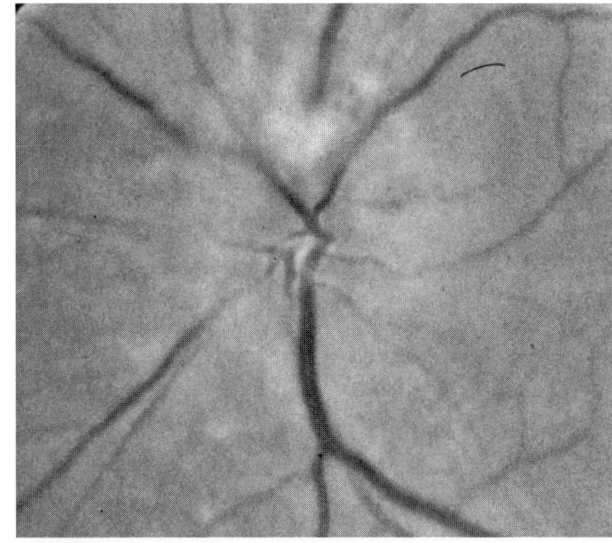

5-18A

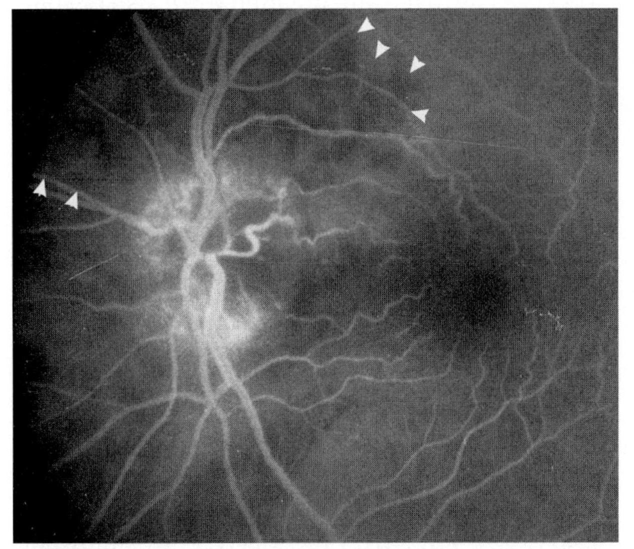

5-18B

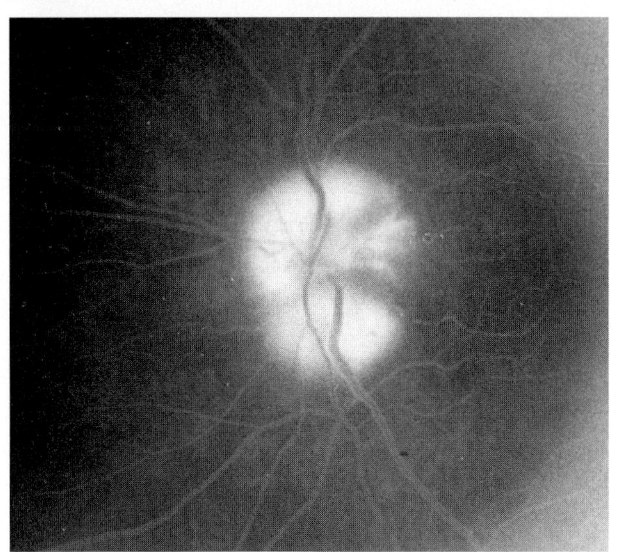

5-18C

Arnold and colleagues showed a significant delay in the onset of dye appearance as well as prolonged time to the filling of the prelaminar optic disc in patients with anterior ischemic optic neuropathy (AION).[14] They also found that other causes of disc swelling, such as optic neuritis, did not have this delay.[15] Hayreh showed that the disc lies in a "watershed" between the lateral and medial posterior ciliary arteries.[2] Lack of flow between these two circulations can sometimes be demonstrated on fluorescein angiography.

Because nonarteritic (NA)-AION and arteritic AION sometimes cannot be differentiated one from the other, a Westergren erythrocyte sedimentation rate is essential. C-reactive protein and fibrinogen testing can also be helpful.[16] In general, the erythrocyte sedimentation rate and C-reactive protein are normal in NA-AION. If they are elevated, a temporal artery biopsy may be needed. Studies have looked at the value of a negative temporal artery biopsy in the face of elevated erythrocyte sedimentation rate and found an association with underlying malignancy, inflammation, and infection.[17–19] Glucose and blood urea nitrogen and creatinine are also of some help. In the young, look for homocystinemia, which has been associated with AION.[20]

Arteritic Anterior Ischemic Optic Neuropathy (Giant Cell Arteritis)

Arteritic AION (giant cell or temporal arteritis) is a disease seen, with only rare exceptions, in older individuals with a lower limit of 50 years of age. Usually, they are older than 65 years, and most are 70–90 years old. Arteritic AION is an important cause of transient monocular vision loss or acute blindness in the elderly. This type of ocular stroke can usually be prevented with steroids; therefore, it is extremely important to know about this cause of disc swelling and to recognize not only the disc appearance, but also the entire clinical syndrome. Here, ophthalmoscopy is key in identifying a medical emergency. Temporal arteritis causes many observable and testable abnormalities.

Table 5-5. Ophthalmologic Findings in Temporal Arteritis

Finding
On the disc
Acute anterior ischemic optic neuritis—acute disc swelling
Posterior ischemic optic neuropathy—no acute swelling, but pallor follows
In the retina
Ischemic retinopathy with cotton-wool spots
Central/branch retinal artery occlusion
Cilioretinal artery occlusion
Ischemic choroidopathy
Orbital ischemia
Orbital cellulitis and pseudotumor
Other eye findings
Corneal edema
Iritis
Hypotony
Pupil
Afferent and efferent defects
Tonic pupil
Cranial nerve ischemia, especially oculomotor nerve
Ocular muscle ischemia

Source: Adapted in part from reference 16.

Although appearance of the disc in arteritic AION is sometimes indistinguishable from NA-AION, there are a few clues in the disc appearance. First, if the disc has a very chalky white appearance, this should suggest arteritis. Second, if you see a concomitant occlusion of the cilioretinal artery, the diagnosis is temporal arteritis until proven otherwise. The combination of retinal cotton-wool spots and AION should lead you to perform a fluorescein angiogram. There is also a characteristic pattern to the fluorescein angiography, including occlusion of posterior ciliary arteries and choroidal nonperfusion.[21]

Figure 5-19. A–C. **Chalky white swollen disc suggests temporal arteritis in these three cases. The chalky white swelling is owing to the complete wipeout of blood flow to these discs due to arteritic occlusion of the posterior ciliary arteries from giant cell arteritis.**

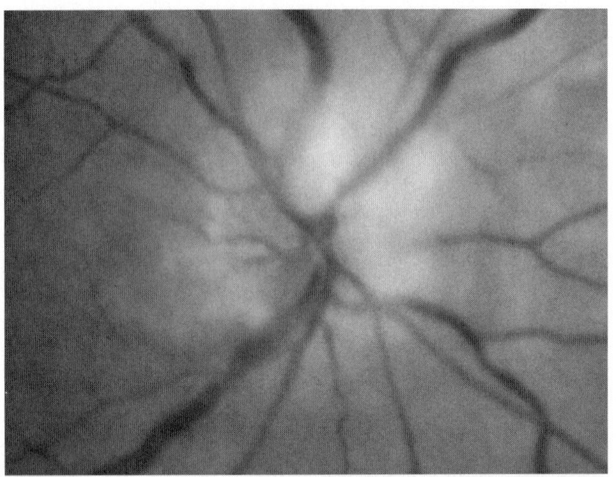

5-19A

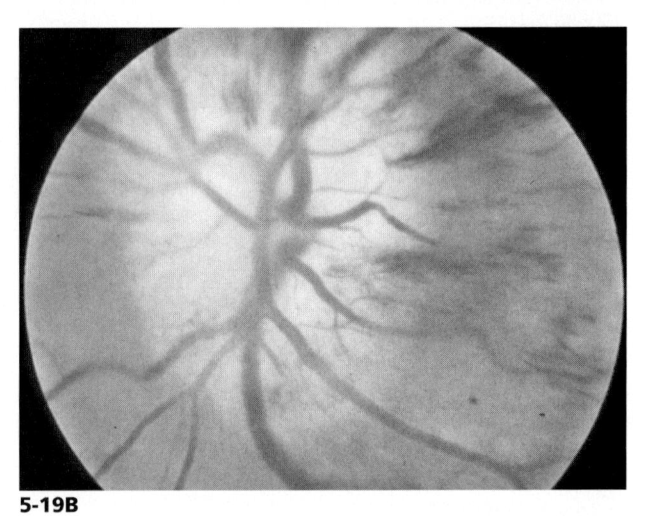

5-19B

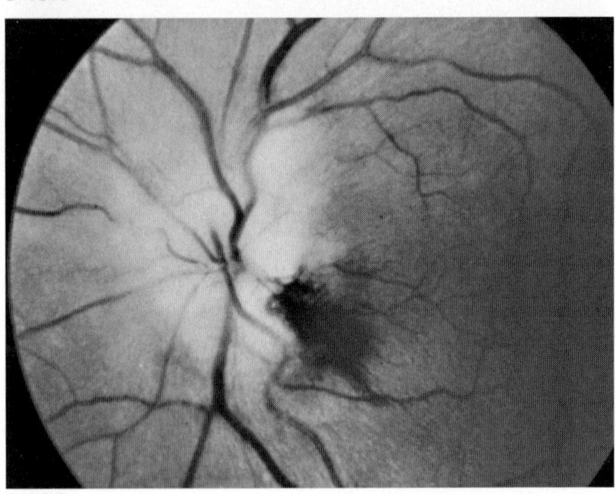

5-19C

Figure 5-20. This man presented with painless vision loss with acuity of 20/60 in the right eye. He had no other symptoms of polymyalgia rheumatica or temporal arteritis. A swollen disc (A, right eye) consistent with early AION and cotton-wool spots owing to retinal microinfarcts (B, left eye) prompted a temporal artery biopsy, confirming the diagnosis of temporal arteritis. A cotton-wool spot occurring in isolation in the right age group should lead to an evaluation for temporal arteritis. C. Fluorescein angiogram shows a typical patchy pattern of posterior ciliary infarction causing poor flow in the choroidal circulation, typical of temporal arteritis, in the same patient. The arrows show areas between nonperfusion and perfusion. D. Fluorescein angiogram in temporal arteritis.

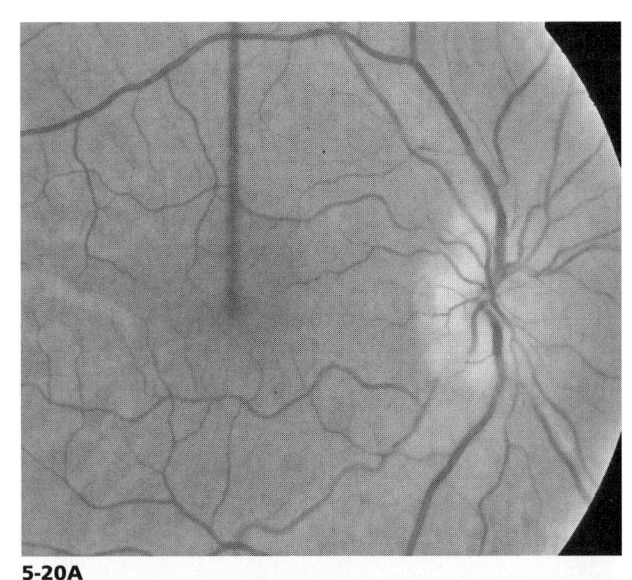

5-20A

5-20B

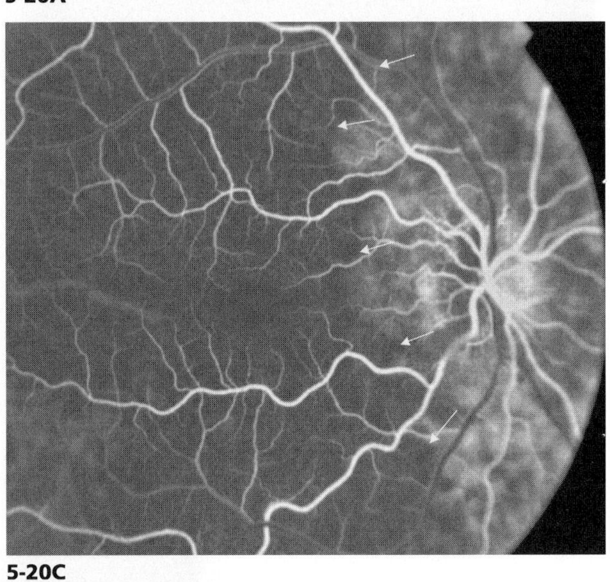

5-20C

5-20D

Learn to differentiate the two types of AION—arteritic and nonarteritic. Although both can be related to posterior ciliary artery occlusion, the pathophysiology of the swelling is different, and so is the treatment. The failure to diagnose arteritic AION can lead to severe, permanent blindness, and the condition is thus a true ophthalmologic emergency. Examination of an eye with arteritic AION shows loss of visual acuity—in fact, in studies comparing NA-AION to arteritic AION, the arteritic form shows much greater immediate loss of visual acuity.

Figure 5-21.

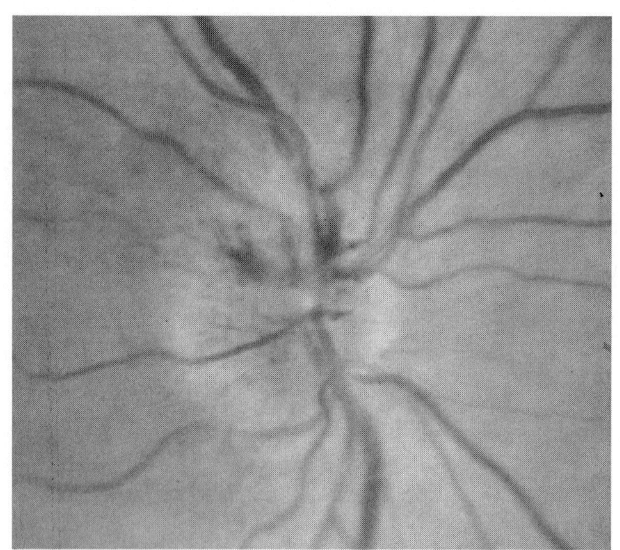

5-21A

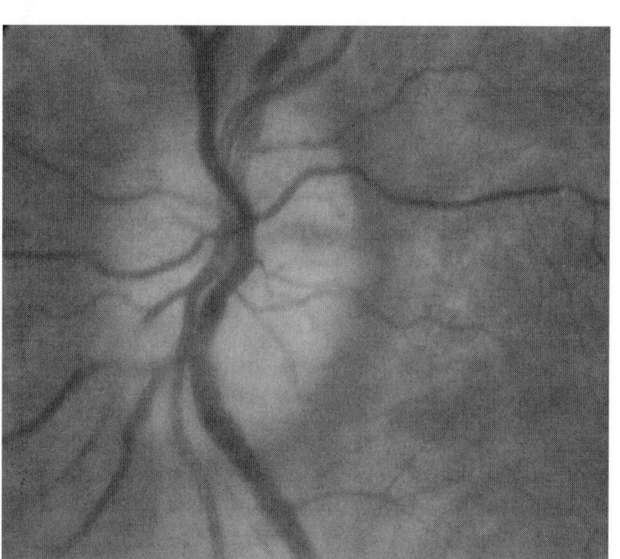

5-21B

Table 5-6. Differentiating Arteritic and NA-AION

Characteristic	NA-AION (see Figure 5-21A)	Arteritic AION (see Figure 5-21B)
Age	Usually older than 45 years	Usually older than 65 years
Sex	Men and women	Women >men
Risk factors	Diabetes, hypertension, smoking, small cup-to-disc ratio, hypotension, anemia	Polymyalgia rheumatica
Symptoms	Visual blurring, dimming	Same
Headache	Absent	Present—new and persistent

Characteristic	NA-AION (see Figure 5-21A)	Arteritic AION (see Figure 5-21B)
Jaw claudication	Absent	Present—the most common symptom
Scalp tenderness	Absent	Present
Temporal artery tenderness	Absent	Present
Weight loss	Absent	Present
Polymyalgia rheumatica—aching but no tenderness in the shoulders and hips, especially neck pain; fatigue, fever, night sweats	Absent	Present
Visual acuity	Variably decreased	Usually severely decreased
Visual field	Variably altitudinal, constriction	Usually severely affected
Disc	Swelling globally or sectorially—may be hyperemic and pale segmentally	Usually very pale swelling, chalk white disc
Fluorescein angiogram	Late disc staining	See patchy choroidal filling around disc
Evaluation	Erythrocyte sedimentation rate usually normal, normal fibrinogen and C-reactive protein	Elevated erythrocyte sedimentation rate in 90%, elevated C-reactive protein, must do temporal artery biopsy
Treatment	Aspirin	Corticosteroids—high dose
Outcome	Usually improves somewhat	Little improvement

Ophthalmic Artery Occlusion: Central Retinal Artery Occlusion and Anterior Ischemic Optic Neuropathy

The combination of a pale retina as seen in CRAO and a swollen disc (AION) indicates an occlusion of the ophthalmic artery—occlusion of the central retinal artery and the posterior ciliary artery. With this combination, there would be no cherry-red spot. Other findings include reduced intraocular pressure and an extinguished electroretinogram. The incidence of ophthalmic artery occlusion is unknown; however, it is uncommon.

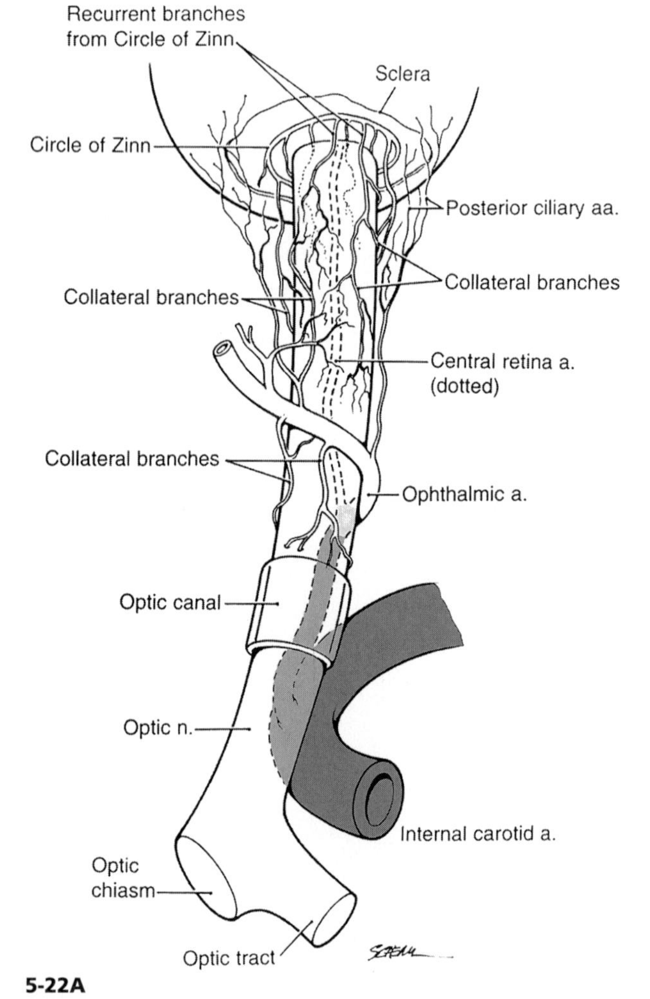

5-22A

Figure 5-22. A. **Diagram of ophthalmic artery occlusion: When the ophthalmic artery is occluded, there is CRAO and a swollen optic disc. Ophthalmic artery occlusion has devastating consequences to the eye.** B. **Notice that an ophthalmic artery occlusion occludes the central retinal artery and the posterior ciliary artery.** ***Continued***

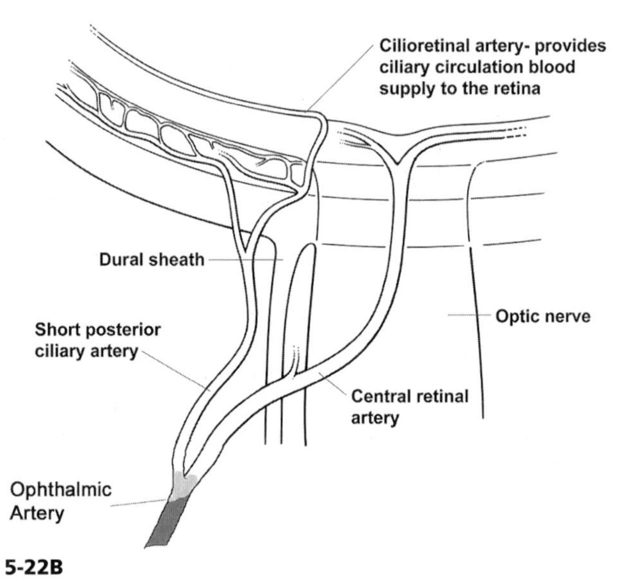

5-22B

Figure 5-22. ***Continued.*** C. **In ophthalmic artery occlusion, you see no cherry-red spot, because the posterior ciliary artery occlusion results in no perfusion of the choroid beneath the macula. A pale, swollen retina and optic disc swelling typical of AION is characteristic.** D. **This man exhibited a complete ophthalmic artery occlusion, showing an opaque retina as well as AION.**

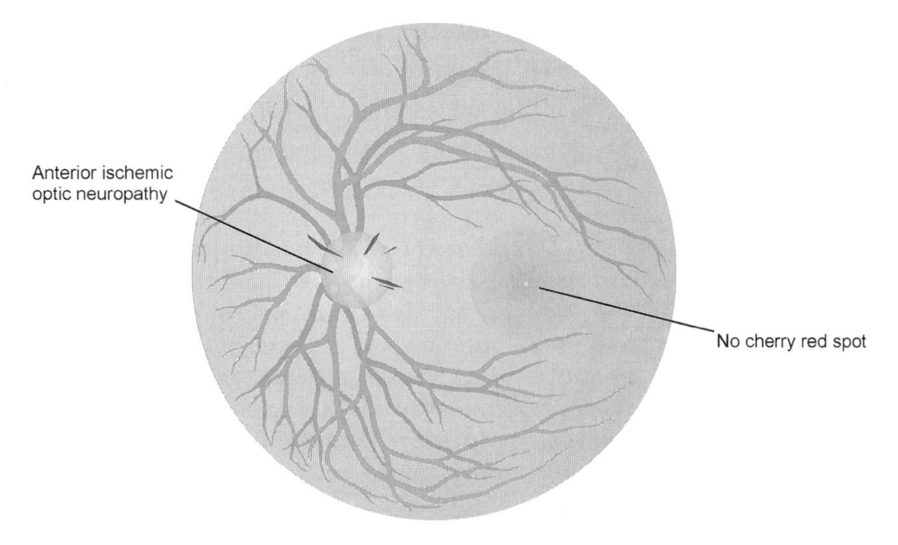

5-22C

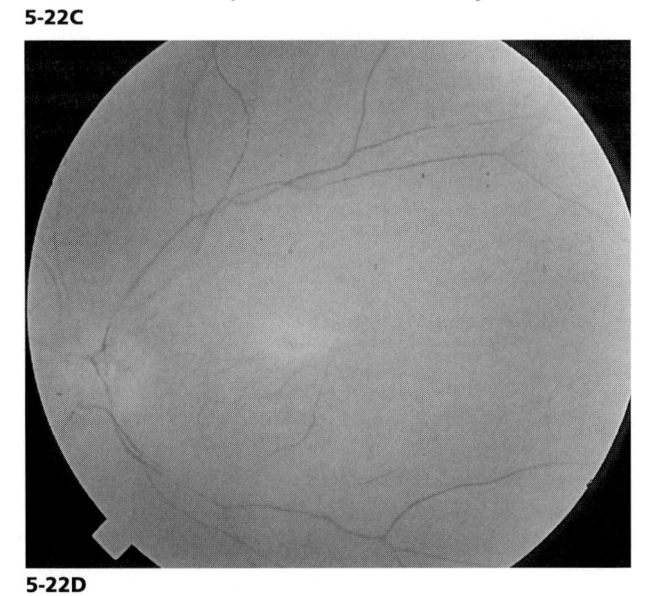

5-22D

Choroidal Artery Occlusion and Ocular Ischemic Syndrome

Choroidal ischemia occurs with severe hypertension. Recall that the choroid is filled by the posterior ciliary arteries (see Chapter 2). These small arterioles are particularly susceptible to acute and accelerated hypertension. See the discussions on hypertensive retinopathy and severe pre-eclampsia (see Chapters 9 and 13).

Figure 5-23. The choroid is filled by posterior ciliary arteries. The arteries form capillary (choriocapillaris) cobblestones that feed the retinal pigment epithelium and cones and rods. A is the arterial end and V is the venous end. (Photograph courtesy of Lee Allen.) (Reprinted from Hayreh SS. Segmental nature of the choroidal vasculature. Br J Ophthalmol 1975;59:631–648, with permission.)

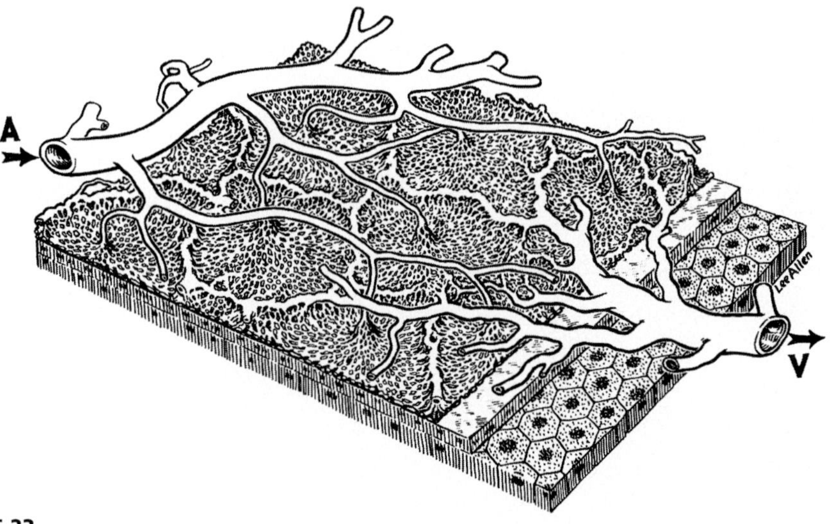

5-23

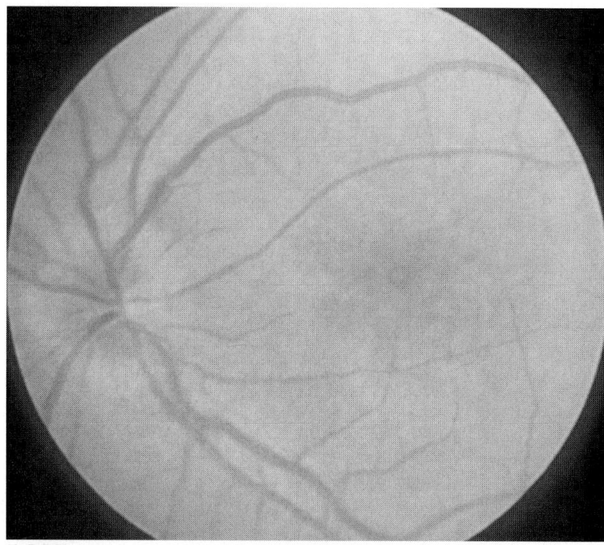
5-24A

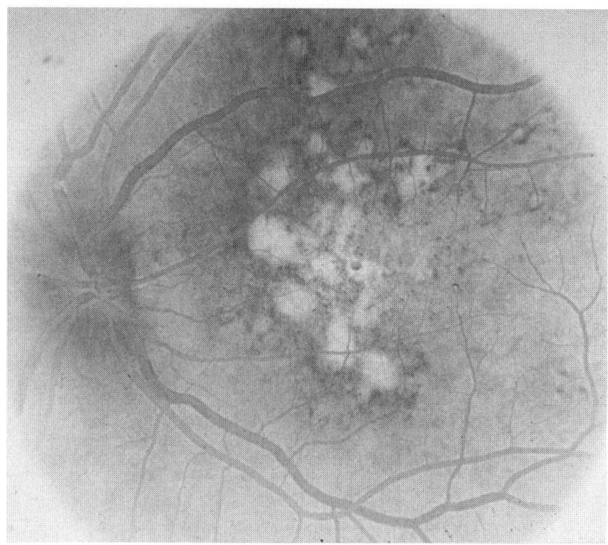
5-24B

Figure 5-24. A. **This 27-year-old man ingested large doses of ephedrine and presented with visual blurring, as well as very high blood pressures. The retinal findings were not impressive, however, except for some subtle changes in the choroid.** B. **The fluorescein angiogram dramatically indicated choroidal infarctions in the grapelike clusters of the choroidal blood supply.**

Ischemic ocular syndrome or *pan-ocular hypoperfusion* occurs with severe carotid artery disease. Described by Knox,[22] ocular ischemic syndrome is severe ischemic disease of the eye caused by reduced direct and collateral perfusion of the ophthalmic artery. Because there is extensive collateral circulation to the eye, most cases of ocular ischemic syndrome reported have been owing to bilateral extensive vascular occlusive disease or, at least, very significant (>90%) carotid stenosis affecting the internal and external carotid systems.

The ocular ischemic syndrome presents insidiously as transient monocular blindness (Wray's type 2). Often, that visual symptom is brought on by exposure to bright light. Bright objects appear brighter and the edges may flicker. Everything may look like an overexposed photograph. Some of the symptoms are postural; that is, they worsen when the patient is upright and improve with recumbency. For example, ischemic pain, which is a constant ache of the orbit, face, or temple may be worse in an upright position. This postural visual problem is said to occur occasionally in Takayasu's disease.

The earliest retinal findings in the ocular ischemic syndrome are intraretinal hemorrhages (usually peripheral dot-and-blot), microaneurysms, and tortuous veins. Fluorescein angiography may show delay in retinal filling as well as choroidal hypoperfusion. Also look for neovascularization of the iris and redness of the eye. Further evidence of this condition is decreased intraocular pressure owing to ciliary body ischemia. Fluorescein angiography shows slow flow and a delay in retinal arterial filling, as well as choroidal hypoperfusion.

Table 5-7. Findings in Ocular Ischemic Syndrome

Conjunctival injection with ciliary flush
Corneal decompensation; edema
Episcleral injection
Cells and flare in the anterior chamber
Spontaneous hyphema
Iris neovascularization
Neovascular glaucoma
Cataract
Cotton-wool spots of retina
Venous stasis retinopathy
Horner's syndrome on the side of the carotid disease

Source: Adapted from JB Mizener, P Podhajsky, SS Hayreh. Ocular ischemic syndrome. Ophthalmology 1997;104:859–864.

Table 5-8. Causes of Ocular Ischemic Syndrome

Cerebrovascular disease:
Carotid stenosis;
External carotid artery disease
With associated:
Diabetes mellitus,
Arterial hypertension,
Coronary artery disease
Takayasu's arteritis

Source: Adapted from JB Mizener, P Podhajsky, SS Hayreh. Ocular ischemic syndrome. Ophthalmology 1997;104:859–864.

Table 5-9. Disc and Retinal Findings with Ocular Ischemic Syndrome*

Optic disc	Cherry-red spot
Pallor	Central retinal artery collapse with gentle pressure on the globe
Neovascularization of the disc	Spontaneous pulsations of central retinal artery
Cupping with/without pallor	Neovascularization of the retina
Disc edema	Nonischemic central retinal vein occlusion
Retina	Multiple embolic plaques
Superficial hemorrhages	Choroid
Box-carring of flow in the blood vessels	Infarction
Retinal arteriolar attenuation or sclerosis	Chorioretinal degeneration

*Findings in descending order of frequency.
Source: Adapted from JB Mizener, P Podhajsky, SS Hayreh. Ocular ischemic syndrome. Ophthalmology 1997;104:859–864.

Table 5-10. Conditions That Cause Neovascularization of the Iris

Ischemic syndromes	Systemic disorders	Surgery/radiation/ trauma (eye)	Ocular disease	Genetic disorders
Central retinal vein occlusion	Diabetes mellitus	Surgery for retinal detachment	Neovascular glaucoma	Neurofibromatosis
Central retinal artery occlusion	Sickle cell disease	Vitrectomy	Uveitis	Marfan's syndrome
Branch retinal artery occlusion	Systemic lupus erythematosus	Cataract surgery	Endophthalmitis	Ehlers-Danlos syndrome
Carotid artery disease	Giant cell arteritis	Radiation	Retinal detachment	
C-C fistula	Metastatic cancer to the eye or orbit	Eye trauma	Persistent hyperplastic vitreous	
Ocular ischemic syndrome			Sympathetic ophthalmia	
			Retinoblastoma	
			Melanoma of choroid, iris	

Source: Adapted from P Lee, CC Wang, AP Adamis. Ocular neovascularization: an epidemiological review. Surv Ophthalmol 1998;43:245–269.

The typical story of an ocular ischemic syndrome is an older individual who notices decreased vision (transient monocular blindness) in an upright posture and also a positional aching above the brow (better lying flat and worse upright). In these cases, look for signs of ischemic retina, including iris neovascularization and hemorrhages in the retina.

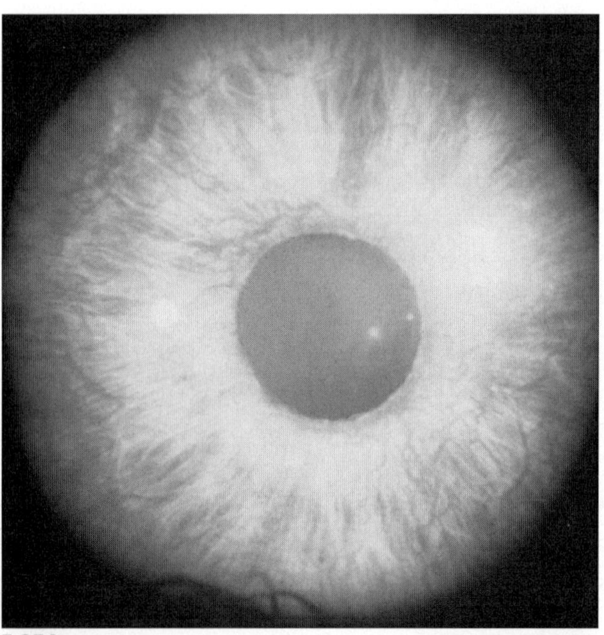

5-25A

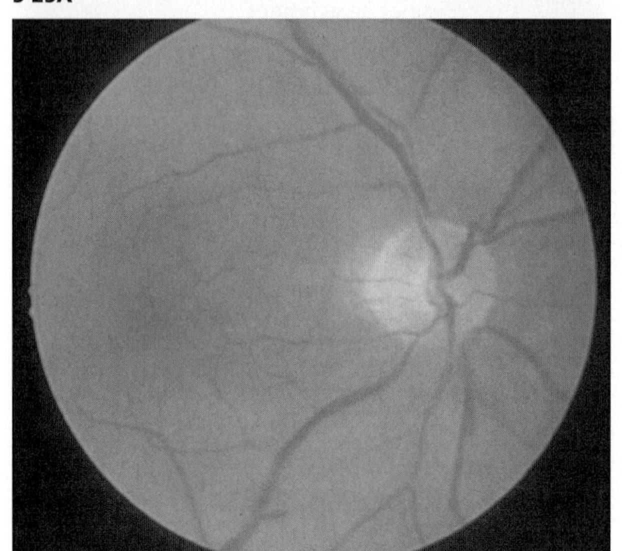

5-25B

Figure 5-25. (A,B left; C–H, opposite page) **Ischemic ocular syndrome.** A. **This individual had severe iris neovascularization characterized by small vessels throughout the iris, rubeosis iridis.** B. **He complained of transient vision loss with discomfort around his right eye. The fundus examination showed a normal disc with slightly attenuated arterioles.** C. **Following the arteries inferiorly, you will detect hemorrhages seen around the inferior branch retinal artery in his right eye. Follow the interior vessels further and note hemorrhages of the dot-and-blot type.** D. **Following the same disc superiorly, you will find other hemorrhages.** E. **The fluorescein angiogram did not show dye in the arteries until 21 seconds (normally it appears at 8–12 seconds and the disc begins to glow first).** F. **At 25 seconds, you see blood only in the arterioles.** G. **At 34.5 seconds, the choroid shows patchy filling, and more blood appears in his arterial circulation.** H. **At 42 seconds, the arteries are finally filled, but the veins are not. The choroid remains dark temporally, indicating that the posterior ciliary arteries are filling slowly and poorly. The disc stains. The cause of this man's ocular ischemic syndrome was severe atherosclerotic disease.**

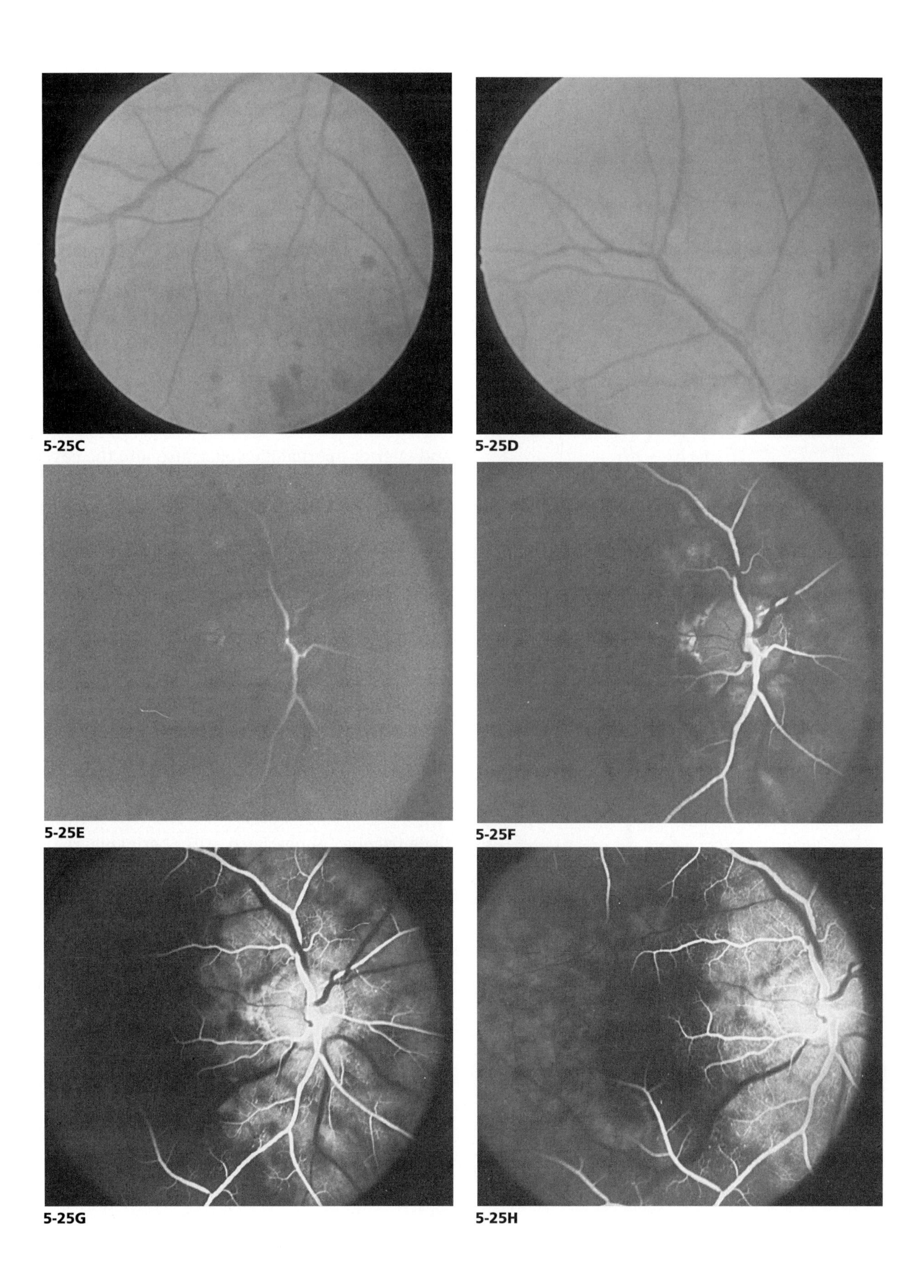

5-25C

5-25D

5-25E

5-25F

5-25G

5-25H

Venous Disease Can Cause Episodic Vision Loss

The venous drainage of the inner retina (the nerve fiber layer and ganglion cell layer) occurs via the central retinal vein, after which the blood passes via the superior ophthalmic vein into the cavernous sinus and out of the skull through the internal jugular vein. The choroidal venous circulation drains through a cobblestone or paving-stone arrangement into the *vortex veins,* thence into the orbit where they exit via the superior ophthalmic and inferior ophthalmic veins, also into the cavernous sinus and then jugular venous system.

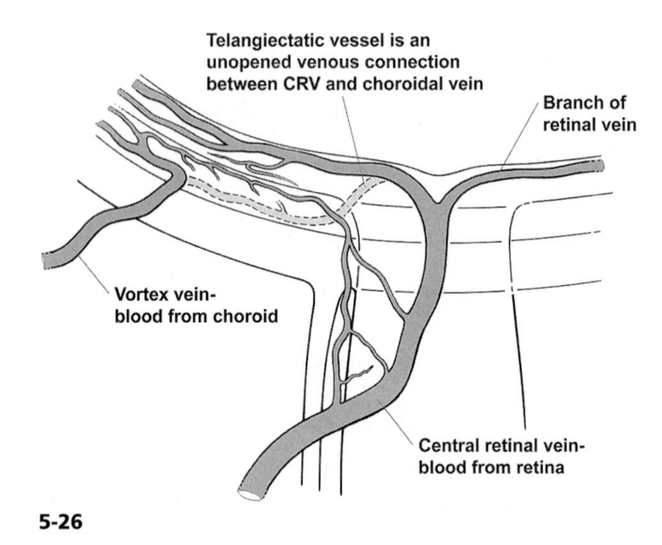

5-26

Figure 5-26. Diagram of the venous drainage: central retinal vein (CRV), vortex vein. Notice the potential unopened venous connection between the CRV and the choroidal vein (light gray).

Veno-occlusive disease usually occurs in the elderly.

Central Retinal Vein Occlusion—Acute/Chronic

Retinal vein occlusion often has a dramatic ophthalmoscopic appearance with peripapillary and peripheral hemorrhages, some of which are massive and can obscure all retinal detail. The hemorrhages in central retinal vein occlusion (CRVO) generally follow the retinal veins and nerve fiber layer. The veins become dilated and tortuous. Just as there can be central and branch retinal *artery* occlusion, there may be central and branch retinal *vein* occlusions. The site of CRVO is usually behind or within the lamina cribrosa (where the central retinal artery and central retinal vein share a single wall). The site of branch retinal vein occlusion (BRVO) is characteristically at an arteriolar/venular crossing. Multiple nerve fiber layer infarcts in addition to the hemorrhages herald a combined CRVO and CRAO. CRVO by itself is limited in visual recovery only by the extent to which the macula has been damaged.

There are two types of CRVO: *Non-ischemic* , the most common form, is associated with relatively little visual morbidity and no relative afferent pupillary defect (RAPD), whereas the *ischemic (hemorrhagic retinopathy*) type is often associated with permanent vision loss and an RAPD. The ischemic form subsequently has associated neovascularization and requires more aggressive treatment. Both forms of these venous occlusions are usually painless.

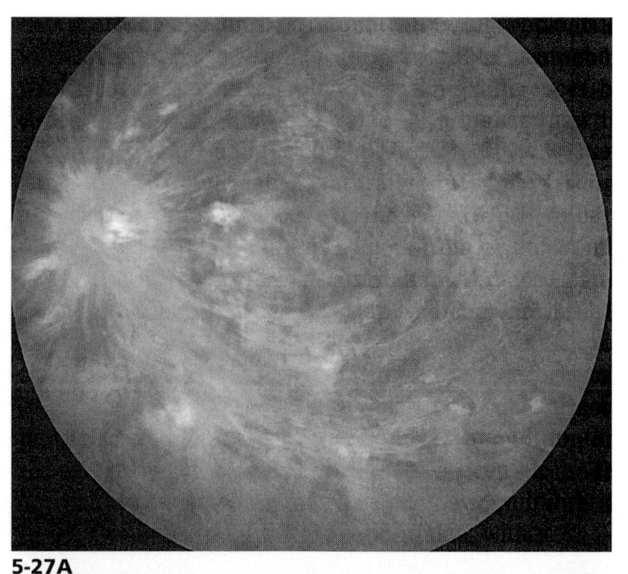

5-27A

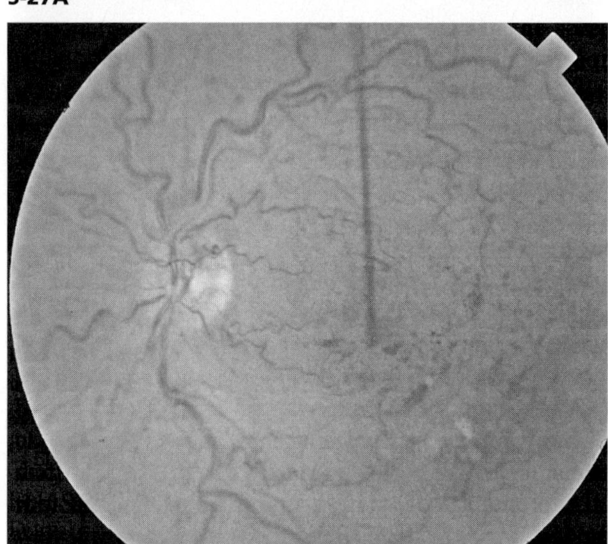

5-27B

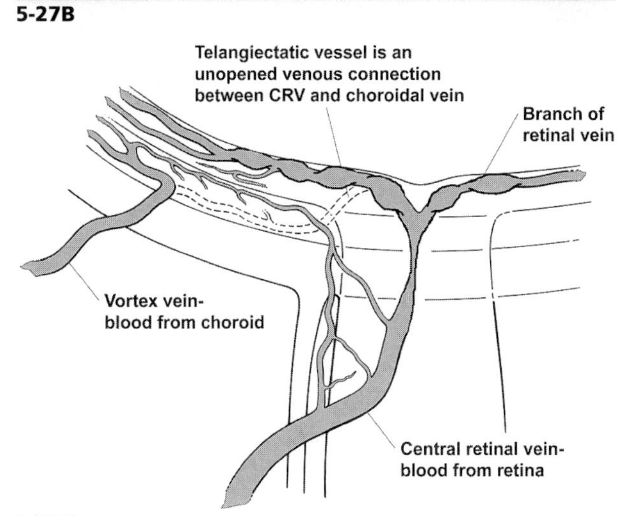

5-27C

Figure 5-27. A. **Typical CRVO shows hemorrhages following the veins and nerve fiber layer. Some have likened it to a "tomato splat" or "blood and thunder"—one look into the fundus, and you see hemorrhages 360 degrees around the disc. In the nonischemic form of CRVO, the vision usually recovers after several weeks, leaving little sign of the dramatic ophthalmoscopic appearance.** B. **This chronic CRVO occurred almost 3 years earlier; notice that fresh hemorrhages and nerve fiber layer hemorrhages are still present, indicating an ongoing slowing of retinal venous drainage. The venules are extremely tortuous.** C. **Notice that when there is a CRVO there is stasis of venous egress. In CRVO, the occlusion is somewhere at the disc or lamina.**

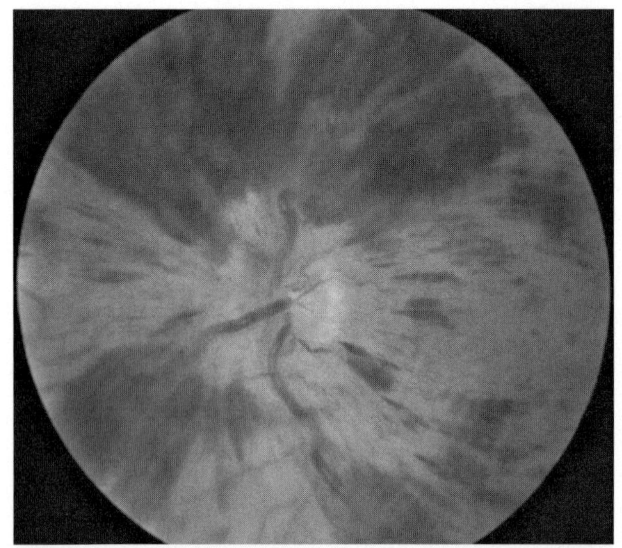
5-28A

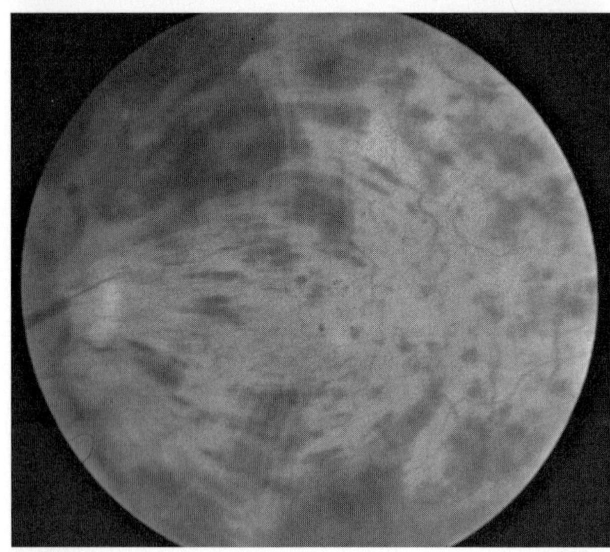
5-28B

Figure 5-28. A. **This man had a severe acute CRVO. He had reduced visual acuity and a large afferent pupillary defect. Ischemic retinal vein occlusion may look similar to the nonischemic version, but you will see an RAPD, indicating significant vision loss. Furthermore, there may be macular edema, which can cause a profound drop in visual acuity.** B. **In macular edema, the foveal reflex is lost.**

Examination of a patient with CRVO should involve measuring visual acuity and an assessment for an RAPD. The presence or absence of an RAPD is important, because ischemic retinal vein occlusion is associated with an RAPD defect of greater than 0.6 log units.[23] No venous pulsations will be present (if one can see the veins at all). Ophthalmoscopic findings include the presence of retinal hemorrhages and cotton-wool spots, usually along a dilated retinal vein. Disc edema can occur. Evaluation of the macula for edema is also important, because macular edema can occur with particularly severe CRVO. Approximately 20% of cases develop venous-venous collaterals of the disc (retinochoroidal or opticociliary shunt vessels).

Complications of CRVO include neovascularization of the retina and angle-closure glaucoma. In fact, 40% of patients developed glaucoma 1 year after severe CRVO.[24]

Although CRVO usually occurs in older adults, young adults may develop the condition. Many terms have been developed to describe CRVO in the young, including *papillophlebitis* , *benign retinal vasculitis*, *optic disc vasculitis* , *nonischemic CRVO* , a variety of the *big blind spot syndrome* , and *phlebitis of the optic disc* . Most young adults do well, with good visual acuity; however, approximately 1 in 5 develops significant vision loss.[25]

All patients with CRVO should be followed by an ophthalmologist because glaucoma, neovascularization, and macular edema may develop and require treatment.

Table 5-11. Causes of Retinal Vein Occlusion

Ocular disease	Sickle cell disease
Glaucoma	Protein C, S
Intraocular hypertension	Antithrombin III
Hypermetropia	Factor V Leiden
Optic nerve/retinal disorders	Platelet abnormalities
Orbital tumor	Cryofibrinogenemia
Graves'	Malignancy
Drusen	Metabolic
Papilledema	Diabetes
Retinal artery occlusion	Hyperuricemia
Hypertension and arteriosclerosis	Infections
Carotid artery disease (slow filling and slow venous drainage)	Sarcoid
Hyperlipidemia	Acquired immunodeficiency syndrome
Vasculitis	Tuberculosis
Systemic lupus erythematosus	Syphilis
Behçet's disease	Toxins/drugs
Hyperviscosity/hypercoagulability	Smoking
Polycythemia	Sympathomimetics
Multiple myeloma	Oral contraceptives
Paraproteinemia	Diuretic use
Hyperglobulinemia	Trauma

Source: Adapted in part from EM Graham. The investigation of patients with retinal vascular occlusion. Eye 1990;4:464–468.

BRVO tends to occur in the setting of systemic hypertension associated with severe vascular crossing changes. Instead of hemorrhages, exudates, and dilated veins throughout the retina, BRVO produces segmental, usually altitudinal nerve fiber layer splinter hemorrhages.

Table 5-12. Evaluation of Retinal Vein Occlusion

Hypertension	Blood pressure
	Urine analysis
	Serum blood urea nitrogen and creatinine
Diabetes	Urine analysis
	Fasting glucose
	2-hour postprandial glucose
Atherosclerosis	Cholesterol
	Triglycerides
Infection	Human immunodeficiency virus; PPD; angiotensin-converting enzyme
Vasculitis	Erythrocyte sedimentation rate, antinuclear antibodies
Viscosity	Complete blood cell count; erythrocyte sedimentation rate; platelet serum protein electrophoresis; anticardiolipin antibody; lupus anticoagulant; protein C, S; Factor V Leiden
Glaucoma	Intraocular pressure

Source: Adapted in part from EM Graham. The investigation of patients with retinal vascular occlusion. Eye 1990;4:464–468.

Table 5-13. Differential Diagnosis of Retinal Vein Occlusion

Features	Retinal vein occlusion	Diabetic retinopathy	Carotid insufficiency
Demographic	Any age, tends to be older	Any age–older	Older
Symptoms	None, blurred vision	None, blurred vision	Transient monocular blindness, positional vision loss, light-induced vision loss, pain around orbit
Signs	Relative afferent pupillary defect, visual acuity variable, poor compression of the central retinal vein	Normal visual acuity until late	Normal visual acuity, slight compression of the globe causes the artery to collapse
Ophthalmoscopic findings	Hemorrhages and exudates along dilated retinal veins	Hemorrhages and cotton-wool spots scattered, unassociated with retinal veins	Similar to central retinal vein occlusion, fewer hemorrhages
Risk factors	Hypertension, hyperlipidemia, diabetes	Diabetes	Severe atherosclerotic disease

Table 5-14. Complications of Central Retinal Vein/Branch Retinal Vein Occlusions

Cystoid macular edema
Neovascularization of the retina, disc, iris
Glaucoma: neovascularization of the iris angle
Retinal-choroidal collaterals
Retinal detachment

Table 5-15. Ischemic versus Nonischemic Central Retinal Vein

	Nonischemic	Ischemic
Age	80% of young adults as well as older patients	Usually older individuals
Symptoms	Visual blurring	Vision loss
Visual acuity	Generally good	Usually reduced
Relative afferent pupillary defect	Not present or < 0.6 log units	Present > 0.6 log units
Fundus examination	Nerve fiber layer splinter hemorrhage, dilated veins, disc swelling; no cotton-wool spots	Nerve fiber layer splinter hemorrhage, cotton-wool spots, disc edema; macular edema
Fluorescein angiogram	Normal capillary perfusion	Capillary nonperfusion
Electroretinogram	Normal B wave	Reduced B wave
Outcome	Good	Poor vision
Complications	Approximately 20% develop some vision loss	Neovascular glaucoma (40%), macular edema, macular hole

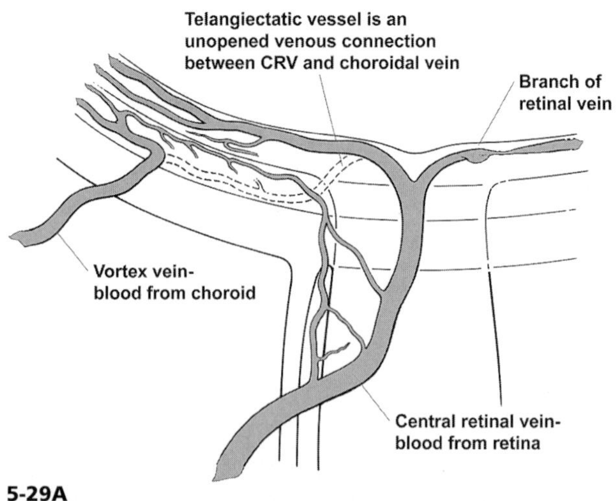

5-29A

Figure 5-29. A. **A BRVO affects one branching vein; the occlusion often occurs at arteriovenous crossings.** B. **An impending BRVO: The artery crosses the vein, and the vein is congested (*arrow*). This is an impending branch vein occlusion.** C. **Some months later, hemorrhages occur in that distribution.** D. **One year later, there are still hemorrhages, and a ghost of a vein appears.** E. **Three years later, there are no hemorrhages, but the vessel appears vacant. (Photographs** B–E **courtesy of Paul Zimmerman, M.D.)** ***Continued***

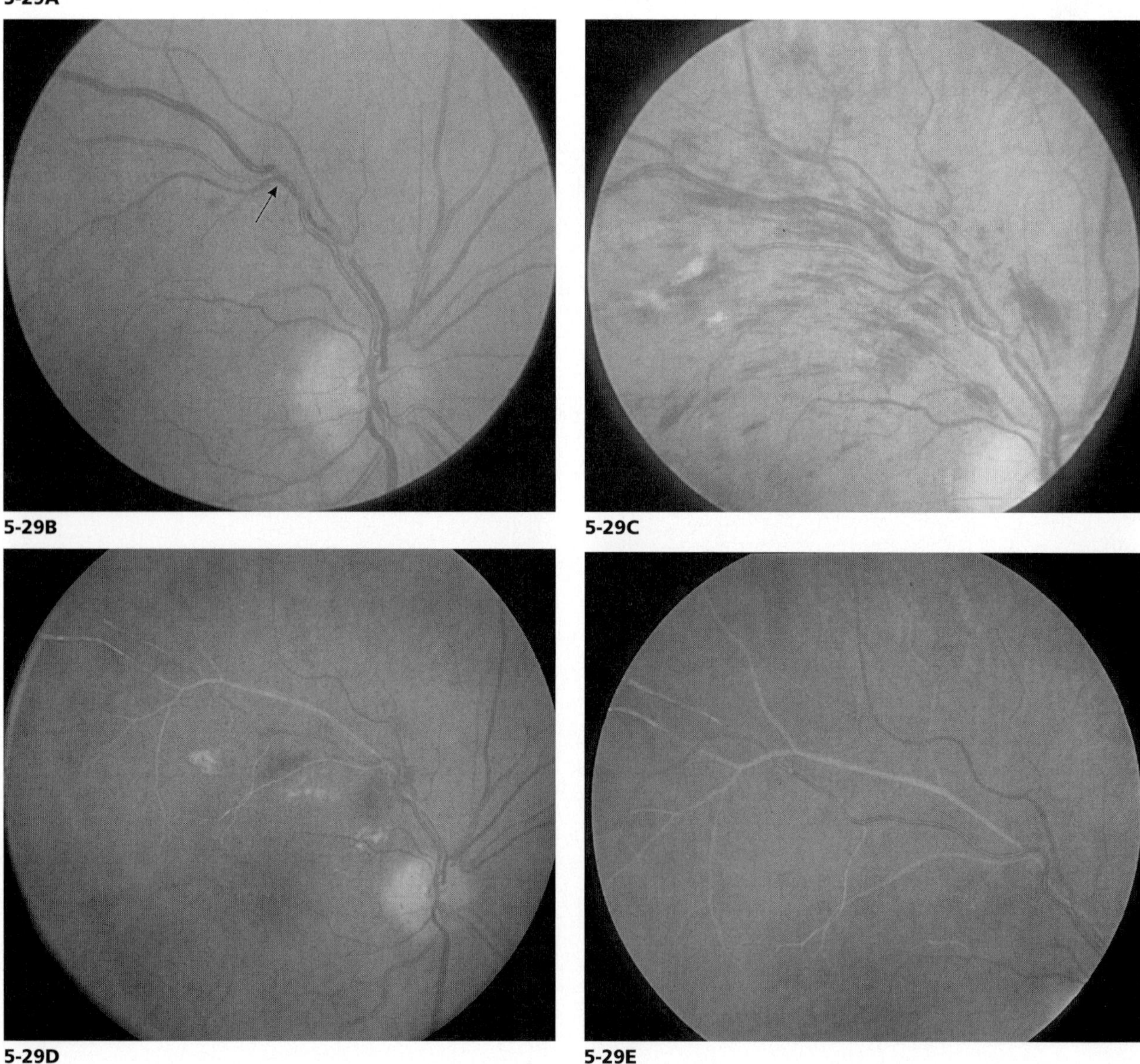

Figure 5-29. *Continued.* F. Although at first glance the fundus may appear as a BRVO, there may be hemorrhages throughout the retina, suggesting that it is actually a CRVO, as in this case. G. The hemorrhages associated with a BRVO. (Photograph courtesy of Paula Morris, CRA.)

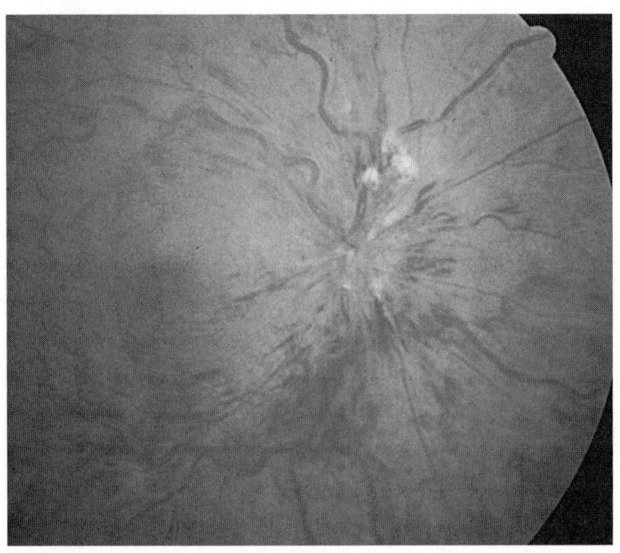

5-29F

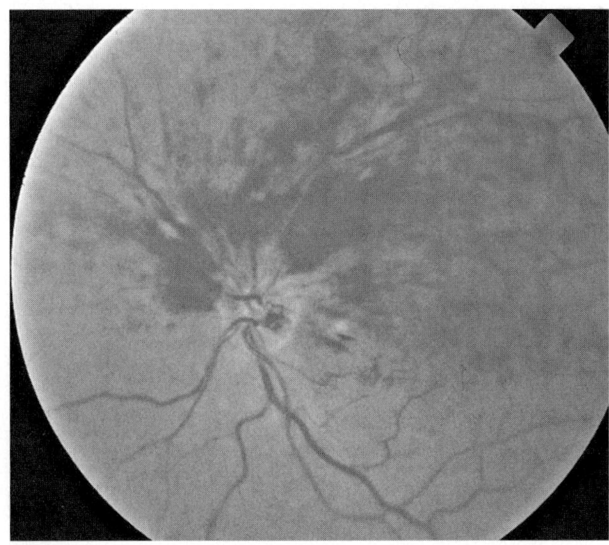

5-29G

Figure 5-30. A. **A BRVO.** B. **If you follow the artery up, you can see that the occlusion involves an entire branch retinal vein.** C. **Fluorescein angiography early on shows arterial filling, but no venous filling in the area of the vein occlusion.** D. **Mid-phase angiogram shows focal areas of staining.** E,F. **Late staining in the area of the BRVO.**

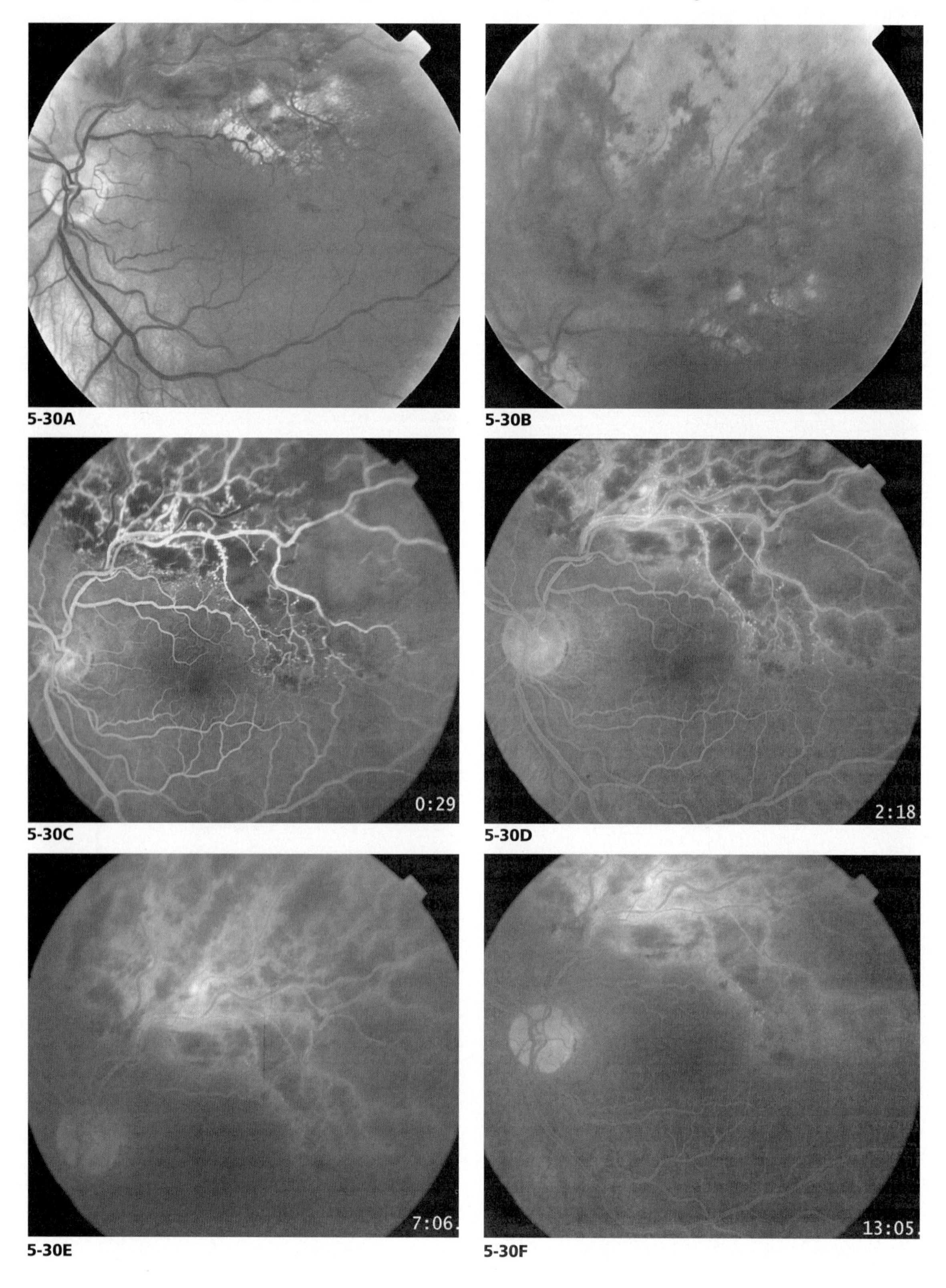

Venous stasis retinopathy is a term to describe mid-periphery dot-and-blot hemorrhages associated with dilated retinal veins as well as arterial narrowing, and it can occur with chronic ocular ischemia. Macular edema and neovascularization of the retina and the disc may be present. Hedges[26] as well as Kearns and Hollenhorst[27] first described venous stasis retinopathy in association with high-grade ipsilateral carotid insufficiency. The feature that distinguishes venous stasis retinopathy from a vein occlusion is that optic disc edema is not a prominent feature of venous stasis retinopathy.

Papillophlebitis has also been called *retinal vasculitis*, *papillary vasculitis*, *benign retinal vasculitis*, *optic disc vasculitis*, and *big blind spot syndrome*. Although some argue that it is a form of CRVO, it is usually visually benign. The most important features of papillophlebitis include unilateral retinal findings in young individuals with vague complaints of vague visual blurring; normal or minimally depressed visual acuity; marked disc swelling; an enlarged blind spot on the visual field; engorged retinal veins with multiple, usually nonconfluent mixed splinter and intraretinal hemorrhages; and spontaneous recovery, usually without therapy. The etiology is unknown, and prognosis is good in more than 80%.

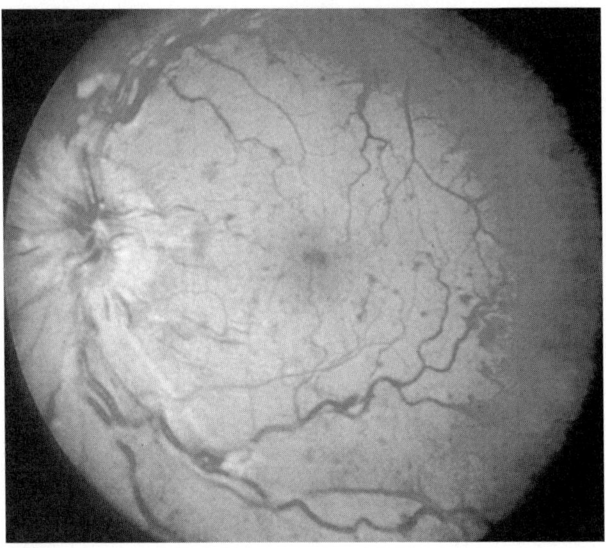

5-31

Figure 5-31. This patient was diagnosed with papillophlebitis. Notice that the optic disc is swollen, and there are hemorrhages that follow the dilated retinal veins.

Other Forms of Venous Disease That Can Cause Symptomatic Vision Loss

RETINOCHOROIDAL COLLATERALS OR OPTICOCILIARY COLLATERAL VESSELS (OPTICOCILIARY VEINS)

Also known as *veno-venous collaterals of the disc* or *ciliary shunt vessels*, retinochoroidal collaterals are telangiectatic connections between the CRV and the vortex vein. Although sometimes called "shunts," these are actually vein-to-vein collateral connections.[28] These collaterals are present congenitally, but normally are not open unless there is obstruction to central retinal venous blood drainage, in which case the collateral veins open, become large and engorged, and drain venous retinal blood out through the vortex veins (see Figure 5-32A). The retinochoroidal collaterals close when the obstruction is removed.

These collaterals arise in a number of clinical circumstances: CRVO; chronic papilledema; and constrictive lesions of the optic nerve, such as meningioma, glioma, and sarcoidosis. Less commonly, these vessels are seen with optic disc drusen, arachnoid cysts, high myopia, glaucoma, and optic nerve glioma.[29] Retinochoroidal collaterals have been recognized to be associated with meningiomas and optic nerve tumors since at least the time of Salzmann (1893) and Elschnig (1898).[30] In patients with end-stage glaucoma, retinochoroidal collaterals occur approximately 25% of the time, probably due to asymptomatic CRVO. Occasionally, individuals are born with retinochoroidal collaterals, which function without apparent cause.

Figure 5-32. A. **Retinochoroidal collaterals formed between the CRV and the vortex vein via unopened telangiectatic vessels are shown in this diagram.** B. **When venous pressure in the CRV drainage increases (constriction of the optic nerve by tumor, increased intracranial pressure, or by venous occlusion), the telangiectatic connection opens, allowing drainage into the cavernous sinus by way of the vortex veins and their venous connections within the orbit. The arrows point to the retinochoroidal collaterals.**

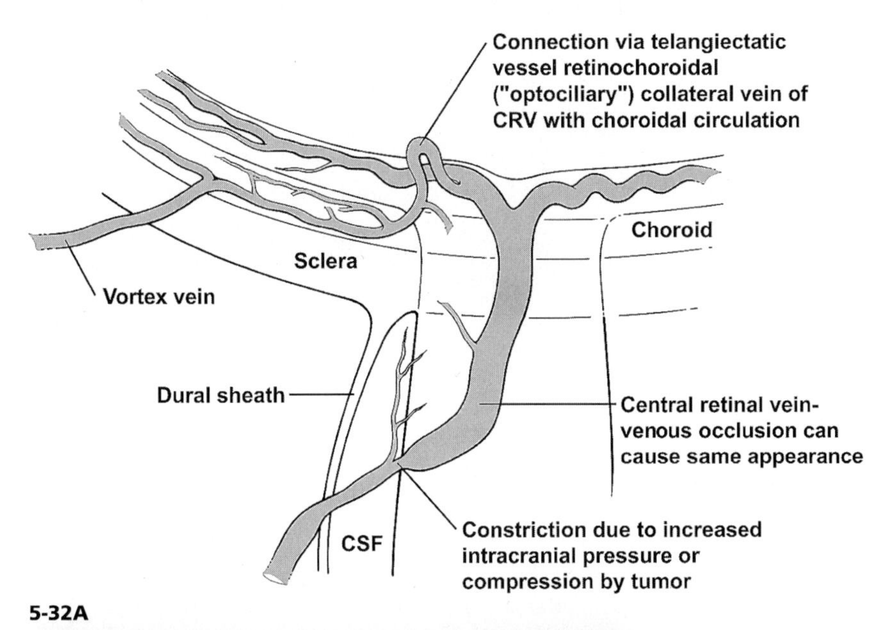

5-32A

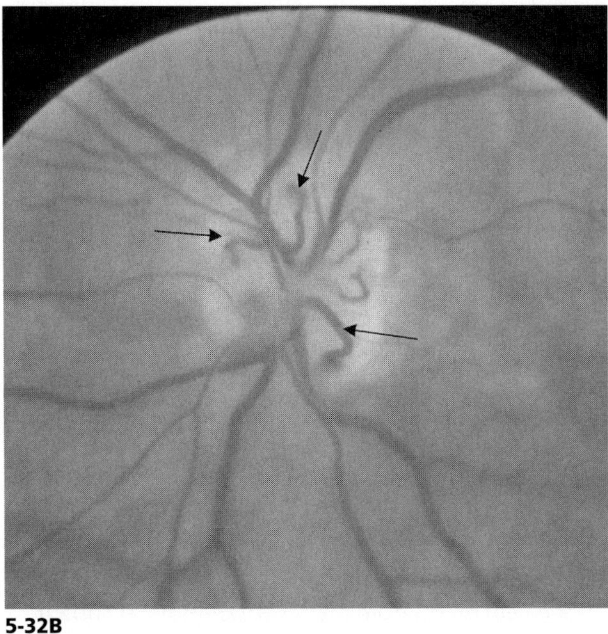

5-32B

Figure 5-33. A. **This man developed a retinochoroidal anastomosis (*arrow*) after a CRVO.** B. **He subsequently developed NA-AION, and after the disc swelling resolved, the retinochoroidal collateral disappeared.**

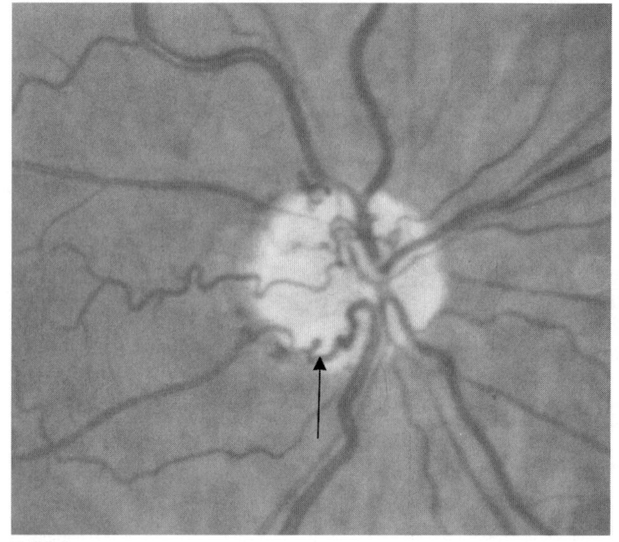

5-33A

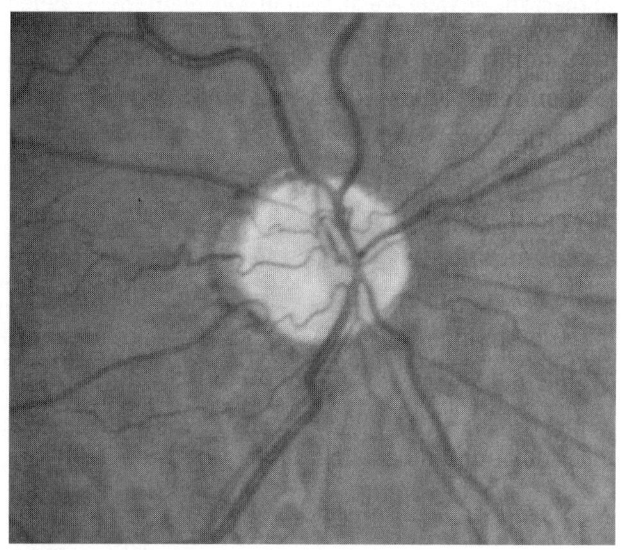

5-33B

Table 5-16. Retinochoroidal Collaterals

Condition	Age	Visual acuity	Ocular findings	Associated findings
Tumors				
Optic nerve meningioma	Middle age	Slowly progressive vision loss	Proptosis, disc pallor/edema; hyperopia	Women; look for neurofibromatosis-1 (NF-1)
Glioma of optic nerve	Childhood	Progressive vision loss	Proptosis, disc pallor/edema	NF-1
Sarcoidosis of the optic nerve	Any age	Slowly progressive vision loss, stepwise vision loss	Sarcoid granule disc, look for Koeppe's and Busacca's nodules	Chest x-ray usually abnormal. Check conjunctival biopsy, gallium scan
Vascular				
CRVO	Middle age	Vision loss is variable	Early: tortuous veins, hemorrhages, swollen disc; late: neovascularization with pale disc	Hypertension, atherosclerosis
Chronic papilledema	Any age	Slowly progressive visual field constriction, acuity affected late	Pale swollen disc, sheathing of vessels	See other evidence of increased intracranial pressure
Chronic open-angle glaucoma (late)	Older	Progressive visual field constriction	Pale disc with cupping	Glaucoma history (possibly also due to subclinical CRVO in this setting)
Congenital opticociliary vessel	Congenital	Normal	See vein going from retina to choroid circulation on fluorescein	None—normal variant

Figure 5-34. A–D. These discs all exhibit retinochoroidal collaterals (*arrows*) owing to optic nerve meningioma.

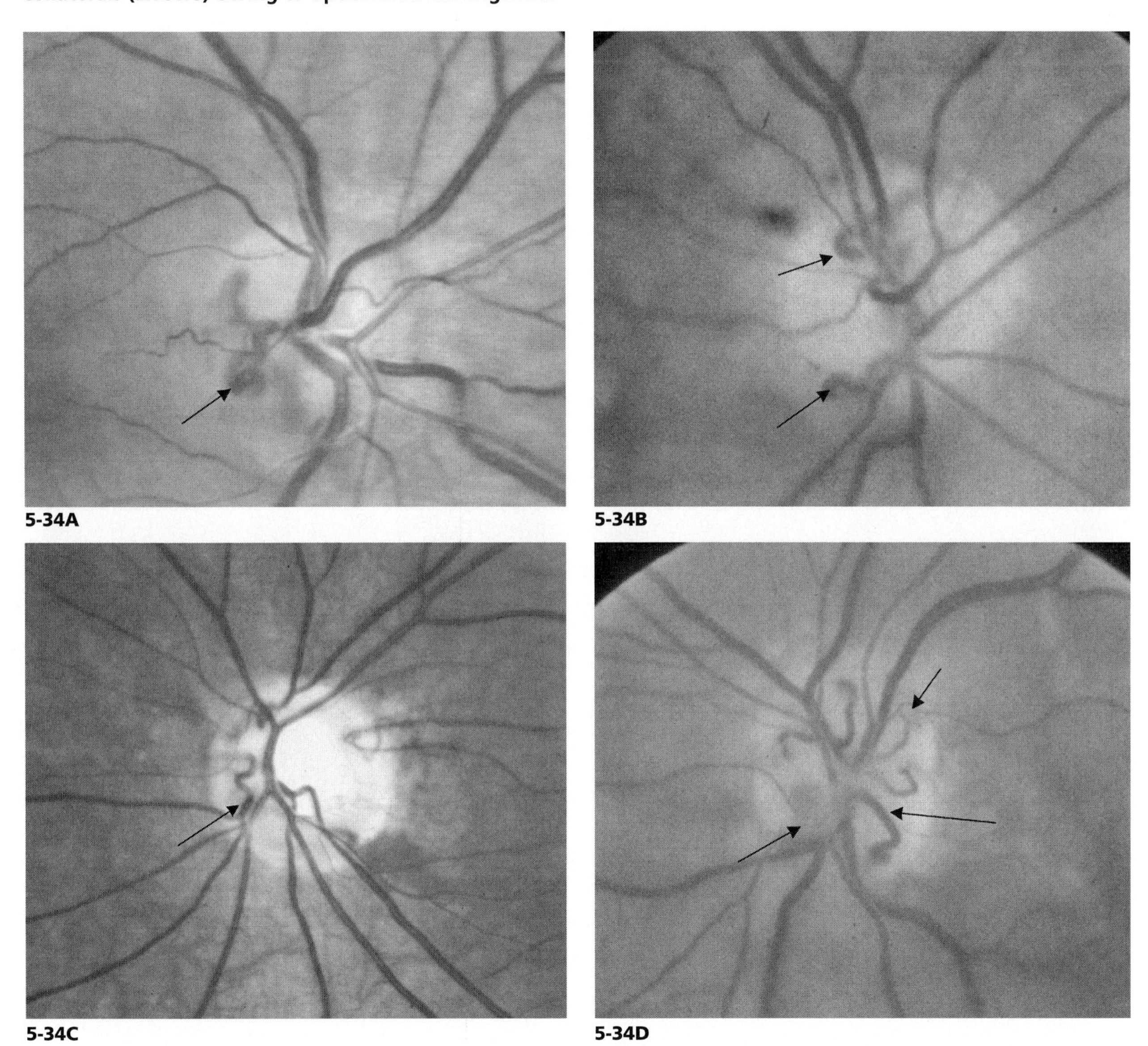

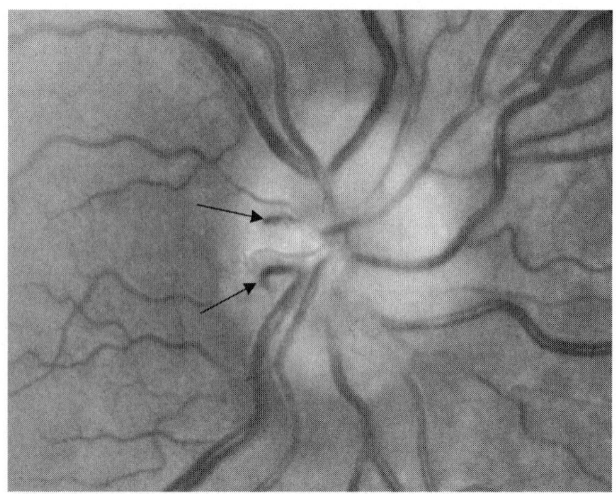

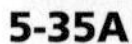

5-35A

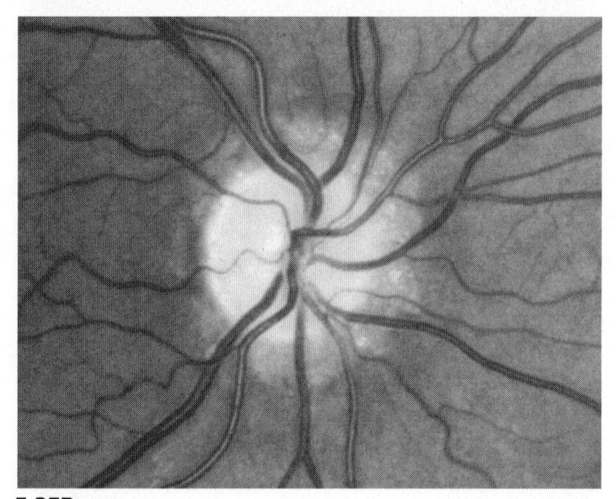

5-35B

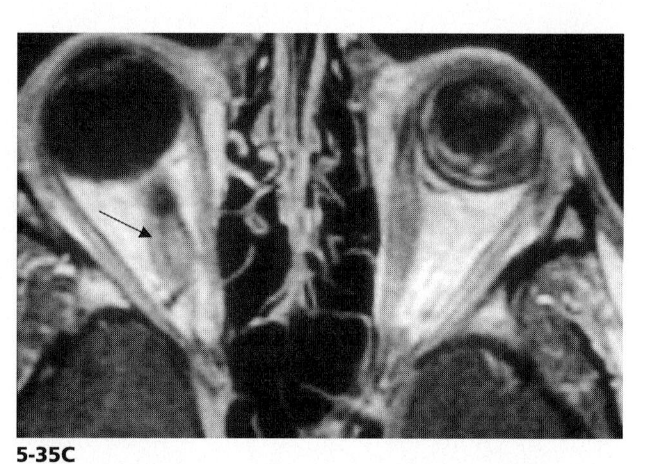

5-35C

Figure 5-35. A. **This man with a previous optic nerve meningioma of the left optic nerve presented with slowly progressive vision loss in his right eye. Retinochoroidal collaterals were observed (*arrows*).** B. **After radiation, the collaterals disappeared.** C. **His MRI reveals the underlying meningioma (*arrow*).**

Figure 5-36. A. **Chronic end-stage glaucoma produces high pressure that interferes with venous drainage from the disc. The arrows point to multiple retinochoroidal collaterals.** B. **Sometimes, broad, smooth venous collaterals drain the disc centrifugally to the disc margin where they drain (*arrow*). (Photographs courtesy of F. Jane Durcan, M.D.)**

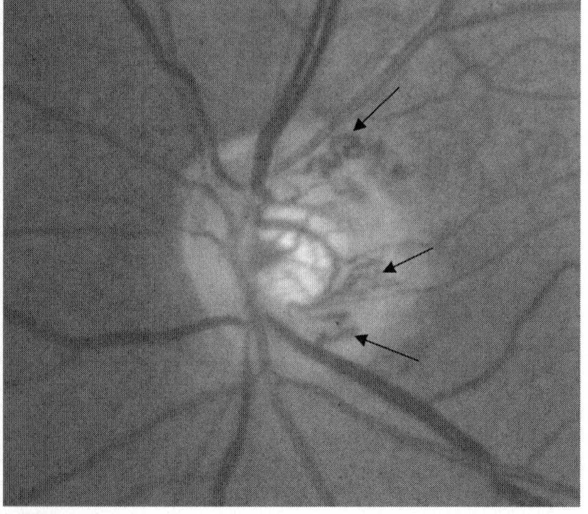

5-36A

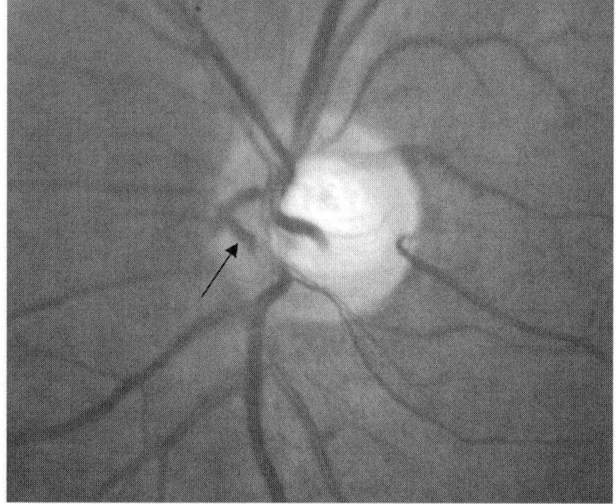

5-36B

Figure 5-37. A. This woman had chronic papilledema owing to a third ventricular glioma. She had a prominent retinochoroidal connection inferiorly on her swollen disc (*arrows*). B. Fluorescein angiography showed filling of the arteries and confirms the collateral (*arrow*). C. Later, the fluorescein angiogram showed that the collateral filled (*arrow*). D. After treatment of the tumor, the patient's optic disc drusen were visible, and the collateral resolved. (Courtesy of Norman Schatz, M.D.)

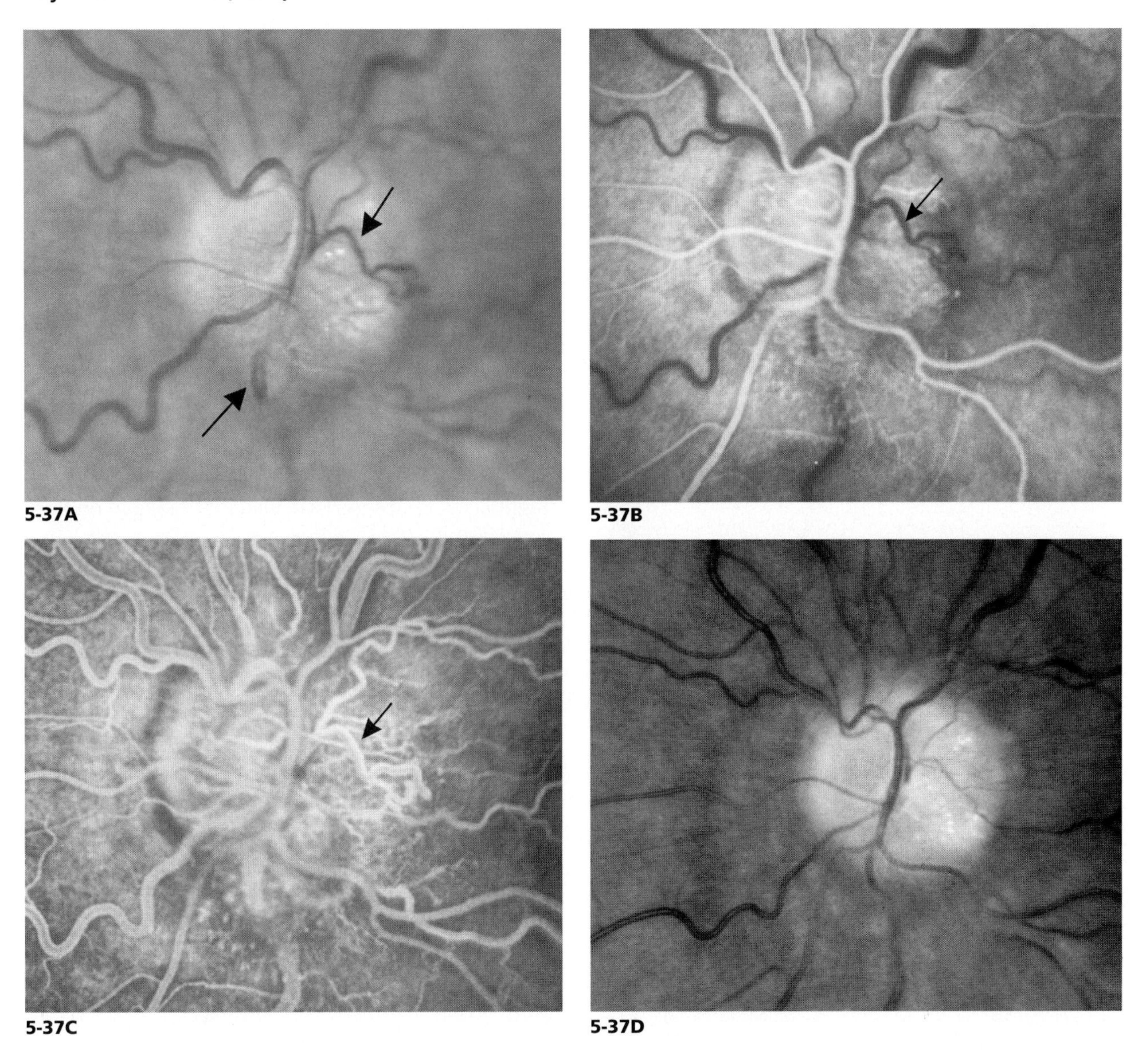

The retinochoroidal vessels with chronic papilledema begin with a "hairnet" of telangiectasias that gradually winnow down to one or more large collateral tortuous draining channels. (See Chapter 3, Figure 3-31A, for the appearance of the hairnet.) The presence of these vessels is evidence of longstanding disc swelling. When the cerebrospinal fluid pressure is lowered, these collaterals close.

ARTERITIS/VASCULITIS

Although giant cell arteritis can cause permanent retinal artery and especially cilioretinal artery occlusion, other vasculitides also affect the retinal vessels. Clues to this diagnosis are sheathing of the vessels and the presence of cells in the vitreous. Cells in the vitreous are best appreciated with a slit lamp, but inability to bring the fundus into clear crisp view, in the absence of a cataract, is indirect evidence that there are cells in the vitreous. Frequently, the disc is swollen. A further clue to the diagnosis is characteristic vascular leakage on fluorescein angiography.

Retinal vasculitis is a broad term for both infectious and noninfectious types of inflammation of the retinal blood vessels. Vasculitis of the blood vessels in the body is associated with immune complex deposition. In the retinal blood vessels there is little evidence of the deposition, but there is evidence of inflammation of the retinal vasculature—sheathing, staining of the vasculature on fluorescein angiography, cotton-wool spots, and, occasionally, inflammation of the retina (retinitis). Posterior uveitis is sometimes used to describe the type of inflammation occurring in the choroidal blood vessels. In this case, you see cells in the vitreous and white spots in the choroid (see Chapter 6). Uveitis is inflammation of the pigmented portions of the eye—iris, choroid, and ciliary body.

Causes of vasculitis include systemic lupus, Eales' disease, sarcoidosis, Behçet's disease, tuberculosis, syphilis, periarteritis nodosa, Churg-Strauss disease, and temporal arteritis.

Symptoms of vasculitis in the retina or disc may be transient monocular blindness, persistent blurring of vision, or permanent vision loss.

Findings on the eye examination include variable visual acuity and visual fields. Ophthalmoscopic findings include cells in the vitreous (vitreous haze is a sign of inflammation), white spots, hemorrhages, narrowing and partial arterial or venous occlusion, sheathing of blood vessels, disc swelling, and macular edema. Fluorescein angiography may demonstrate perivascular staining, signifying a breakdown of the blood-retinal barrier. Certain autoimmune conditions are associated with retinal and optic disc vasculitis. Another uveitis/vasculitis meningeal vasculopathy to consider is Vogt-Koyanagi-Harada disease, which includes *p*oliosis of lashes, *u*veitis (anterior and posterior), *v*itiligo, *a*lopecia, and *d*eafness, or the mnemonic PUVAD (an old mnemonic device from J. Lawton Smith, M.D., Professor of Ophthalmology at the Bascom Palmer Eye Institute, Miami: "Too bad if you have PUVAD").

Table 5-17. Optic Disc and Retinal Vasculitis

	Behçet's disease	Systemic lupus erythematosus	Sarcoidosis	Vogt-Koyanagi-Harada disease
Etiology	Autoimmune	Autoimmune	Unknown	Unknown
Characteristic features	Aphthous mouth ulcers, genital ulcers, uveitis, pathergy	Arthritis, skin rash	Pulmonary symptoms, lymphadenopathy	PUVAD, cerebrospinal fluid pleocytosis, increased protein
Visual symptoms	Visual blurring	Dry eyes, visual blurring	Visual blurring	Visual blurring
Ocular findings	Uveitis—cells in the anterior and posterior chambers	Uveitis	Uveitis	Uveitis
Optic disc findings	Disc edema, papilledema	Optic disc edema—AION	Optic disc swelling, granulomas	± Disc swelling
Retinal findings	Retinal vein occlusion, white patches around blood vessels	Vascular irregularity with staining of the vessel walls, choroidopathy	Vascular irregularity and staining of vessel walls on fluorescein angiography	Retinal vasculitis
Neurologic findings	Headache	Lupus cerebritis	Neurosarcoid is variable	Decreased hearing
Diagnostic test	Pathergy skin testing, magnetic resonance imaging	Antinuclear antibodies, anticardiolipin antibodies, decreased platelets	Angiotensin-converting enzyme, gallium scan, cerebrospinal fluid examination, magnetic resonance imaging	Light perception, audiometry

PUVAD = *p*oliosis of lashes, *u*veitis (anterior and posterior), *v*itiligo, *a*lopecia, and *d*eafness.

Figure 5-38. A. This disc is somewhat swollen due to sarcoid. The vessels show narrowing and sheathing typical of vasculitis. B. Fluorescein angiogram shows staining of the retinal arteries indicating inflammation of the blood vessels consistent with vasculitis. C. The vessels are sheathed and narrow (*arrows*). (Photograph courtesy of Paul Zimmerman, M.D.)

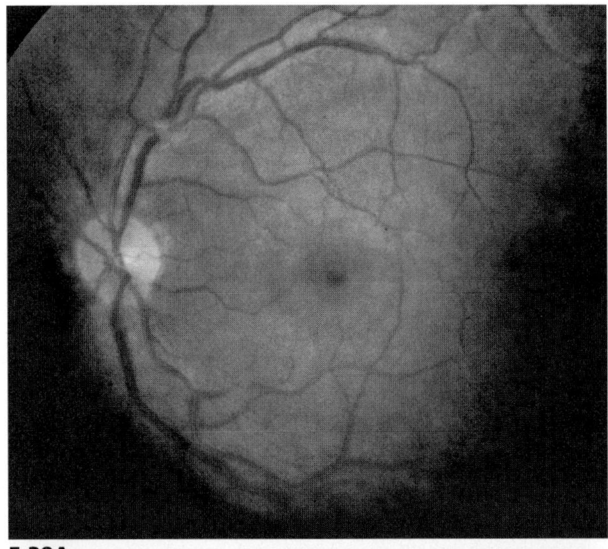

5-38A

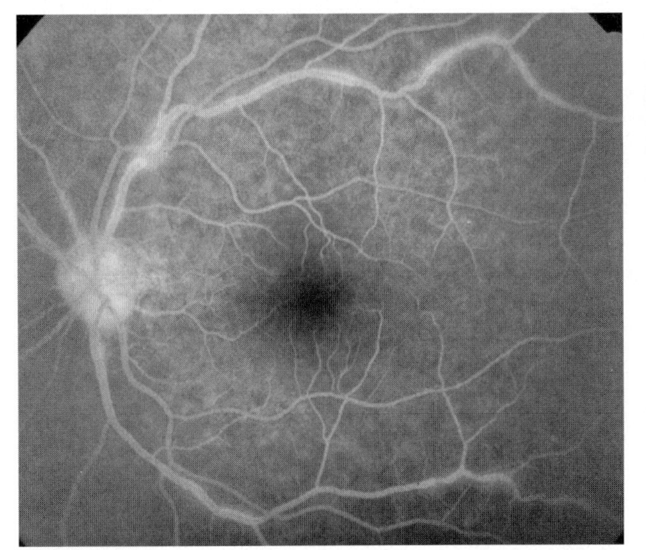

5-38B

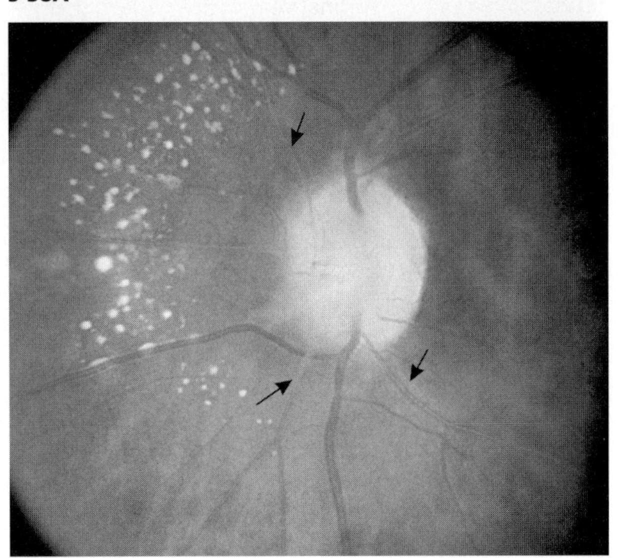

5-38C

SUSAC'S SYNDROME: MICROANGIOPATHY OF THE DISC AND RETINA

In 1979, John Susac et al. reported a microangiopathy affecting the brain and retina. These individuals had multiple BRAOs as well as a microangiopathy of the brain. Tests for systemic lupus erythematosus are frequently negative.[31] Since then, other reports have described many other cases; many are also associated with microangiopathy of the ear, leading to hearing loss. *Susac's syndrome* includes microangiopathy of the eye (multiple BRAOs), ear (hearing loss), and brain (encephalopathy).[32]

Figure 5-39. Susac's syndrome. This 24-year-old man developed headaches, visual changes, and memory loss. Examination revealed BRAO. He then developed vertigo, tinnitus, and hearing loss. His workup was extensive. MRI showed evidence of small infarcts. Fluorescein angiogram showed multiple occlusions. He was treated with anticoagulation, and did very well without further sequelae. A full discussion of this case is reported in reference 33. A. **When first seen, he had symptoms only in his left eye, but notice the vessel irregularity (*arrow*) in his right eye.** B. **At his first visit, he had suffered a BRAO (*arrow*) in the left eye.** C. **You can appreciate pallor of the retina and a vascular occlusion (*arrows*); there is also a cotton-wool spot (*arrowhead*).** D. **Still later, another vessel occluded (*arrow*).**

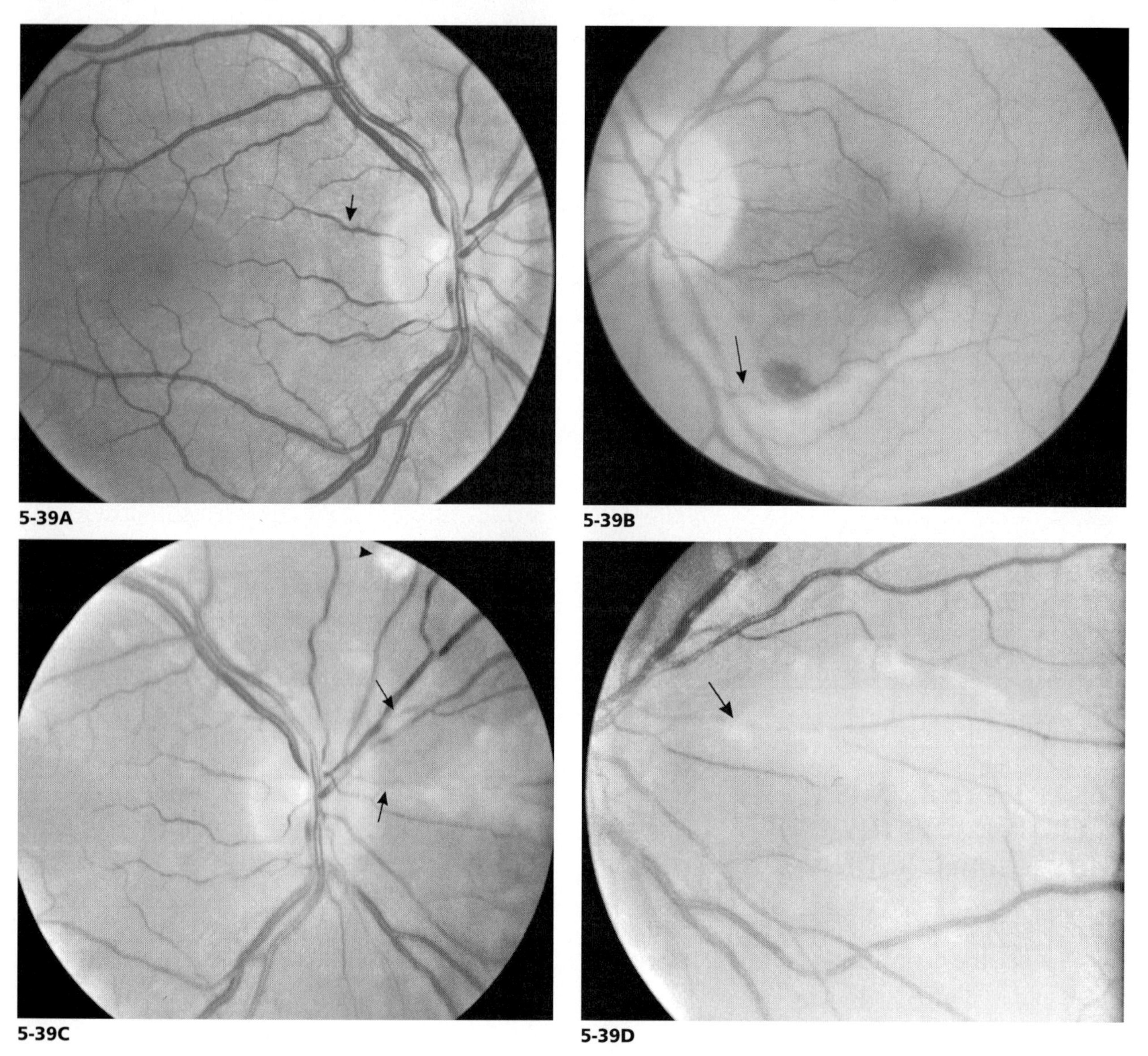

VASOSPASM OF THE ARTERIES

Wray's type 3 amaurosis fugax is caused by vasospasm of the retinal arteries. In this type, the veins also constrict during the vasospasm because reduced flow goes through the retina. This has been documented several times recently in the literature. Typically, only the history tells the story, as rarely is vasospasm observed. The importance of recognizing this type of transient monocular vision loss is that it is treatable with calcium channel blockers.

Figure 5-40. This individual experienced recurrent episodes of vision loss and was photographed in the middle of an episode. A. **Before the attack, notice the color and caliber of the vessels.** B. **During the attack, notice the arterial and venous narrowing and darkening of the blood column.** C. **After the attack, the blood vessels are ever so slightly engorged. (Photographs courtesy of Robert Saul, M.D.)** ***Continued***

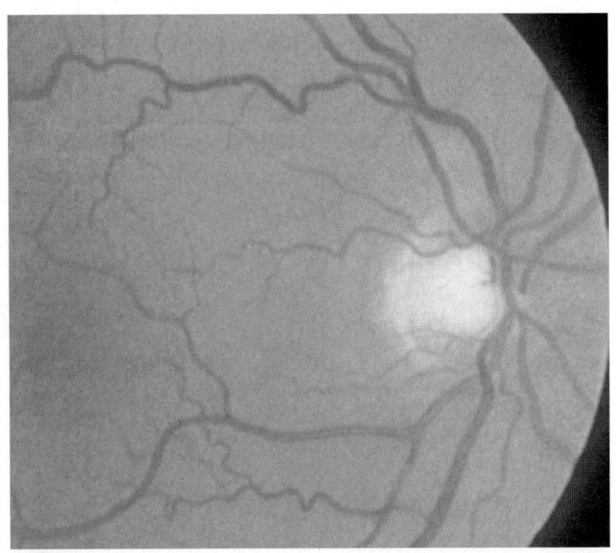

5-40A

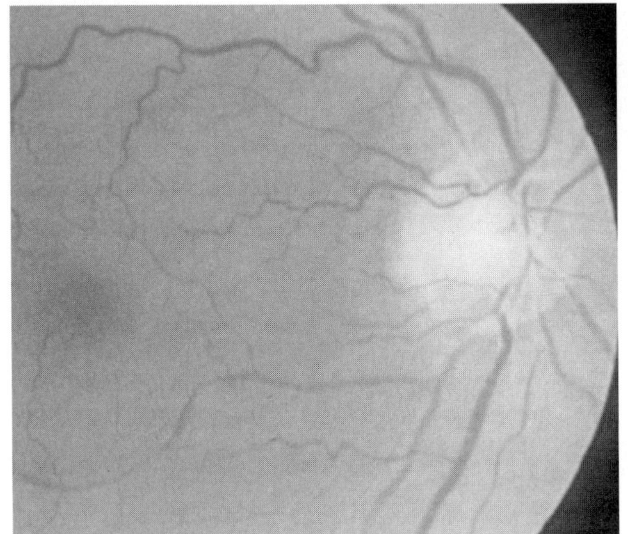

5-40B

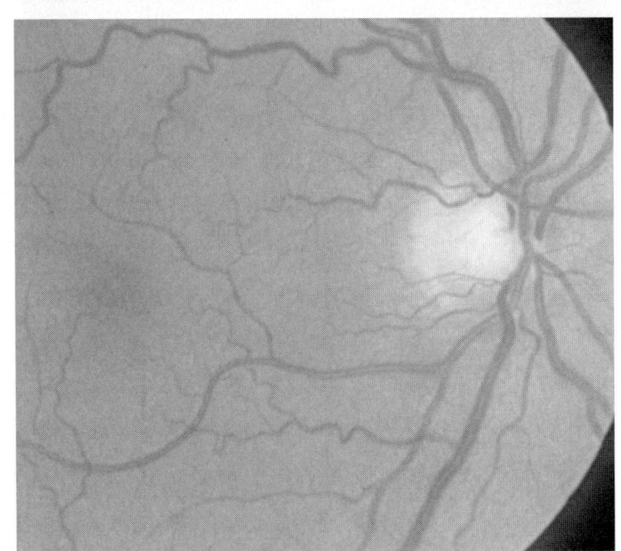

5-40C

Figure 5-40. *Continued*. D. Another case of vision loss associated with unilateral cluster headache. The panel on the left shows the vessel in its normal state. On the right, arterial and venular narrowing occurs with the vision loss. E. On the left panel, the vascular spasm is present, and on the right, the attack is over and the vessels have returned to normal. (Photographs courtesy of Lanning Kline, M.D.)

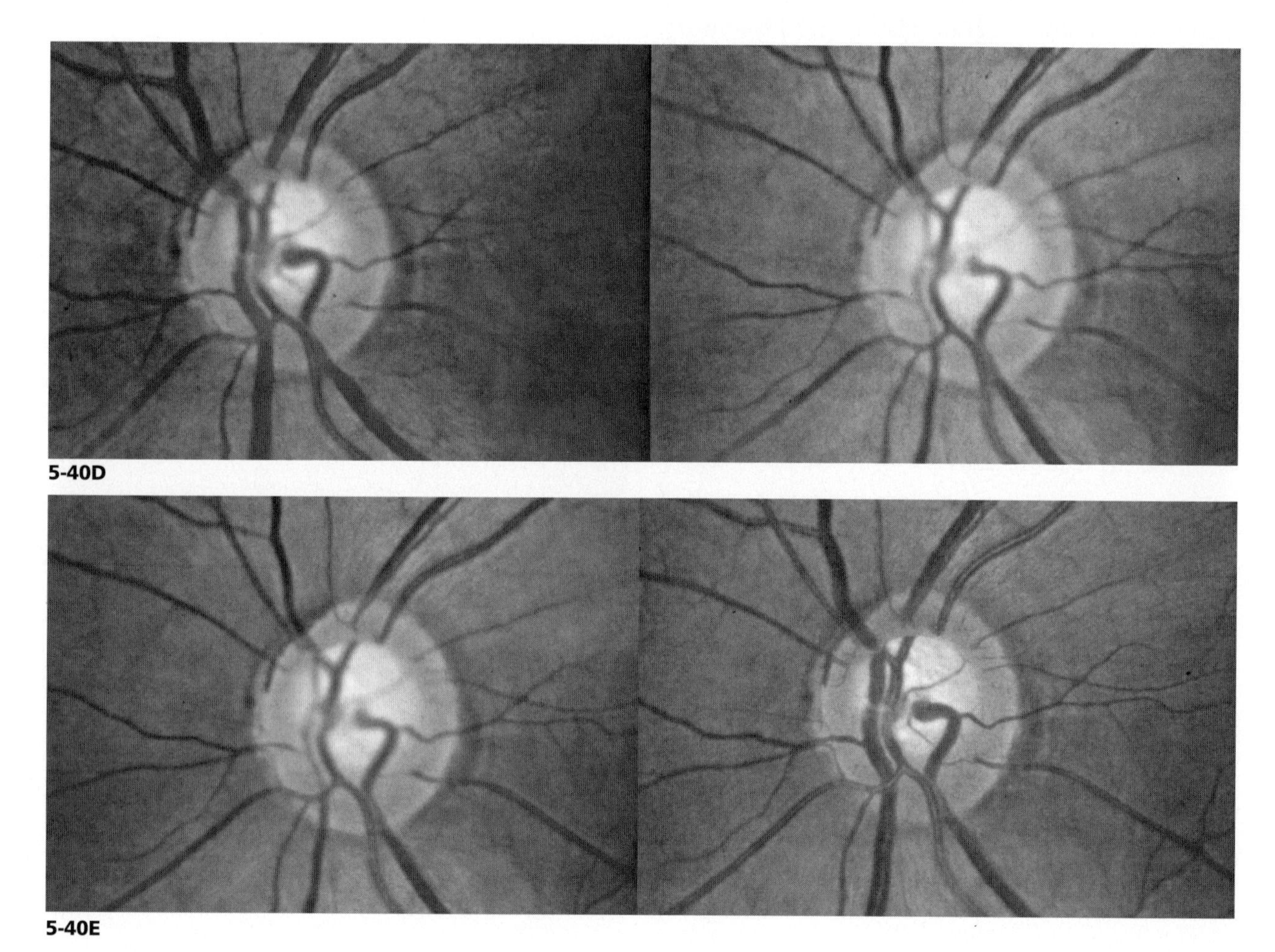

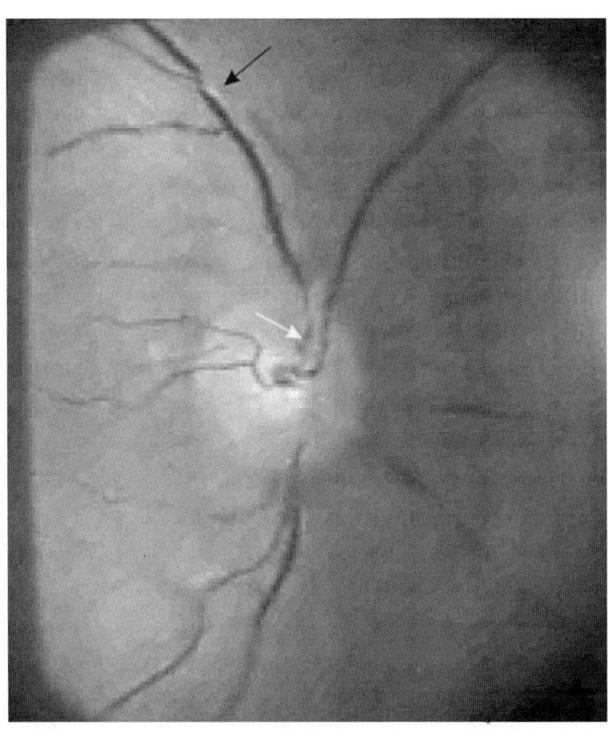

5-41

Figure 5-41. This man had repeated episodes of total monocular blindness lasting seconds to minutes, often brought on by Valsalva maneuver. During his blindness, the central retinal artery would occlude and the retina would become pale. There was almost no blood flow through the retinal vessels. The blood column darkened. When blood flow returned, the vessels had a dilated appearance. This photograph shows the pale retina with severely attenuated arterial circulation. You can appreciate box-carring of the arteriolar vessel (*black arrow*) and occlusion of the central retinal artery with narrowing of the vein (*white arrow*). There are small cilioretinal arteries that continue to perfuse the retina (*small arrows*). The video (see Video 5-V-2 on the accompanying CD-Rom) shows the loss of blood flow with subsequent return. Notice first that the spasm occurs fairly abruptly and the vein becomes darker as the retinal transit time is prolonged and more oxygen is extracted from the blood. When the blood supply returns to the retina again, it also returns abruptly. The venous system is slightly engorged from the preocclusion state.

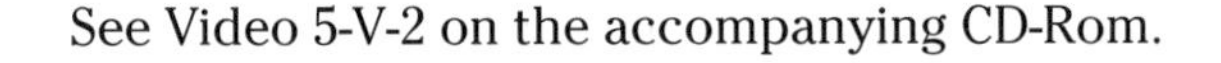

See Video 5-V-2 on the accompanying CD-Rom.

Practical Viewing Essentials

1. Remember that the eye is very vascular, and there are multiple communications between the internal and external carotid arteries.
2. When the patient complains of transient monocular blindness, consider all possible causes, including local disc disease as well as vascular problems. Do not let the term *amaurosis fugax* arrest your ability to think clearly of alternative explanations.
3. Branch and central retinal artery occlusions are embolic until proven otherwise.
4. The presence of a cilioretinal artery frequently improves visual outcome in CRAO.
5. The occlusion of a cilioretinal artery in an older individual strongly suggests giant cell arteritis.

6. If you see an embolus, always look downstream (in the periphery) for more emboli.
7. Posterior ciliary artery occlusions cause ischemic optic neuropathy.
8. Learn to look for the historical, physical, and laboratory clues for arteritic AION.
9. Swelling of the disc due to AION in addition to a CRAO is caused by occlusion of the more proximal ophthalmic artery.
10. Ocular ischemic syndrome is associated with severe internal and external carotid artery disease.
11. Retinal vein occlusions in the young require an evaluation of the cause.
12. Retinochoroidal collaterals are caused by obstruction to central venous drainage.

References

1. Gowers W. A Manual and Atlas of Medical Ophthalmoscopy. London: J & A Churchill, 1879.
2. Hayreh SS, Kolder HE, Weingeist TA. Central retinal artery occlusion and retinal tolerance time. Ophthalmology 1980;87:75–78.
3. Barroso LH, Hoyt WF, Narahara M. Can the arterial supply of the retina in man be exclusively cilioretinal? J Neuroophthalmol 1994;14(2):87–90.
4. Kestenbaum A. Clinical Methods of Neuro-Ophthalmologic examination. New York: Grund and Stratton, 1947.
5. Cogan D. Neurology of the Visual System. Springfield, IL: Thomas, 1967.
6. David NJ, Saito Y, Heyman A. Arm to retina fluorescein appearance time. Arch Neurol 1961;5:165–170.
7. Hollenhorst RW, Kearns TP. The fluorescein dye test of circulation time in patients with occlusive disease of the carotid arterial system. Proc Staff Meeting Mayo Clinic 1961;36:457–465.
8. Jonas JB, Hayreh SS. Optic disk morphology in experimental central retinal artery occlusion in rhesus monkeys. Am J Ophthalmol 1999;127:523–530.
9. Digre KB, Blodi C, Bale J. Recurrent branch retinal artery occlusion associated with CMV infection. Retina 1987;7:230–232.
10. Duker JS, Magaragal LE, Stubbs GW. Quadrantic venous-stasis retinopathy secondary to an embolic branch retinal artery obstruction. Ophthalmology 1990;97:167–170.
11. Hollenhorst RW. Significance of bright plaques in the retinal arterioles. Trans Am Ophthalmol Soc 1961;59:252–273.
12. Savino PJ, Glaser JS, Cassady J. Retinal stroke. Is the patient at risk? Arch Ophthalmol 1977;95:1185–1189.
13. Chuang EL, Miller FS, Kalina RE. Retinal lesions following long bone fractures. Ophthalmology 1985;92:370–374.
14. Arnold AC, Hepler RS. Fluorescein angiography in acute nonarteritic anterior ischemic optic neuropathy. Am J Ophthalmol 1994;117:222–230.
15. Arnold AC, Badr MA, Hepler RS. Fluorescein angiography in nonischemic optic disc edema. Arch Ophthalmol 1996;114:293–298.
16. Ghanchi FD, Dutton GN. Current concepts in giant cell (temporal) arteritis. Surv Ophthalmol 1997;42:99–123.
17. Hedges TR 3rd, Gieger GL, Albert DM. The clinical value of negative temporal artery biopsy specimens. Arch Ophthalmol 1983 Aug;101(8):1251–1254.
18. Gonzalez-Gay MA, Garcia-Porrua C, Llorca J, et al. Biopsy-negative giant cell arteritis: clinical spectrum and predictive factors for positive temporal artery biopsy. Semin Arthritis Rheum 2001;30(4):249–256.
19. Duhaut P, Pinede L, Bornet H, et al. Biopsy proven and biopsy negative temporal arteritis: differences in clinical spectrum at the onset of the disease. Groupe de Recherche sur l'Arterite a Cellules Geantes. Ann Rheum Dis 1999;58(6):335–341.
20. Kawasaki A, Purvin VA, Burgett RA. Hyperhomocysteinaemia in young patients with non-arteritic anterior ischaemic optic neuropathy. Br J Ophthalmol 1999;83:1287–1290.
21. Hayreh SS. Anterior ischaemic optic neuropathy. Differentiation of arteritic from non-arteritic type and its management. Eye 1990;4:25–41.
22. Knox DL. Ischemic ocular inflammation. Am J Ophthalmol 1965;60:995–1002.
23. Servais GE, Thompson HS, Hayreh SS. Relative afferent pupillary defect in central retinal vein occlusion. Ophthalmology 1986;93:301–303.
24. Hayreh SS, Rojas P, Podhajsky P, et al. Ocular neovascularization with retinal vascular occlusion—III. Incidence of ocular neovascularization with retinal vein occlusion. Ophthalmology 1983;90:488–506.
25. Fong AC, Schatz H. Central retinal vein occlusion in young adults. Surv Ophthalmol 1993;37:393–417.
26. Hedges TR Jr. Ophthalmoscopic findings in internal carotid artery occlusion. Bull Hopkins Hosp 1962;3:89–97.
27. Kearns TP, Hollenhorst RW. Venous-stasis retinopathy of occlusive disease of the carotid artery. Mayo Clin Proc 1953;38:304–312.
28. Schatz H, Green WR, Talamo JH, et al. Clinicopathological correlation of retinal to choroidal venous collaterals of the optic nerve head. Ophthalmology 1991;98:1287–1293.

29. Masuyanma Y, Kodama Y, Matsuura Y, et al. Clinical studies on the occurrence and the pathogenesis of optociliary veins. J Clin Neuroophthalmol 1990;10:1–8.
30. Frisén L, Hoyt WF, Tengroth BM. Optociliary veins, disc pallor and visual loss. A triad of signs indicating spheno-orbital meningioma. Acta Ophthalmol (Copenh) 1973;51(2):241–249.
31. Susac JO, Hardman JM, Selhorst JB. Microangiopathy of the brain and retina. Neurology 1979;29:313–316.
32. Susac JO. Susac's syndrome. Neurology 1994;44:591–593.
33. Turner BW, Digre KB, Shelton C. Susac syndrome. Otolaryngol Head Neck Surg 1998;118:866–867.

6 White Spots—What Are They?

Since the white spots in the retina which have been described, are present in many forms of retinal disease which occur secondarily to, and are significant of general disease, it is of great importance to distinguish them from other appearances which have a different significance. First it is necessary to distinguish whether the white spot is in the retina or in the choroid.

William Gowers[1]

What would cause a white spot in the retina, choroid, or optic disc, and what is "white?" The only inherently "white" structure in the eye is the sclera. When there is atrophy of the retina and retinal pigment epithelium (RPE), the sclera can be seen. Although we are labeling spots as "white," some have a distinctly yellow appearance, such as hard exudates.

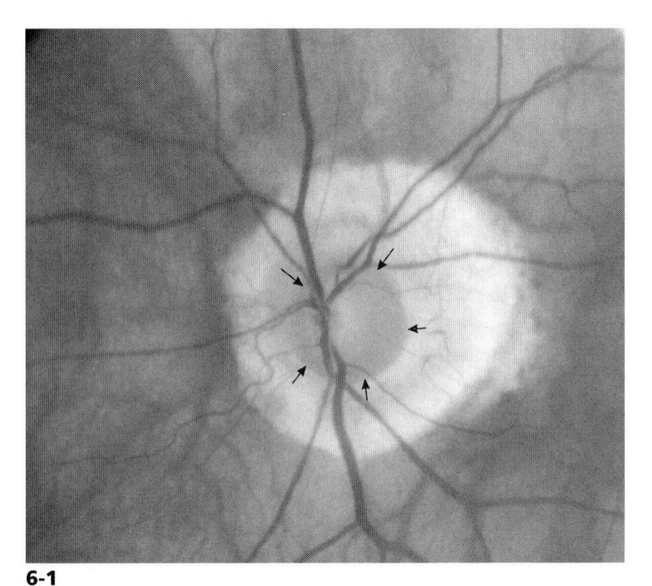

6-1

Figure 6-1. The disc is surrounded by white sclera in this photograph. The arrows point to the true margin of the disc. This kind of disc is seen in myopia.

The second "white" structure is the optic nerve. Most of the time, the optic disc is not really white, but pink from all of the capillaries on the surface of the disc as well as the light off of the nerve fiber layer (recall Figure 2-41A). We have seen why a disc can be pale or "white" in Chapter 4. Within the optic nerve, especially in patients with large cups, the lamina cribrosa is seen as white. Finally, any extra glial tissue in the eye looks white. In pathologic states (e.g., ischemia, fluid, inflammation, and atrophy), "white" may appear. The inside of the eye and the disc really have only a few ways to respond—turning white or becoming pigmented. When is a white spot a variant of normal?

A scleral crescent (not really a "spot") is seen around the disc. The cause of this crescent is that the choroid and retina do not abut the edge of the disc (see discussion in Chapter 2, Figure 2-10). This "white" is usually around the central aspect of the disc. There may also be pigment associated with the crescent.

Figure 6-2. A,B. **An extensive scleral crescent almost around each disc is shown here. The arrows mark the outside of the crescent, and the arrowheads mark the edge of the disc.**

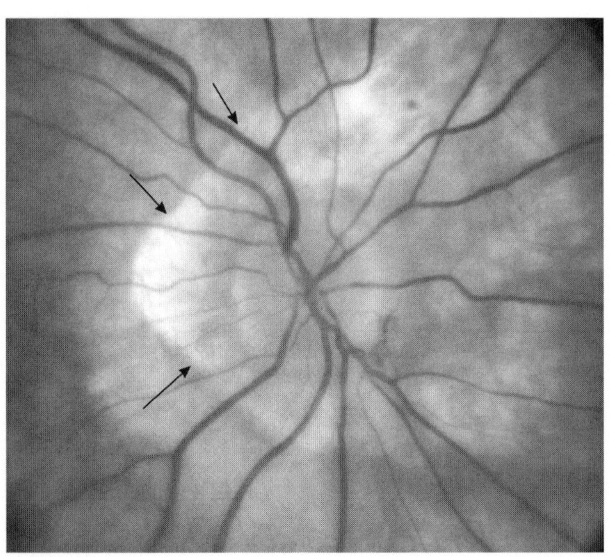

6-2A

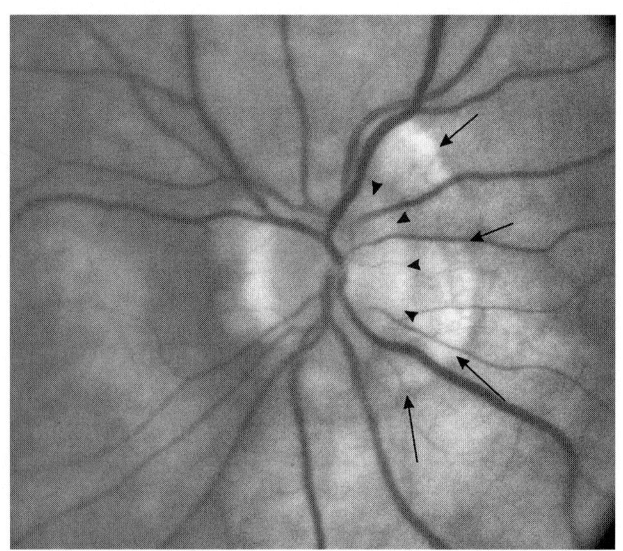

6-2B

Medullated or myelinated nerve fiber layer may appear white on the disc or just off of the disc (see discussion in Chapter 2, Figure 2-17). Sometimes this can be mistaken for optic disc swelling or inflammation. Examination, however, shows a characteristically feathery edge. There are no cells or inflammatory debris. These myelinated nerve fibers may be seen distally in the retina as well. Myelinated fibers have a very different appearance from the "cumulus cloud" of a nerve fiber layer infarct or cotton-wool spot.

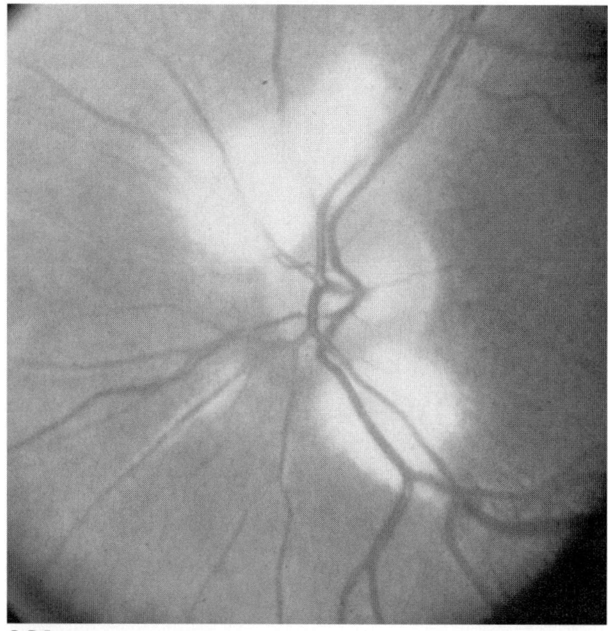

6-3A

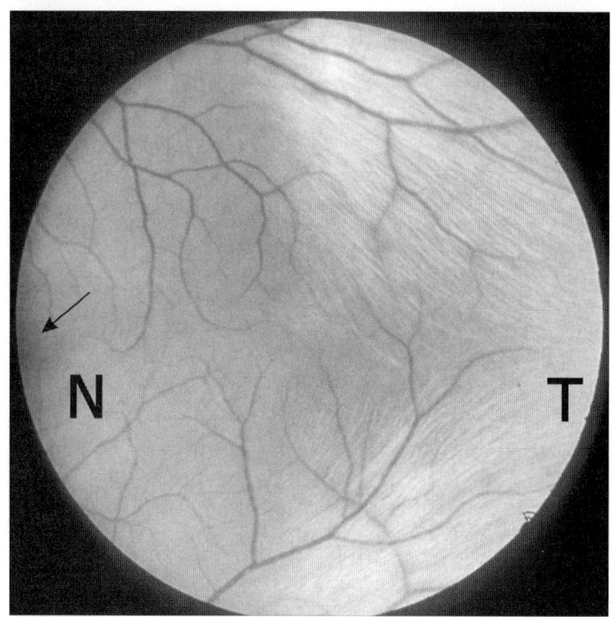

6-3B

Figure 6-3. A. **The myelinated nerve fibers shown here are just off of the disc. Notice that they cover the vessels, and also that they have the feathery edge without evidence of the "cumulus cloud" of a nerve fiber layer infarct. Furthermore, the vessels are well seen.** B. **These medullated or myelinated nerve fibers are in the temporal (T) peripheral retina. The arrow points toward the macula on the nasal (N) side. Notice the feathery appearance.**

Epipapillary membranes and Bergmeister papillae (see Figure 2-19) may be white and are congenitally present. Again, there should be no change in vision, the appearance is stable, and there are no signs of inflammation.

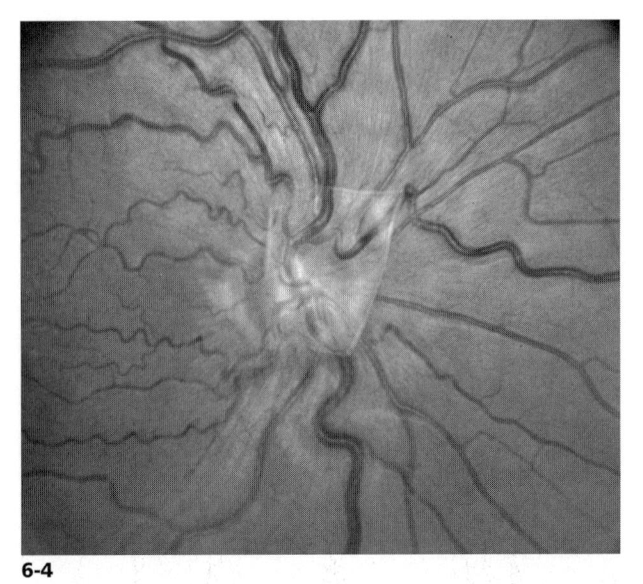

6-4

Figure 6-4. A Bergmeister papilla, present since birth, has no effect on vision in this individual, but may be confusing when first encountered. Here you see the white glial tissue on the disc.

Other white spots in and around the disc may be pathologic.

The possibilities for white spots include lipoproteinaceous deposits, infarcted tissue, and proliferative tissue[2]:

Deposits: Edema (with and without protein), edema which has changed to lipid, calcium, hyaline, or cellular deposits.

Tissue that has infarcted: A section of the retina or cells within a layer that have degenerated (e.g., nerve fiber layer—cotton-wool spot)

Tissue that has proliferated: Connective tissue, blood vessels, glial tissue, pigmented epithelium, and tumors

---

White Spots on the Disc

Optic disc drusen appear as white elevated variably refractile lumps in the disc. See the discussion on optic disc drusen (Chapter 3). You can verify the presence of disc drusen by examining with B-scan ultrasonography or by computed tomography scan of the disc, or by looking for late focal fluorescence on fluorescein angiography.

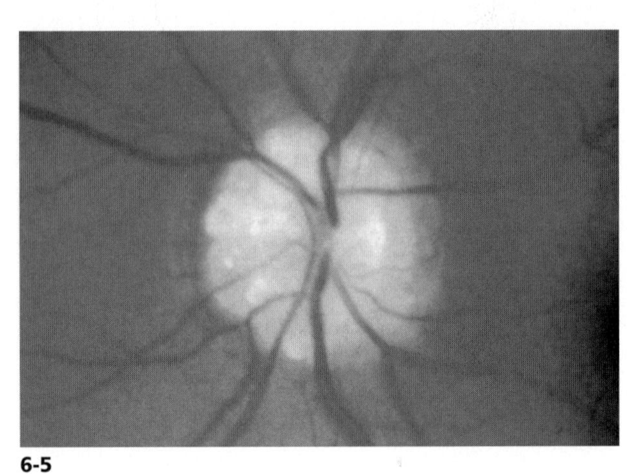

6-5

Figure 6-5. Visible drusen appear as mineralized concretions in and on the disc.

(Sarcoid granules may appear to be a "white spot" on the disc. See discussion of sarcoid under disc swelling [see Figure 6-13 and Chapter 3, Figure 3-64].)

White Spots Around the Disc

Peripapillary retinal atrophy seen in myopia is common. Sometimes, however, the atrophy can be quite dramatic and can even progress (see Figure 11-24).

White Spots in the Peripapillary Retina

White or yellowish spots around blood vessels can be owing to glial or cellular sheathing. Sheathing may be around veins or arteries. Venous sheathing may involve one or both sides of the vein. In addition, the entire vein may be broad and white. *Apparent sheathing* is associated with deposition of lipid and fibrosis of the intima of the vein. *True extravascular sheathing* may not be readily visible without viewing a fluorescein angiogram, which can show staining of blood vessels. *Taches de bougie* (candle wax spots) are discrete, perivascular chorioretinal infiltrates associated with sarcoidosis.[3] These spots are frequently mistaken for birdshot retinochoroidopathy and multifocal choroiditis.

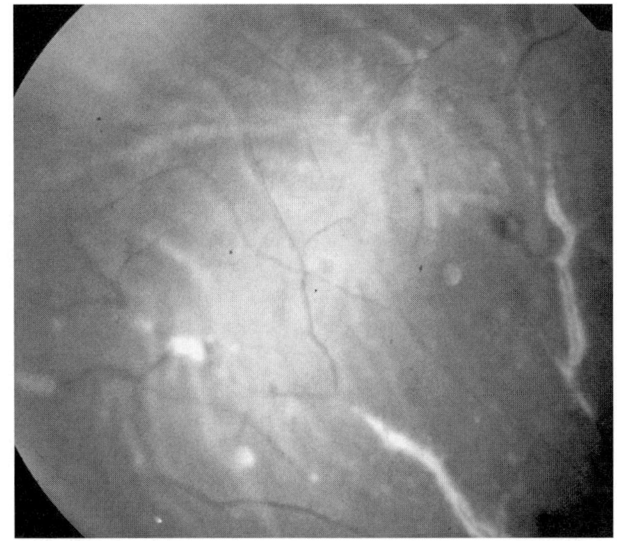

Figure 6-6. Venous sheathing may involve one or both sides of the vein. In addition, the entire vein may be broad and white. "Sheathing" is associated with deposition of lipid and fibrosis of the intima of the vein. The sheathing in this case is owing to sarcoidosis.

6-6

Cotton-Wool Spots

Soft exudates, or *cotton-wool spots*, can appear as a white, gray, or yellow fluffy, feathery area around or on the disc and in the retina. The term *cotton-wool* comes from the light appearance of absorbent cotton: It has the appearance of a cumulus cloud. A cotton-wool patch is actually a nerve fiber layer infarct, and is not the result of any vascular exudation. These are known pathologically as *cytoid bodies*.

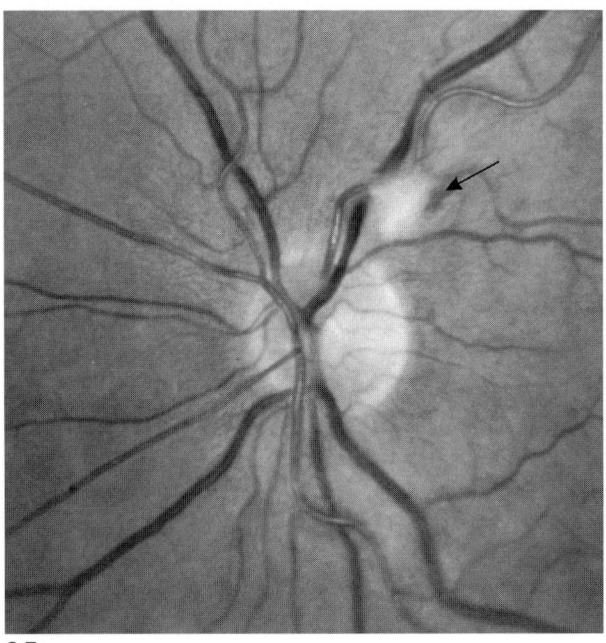

Figure 6-7. This is a single cotton-wool spot in a woman who is on interferon alpha (recombinant) for hepatitis C. Notice the "cloudlike" appearance. You can tell that the cotton-wool spot is in the nerve fiber layer because the retinal vessels are obscured. Notice the small nerve fiber hemorrhage (*arrow*) next to the cotton-wool spot.

6-7

Figure 6-8. A. **The cotton-wool spot (or soft exudate) is a nerve fiber layer infarct. Therefore, you see the fluffy exudate at the level of the nerve fiber layer.** B. **This is a giant cotton-wool spot just off of the disc.**

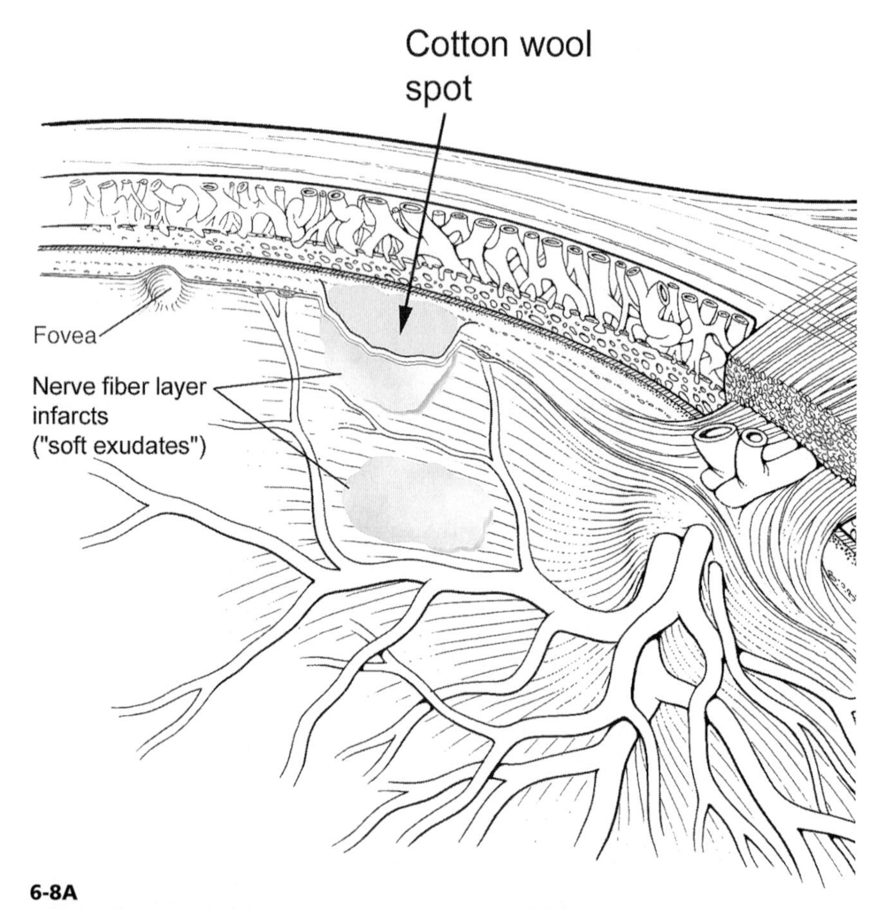

6-8A

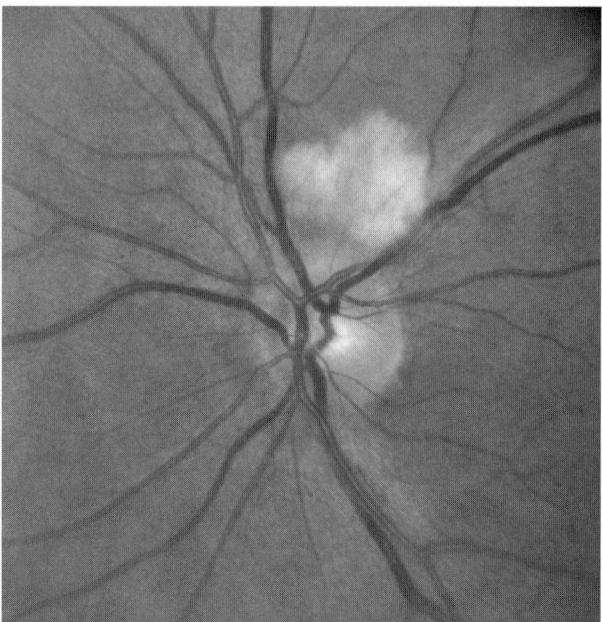

6-8B

The following are visual characteristics of cotton-wool spots:

- Fluffy-appearing white, yellow, or gray patches that have striate borders that radiate in the direction of the nerve fiber layer.
- The shape is round or oval.
- They may be single or multiple.
- There may be a small linear or "flame-shaped" hemorrhage seen in the same area.
- The cotton-wool spot tends to obscure the retinal vessels because the ganglion cell and nerve fiber layer, where the infarct occurs, overlies most of the blood vessels of the retina.
- Cotton-wool spots usually are seen within the posterior pole—near the disc, not in the peripheral retina.

So, look for cotton-wool spots and you will frequently find them in individuals who are predisposed.

Figure 6-9. A. **Acute disc swelling with cotton-wool spots (*arrows*).** B. **Pathologic changes with cytoid bodies. Cytoid bodies are seen histologically as round or oval eosinophilic bodies (*arrows*) on hematoxylin and eosin stains in the nerve fiber and ganglion cell layer of the retina.** C. **Pathologic changes of nerve fiber layer infarct with disc swelling of cytoid bodies.**

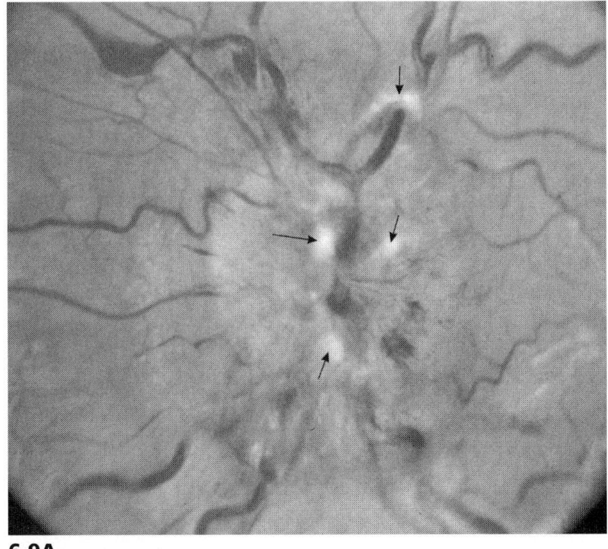

6-9A

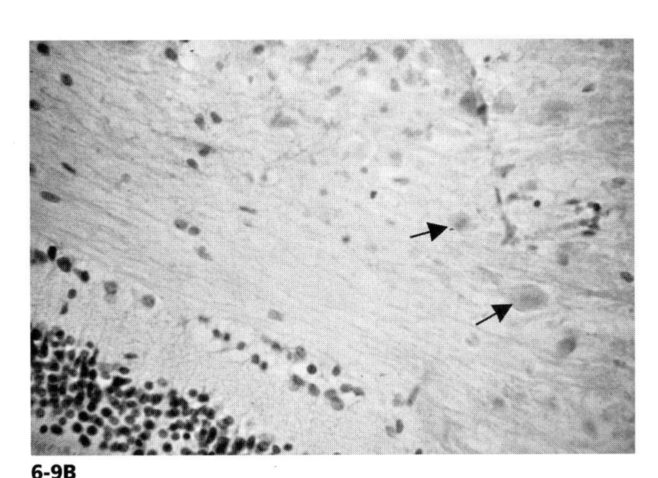

6-9B

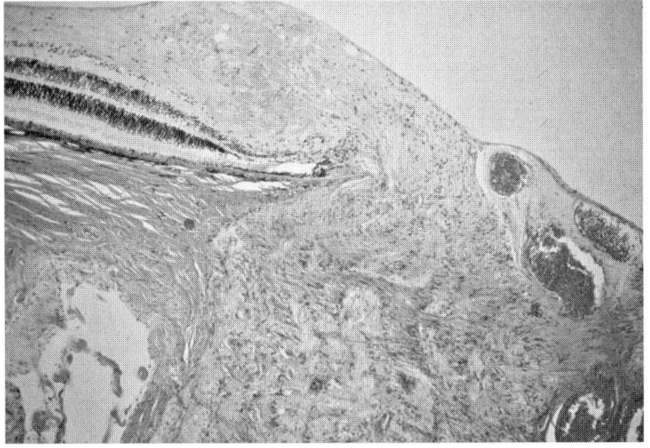

6-9C

Pathologically, cotton-wool spots are micro-infarctions of axons that then swell. The swelling is owing to the continued production of axoplasm by ganglion cells. The axoplasm is then carried to the ischemically damaged area and cannot flow past; it is dammed up at the locus of the infarct, creating the fluffy nerve fiber layer infarct. The infarcts are known pathologically as *cytoid bodies*. Cytoid bodies are seen histologically as round or oval eosinophilic bodies on hematoxylin and eosin stains in the nerve fiber and ganglion cell layer of the retina.[4] The cytoid body is composed of lipid and swollen mitochondria.[5] The cotton-wool patch has been reproduced experimentally by specific occlusion of arterioles in experimental animal models.[6]

The importance of a cotton-wool spot is that it represents occlusion of a retinal arteriole or capillary. Continued new appearance of cotton-wool spots may represent progression of a serious underlying condition affecting small vessels.

Cotton-wool spots are highly significant, and a single cotton-wool spot should lead to a thorough evaluation of possible causes. Although diabetes is the most common cause of a cotton-wool spot, other conditions to think of when seeing a cotton-wool spot include hypertension, emboli, vasculitis, collagen vascular disease, hypercoagulable states, anemia, and leukemia.

The natural history of cotton-wool spots is that they usually resolve within days to weeks. Once the cotton-wool spot is gone, the retina appears normal.

Table 6-1. Cotton-Wool Spots—What to Think of

Condition	Symptoms	Signs	Funduscopic findings
Hypertension—especially accelerated or malignant forms seen with renal disease; eclampsia	Headache, blurred vision; sometimes none	Elevated blood pressure	Hypertensive retinopathy (see also Figure 9-22A–D)
Diabetes	Blurred vision; fluctuating vision	Peripheral neuropathy	Diabetic retinopathy (see also Table 9-3)
Embolic disease: endocarditis, rheumatic heart disease; valvular disease	Episodic vision loss; strokelike symptoms	Splinter hemorrhages; focal neurologic deficit; heart murmur	Embolic material in retinal vessels (see also Figures 5-13–5-15)
Vascular: Carotid artery disease (severe stenosis or occlusion); retinal vessel (e.g., artery, vein) occlusion; aortic arch disease	Episodic neurologic events; amaurosis fugax	Carotid bruit; neovascular iris; murmur	See Chapter 5, Figure 5-25
Acute blood loss	History of blood loss	Possible posterior ischemic optic neuropathy	Pale disc (see also Figure 4-46)
Vasculitis, temporal arteritis[7]	Headache, sensory disturbances; fatigue; jaw claudication	Livedo reticularis; skin lesions	Possible vessel narrowing; sheathing of blood vessels (see Table 5-17)
Collagen vascular diseases: systemic lupus erythematosus; scleroderma; dermatomyositis; polyarteritis nodosa	Arthralgias, myalgias fatigue	Butterfly rash; skin lesions	See cotton-wool spots, Figure 6-11
Blood dyscrasias: anemia; leukemia; thrombocytopenic purpura; multiple myeloma;[8] dysproteinemia; macroglobulinemia; sickle cell disease	Fatigue; arthralgias	Pale; tachycardia	Tortuosity of retinal vessels; intraretinal hemorrhage
Infections: septicemia; virus: acquired immunodeficiency syndrome; leptospirosis; Rocky Mountain spotted fever	Fever; malaise	Rash	Disc swelling; Roth's spots; retinopathy (see also Figures 7-17 and 9-32)
Acute pancreatitis	Abdominal pain	Epigastric tenderness	Cotton-wool spots and hemorrhages (see also Figure 5-16)
High altitude	History	Nausea; disorientation	May see hemorrhages
Trauma; Purtscher's retinopathy	History; especially chest crush injuries	Other signs of trauma	May see hemorrhages (see also Figure 14-8)
Neoplasia: leukemia; lymphoma; metastases	Fatigue	Anemia	Disc swelling (see also Figure 3-66)
Radiation retinopathy	History	—	Hemorrhages; optic neuropathy (see also Figure 9-25)
Drugs: intravenous drug abuse; interferon-alpha	History	Splinter hemorrhages	Look for talc; cotton-wool spot (see Figure 6-7)

Source: Adapted from reference 5 and GC Brown, MM Brown, T Hiller, et al. Cotton-wool spots. Retina 1985;5(4):206–214.

Figure 6-10. A. **Diabetes is the classic retinopathy that is associated with cotton-wool spots (*arrows*) and hemorrhages.** B. **Another diabetic with a large single cotton-wool spot (*arrow*) associated with a hemorrhage.**

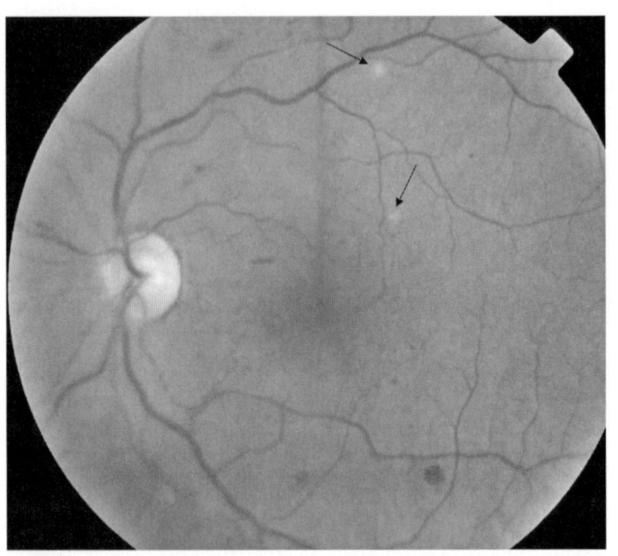

6-10A

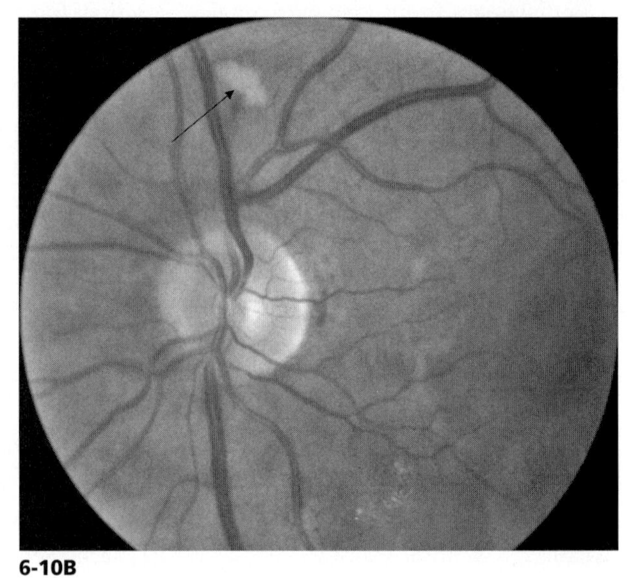

6-10B

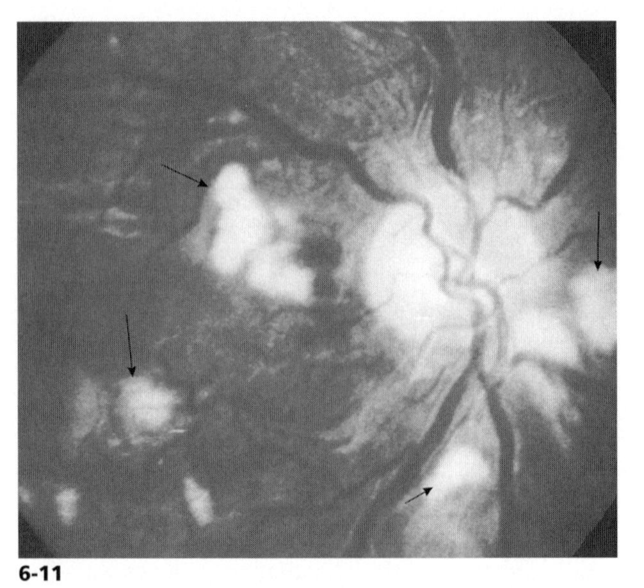

6-11

Figure 6-11. **This woman had systemic lupus and a complaint of blurred vision. The retinal examination showed many cotton-wool spots (*arrows*).**

Figure 6-12. This man presented with fatigue and blurred vision. On examination he had only cotton-wool spots (*arrows*). His erythrocyte sedimentation rate was 25 mm/hr. A temporal artery biopsy revealed findings consistent with giant cell arteritis. Cotton-wool spots, single or multiple, in an older individual without diabetes or hypertension should prompt an evaluation for temporal arteritis.[7] (See the discussion of temporal arteritis in Chapter 5, Figure 5-20.)

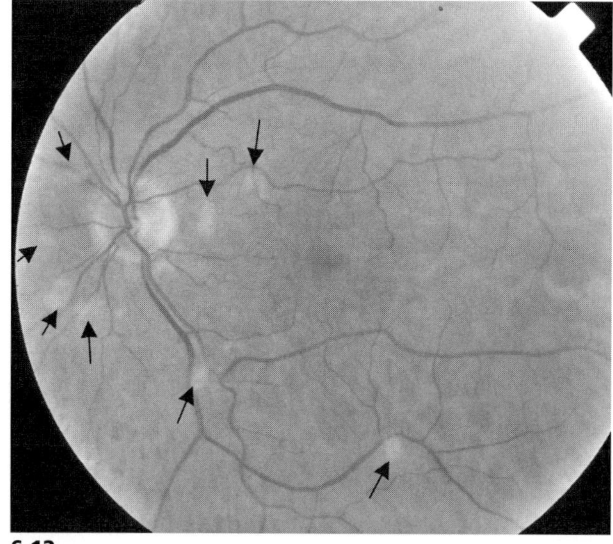

6-12

White Spots Owing to Deposits (Cellular: Sarcoid Granulomas)

Figure 6-13. This woman has biopsy-documented sarcoidosis. She presented with a steroid-responsive optic neuropathy. She had a sarcoid granuloma superior to the optic disc. Notice how the white spot (*arrow*) elevates the blood vessel above it. At first blush, these granulomas can appear to be myelinated nerve fibers, but they do not obscure the blood vessels because they are deep to the nerve fiber layer and beneath the blood vessels. Notice how the blood vessel drapes over the granuloma. See also the discussion of disc swelling with sarcoid (Chapter 3, Figure 3-64).

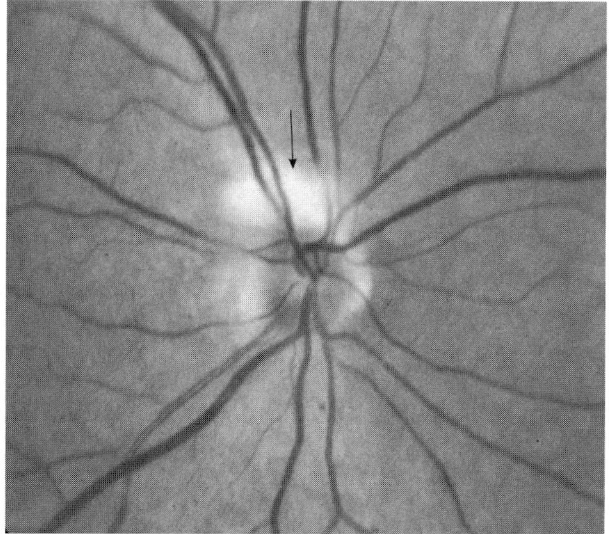

6-13

HARD EXUDATES

Hard exudates may be yellow or white. They are small, discrete hard-edged lesions or may coalesce in larger masses. They are sometimes described as "waxy or glistening." The level of the retina in which these occur is beneath the retinal vessels in the nuclear layers or outer plexiform layer, in the outer- to mid-level retina. How hard exudates accumulate is unclear. Some report that initially, fluid pools from vessels in the retina, attracting macrophages and depositing fibrin in the retina, whereas others report there is actual neuronal damage at the level of the outer plexiform layer.[6] Most believe that because soft exudates (cotton-wool spots) are seen often in conjunction with hard exudates, the process must be similar. The vessels responsible for blood supply to the outer plexiform layer are choroidal. Thus, diseases that affect the choroidal circulation presumably also cause hard exudates; the two most common are accelerated hypertension and diabetes.

Hard exudates consist of lipids and fat in macrophages, and may be difficult to differentiate from drusen of the retina. Hard exudates do not always regress (and if they do, it takes many months to years), although treatment of an underlying condition such as diabetes or hypercholesterolemia has been associated with regression.

Figure 6-14. A. **Hard exudates are found in the nuclear layer or outer plexiform layer—mid-level retina. Hard exudates are mostly lipid and fat in macrophages. The classic example of hard retinal exudate is the macular star found in Henle's layer.** B. **Here you see hard exudates (*arrows*) and cotton-wool spots (*arrowheads*).**

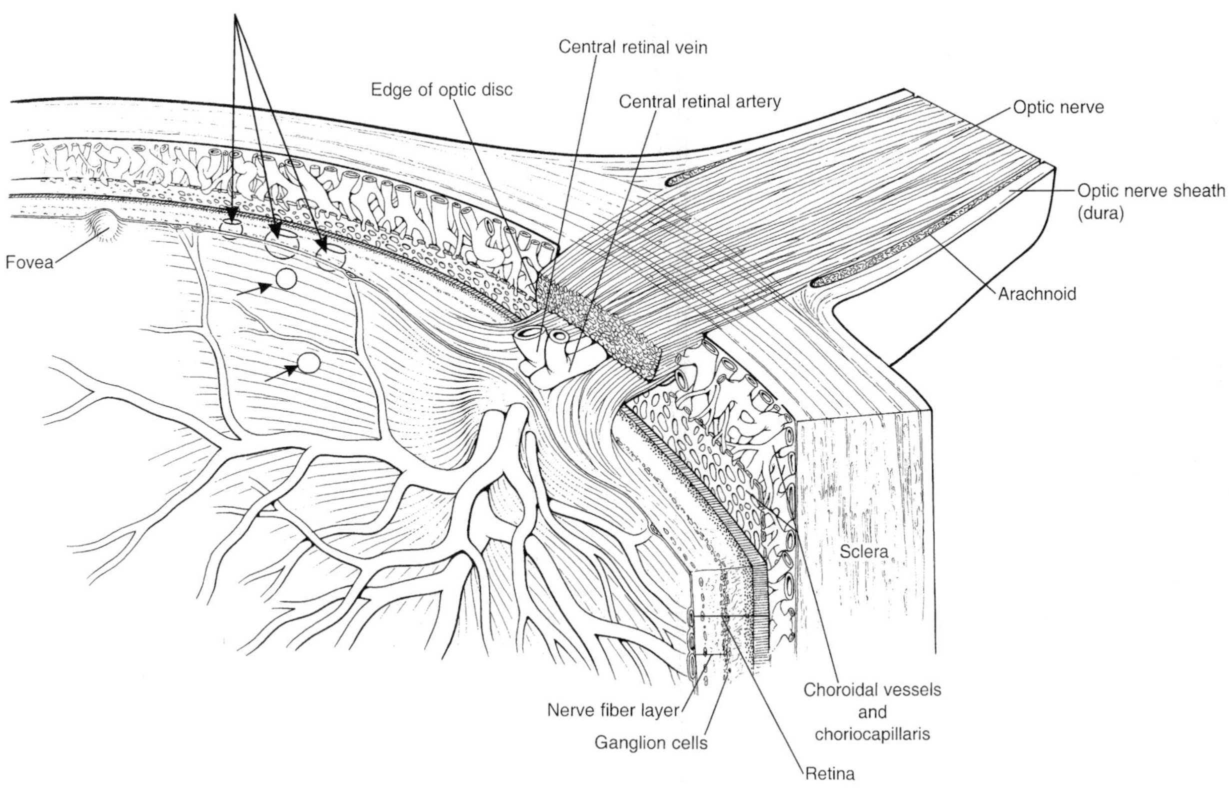

6-14A

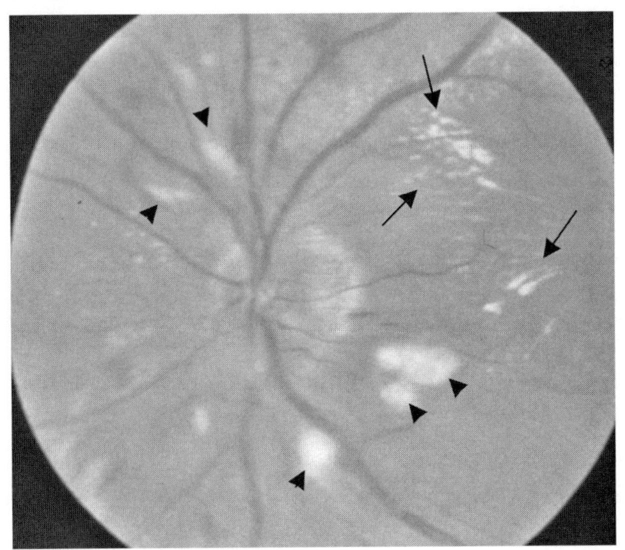

6-14B

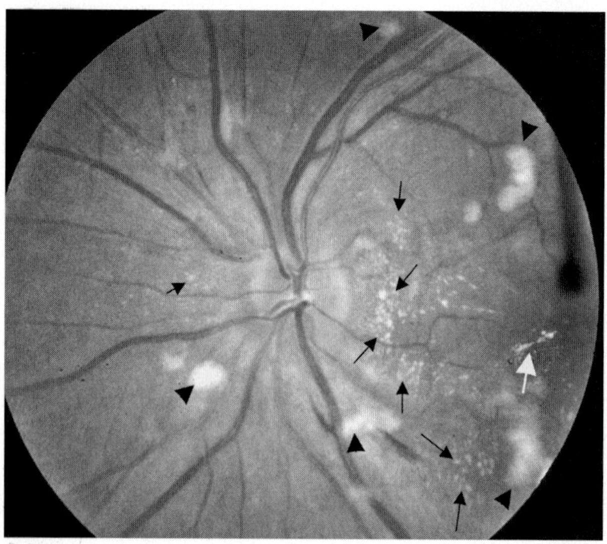

6-15

MACULAR STAR

The outer plexiform layer (or Henle's layer) of the macula is produced by nerve fibers in a radiating pattern away from the center of the fovea, like spokes of a bicycle tire. When hard exudates accumulate in this region, a starlike appearance is produced. When the star is associated with focal optic disc swelling, a search for a cause must be undertaken. See the full description in the chapter on macula (Chapter 10, Figures 10-17–10-19).

Figure 6-15. This boy had retinopathy owing to a viral infection. Notice the cotton-wool spots (*arrowheads*) and hard exudate patches (*arrows*). He also has a partial macular star (*white arrow*).

RETINAL DRUSEN (OR COLLOID BODIES)

Drusen are commonly seen in many older persons. There are two types of retinal drusen: *Hard drusen* are small, discrete, round, yellow spots, whereas *soft drusen* are larger and have indistinct edges. Both types most frequently are found in the macula. Drusen appear as yellow-white, and sometimes a "thin line of pigment" can be seen around them.[9] Pathologically, drusen are outgrowths of Bruch's membrane. As they accumulate, they elevate the outer nuclear layer of the retina. They lie deep in the retina—just above the RPE. Drusen contain mucopolysaccharides and lipids, and probably represent degeneration of pigment cells.[10] When Bruch's membrane is affected with drusen cracks, choroidal upgrowth, subretinal neovascularization, and subsequent hemorrhage occur. When this condition occurs in the macula, it is known as *aging macular degeneration*. It is a common cause of vision loss in the elderly (see Chapter 12). Although retinal drusen are most frequently associated with macular degeneration, the relationship is not absolute. There is also an inherited form of retinal drusen.

Viewing drusen is best done with a red-free (green) light. In addition, fluorescein angiography may show drusen well.

Figure 6-16. A. Drusen are yellow-white deposits deep in the retina. Both hard and soft drusen are seen in the macula, especially in macular degeneration. B. The arrows point to "crops" of hard drusen. C. Notice the soft drusen (*arrows*) seen just temporal to the disc around the macula (M).

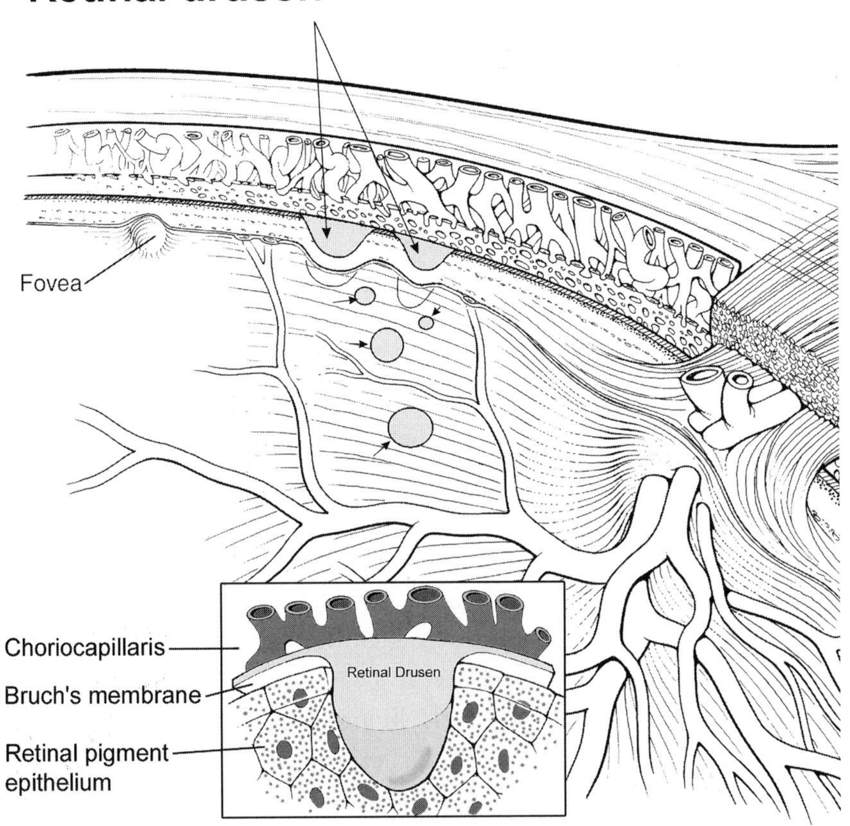

6-16A

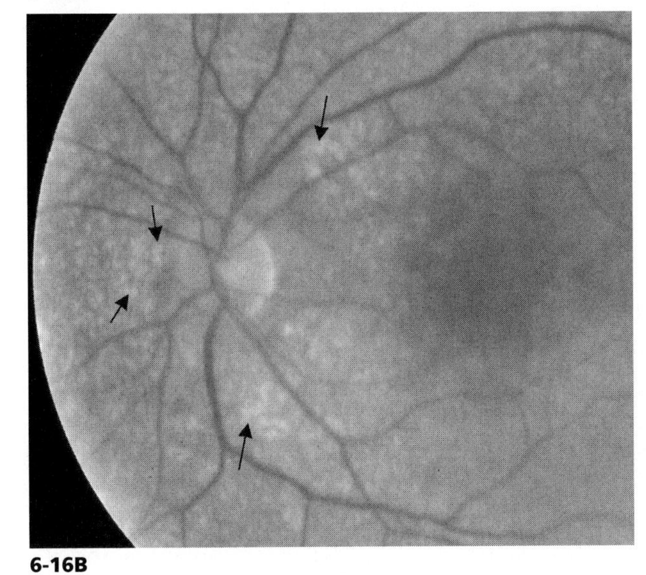

6-16B

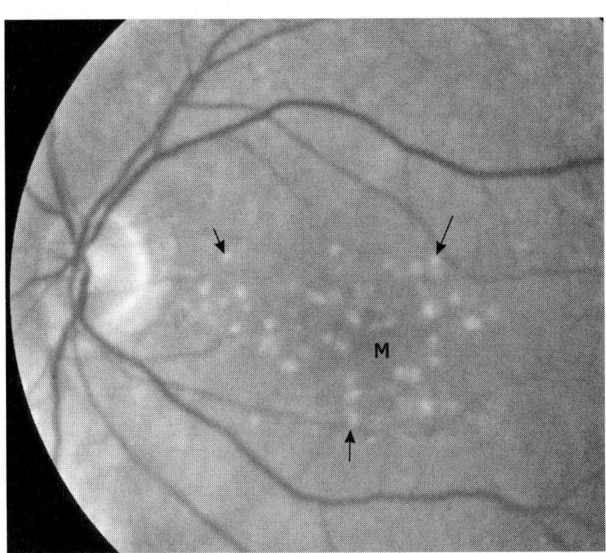

6-16C

Table 6-2. Distinguishing Hard Exudates and Drusen

Characteristic	Hard exudate	Drusen
Depth of retina	More superficial—outer to mid-retina	Deeper—at the level of the retinal pigment epithelium, at or anterior to Bruch's membrane
Position	Found in proximity to microaneurysms and retinal edema	Usually around the macula
Shape	Irregular shapes	Round
Appearance	Shiny	Dull
Border	No pigment border	May show faint pigment border

Source: Adapted from reference 9.

CALCIFICATION OF THE CHOROID

Sclerochoroidal calcification is an uncommon cause of yellow, flat lesions found, often incidentally, in usually asymptomatic people. The retinal tumors, such as choroidal melanoma or metastases, are often diagnosed initially. These calcifications are usually seen in older individuals and can be bilateral or unilateral. The appearance of the fundus is usually of well-circumscribed yellow plaques seen in the posterior pole. Ultrasonography (orbital) and computed tomography scanning can show calcification in the sclera. It is important to diagnose these calcifications because there are several known systemic associations, including parathyroid-related disorders such as primary hyperparathyroidism and secondary hyperparathyroidism, calcium pyrophosphate deposition disease (pseudogout), Vitamin D intoxication, sarcoidosis, renal disease (primary renal tubular hypokalemic metabolic alkalosis syndromes or Bartter syndrome), Gitelman syndrome, and chronic renal failure.[11]

Acute Retinal Necrosis

Acute retinal necrosis (ARN) causes inflammation and subsequent retinal detachment. ARN usually presents in healthy patients with a periorbital pain, red eye (scleritis), and anterior uveitis (inflammation of the anterior chamber or in front of the iris), then progresses to peripheral retinal white/yellow spots, an optic neuropathy, and retinal detachment. The cause of ARN is frequently the herpes family of viruses, especially varicella-zoster (e.g., primary varicella, varicella-zoster) infection, and may be seen as part of the "uveomeningeal syndromes" (e.g., uveitis and meningitis). Age also plays a role: In patients older than 25 years, the varicella-zoster and herpes simplex virus types are more common, but in patients younger than 25 years, herpes simplex virus type 2 is more common. When there is a history of nervous system findings with ARN, herpes simplex virus is most likely.[12] Because it is treated with intravenous acyclovir, ARN is a diagnosis that needs prompt attention and treatment by an ophthalmologist or retinal specialist.[13] Viewing retinal necrosis is difficult: Most of the time, your view into the fundus with the direct ophthalmoscope is obscured by the cellular response in the vitreous and anterior chamber.

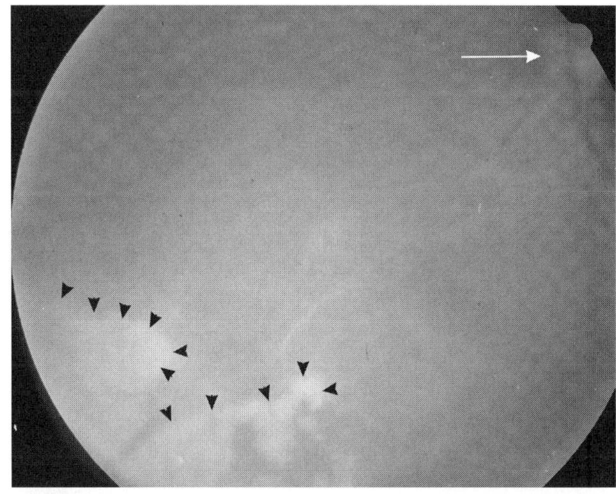
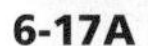

6-17A

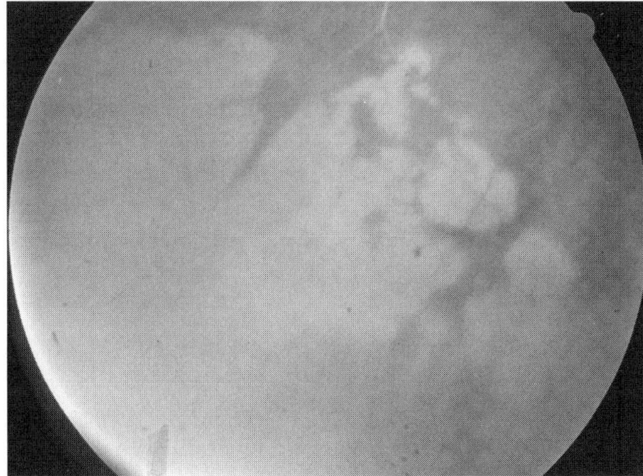

6-17B

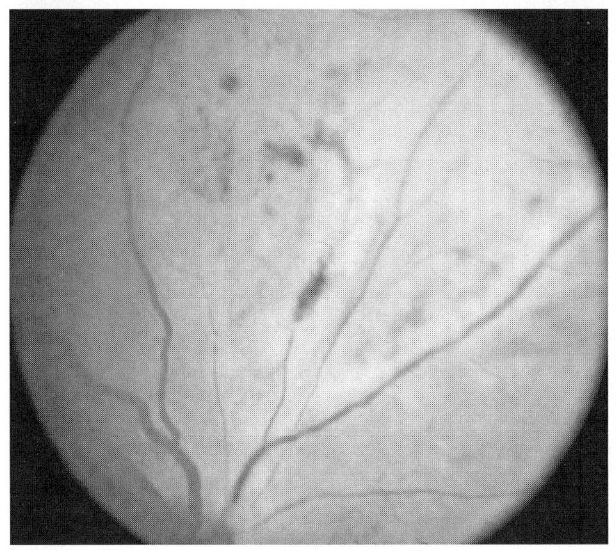

6-17C

Figure 6-17. A–C. **ARN is associated with pain around the eye, inflammation of the eye (uveitis), and white/yellow patches in the retina that can progress to retinal detachment. The primary virus seen with the condition is varicella-zoster.** A. **The white arrow points to the optic disc. The arrowheads outline the area of necrosis in the retina.** B. **ARN due to varicella-zoster infection. The white areas are retinal necrosis.** C. **ARN caused by varicella-zoster infection. Here you see hemorrhages and white areas associated with ARN. (Photographs courtesy of Paul Zimmerman, M.D.)**

Infections of the choroid and retina can also produce fuzzy white spots that are clumps of mycelia in the retina and vitreous: These are fungus balls, and also should be referred immediately to the ophthalmologist for diagnosis and treatment. Fungus in particular can produce white spots. Risk factors for developing intraocular fungal infections include recent surgery (especially gastrointestinal), bacterial sepsis with systemic antibiotic use, intravenous drug abuse, intravenous catheters, and debilitating disease.[14]

Table 6-3. Fungus Causing White Spots

Fungus	Characteristic features	Other
Candida	White spot < 1 mm; overlying vitreous haze	Most common fungal infection; associated with candidemia (1/3)
Aspergillosis	Invades blood vessels; therefore occludes choroidal vessels and causes retinal necrosis with retinal detachment	Common in intravenous drug users, organ transplant patients
Cryptococcosis	Presents as multifocal choroiditis	Occurs also with cryptococcal meningitis; common in acquired immunodeficiency syndrome
Histoplasmosis	Most often seen after subacute pulmonary infection as a pigmented peripapillary scar; active infection can cause retinitis	Associated with lung infections in the central United States (Mississippi Valley) (see Figure 6-23)
Coccidioidomycosis	Looks like multifocal choroiditis with small, yellow-white lesions	Soil borne—pulmonary infection in the southwestern United States (see Figure 6-18)
Sporotrichosis	Chronic uveitis and massive inflammation of choroid and retina	Skin infection; rose bushes; common in France
Blastomycosis	Severe inflammation of choroid and retina	Skin infection—frequent in southeastern United States

Source: Adapted from reference 14.

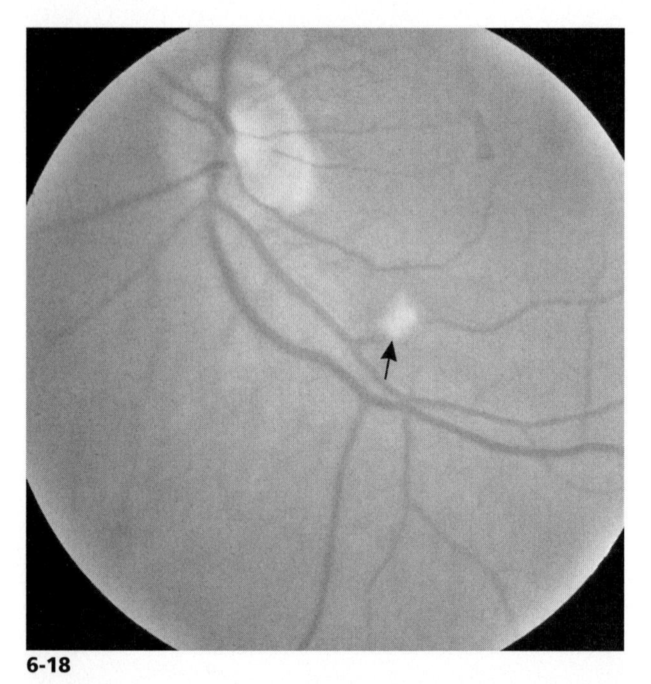

6-18

Figure 6-18. This woman contracted systemic coccidioidomycosis while on an archeological dig in the southwestern United States. The white spot (*arrow*) is a cotton-wool spot.

Sarcoidosis

Sarcoidosis causing disc swelling was discussed in Chapter 3, Figure 3-64. However, sarcoid can cause white spots in many ways. Sarcoid is associated with white spots on the disc (see Figure 6-13), in the retina, in the sheathing along vasculature (see Figure 6-6), and even in the choroid (Figure 6-19).

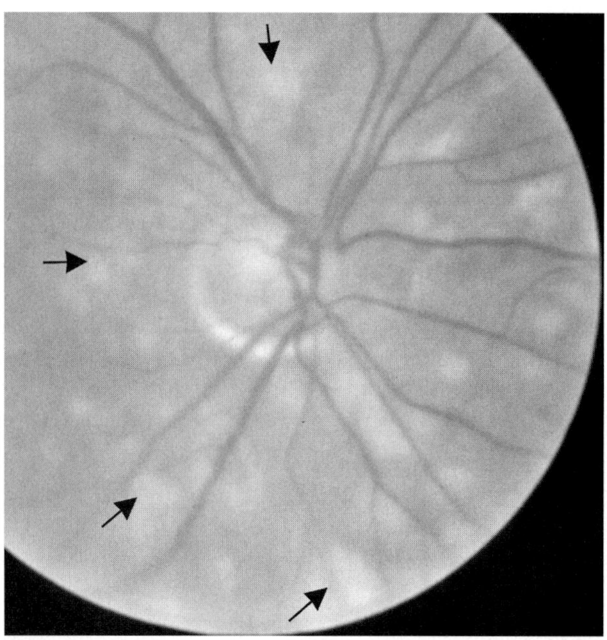

6-19

Figure 6-19. This woman has sarcoid diagnosed involving the choroid and presenting with choroidopathy. Note that the white spots in the posterior pole are deep to the retinal vessels, unlike cotton-wool spots. The arrows point to some of the white spots in the choroid. Sarcoid affects all parts of the eye.

Figure 6-20. A. **Sarcoid vasculitis is seen as white blood vessels and *tache de bougie* (candle wax drippings).** B. **The fluorescein angiogram shows areas of hypofluorescence (dark areas) and staining of blood vessels (fuzzy white blood vessels) consistent with sarcoid vasculitis. Vasculitis may occur owing to many inflammatory conditions such as sarcoid. The hallmark of vasculitis is vessel sheathing or occlusion (especially seen on fluorescein angiogram), cotton-wool spots, and hemorrhages. Although the direct view of the blood vessels** (C) **does not show obvious vasculitis, the fluorescein angiogram** (D) **demonstrates perivenous staining. (Photographs courtesy of Paul Zimmerman, M.D.)**

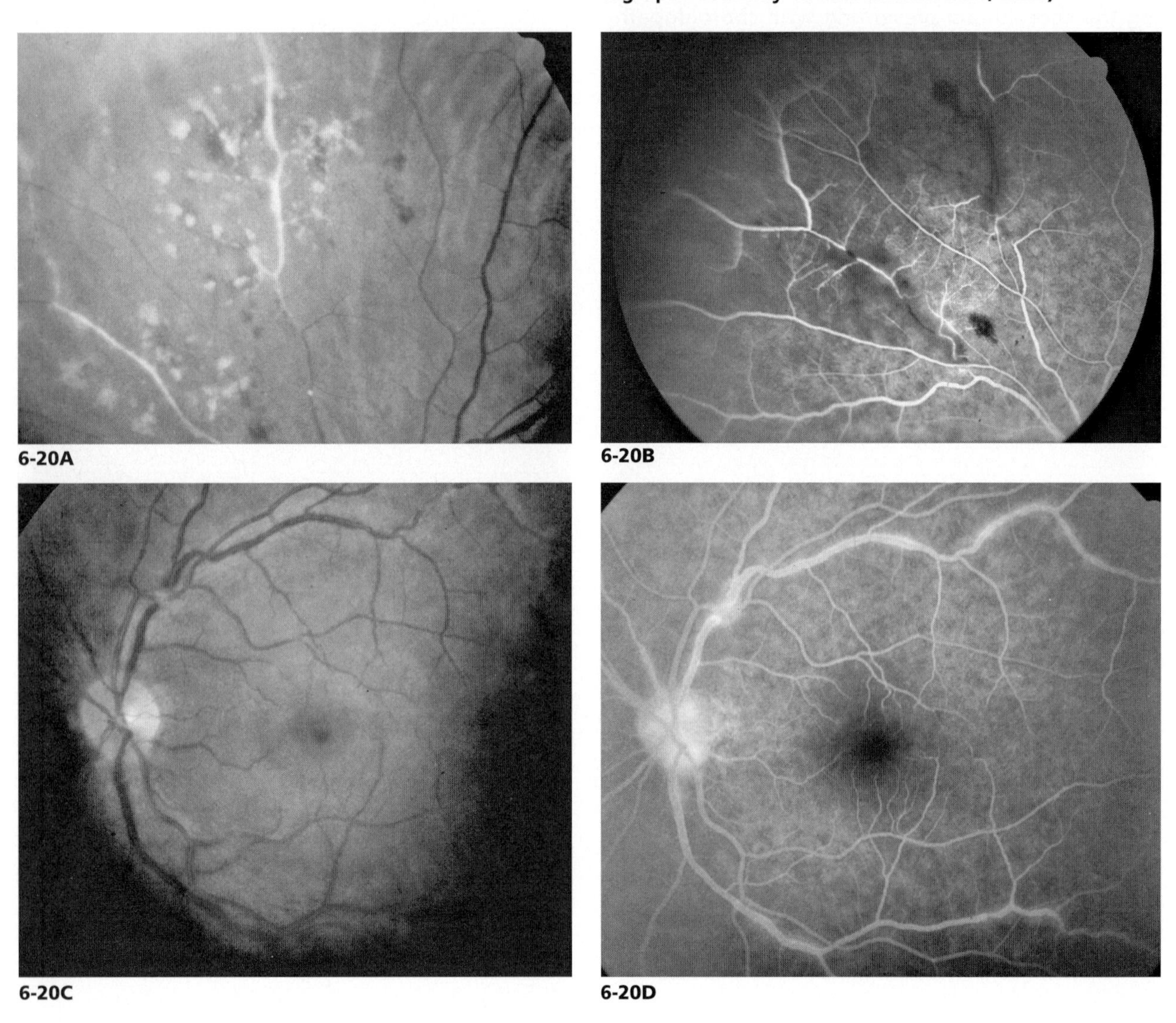

6-20A **6-20B** **6-20C** **6-20D**

Pars Planitis

Pars planitis is an inflammatory condition seen in children and young adults. It is associated with an inflammation of the pars plana, which is in the far periphery of the retina and therefore rarely seen by neurologists, internists, and primary care physicians. Pars planitis is difficult to see with the direct ophthalmoscope and full pupil dilation. Along with white spots over the pars plana, retinal phlebitis and macular edema may be present. The vitreous is usually hazy owing to cells, which further impairs peripheral visualization of the pars plana. Although most cases are idiopathic, multiple sclerosis and sarcoidosis are the most common identifiable causes.[15]

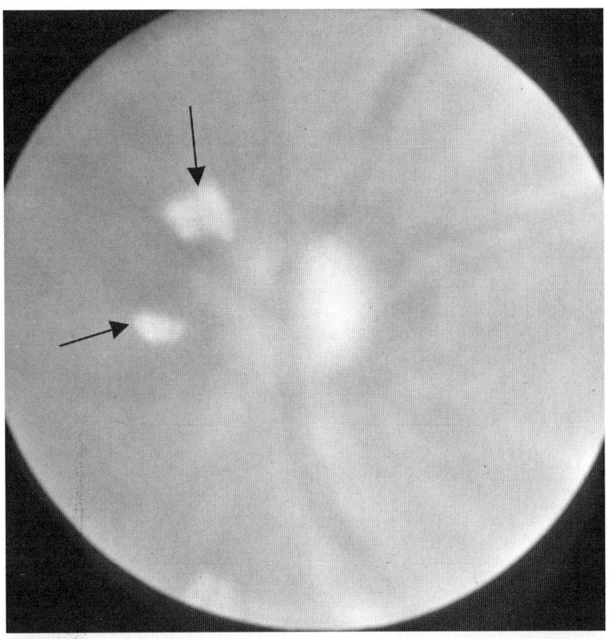
6-21A

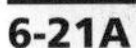

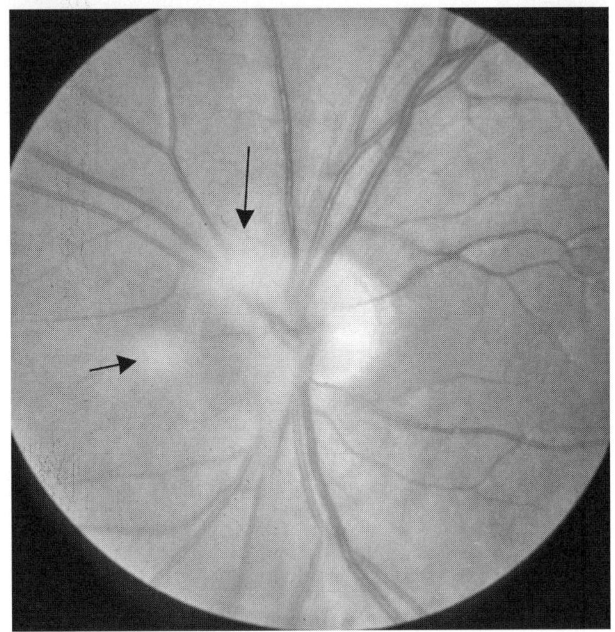
6-21B

Figure 6-21. A,B. **Pars planitis is a common inflammatory condition in children and young adults. Although it is difficult to see "snow banking" in the periphery with the direct ophthalmoscope, you can see signs of inflammation near the disc. Not only can there be venous sheathing, but, also, "vitreous snowballs" can be present:** (A) **focuses on the snowball of inflammation (*arrows*) and the disc is out of focus;** (B) **focuses on the disc, the inflammation is out of focus (*arrows*). (Photographs courtesy of Paul Zimmerman, M.D.)**

Presumed Ocular Histoplasmosis Syndrome

Although histoplasmosis, a fungus, can present acutely with a systemic condition, common chorioretinal atrophic scars seen around the disc and macula are thought to be owing to previous histoplasmosis, but this has never been satisfactorily demonstrated with histology. Because most infections are not symptomatic, presumed ocular histoplasmosis syndrome can be a common finding, especially in the Mississippi Valley, where there is a 1.6% prevalence.

According to Nussenblatt and Palestine, there are four distinct clinical pictures with ocular histoplasmosis: The first, disseminated choroiditis, produces typical "histo spots." These appear to be circular, atrophic, punched-out scars, with variable amounts of pigment centrally.[16] In addition, peripapillary scarring can also be present.[17] The second, a less common finding, is a maculopathy that can decrease visual acuity. Early on, the macular lesion may be raised; it hemorrhages easily, and a scar forms.[16] Thirdly, a peripapillary pigmentary change from choroiditis is common in ocular histoplasmosis. Finally, in ocular histoplasmosis, the vitreous is usually clear, so you can get a good view in. If the vitreous is hazy, think of other inflammatory conditions.[16]

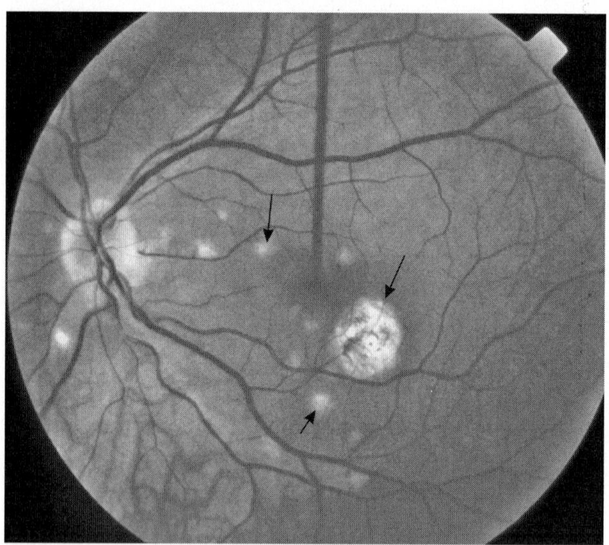
6-22

Figure 6-22. Presumed ocular histoplasmosis: There are white, punched-out lesions (*arrows*) in the posterior pole around the disc and macula. There is variable amount of pigment associated with these white lesions.

Infiltrating Lesions in the Choroid Caused by Metastatic Malignancy

Infiltrating lesions, such as leukemia and lymphoma, can be difficult because they will often look like a choroiditis, retinopathy, or choroidal white spots. Vitreal aspirates are necessary to make the correct diagnosis.

Table 6-4. Diagnosing White Spots

Type of white spot	Appearance	Level of the retina	Time course	Significance	Associations/ Treatment
Soft exudate (cotton-wool spot)	Fluffy, white, yellow—often associated with hemorrhages; larger than hard exudates; fluorescein stains gradually, surrounded by leaking capillaries and microaneurysms	Nerve fiber layer; often around the disc where nerve fibers are more prevalent	Appears shortly after occlusion and lasts for weeks; usually resolves in 4–8 weeks	Small arteriole occlusion—retinal artery circulation	Hypertension, diabetes, collagen vascular disease, anemia, leukemia
Hard exudate	Discrete shiny or conglomerate white or yellow; distinct, irregular border; forms rings, clusters, or stars; can be associated with cotton-wool spots and hemorrhages; fluorescein produces hypofluorescent spots under retinal blood vessels	Junction of inner nuclear and outer plexiform layer	Lasts a long time—months to indefinite	Vascular occlusive disease—choroid	Hypertension, diabetes, collagen vascular disease, anemia
Drusen of the retina	Small yellow; may coalesce	Between Bruch's membrane and the retinal pigment epithelium—form in the macula	Usually accumulates	Unknown	Macular degeneration treatment; vitamin trials have been recommended
Chorioretinitis—infiltrates	Yellow and white lesions deep to retinal vessels	Choroid—can see exudative retinitis	Early yellow and white; become pigmented with time	Chorioretinal infection—including fungal infection, white dot syndromes, malignant infiltrates, sarcoid	Treat the infection
Diffuse unilateral subacute neuroretinitis	White, gray-white, yellow-white; disc swelling	Deep retina, retinal pigment epithelium	Later see depigmentation of the retinal pigment epithelium, optic atrophy, retinal arteriole narrowing	Associated with nematodes	Laser treatment direct; antihelminthic thiabendazole

White Dot Syndromes—White Spots in the Choroid

There are several conditions to consider when the inflammation takes place in the choroid. In general, retinitis causes inflammation of the vitreous, which tends to obscure the view of the fundus, whereas choroiditis does not. Many of these choroidal inflammations have been termed *white dot syndromes*. After evaluating for infectious causes of chorioretinitis, what other conditions could cause "white spots?"

In general, most would recommend a more thorough evaluation if there are any atypical features. Patients with white spots in the choroid should be seen by an ophthalmologist and followed carefully, because the findings can be subtle and the effect on vision may be great. Electroretinography, electrooculography (which tests the function of the RPE), and fluorescein angiography can be helpful.

Acute (posterior) multifocal placoid pigment epitheliopathy (AMPEE) is a condition seen in younger individuals (usually teens and those younger than 30) that can follow a viral illness. On occasion, papillitis (disc swelling) may be seen. Although visual acuity may be affected, spontaneous recovery without treatment is usual. There may be associated immune diseases, such as erythema nodosum, episcleritis, cerebral vasculitis, seizures, stroke, and sensorineural hearing loss.[16] Recently, partial choroidal vascular occlusion owing to occlusive vasculitis has been postulated.[22]

6-23A

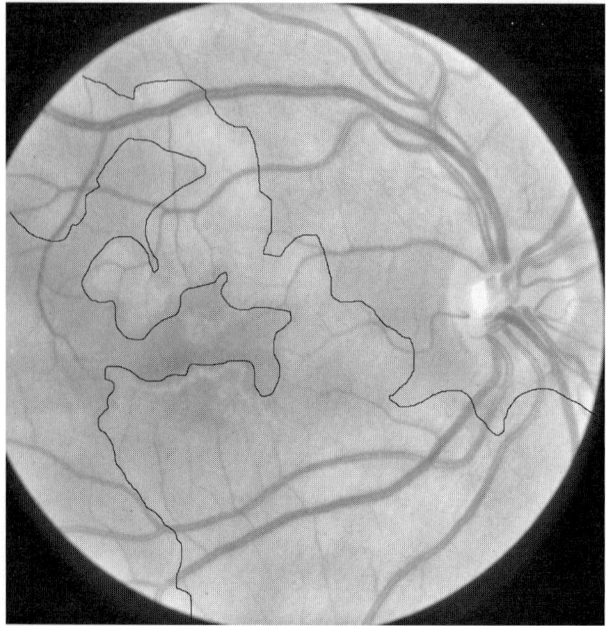

6-23B

Figure 6-23. A. **The appearance of acute multifocal placoid pigment epitheliopathy is usually of flat, yellow-white or cream-colored plaques at the level of the RPE.** B. **Here we have outlined the area of the retinal lesion in the RPE so that you can see where the abnormality is. (Photographs courtesy of Paul Zimmerman, M.D.)**

Table 6-5. White Dot Syndromes—Features

Characteristic	Acute multifocal placoid pigment epitheliopathy[21,22,29]	Vogt-Koyanagi-Harada syndrome[31]	Serpiginous choroidopathy (geographic choroidopathy)[32]	Multifocal choroiditis[23,24]	Punctate inner choroidopathy[23,33]	Multiple evanescent white dot syndrome[25]	Birdshot choroidopathy[26,27]
Age (yrs)	Teens to 40	20–40	30–40	20–50	20–40	17–47	40–60
Gender-based incidence	M = F	F > M	M = F	F > M	F >> M	F >> M	F > M
Symptoms epitheliopathy	Sudden loss of vision in both eyes; flulike episode in one-third	Headache, aseptic meningitis, flulike illness; visual blurring	Blurred vision in one eye; no prodrome	Blurring of vision	Acute onset photopsias and scotomas, metamorphopsia	Acute vision loss; photopsias; prodrome viral illness;	Blurred vision and floaters; night blindness and color blindness; glare; photopsias
Appearance	White to gray-white lesions deep at level of RPE around the posterior pole and mid-periphery; late: depigmented RPE and pigment clumping	Optic nerve swelling; yellow-white lesions in the retina and choroid	White to gray at level of RPE and choroid—distinct borders around the optic nerve and macula; retinal veins can be inflamed/occluded; late: deep scars in the RPE	White to yellow to gray-white lesions at choroid or RPE—especially inferiorly and peripherally	Small yellow or gray spots in the choroid; serous retinal detachment possible	Small, white-gray dots temporal to macula; patches and even smaller white dots at level of RPE; macula may look granular	White-yellow depigmented spots in choroid and RPE
Fluorescein angiography	Hypofluorescence early and diffuse staining or hyperfluorescence late of the lesion	Many areas of leakage; disc leakage; neovascularization common	Acute nonfluorescent lesions; late diffuse staining	Variable—acute may block fluorescein or fluoresce early	Leakage late	Early hyperfluoresescence; late staining	Delayed filling of the retinal circulation and arterioles; late retinal leakage (mild), macular edema, and disc leakage

continued

Table 6-5. *Continued*

Characteristic	Acute multifocal placoid pigment epitheliopathy[21,22,29]	Vogt-Koyanagi-Harada syndrome[31]	Serpiginous choroidopathy (geographic choroidopathy)[32]	Multifocal choroiditis[23,24]	Punctate inner choroidopathy[23,33]	Multiple evanescent white dot syndrome[25]	Birdshot choroidopathy[26,27]
Other eye findings	Mild vitreous inflammation	Uveitis; nodules on pupillary margin; vitiligo	Vitreal and anterior segment inflammation; Amsler's grid can help to mark scotoma	Vitreal inflammation	No or little vitreal inflammation; Amsler's grid can help to mark scotoma	Optic nerve head swelling and enlarged blind spot; vitreal cell; occasional venous sheathing; ? related to acute idiopathic blind spot enlargement	Prominent vitreal inflammation; optic disc edema in 14% of patients; optic atrophy; macular star; neovascularization; electroretinogram shows reduced B and A waves
Associations	HLA-B7; HLA-DR2; vasculitis	Japanese, Asian, and Native American heritages	Elevated factor VIII; no known systemic associations	Epstein-Barr virus occasionally	Myopia	Possible viral illness	HLA-A29
Evaluations	VDRL, CBC, CXR; electro-oculogram impaired	Lumbar puncture shows elevated white cells in the cerebrospinal fluid	VDRL, CBC, CXR	VDRL, CBC, CXR; look for sarcoid	VDRL, CBC, CXR	VDRL; electroretinogram-reduced A wave; visual field: enlarged blind spot	VDRL, CBC, CXR
Neurologic involvement	Headache, cerebrospinal fluid pleocytosis; cerebral vasculitis; tinnitus	Meningitis, headache; hearing loss	Unknown	Unknown	Unknown	None	Unknown; disc swelling reported; possible increased vascular disease

Treatment	None or some suggest oral corticosteroids	IV pulse steroids	Injection of periocular corticosteroids; oral corticosteroids; photocoagulation of membranes; other immunosuppression	Oral or periocular steroids	Photocoagulation of membrane	None	Periocular or oral corticosteroids; immunosuppression—cyclosporine
Outcome	Good without treatment, although retinal findings persist	Can be chronic	Can be recurrent, with new lesions extending from the old ones; scars leave scotomas and field loss	Fair outcome	Good; leaves scars that look like histoplasmosis	Good; recovers in 3–10 wks	Chronic condition; late looks like "blonde fundus"
Complications	Usually none	Vascular complications possible; glaucoma	Vision loss, neovascular membranes	Vision loss; membranes	Good unless sub-retinal neovascularization occurs	Rare recurrence; rare membranes	Vision loss due to cystoid macular edema; optic disc edema and epiretinal membrane

>> = much greater than; CBC = complete blood cell count; CXR = chest x-ray; RPE = retinal pigment epithelium.
Source: Adapted in part from references 18–20; with greatest contribution from 18.

Vogt-Koyanagi-Harada syndrome[31] consists of (1) a uveitis affecting the choroid, iris, or ciliary body; (2) systemic findings of alopecia, vitiligo, and poliosis (whitening of the lashes and hair); (3) central nervous system findings of headache and hearing loss; and (4) cerebrospinal fluid showing pleocytosis with occasionally increased intracranial pressure. The etiology is unknown, but may be an immune reaction against melanocytes. Dr. J. Lawton Smith's acronym PUVAD (*p*oliosis, *u*veitis, *v*itiligo, *a*lopeica, and *d*ysacousis) has been used to remember the major features of this syndrome (see also Table 5-17).

6-24A

Figure 6-24. A. **Here you see the typical serous retinal detachment changes associated with the choroidopathy of Vogt-Koyanagi-Harada syndrome. The arrows outline where the detachment is.** B. **The posterior pole shows a mottled appearance with loss of pigmentation characteristic of Vogt-Koyanagi-Harada syndrome. Although the fundus changes here are fairly mild, there can be dramatic fibrosis in severe cases.[16]** C. **The optic disc may be swollen as well. The disc shown here is a swollen disc with retinal striae. (Photographs courtesy of Paul Zimmerman, M.D.)**

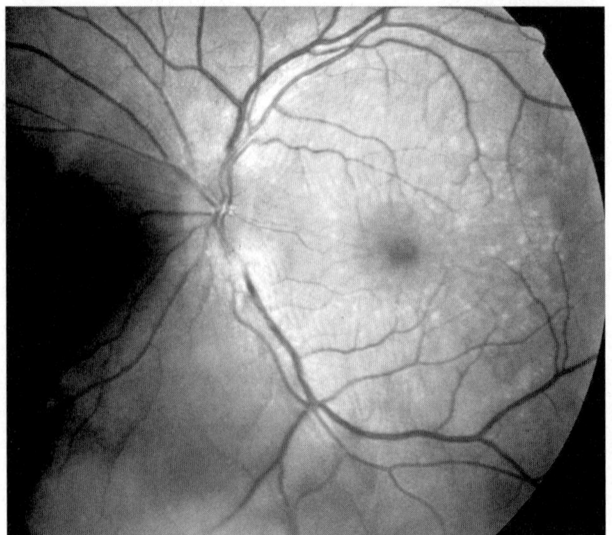

6-24B

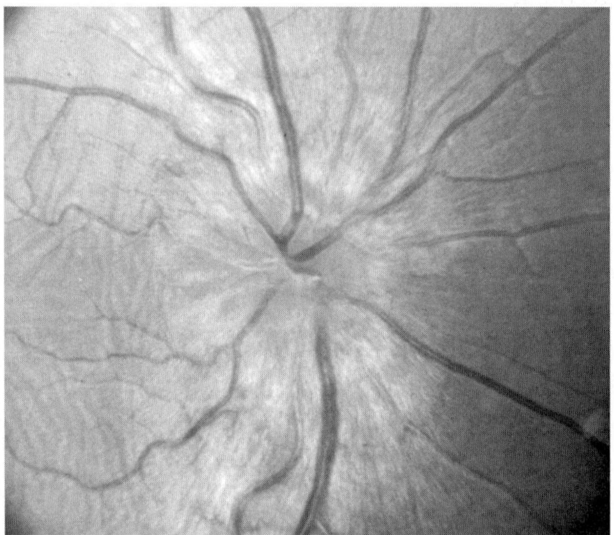

6-24C

Figure 6-25. A,B. ***Serpiginous choroidopathy*** **(also known as *geographic choroidopathy*)[20] usually affects the choroid, the choriocapillaris, and the RPE in both eyes. The process begins around the disc, and new lesions that are usually white or yellow in appearance are seen near an old lesion. There is usually a rapid progression, and in a few weeks pigment and punched-out areas are present. The name comes from the serpentine course of the edge of the lesions. In** (A) **and** (B) **you can appreciate the peri-disc lesions extending in a characteristic "centripetal" pattern. In** (A) **you see old lesions more distally and newer lesions extending from the disc, whereas in** (B) **you see acute lesions around the disc. The condition can be chronic. Visual acuity may decrease in an acute attack, but usually returns to the previous level. Treatment has been variable with immunosuppression.[16] (Photographs courtesy of Paul Zimmerman, M.D.)**

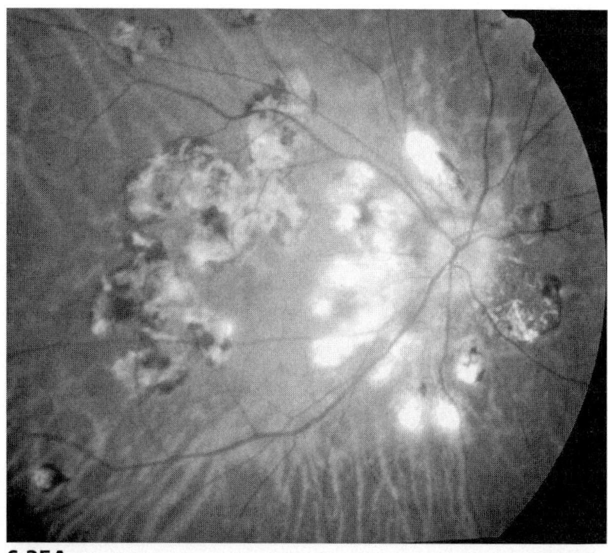

6-25A

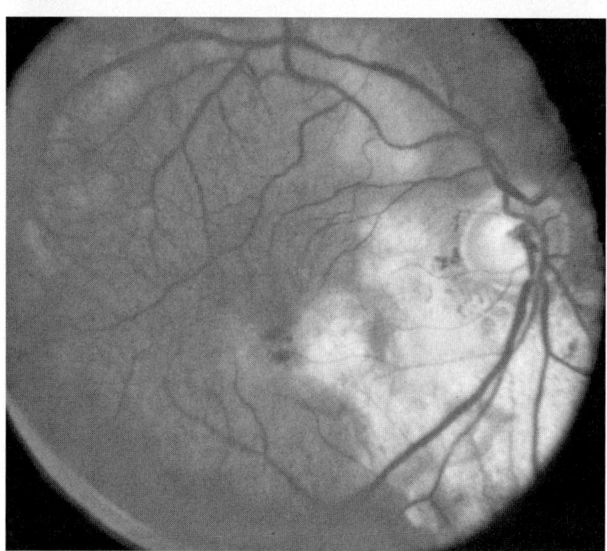

6-25B

Multifocal choroiditis[24,33,34] is usually a bilateral choroidopathy seen more frequently in women associated with punched-out–appearing lesions and, occasionally, with pigment around the edges. It can appear similar to ocular histoplasmosis. Mild disc swelling may be present. Pathologically, there is no granulomatous inflammation, but only B-cell lymphocytes.[24] The etiology is unknown but thought to be related to the Epstein-Barr virus. Treatment is usually steroids, and vision is usually good.

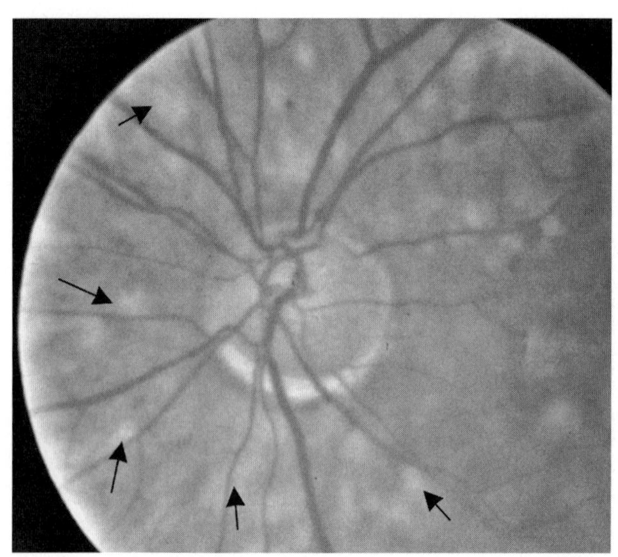
6-26

Figure 6-26. In this photograph you see distinct creamy-colored lesions (*arrows*) within the choroid appearing prominently in the posterior pole. Sometimes multifocal choroiditis is lumped with other white dot syndromes.[16] (Photograph courtesy of Paul Zimmerman, M.D.)

Multiple evanescent white dot syndrome (MEWDS) was described by Jampol et al. in women with "white dots" at the level of the RPE.[35] Fletcher et al. in 1988 then described (acute) idiopathic blind spot enlargement (AIBSE) to indicate a condition in patients with positive photopsias, enlarged blind spot on visual fields, little disc swelling, and no obvious choroiditis or white dots.[36] MEWDS and AIBSE have often been lumped together as *big blind spot syndrome*, which has been used to describe several conditions that cause enlargement of the blind spot with or without disc swelling. Some have even lumped MEWDS and AIBSE with acute macular neuroretinopathy and pseudo–presumed ocular histoplasmosis syndrome together into *acute zonal occult outer retinopathy* (AZOOR) because these conditions present with vision loss and many ocular symptoms such as spots, dots, and colors. Also, all of these conditions are typically seen in young women. There is often acute blind spot enlargement, which may be symptomatic. There are electroretinogram (ERG) findings, and visual acuity is usually good. The conditions go away without treatment.[37,38] Jampol et al. and Volpe et al. maintain that AIBSE is distinct from the others in that the visual field findings did not resolve, there was disc swelling and often permanent peripapillary pigmentary changes around the optic nerve, and, finally, the focal ERG was invariably positive.[39,40]

In MEWDS, the lesions are usually seen unilaterally, deep in the retina or RPE, and especially around the fovea and posterior pole. If you suspect this syndrome, be sure to look around the macula, in which granular pigmentary changes have been reported. The disc may also be swollen. The visual field shows an enlarged blind spot. The ERG shows an abnormal A wave, and multifocal ERG also shows abnormalities. The fluorescein angiogram shows early hyperfluorescence and late staining of the lesions and the disc. There is no treatment, and spontaneous resolution is common.[16]

Figure 6-27. A. **The fundus of a woman with multiple evanescent white dot syndrome. There are small, creamy-colored lesions deep in the choroid scattered around the disc and macula.** B. **The fluorescein angiogram shows that the disc stains late. (Photographs courtesy of Paul Zimmerman, M.D.)** C. **Another multiple evanescent white dot syndrome in which the choroidal lesions are more prominent (*arrow*).**

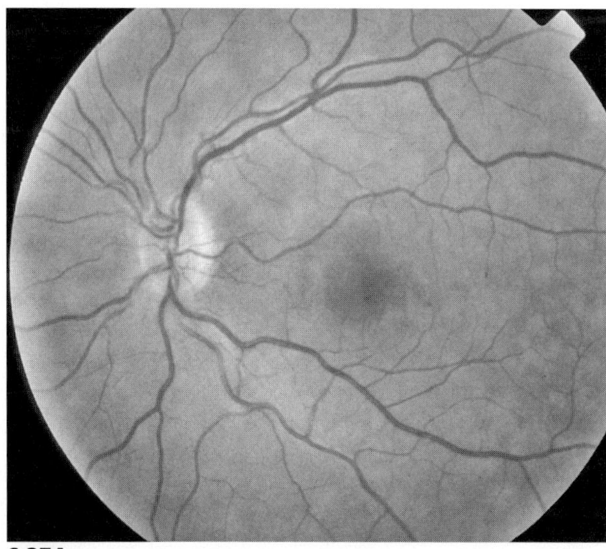

6-27A

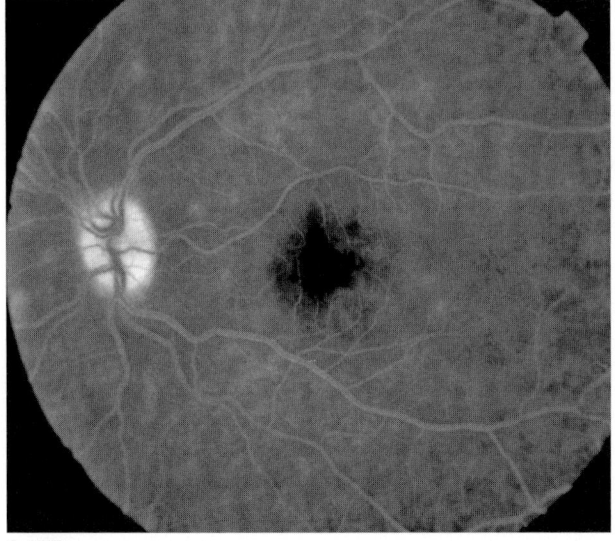

6-27B

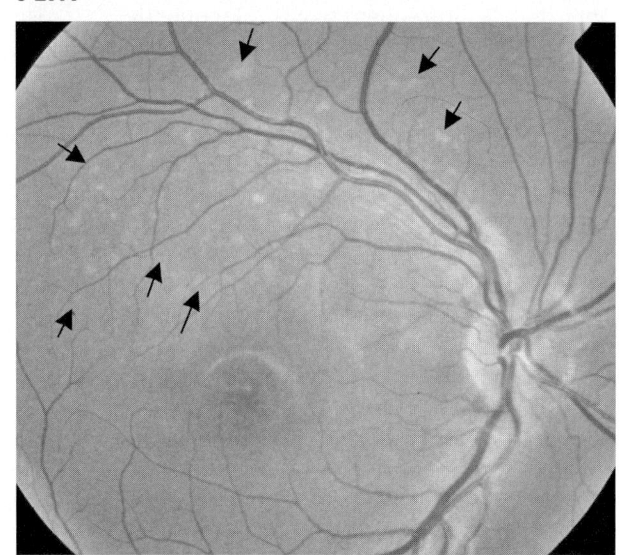

6-27C

Table 6-6. Sorting Out Big Blind Spot Syndromes[40,41]

	Acute idiopathic blind spot enlargement	**Multiple evanescent white dot syndrome (MEWDS)**	**Acute zonal occult outer retinopathy (AZOOR)[38]**	**Acute macular neuroretinopathy[42]**	**Multifocal choroiditis[41]**
Patients	F	M = F	F > M	F > M	F > M
Symptoms	Photopsias; unilateral	Flulike illness before symptoms; photopsias	Flulike illness often before symptoms; second eye; chronic photopsias	Positive scotomas	Blurred vision; photopsias; floaters
Visual fields	Enlarged blind spot	Enlarged blind spot	Progressive visual field loss	Normal except enlarged blind spot	Enlarged blind spot; central/paracentral scotomas
Optic disc	Infrequent swelling followed by peripapillary pigmentary changes	Frequently swelling is present	Normal	Normal	Occasionally mild swelling
Retina	May see white dots	White dots around the disc and macula	Late retinal pigment epithelium atrophy	Normal	Small pigmentary changes in the choroid
Macula	Normal	Macular pigmentary granularity	Normal	Reddish-brown, wedge-shaped lesion	Normal
Electroretinogram	Focal electroretinogram shows abnormality in peripapillary area	Abnormal	Abnormal; moderate reduction in rod and cone amplitude	Normal full fields	Normal in mild cases; moderate to severe showed poor oscillatory potentials
Fluorescein/Indocyanine green	Disc staining; peripapillary hyper-fluorescence	Peripapillary hyperfluorescence; disc staining	Increased circulation time in areas affected; narrowing of retinal vessels in active areas; CME	Normal	One-third of cases have disc staining; CME; leakage of lesions; choroidal neovascular membrane may form
Outcome	Permanent enlargement of the blind spot	Usually full recovery	Permanent visual field defects can occur	Not always complete recovery	Recurrent inflammation possible; 55% better than 20/40

Source: Adapted from references 40–42.

Birdshot retinochoroidopathy is a chronic, posterior uveitis seen in women 30–60 years of age who present with increased floaters, changes in color vision, and difficulty with night vision. It is called *birdshot* after the appearance of the skin of a duck shot with pellets from a shotgun.[20] They are small, equal in size, and diffusely distributed. Criteria for the diagnosis are minimal anterior uveitis or inflammation; vitreitis; retinal vascular leakage that can be seen with macular edema or optic disc swelling; discrete, cream-colored, or depigmented spots; and no pain.[27] Examination shows little anterior inflammation, but cells in the vitreous, cream-colored spots throughout the fundus, macular edema, and, occasionally, disc edema are present in both eyes. As the disease progresses, the fundus becomes progressively and strikingly more like a "blonde" fundus, with little pigmentation. Visual fields show enlargement of the blind spot, paracentral scotomas, and visual field constriction. In a few cases, the visual fields can be normal. The ERG shows reduction of the B wave, and the electro-oculogram is also abnormal. Vision remains good unless there is significant cystoid macular edema. Treatment with steroids has sometimes been recommended.

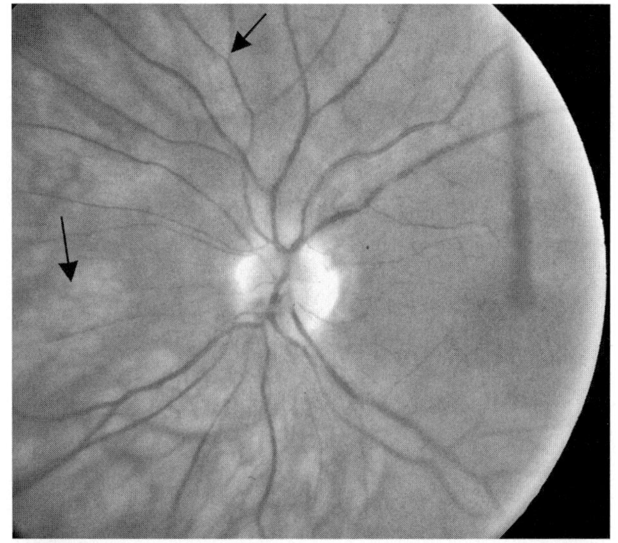

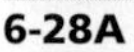

6-28A

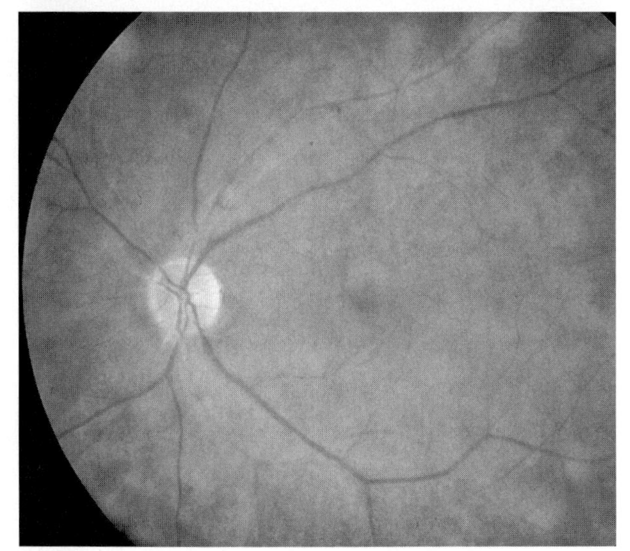

6-28B

Figure 6-28. A. **Long-standing birdshot retinopathy in a woman with slight disc swelling. You can see the depigmentation in the retina and choroid, especially nasal to the disc (*arrows*).** B. **Typical depigmentation of birdshot retinopathy; the vasculature is somewhat attenuated. (Photograph courtesy of Paul Zimmerman, M.D.)**

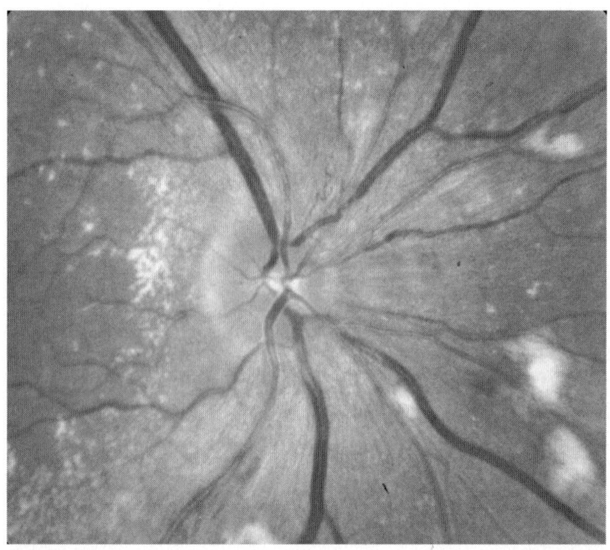

6-29

Practical Viewing Essentials

1. Determine the region in which the white spot is occurring—is it at the disc, on the retina, or in the choroid?
2. Try to determine in what layer of the retina or choroid the white spot resides.
3. If there is a single cotton-wool spot and diabetes or hypertension is not present, an extensive systemic evaluation is warranted.
4. When you see perivascular white spots, sarcoid should be in the differential diagnosis.
5. White spots in the choroid have a number of causes, and, if symptomatic, they need to be evaluated by an ophthalmologist.

References

1. Gowers W. A Manual and Atlas of Medical Ophthalmoscopy. London: J & A Churchill, 1879.
2. Ballantyne AJ, Michaelson IC. Textbook of the fundus of the eye. Baltimore: Williams & Wilkins, 1970.
3. Vrabec TR, Augsburger JJ, Fischer DH, et al. Taches de bougie. Ophthalmology 1995;102(11):1712–1721.
4. Wolter JR. Pathology of a cotton-wool spot. Am J Ophthalmol 1959;473–485.
5. Brown G. Retinal arterial obstructive disease. In AP Schachat, RB Murphy (eds), Retina. St. Louis: Mosby, 1994;1361–1377.
6. Chester EM. The Ocular Fundus in Systemic Disease. Chicago: Year Book, 1973.
7. Melberg NS, Grand MG, Dieckert JP, et al. Cotton-wool spots and the early diagnosis of giant cell arteritis. Ophthalmology 1995;102:1611–1614.
8. Shami MJ, Uy RN. Isolated cotton-wool spots in a 67-year-old woman. Surv Ophthalmol 1996;40:413–415.
9. Early Treatment Diabetic Retinopathy Study Research Group. Grading diabetic retinopathy from stereoscopic color fundus photographs—an extension of the modified Airlie House classification. ETDRS report number 10. Ophthalmology 1991;98(5 Suppl): 786–806.
10. Sarks SH, Sarks JP. Age-related macular degeneration: atrophic form. In AP Schachat, RB Murphy (eds), Retina. St. Louis: Mosby, 1994;1071–1102.
11. Honavar SG, Shields CL, Demirici H, Shields JA. Sclerochoroidal calcification. Arch Ophthalmol 2001; 119:833–840.
12. Ganatra IB, Chadler D, Santos C, et al. Viral causes of acute retinal necrosis syndrome. Am J Ophthalmol 2000;129:166–172.
13. Pepose J. Acute retinal necrosis syndrome. In AP Schachat, RB Murphy (eds), Retina. St. Louis: Mosby, 1994;1597–1605.
14. Holland GN. Endogenous fungal infections of the retina and choroid. In AP Schachat, SJ Ryan (eds), Retina. St. Louis: Mosby, 2001;1632–1646.
15. Dugel PU, Smith RE. Pars planitis. In AP Schachat, SJ Ryan (eds), Retina. St. Louis: Mosby, 2001;1647–1657.
16. Nussenblatt RB, Palestine AG. Uveitis Fundamentals and Clinical Practice. Chicago: Year Book, 1989;379–387.
17. Hawkins BS, Alexander J, Schachat AP. Ocular histoplasmosis. In AP Schachat, RB Murphy (eds), Retina. St. Louis: Mosby, 1994;1661–1675.
18. Folk J, Pulido J, Wolf MD. White dot chorioretinal inflammatory syndromes. In NT Shults (ed), Focal Points (vol. 7, mod. 7). San Francisco, American Academy of Ophthalmology, 1990.
19. Polk TD, Goldman EJ. White-dot chorioretinal inflammatory syndromes. Int Ophthalmol Clin 1999;39:33–53.
20. Jones NP. Uveitis. An illustrated manual. Oxford: Butterworth–Heinemann, 1998;322–341.
21. Bird AC. Acute multifocal placoid pigment epitheliopathy. In AP Schachat, RB Murphy (eds), Retina. St. Louis: Mosby, 1994;1713–1720.
22. Park D, Schatz H, McDonald R, Johnson RN. Indocyanine green angiography of acute multifocal posterior placoid pigment epitheliopathy. Ophthalmology 1995; 102:1877–1883.
23. Reddy CV, Folk JC. Multifocal choroiditis with panuveitis, diffuse subretinal fibrosis, and punctate inner choroidopathy. In AP Schachat, RB Murphy (eds), Retina. St. Louis: Mosby, 1994;1687–1698.
24. Dunlop AA, Cree IA, Hague S, et al. Multifocal choroiditis: clinicopathologic correlation. Arch Ophthalmol 1998;116(6):801–803.
25. Jampol LM, Tsai L. Multiple evanescent white dot syndrome. In AP Schachat, RB Murphy (eds), Retina. St. Louis: Mosby, 1994;1699–1703.
26. Ryan SJ, Dugel PU, Sout JT. Birdshot retinochoroidopathy. In AP Schachat, RB Murphy (eds), Retina. St. Louis: Mosby, 1994;1677–1685.
27. Gasch AT, Smith JA, Whitcup SM. Birdshot retinochoroidopathy. Br J Ophthalmol 1999;83:241–249.
28. Cunningham ET Jr, Schatz H, McDonald HR, Johnson RN. Acute multifocal retinitis. Am J Ophthalmol 1997;123(3):347–357.
29. Park D, Schatz H, McDonald HR, Johnson RN. Acute multifocal posterior placoid pigment epitheliopathy: a theory of pathogenesis. Retina 1995;15(4):351–352.
30. Park D, Schatz H, McDonald HR, Johnson RN. Indocyanine green angiography of acute multifocal posterior placoid pigment epitheliopathy. Ophthalmology 1995;102(12):1877–1883.
31. Moorthy RS, Inomata H, Rao NA. Vogt-Koyanagi-Harada syndrome. Surv Ophthalmol 1995;39(4): 265–292.

32. Ciulla TA, Gragoudas ES. Serpiginous choroiditis. Int Ophthalmol Clin 1996;36(1):135–143.
33. Brown J Jr, Folk JC. Current controversies in the white dot syndromes. Multifocal choroiditis, punctate inner choroidopathy, and the diffuse subretinal fibrosis syndrome. Ocul Immunol Inflamm 1998;6(2): 125–127.
34. Hershey JM, Pulido JS, Folberg R, et al. Non-caseating conjunctival granulomas in patients with multifocal choroiditis and panuveitis. Ophthalmology 1994;101(3):596–601.
35. Jampol LM, Sieving PA, Pugh D, et al. Multiple evanescent white dot syndrome, part I: clinical findings. Arch Ophthalmol 1984;102:671–674.
36. Fletcher WA, Imes RK, Goodman D, Hoyt WF. Acute idiopathic blindspot enlargement: a big blind spot syndrome without optic disc edema. Arch Ophthalmol 1988;106:44–49.
37. Callanan D, Gass JD. Multifocal choroiditis and choroidal neovascularization associated with the multiple evanescent white dot and acute idiopathic blind spot enlargement syndrome. Ophthalmology 1999; 99:1678–1685.
38. Gass JD. Acute zonal occult outer retinopathy. J Clin Neuroophthalmol 1993;13:79–97.
39. Jampol LM, Wiredu A. MEWDS, MFC, PIC, AMN, AIBSE, and AZOOR: one disease or many? Retina 1995;15:373–378.
40. Volpe NJ, Rizzo JF, Lessell S. Acute idiopathic blind spot enlargement syndrome. Arch Ophthalmol 2001; 119:59–63.
41. Reddy CV, Brown J Jr, Folk JC, et al. Enlarged blind spots in chorioretinal inflammatory disorders. Ophthalmology 1996;103(4):606–617.
42. Rush JA. Acute macular neuroretinopathy. Am J Ophthalmol 1977;83:490–494.

7 Hemorrhage

Rupture of retinal vessels and consequent extravasation of blood are very common in morbid states and are frequently of important general significance. . . .

[Hemorrhages'] shape and aspect depend very much on their position in the substance of the retina. The commonest seat is in the layer of nerve fibers . . . hence the smaller haemorrhages are linear and the larger striated in part or altogether, and they often radiate from the disc. . . . The next most frequent seat is the inner nuclear layer. Here there is no tendency to striation; the extravasations are round or irregular.

William Gowers[1]

Is It a Hemorrhage?

Hemorrhage in the eye is another sign that something serious may be wrong. Look for hemorrhages with the green (red-free) filter. This helps to bring them into relief against the background red retina. The first thing to decide, however, is this: Is it really a hemorrhage, or could it be a normal structure? What can mimic a hemorrhage?

Normal structures that are red are blood vessels (blood columns within vessels). Vessels should be fairly easy to recognize. Vascular loops in and around the disc may look like hemorrhages, however.

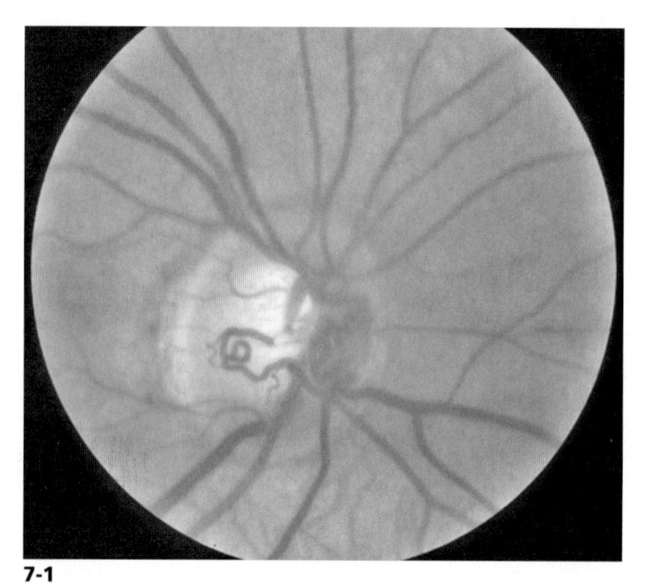

7-1

Figure 7-1. This preretinal loop off of the optic disc could look like a hemorrhage. The shape and appearance are the tip-off.

Widening of retinal veins may also mimic a hemorrhage at the disc.

Figure 7-2. A. **This widened vessel looks like a superior disc hemorrhage (*arrow*).** B. **Widened retinal vein along the inferior disc margin could be mistaken for a hemorrhage.**

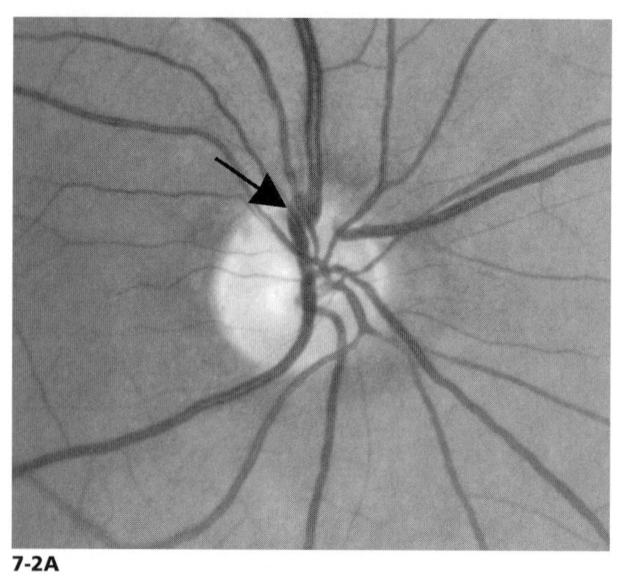

7-2A

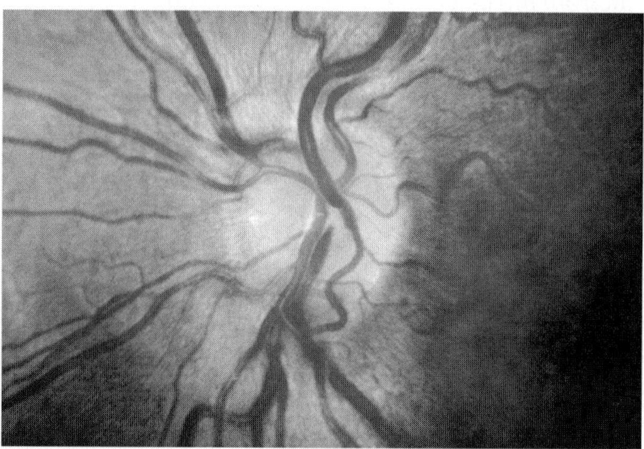

7-2B

Pathologic changes in the retina may also look like a hemorrhage. For example, a choroidal melanoma deep under the retina may mimic a choroidal hemorrhage.[2]

Microaneurysms, common in diabetes, also may need to be differentiated from small round hemorrhages, or small red dots. Commonly, microaneurysms are more apparent between the disc and the macula. Sometimes a microaneurysm dot is easy to mistake for a dot hemorrhage. One way to determine the difference between a microaneurysm and a dot hemorrhage is to do a fluorescein angiogram. Fluorescein stains the aneurysm and makes it look like a bright white dot. A small hemorrhage blocks any background fluorescence if large enough, or appears black on a red-free pre-fluorescein angiogram.

Table 7-1. Distinguishing Hemorrhages from Microaneurysms

Characteristic	Hemorrhage (see Figure 7-3A, *arrows*)	Microaneurysm (see Figure 7-3C, *arrows*)
	Fluorescein of hemorrhage (see Figure 7-3B, *arrows*)	Fluorescein of microaneurysm (see Figure 7-3D, *arrows*)
Size	Variable size, small–large	Usually very small
Border	Less distinct	More distinct
Location	Around disc; throughout retina	Between disc and macula; central retina
Associated lesions	Often seen with cotton-wool spots	No associated lesions
Associated conditions	Hypertension, diabetes, blood disorders	Diabetes, retinal vein occlusion, neovascularization, hypertension
Fluorescein angiogram	Does not fluoresce (Figure 7-3B, *arrows*); in fact, blocks fluorescence; not attached to blood vessel	Associated with blood vessel; bright fluorescence (Figure 7-3D, *arrows*); fluorescein shows many more microaneurysms than are seen on the photograph (*arrowheads*)
Natural history	Disappears within weeks; no trace left	Persists for months; may develop a white halo or become a white dot

Source: Adapted from reference 3.

Figure 7-3. A. **Photograph of dot hemorrhages (*arrows*).** B. **Fluorescein angiogram shows blockage of fluorescein by the hemorrhage.** C. **Photograph of microaneurysm looking like a dot hemorrhage (*arrows*).** D. **Fluorescein staining of a microaneurysm (*arrows*). More aneurysms are present (*arrowheads*) than seen on fundus photograph.**

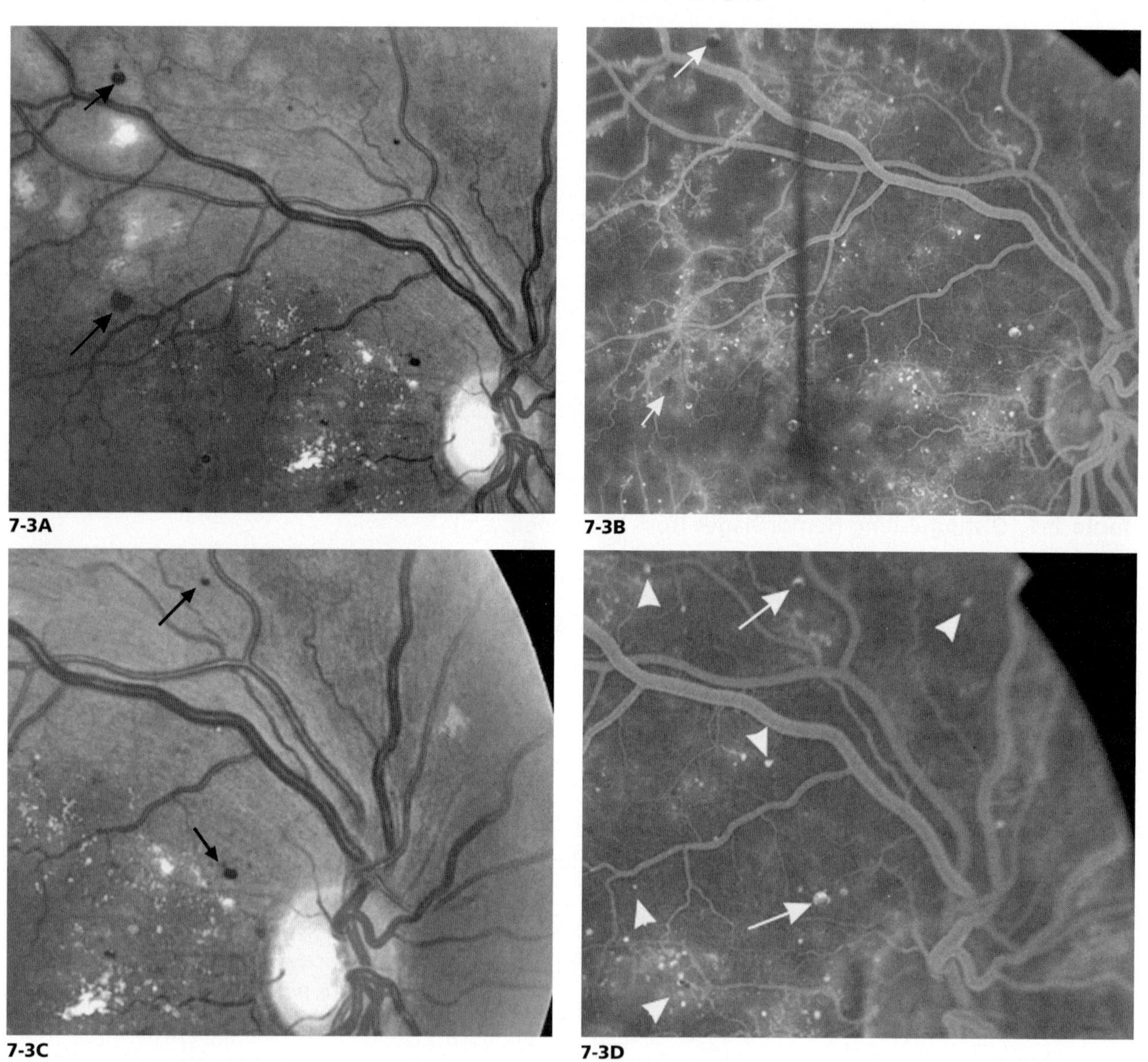

What Causes Hemorrhages to Occur?

Hemorrhages occur in poor perfusional states in which there is retinal hypoxia. The bleeding can occur owing to arterial, capillary, or venous disease (e.g., retinal vein occlusion).

Hemorrhages are commonly associated with systemic diseases (e.g., hypertension, diabetes mellitus, general arteriosclerosis, renal disease), trauma, hematologic disorders (e.g., hypercoagulable state, anemia, thrombocytopenia), infections and sepsis, autoimmune conditions (e.g., systemic lupus erythematosus and idiopathic thrombocytopenic purpura),[4] and in cases with increased intracranial pressure.

Hemorrhages occur most frequently in the eyes of patients with hypertension and diabetes. Why would this occur? First, the blood vessels can undergo sclerotic changes and fibrinoid necrosis, which may cause breaks in vessel walls and allow the egress of red blood cells. Furthermore, if there is neovascularization, the new vessels are more likely to hemorrhage. Increased blood pressure transmitted to pathologic vessels may contribute. Finally, intracranial hypertension can produce intraocular hemorrhages by impeding venous return and increasing capillary pressure.

Table 7-2. Causes of Peripapillary Hemorrhage

Types of conditions	Cause	Notes
Most common types	Diabetes, hypertension	
	Ischemic ocular syndrome	
	Trauma	
	Choroidal/retinal tumor	
Subretinal neovascularization	Idiopathic	
	Optic nerve drusen, angioid streaks	Causes of angioid streaks: pseudoxanthoma elasticum, Paget's disease, sickle cell hemoglobinopathies, thalassemia, Ehlers-Danlos syndrome, acanthocytosis (abetalipoproteinemia; Bassen-Kornzweig syndrome), congenital idiopathic hyperphosphatemia (juvenile Paget's disease), hereditary spherocytosis, calcinosis, acromegaly
	Peripapillary choroiditis	Caused by histoplasmosis, toxoplasmosis, toxocariasis, syphilis
	Sarcoid	
	Senile macular degeneration	
	Serpiginous choroiditis	
Vascular abnormalities within the eye	Hemangiomas	
	Wyburn-Mason	
	Sturge-Weber	
	von Hippel-Lindau	
Elevated intracranial pressure/ elevated perineural pressure	Idiopathic intracranial hypertension; Valsalva maneuver; subarachnoid hemorrhage; brain tumor	
Myopia	Unclear	
Ischemic optic neuropathy	Unclear	
Carcinomatous meningitis	Malignancy elsewhere in the body	
Other systemic conditions	Anemia, thrombocytopenia, hypertension, immune disorders like systemic lupus erythematosus, idiopathic thrombocytopenic purpura, vasculitis	

Source: Adapted in part from reference 5.

It Appears to Be a Hemorrhage

Whenever you see "red," four questions come to mind:

1. Is it really a hemorrhage?
2. If it is a hemorrhage, where, in which retinal layer, is it located?
3. What disease process may have produced the hemorrhage?
4. What do I need to do about it?

Locating the depth of the hemorrhage in the eye can be difficult unless you know the layers and characteristics of hemorrhage in the various layers of the retina or vitreous. The architecture of the retina usually dictates the shape of the hemorrhage. The most common form of hemorrhage is the "splinter hemorrhage." *Splinter hemorrhages* are lines of beading radiating away from the disc between the nerve fiber layer. The second most common hemorrhage is in the deeper retina and appears as circular dots and "blots." Each layer has a characteristic appearance. In general, almost all hemorrhages are round, except for splinter hemorrhages in the nerve fiber layer and scaphoid preretinal hemorrhages.

Table 7-3. Hemorrhages in the Fundus of the Eye

Layer	Characteristics of the layer	Shape of hemorrhage	Other characteristics	Types of diseases causing the hemorrhage
Intravitreous				
Vitreous	No boundaries; breaks through the hyaloid membrane; may obscure all of the normal red reflex and retina	Acutely is within the vitreous gel; later, because of gravity, the blood settles inferiorly	Vision is usually affected	Proliferative retinopathy; trauma, surgery, angiomas of the retina, Eales' disease, retinal detachment
Preretinal or subhyaloid				
Space between vitreous and ILM	Potential space between the vitreous and ILM	Subhyaloid hemorrhage looks like a crescent, teardrop, or boat; scaphoid	Obscures retinal vessels	Diabetes, hypertension, bacterial endocarditis, subarachnoid hemorrhage; subdural hemorrhage and shaken baby syndrome; sickle cell
ILM	Space between the nerve fiber layer and the ILM appears like a subhyaloid hemorrhage; sometimes they can appear as concentric striae in papilledema around the disc*	Like subhyaloid hemorrhage—crescent or teardrop shape; scaphoid	Obscures retinal vessels	Diabetes, hypertension, subarachnoid hemorrhage, any sudden increase in intracranial pressure; trauma; neovascularization; shaken baby syndrome
Intraretinal (superficial)				
Nerve fiber layer	Hemorrhages are generally horizontal; more blotchy in the peripheral retina owing to fewer fibers	Linear; flame-shaped or splinter; the shape is dictated by the orientation of the nerve fibers	Location around the disc; hemorrhages overlie blood vessel, obscuring its view	Hypertension, diabetes, anemia, blood disorders like hemoglobinopathies
Ganglion cell layer	—	Round	—	—
Inner plexiform layer	—	Round	—	—

Deep retina				
Inner nuclear layer	—	Dot: cluster of red cells, may look like microaneurysm, round; blot type larger, more full-thickness	—	Venous occlusion and retinal ischemia
Blood vessels	Lie between inner nuclear and outer plexiform layer	—	Hemorrhages above this layer obscure vessels; below this level, appear behind vessels	—
Outer plexiform layer	Horizontal vertical fibers; when in the macula (Henle's layer) appear like a star	Round hemorrhages—usually less than one-third of disc diameter; dot and blot	Hemorrhages are "cylinders" viewed on end; often lie behind retinal blood vessels	Venous stasis, diabetes, carotid artery disease, hypercoagulable state
Outer nuclear layer	—	Round	—	—
External limiting membrane	—	Round	—	—
Rods and cones	—	Round	—	—
Subretinal				
Anterior to the RPE	Below the retina and above the RPE is a potential space	Blotch of red with elevation of the retina	Can be associated with neovascularization	Various retinopathy; Coats' disease, sickle cell disease, leukemia, retinopathy of prematurity
Below the RPE	Blood usually originates in the choroid in the space above the choroid, below the RPE	Elevated RPE; color very dark	—	—
Choroidal				
Choroid	Irregular dark red, purple, or black spot—deep; may look like a choroidal melanoma	Irregular; can be large	Does not obscure the retinal vessels; fluorescein angiography can distinguish between a choroidal melanoma and a hemorrhage	Head/orbital trauma; post-operative cataract

ILM = internal limiting membrane; RPE = retinal pigment epithelium.
*From AJ Ballantyne, IC Michaelson. Textbook of the Fundus of the Eye. Baltimore: Williams & Wilkins, 1970.
Source: Adapted from references 3,6.

On fluorescein angiography, hemorrhages block the background fluorescence and appear as black spots.

Figure 7-4. By knowing the architecture of the eye, you can tell the layer of the hemorrhage.

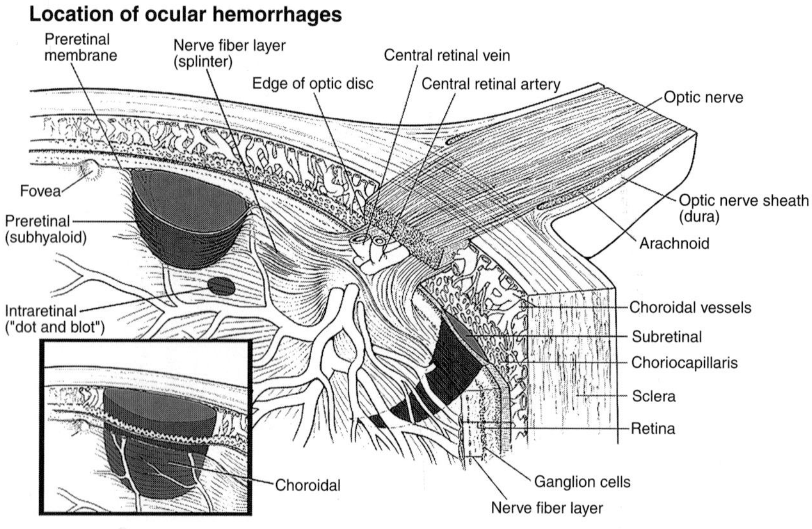

7-4

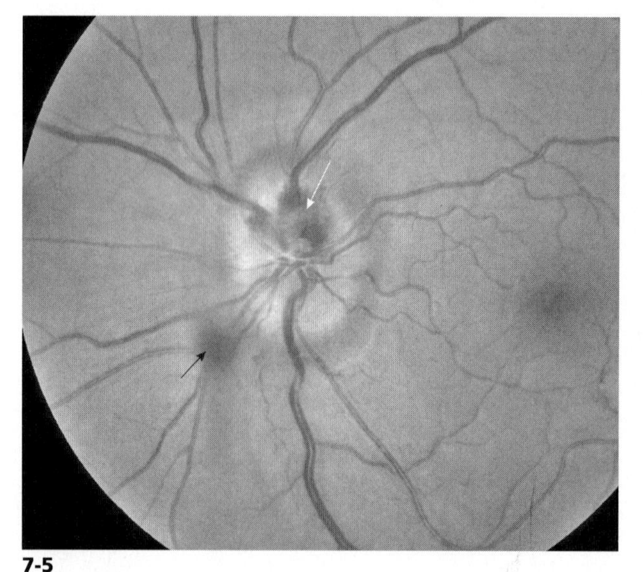

7-5

Figure 7-5. A vitreous hemorrhage obscures the disc and retina. You may need to focus within the vitreous with a +10 lens to see this hemorrhage. Here, the vitreous face has come off of the optic disc (the *white arrow* points to that hemorrhage), which also has optic disc drusen. The vitreous hemorrhage is the indistinct blob (*black arrow*) that obscures the vascular detail at approximately 8 o'clock. The postulated mechanism for the vitreous hemorrhage in this case is a vitreous detachment from the optic disc.[7]

Figure 7-6. A. **Diagram of preretinal subhyaloid hemorrhage. This represents a hemorrhage beneath the preretinal membrane and above the nerve fiber layer.** ***Continued***

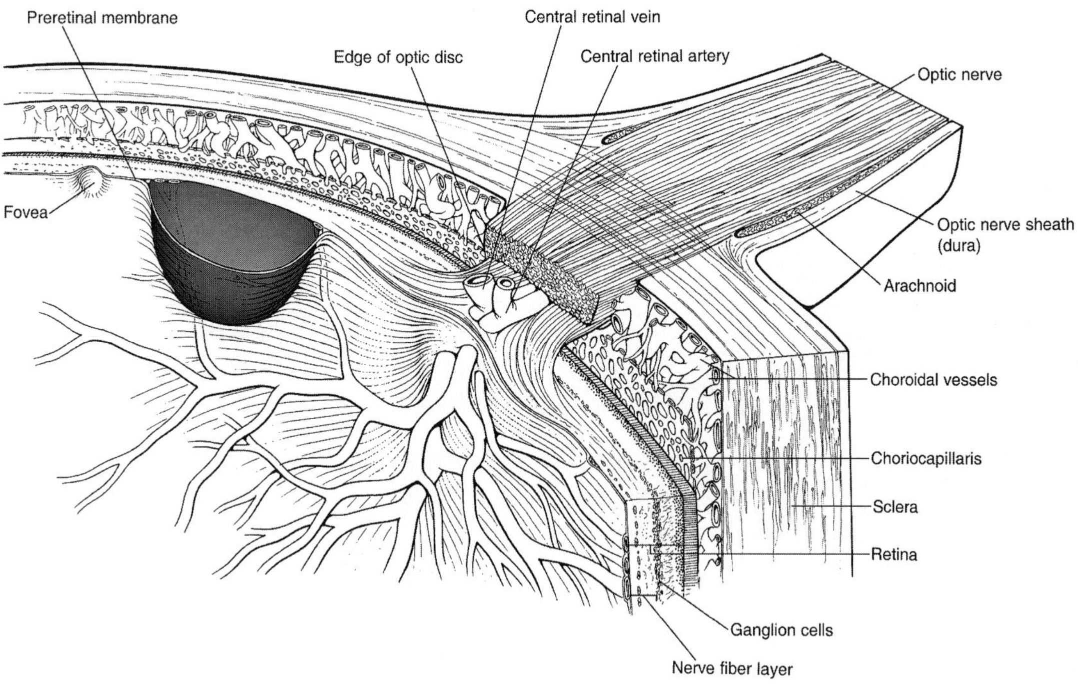

7-6A

Figure 7-6. *Continued.* The women in the following figures have increased intracranial pressure. B. This woman had optic disc drusen and developed a large subhyaloid hemorrhage in the right eye when she struck her head falling off of her horse. She had increased intracranial pressure owing to the closed head injury. C. Two weeks later, you can see the clot organizing and the blood layering out (*arrows*). (Photograph courtesy of H. Stanley Thompson.) D. This woman had idiopathic intracranial hypertension. Seen below the disc is a boat-shaped subhyaloid hemorrhage, as well as numerous nerve fiber layer hemorrhages, linear-shaped and radiating around the optic disc.

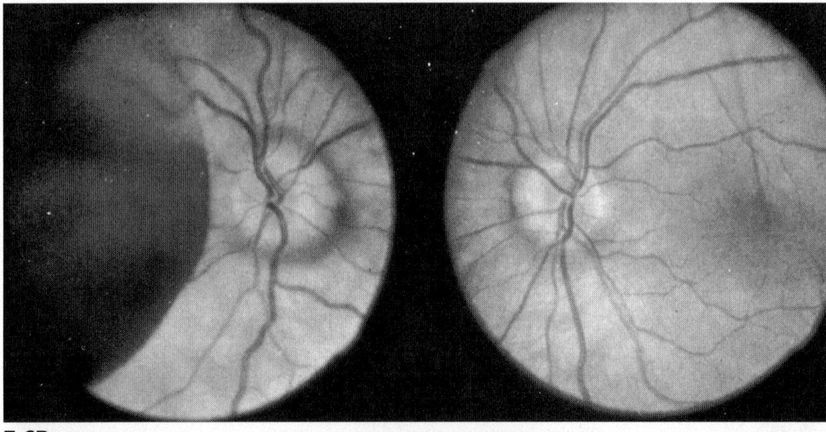

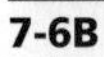

7-6B

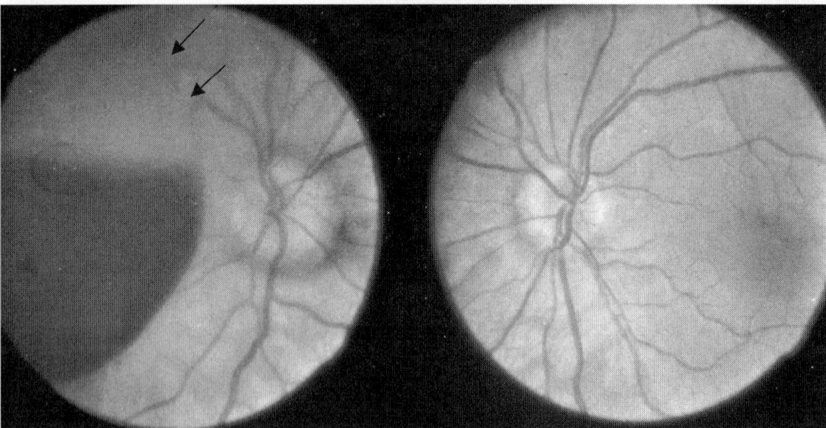

7-6C

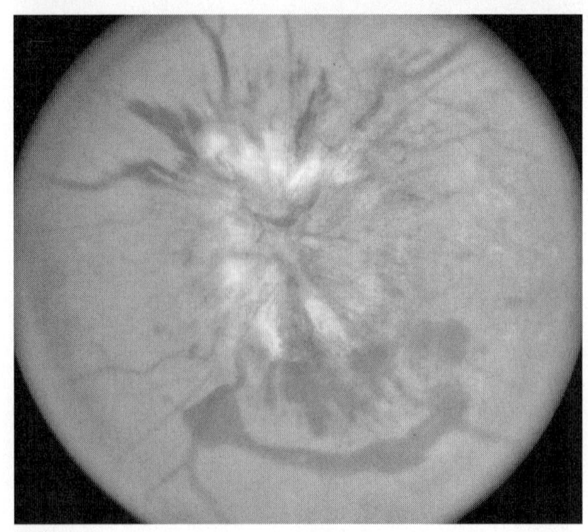

7-6D

Figure 7-7. A. Diagram of nerve fiber layer hemorrhage. B. Nerve fiber layer hemorrhages are common and usually easy to recognize. They follow the nerve fiber layer, are linear, and look like "splinters," hence the term *splinter hemorrhages*. The usual location is around the disc. This patient has extensive nerve fiber layer hemorrhages in association with idiopathic intracranial hypertension. Notice how the hemorrhage patterns itself after the nerve fiber layer. C. There are small splinter hemorrhages at the disc margin (*arrows*).

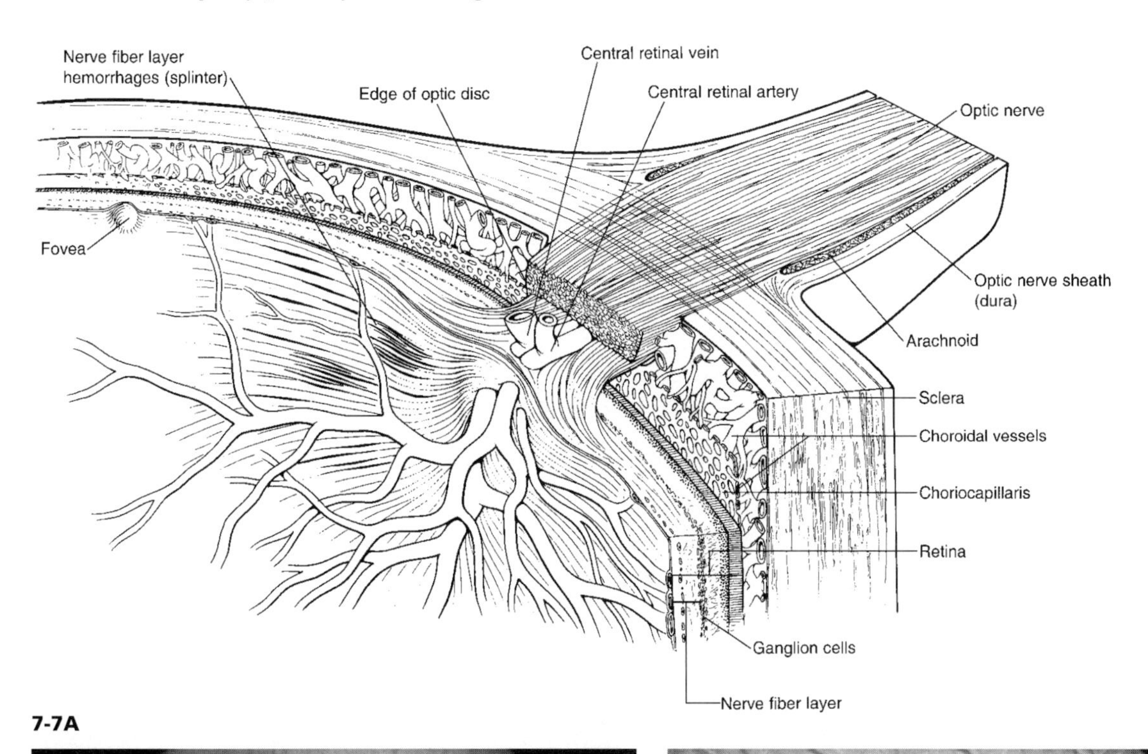

7-7A

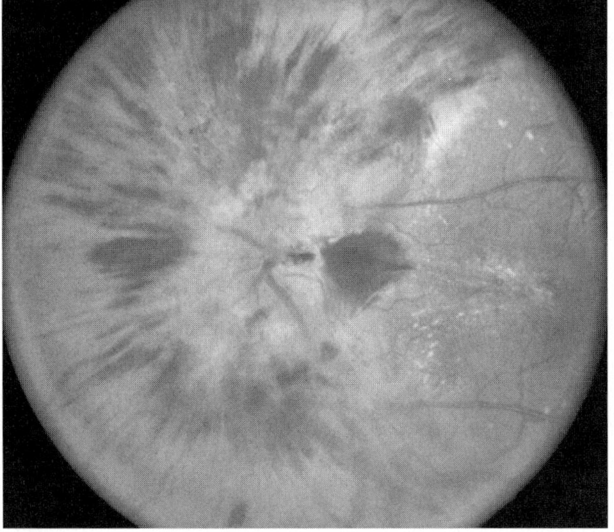

7-7B

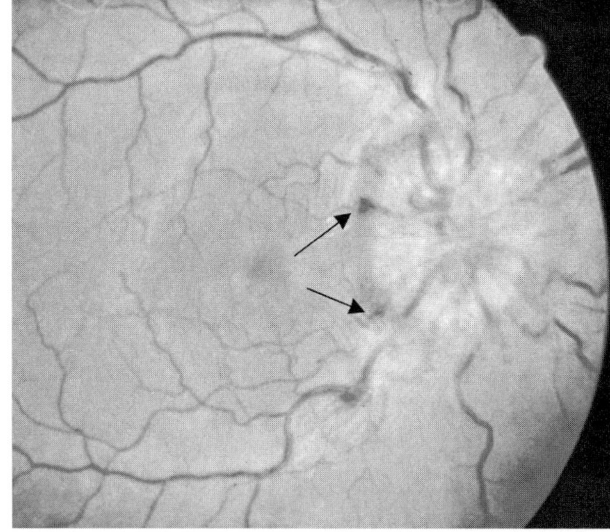

7-7C

Figure 7-8. A. **Diagram of intraretinal hemorrhage. Dot-and-blot hemorrhages are found beneath the nerve fiber layer in the retina.** B. **Intraretinal hemorrhages are most frequently found in the mid-peripheral retina.**

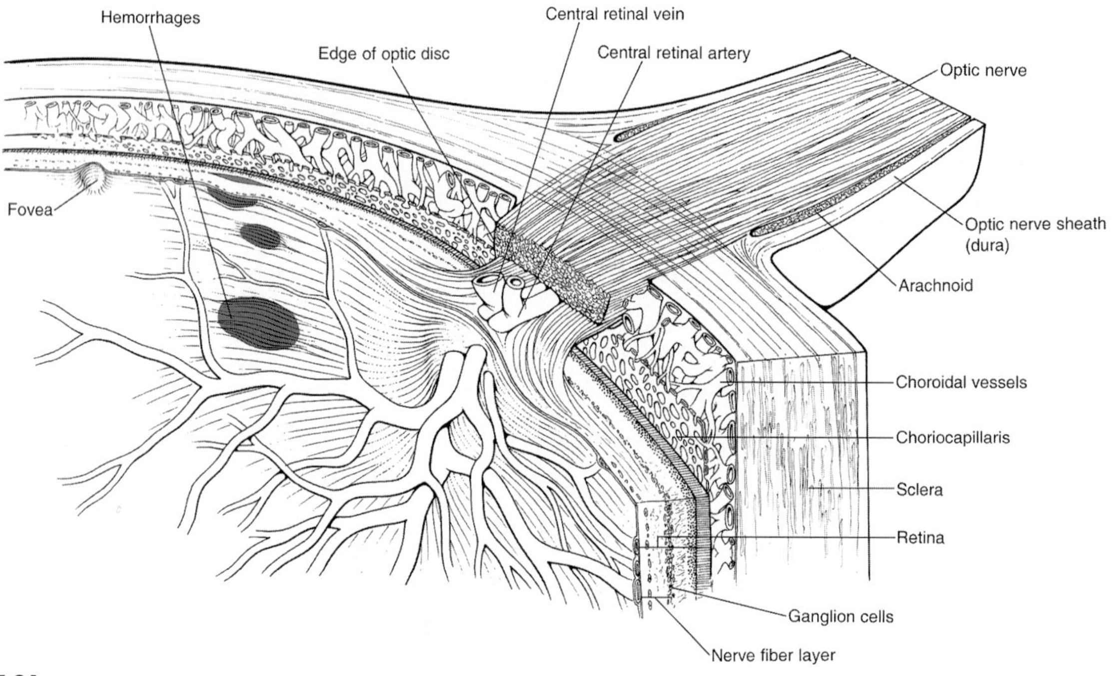

7-8A

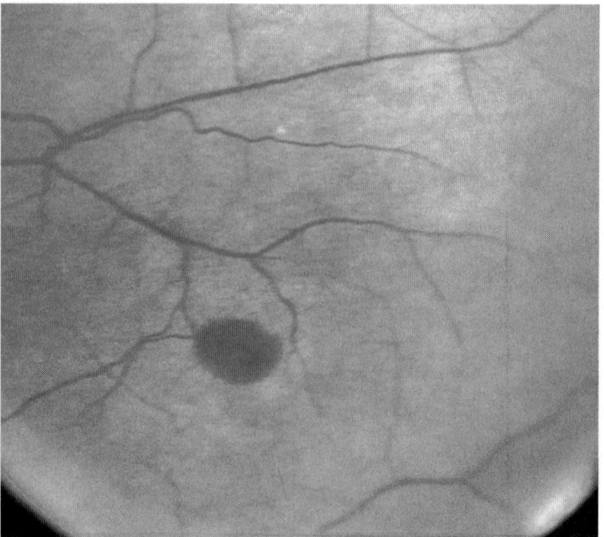

7-8B

Figure 7-9. A. This woman has a low-flow, dural-cavernous fistula presenting with a red eye and retinal venous hypertension. B. Notice that most of the hemorrhages are dot and blot (*arrows*) below the blood vessels; some are nerve fiber layer (*arrowhead*), and the veins are slightly dilated and tortuous.

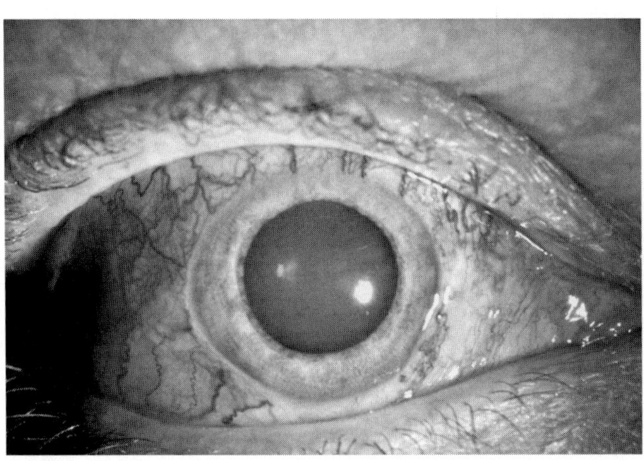

7-9A

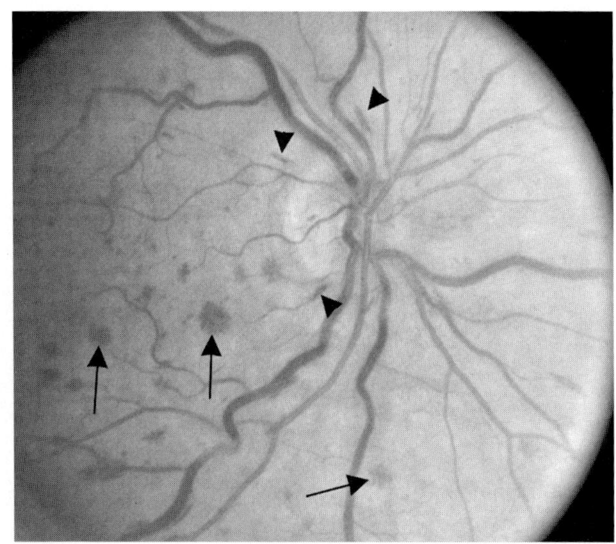

7-9B

Figure 7-10. A. **Notice that in a subretinal hemorrhage the blood is below the retina.** B. **This patient also has optic disc drusen. The subretinal hemorrhage (*arrow*) is deep to the blood vessels and has a typical dark color around the disc.** C. **Here is an anomalous disc with another subretinal hemorrhage around the disc (*arrow*).**

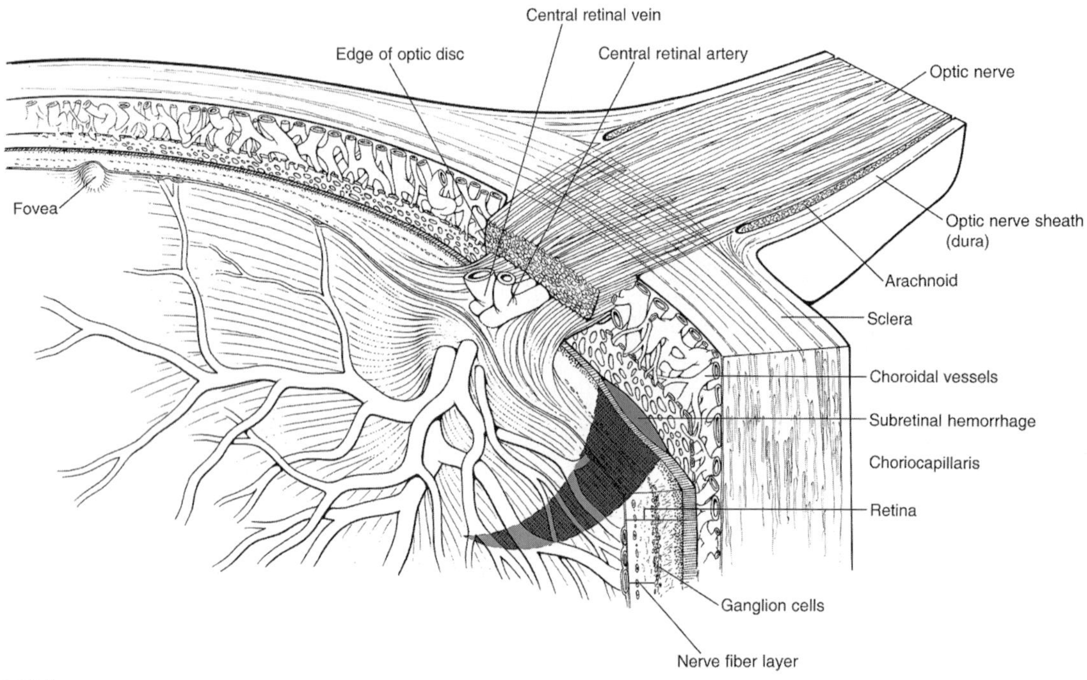

7-10A

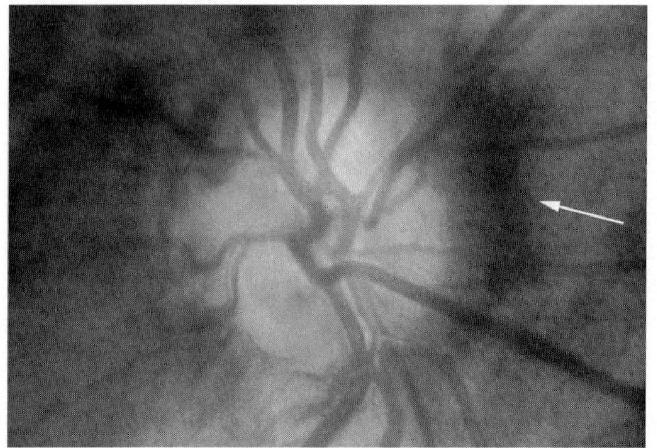

7-10B

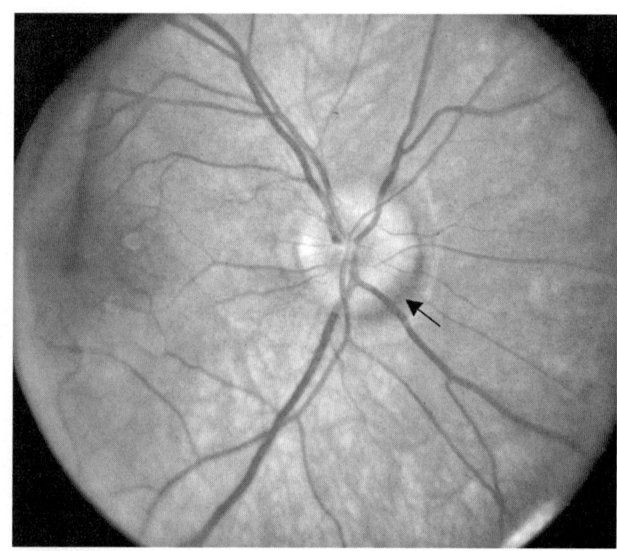

7-10C

Figure 7-11. A. **A choroidal hemorrhage is frequently flat, unlike this enormous choroidal hemorrhage. You can see the vessels and nerve fiber layer above it. Sometimes these are so dark and purple or red-black that they mimic a choroidal nevus.** B. **The diagram shows that a choroidal hemorrhage is beneath the RPE and in the choroid.**

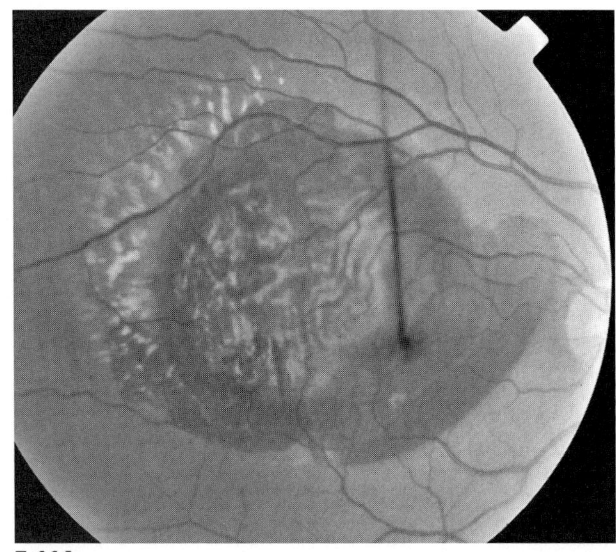

7-11A

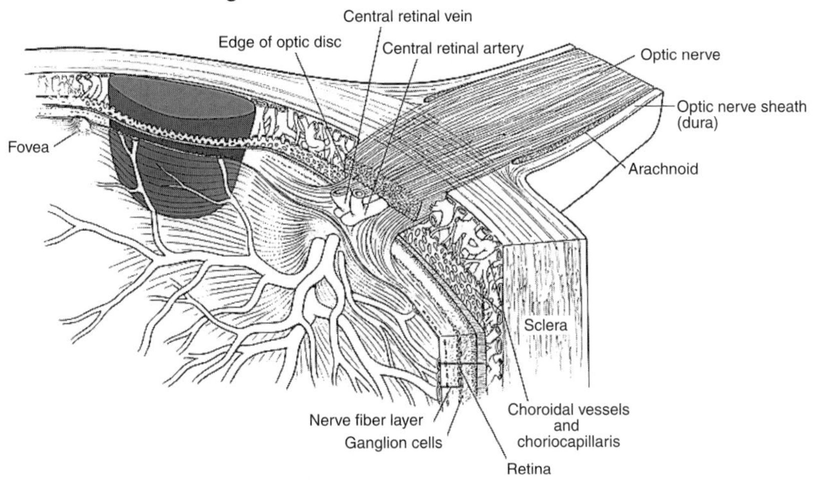

7-11B

Where Hemorrhages Occur

Table 7-4. Hemorrhages by Location

Cause	Papillary	Peripapillary	Macular	Mid-periphery	Periphery
Metabolic					
Diabetes	x	x	—	xx	xx
Hypertension	x	x	—	x	x
Wernicke's encephalopathy	xx	xx	—	—	—
Vascular					
Retinal artery occlusion	x	x	—	x	x
Retinal vein occlusion	x	x	—	xx	—
Ocular ischemic syndrome	—	x	—	xx	xxx
Disc disease	xxx	x	—	—	—
Papilledema	xxx	xxx	—	—	—
Ischemic optic neuropathy	xxx	xxx	—	—	—
Glaucoma	x	—	—	—	—
Drusen	x	xxx	—	—	—
Trauma					
Optic nerve	x	xx	—	—	—
Retina	—	x	x	x	x
Shaken baby syndrome	—	x	x	xx	x

Source: Adapted from reference 9.

Hemorrhages occurring in the nerve fiber layer of the disc are common. The prevalence of optic nerve head hemorrhage is less than 1 per 661 eyes evaluated. In patients with suspected glaucoma or glaucoma, the prevalence increases.[8] Although many have disc hemorrhages with glaucoma, one study found that 70% of patients with optic disc hemorrhages did not have glaucoma. Furthermore, optic disc hemorrhages in general were associated with normal tension glaucoma, discs with large vertical cups, and migraine.[9] Hemorrhages occur anywhere in the retina: on the disc (papillary), around the disc (peripapillary), mid-periphery, and macula.

Table 7-5. Causes of Disc Hemorrhages

Glaucoma (both normal pressure and elevated pressure types)
Diabetic retinopathy
Retinal vein occlusion
Blood vessel abnormalities: retinochoroidal collateral vessels, abnormal disc vessels
Optic nerve disease: ischemic optic neuropathy, papilledema, papillitis
Disc pigment abnormalities
Migraine—rare
Disc drusen

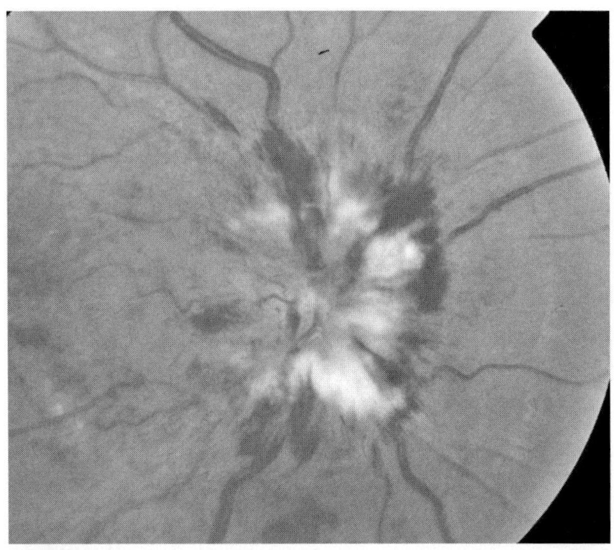

7-12A

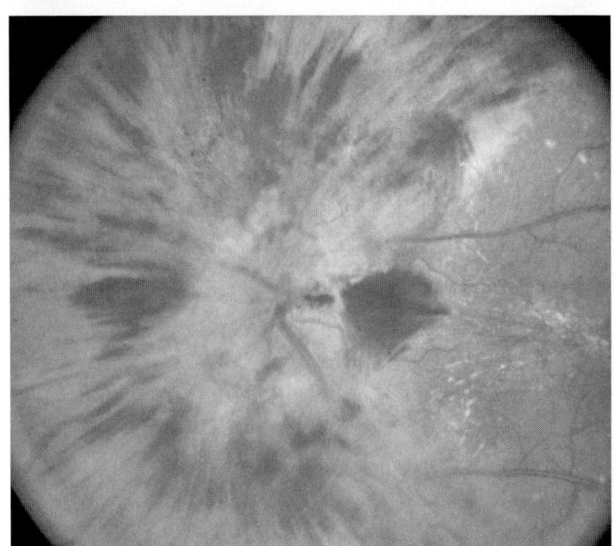

7-12B

Figure 7-12. A. **This swollen disc exhibits nerve fiber layer hemorrhages and cotton-wool spots.** B. **This swollen disc has nerve fiber layer hemorrhages and retinal hemorrhages. Can you pick out each of them?**

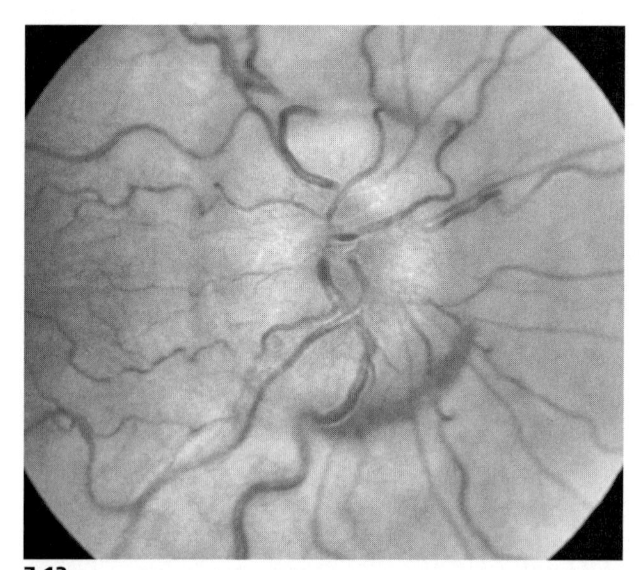
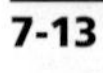

7-13

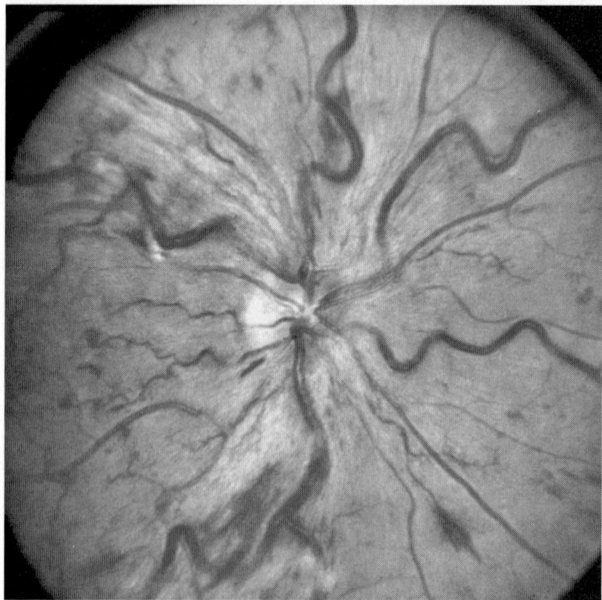

7-14

Figure 7-13. *Peripapillary hemorrhages* occur around, not on, the disc. This swollen disc exhibits a peripapillary subretinal hemorrhage.

Figure 7-14. *Dot hemorrhages in the mid-periphery* typical of early retinal vein thrombosis in diabetic papillophlebitis. Notice that the veins are dilated as well. There are also small papillary nerve fiber layer hemorrhages.

Figure 7-15. A. ***Peripheral hemorrhage*** **in a diabetic.** B. **Dot hemorrhages in the mid-periphery and periphery in a diabetic.**

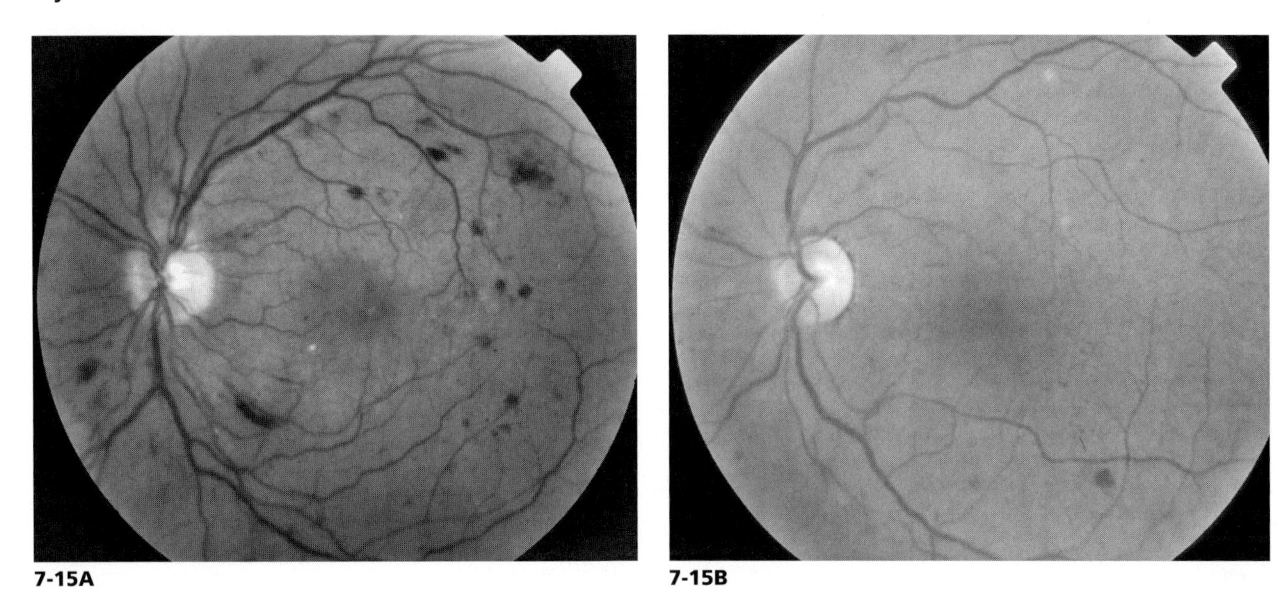

Figure 7-16. ***Macular hemorrhage*****.** A. **This diabetic had increased intracranial pressure and bilateral macular hemorrhages.** B. **Notice not only the macular hemorrhage (*white arrow*) but also the partial macular star formation (*black arrows*).**

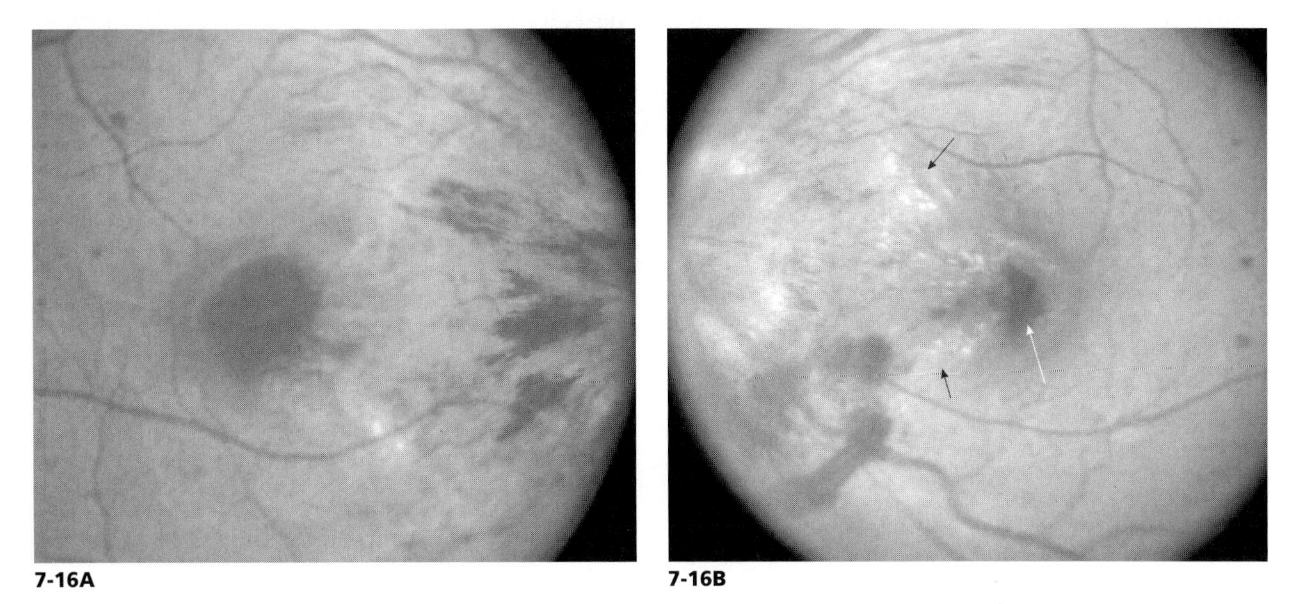

Special Kinds of Hemorrhages

ROTH'S SPOTS

Roth's spots are named for Dr. Moritz von Roth, who described the hemorrhage in 1872, but the connection with endocarditis was later made by Dr. Moriz Litten in 1902.[10,11] von Roth said the following:

In case 5 we have before us a mixed septic and embolic process, putrefication of the lesions in the lower extremities associated with multiple metastatic purulent foci. . . We may therefore more closely associate the present retinitis with the systemic process and from an etiologic point of view we can speak of septic retinitis as we do of leukemic or abluminuric retinitis.[10]

Roth's spots are "white-centered" hemorrhages that occur in round hemorrhages or flame-shaped hemorrhages—that is, either in the nerve fiber layer or in the outer plexiform layer. Histologically, a central core of inflammatory cells or glial tissue characterizes these hemorrhages. Roth's spots at one time were believed to be pathognomonic for bacterial endocarditis; it is now known, however, that these white-centered hemorrhages can be caused by diabetes, hypertension, anemia, anoxia, pernicious anemia, prolonged intubation, myeloma, sickle cell anemia, and leukemia, as well as trauma (especially in battered children and birth trauma) and emboli.

Hemorrhages are common with septicemia. In fact, in a prospective study of 100 septicemic patients, Neudorfer et al. found that approximately one-fourth had hemorrhages, cotton-wool spots, or Roth's spots. The source of the infection was not significant, although bacterial endocarditis and respiratory tract infections led the list. Organisms associated with hemorrhages or Roth's spots were

Staphylococcus aureus, *Klebsiella pneumoniae*, and *Pseudomonas aeruginosa*. All patients were asymptomatic, except for one who developed infection in the eye (endophthalmitis). There were no other findings of septicemia except for splinter hemorrhages and conjunctival petechiae in one patient. Neudorfer et al. recommend routine examination of the fundus in patients with septicemia. All patients examined in follow-up had lesions that resolved within weeks without serious visual morbidity.[12]

Figure 7-17. A. **A typical Roth's spot, close up.** B. **These are typical Roth's spots seen in a baby who presented, comatose, to the emergency room. Although septicemia is a common cause, remember that Roth's spots can be caused by a wide range of pathologies.**

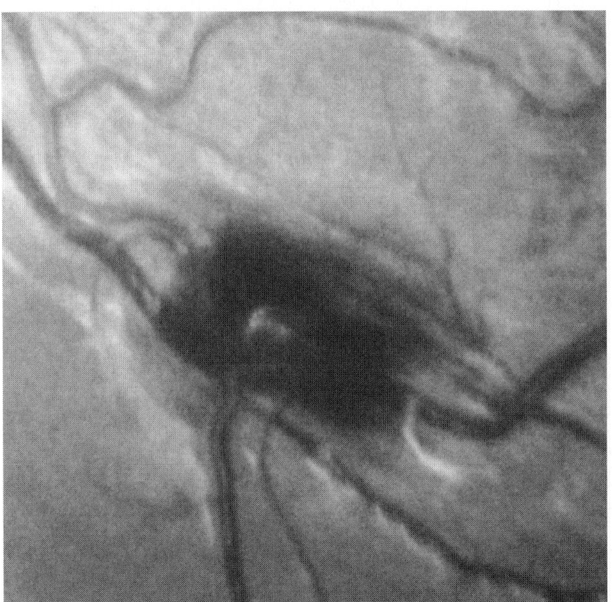

7-17A

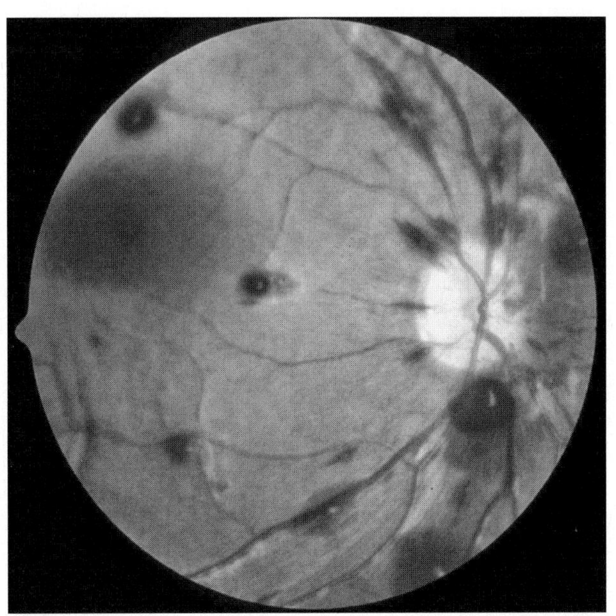

7-17B

TERSON'S SYNDROME

Terson's syndrome involves hemorrhage in the vitreous associated with subarachnoid hemorrhage. This syndrome is named for Albert Terson, a French ophthalmologist, who first described the finding of vitreal hemorrhage associated with subarachnoid hemorrhage.[13,14] Because hemorrhages occur in the vitreous, behind the internal limiting membrane, if these hemorrhages are large, the retina and disc may not be visible. If the retina is visible, multiple hemorrhages may be seen at various levels (e.g., vitreal, subhyaloid, and intraretinal). Subretinal hemorrhages have been reported, but are probably rare.[15] Similarly, hemorrhages may rarely be within the retina (intraretinal), and appear more commonly in the subhyaloid, breaking through or occurring in the vitreous cavity. Terson's syndrome technically is hemorrhage within the vitreous cavity.[14] The blood forms a flat-topped layer owing to gravity with the patient upright; these are "scaphoid" or boat-shaped hemorrhages, such as is pictured in Figure 7-6. Sometimes, you have to sit the patient upright and wait for several minutes to see the hemorrhage "layer out."

7-18A

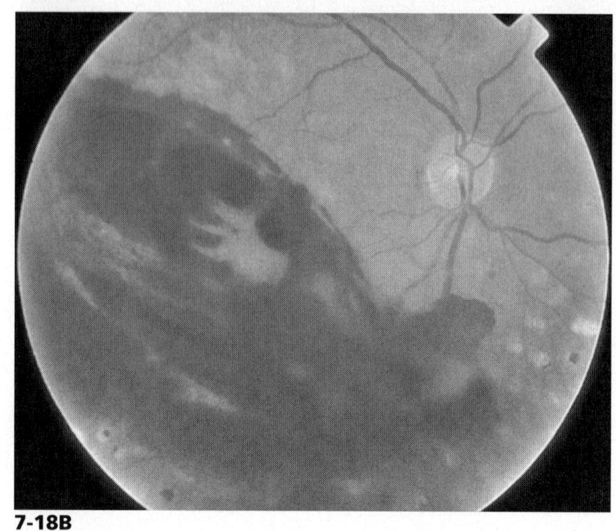

7-18B

Figure 7-18. A. **This man had a serious intracranial hemorrhage after head trauma. When he became conscious, he complained of decreased vision in his left eye. Examination of the red reflex revealed loss of the red reflex on the left, indicating something obscuring the retina. On dilated examination, he had blood throughout his vitreous, obscuring the disc and retina.** B. **Subhyaloid, vitreal hemorrhage typical of Terson's syndrome from another patient. (Photograph courtesy of Paul Zimmerman, M.D.)** ***Continued***

Figure 7-18. *Continued.* C. You can see evidence of the hemorrhage in the vitreous from the patient on the computed tomographic scan (*arrow*). D. This patient had obvious subarachnoid hemorrhage on these non-contrast-enhanced scans. The aneurysm clip is seen (*arrow*). The arrowheads point to the subarachnoid hemorrhage.

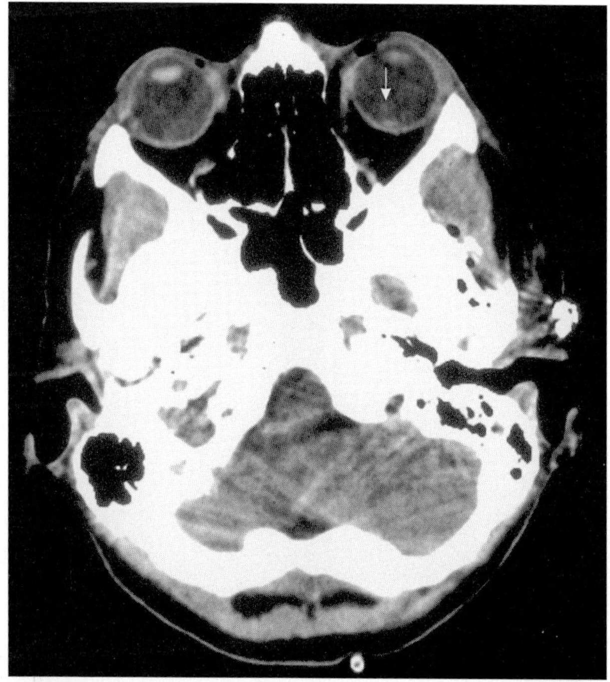

7-18C

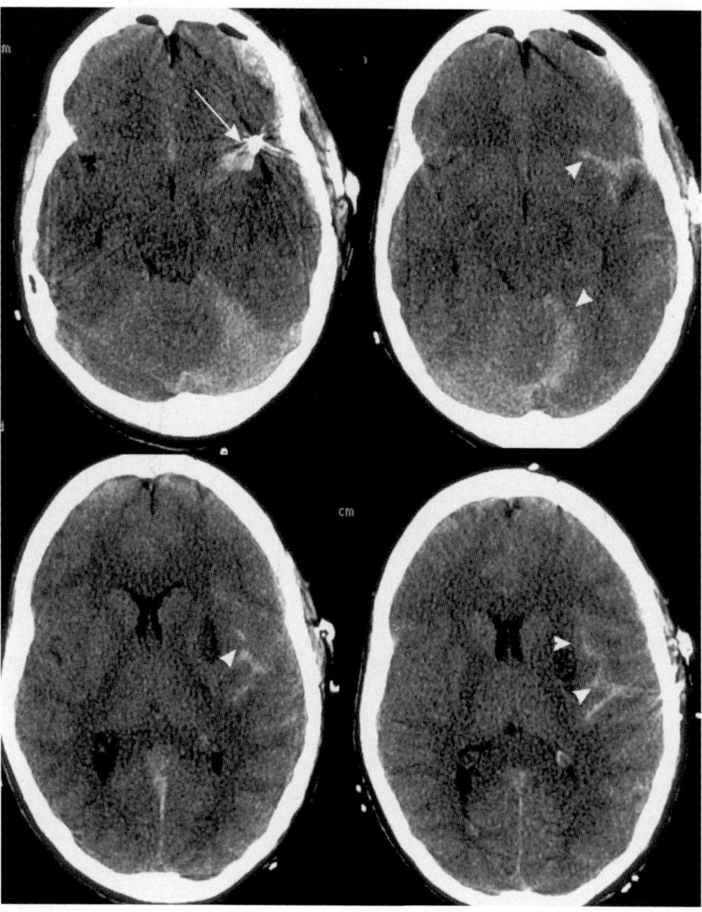

7-18D

The cause of hemorrhages within the eye associated with subarachnoid and other hemorrhages in the brain is unknown. Some hypothesize that the sudden rise of intracranial pressure can cause an increase in intraretinal venous pressure and, hence, the hemorrhage. In addition, a rise in cerebrospinal fluid pressure around the optic nerve may compress retinal and choroidal vasculature and increase retinal vein pressure to cause rupture of small veins.

Hemorrhages occur in approximately 20–30% of patients with an acute subarachnoid hemorrhage owing to aneurysm or arteriovenous malformation.[16] Shaw also found that intraocular hemorrhages had prognostic value. Those with intraocular hemorrhage and a subarachnoid hemorrhage had mortality rates of 54%, compared with 20% in patients without intraocular hemorrhage.[15]

The patient may complain of decreased vision but at times is asymptomatic. The examination shows no afferent pupillary defect. The importance of recognizing this type of hemorrhage is as follows: First, it may be the clue that goes along with the history of a sudden headache to diagnose an aneurysm. Other causes of intravitreal hemorrhage include subdural hemorrhage and increased intracranial pressure from other conditions. Also, intraocular hemorrhage is a treatable cause of vision loss.

Evaluation should include a dilated examination and a follow-up if there is diminished vision, because epiretinal membranes can form after the hemorrhage and may be associated with long-term visual changes. A subhyaloid hemorrhage alone with an appropriate history of a new headache, even with a negative scan, is highly suspicious for subarachnoid hemorrhage.[17] Computed tomography imaging of the orbits reveals the hemorrhage within the globe (see Figure 7-18C).[18] Complications of subhyaloid hemorrhage include increased intraocular pressure, epiretinal membrane, retinal detachment, and macular hole.

HEMORRHAGES IN AN INFANT

For hemorrhages occurring in an infant, consider shaken baby syndrome (Figure 7-19). See Chapter 11, Figure 11-33, Practical Viewing in Children, for more information.

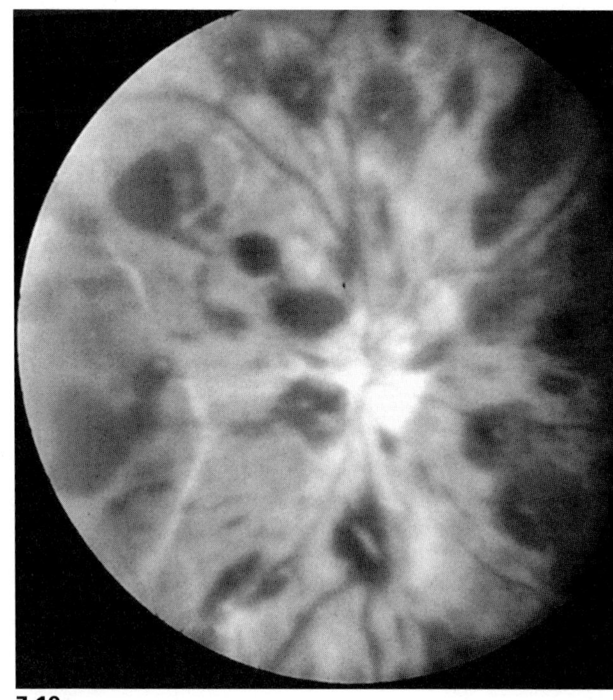

7-19

Practical Viewing Essentials

1. Use the red-free light to see hemorrhages—they appear black on the green background.
2. The newer the hemorrhage, the brighter red it is; the older the hemorrhage, the darker red it is.
3. Try to determine the level in the retina of the hemorrhage.
4. Look on the disc, around the disc, and in the periphery for hemorrhage.
5. Hemorrhage is a sign that something may be seriously wrong—you need an explanation for it.
6. Look for special hemorrhages like Roth's spots and Terson's hemorrhage in the appropriate conditions.

References

1. Gowers W. A Manual and Atlas of Medical Ophthalmoscopy. London: J & A Churchill, 1879.
2. Reinke MH, Gragoudas ES. Unusual hemorrhagic lesions masquerading as choroidal melanoma. Int Ophthalmol Clin 1997;37:135–147.
3. Chester EM. The Ocular Fundus in Systemic Disease. Chicago: Year Book, 1973.
4. Rubenstein RA, Yanoff M, Albert DM. Thrombocytopenia, anemia, and retinal hemorrhage. Am J Ophthalmol 1968;65:435–439.
5. Winterkorn JM. Peripapillary hemorrhage. Surv Ophthalmol 1993;37:362–372.
6. Kaur B, Taylor D. Fundus hemorrhages in infancy. Surv Ophthalmol 1992;37:1–17.
7. Katz B, Hoyt WF. Intrapapillary and peripapillary hemorrhage in young patients with incomplete posterior vitreous detachment. Ophthalmology 1995; 102:349–354.
8. Diehl DL, Quigley HA, Miller NR, et al. Prevalence and significance of optic disc hemorrhage in a longitudinal study of glaucoma. Arch Ophthalmol 1990; 108:545–550.
9. Healey PR, Mitchell P, Smith W, Wang JJ. Optic disc hemorrhages in a population with and without signs of glaucoma. Ophthalmology 1998;105(2): 216–223.
10. Doherty WB, Trubek M. Significant hemorrhagic retinal lesion in bacterial endocarditis (Roth's spots). JAMA 1931;97:308–313.
11. Khawly JA, Pollock SC. Litten's sign (Roth spots) in bacterial endocarditis. Arch Ophthalmol 1994;112: 683–684.
12. Neudorfer M, Barnea Y, Geyer O, Siegman-Igra Y. Retinal lesions in septicemia. Am J Ophthalmol 1993; 116:728–734.
13. Schultz PN, Sobol WM, Weingeist TA. Long-term visual outcome in Terson Syndrome. Ophthalmology 1991;98:1814–1819.
14. Weingeist TA, Goldman EJ, Folk JC, et al. Terson's syndrome. Clinicopathologic correlations. Ophthalmology 1986;93:1435–1442.
15. Shaw HE, Landers MB. Vitreous hemorrhage after intracranial hemorrhage. Am J Ophthalmol 1975; 80:207–213.
16. Keane JR. Retinal hemorrhages. Arch Neurol 1979; 36:691–694.
17. Edlow JA, Caplan LR. Avoiding pitfalls in the diagnosis of subarachnoid hemorrhage. N Engl J Med 2000;342:29–36.
18. Swallow CE, Tsuruda JS, Digre KB. Terson syndrome: CT evaluation in 12 patients. Am J Neuroradiol 1998;9:743–747.

8 Pigment

The common changes [in the choroid] consist of white spots and the disturbance of the choroidal pigment, which so constantly results from any changes in its structure...It must be remembered that this pigment frequently occupies only or chiefly the peripheral portions of the choroid, and an examination confined to the neighbourhood of the optic disc may be insufficient to discover it.

William Gowers[1]

Seeing pigment is like seeing white spots. There are only a few things that cause black spots or pigment changes. There are three questions you may want to answer about any pigment you see: What causes this pigment? What layer is the pigment in? What does pigment mean?

How do you look for pigment? In general, pigment just stands out—it is black against a red/orange background. Furthermore, pigment often is seen next to sclera—it is high contrast. Unlike other changes in the retina and blood vessels, the best place to see pigment is not always around the optic disc, thus you want to look through a dilated pupil. Sometimes indirect illumination of a pigmented spot enhances its visibility. A dilated, indirect ophthalmoscopic examination may be required to see pigment in the periphery.

What Can Look Like Pigment, But Really Isn't?

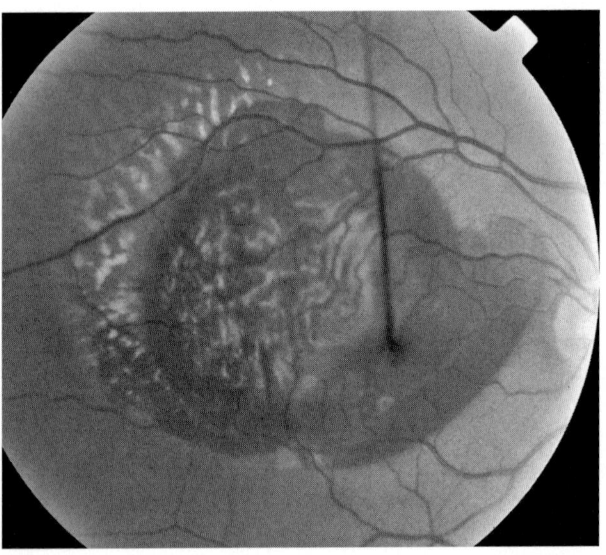

8-1

Figure 8-1. Hemorrhages deep within the choroid can have a dark green, dark blue, slate-gray, or black appearance. Occasionally they may be mistaken for a choroidal nevus. How can you tell the difference? The fluorescein angiogram should be helpful. If there is any doubt, the patient should be referred to an ophthalmologist.

What causes pigment? There really are only two sources of pigment in the fundus. One source is the retinal pigment epithelium (RPE), which is a layer of cells containing pigment that rests on Bruch's membrane at the base of the retina, just below the rods and cones. The second source of pigment is from melanocytes in the choroid. It is the amount of pigment in the RPE that gives the retina its color, so that when there is little pigment in the RPE, the fundus develops a tessellated appearance. This is discussed in Chapter 2, Figure 2-29, in which you see choroidal vessels and black islands of melanin in between the choroidal vessels, whereas a uniform layer of pigment in the RPE gives the uniform, dark red or brown-red fundus, hiding the choroid and its vessels. The RPE's job is to modify the entrance of light and to detoxify the primary photoreceptors (rods and cones). The RPE is alive with metabolic activity, full of mitochondria and active transforming vitamin A for the photoreceptors. The RPE is not often the seat of disease that causes pigmentary changes, but the RPE responds to any disturbance of neighboring retinal/choroidal elements by laying down pigment. When under attack by a pathologic process like inflammation, trauma, or laser treatment, the RPE proliferates wildly. Furthermore, any disorder that disrupts the rods and cones can affect the RPE (e.g., retinitis pigmentosa [RP]). Sometimes the pigment may hypertrophy on its own.

Figure 8-2. Pigment in the retina comes from the retinal pigment epithelium or the melanocytes interspersed in the choroid. The gray pigment in this diagram represents melanocytes interdigitated between the choroidal vessels (shown in the inset is a segment of choroidal circulation). The pigment epithelium lies below the retina and is lightly colored gray to represent the pigment within the retinal pigment epithelium. (See the corresponding color figure on the accompanying CD-Rom.)

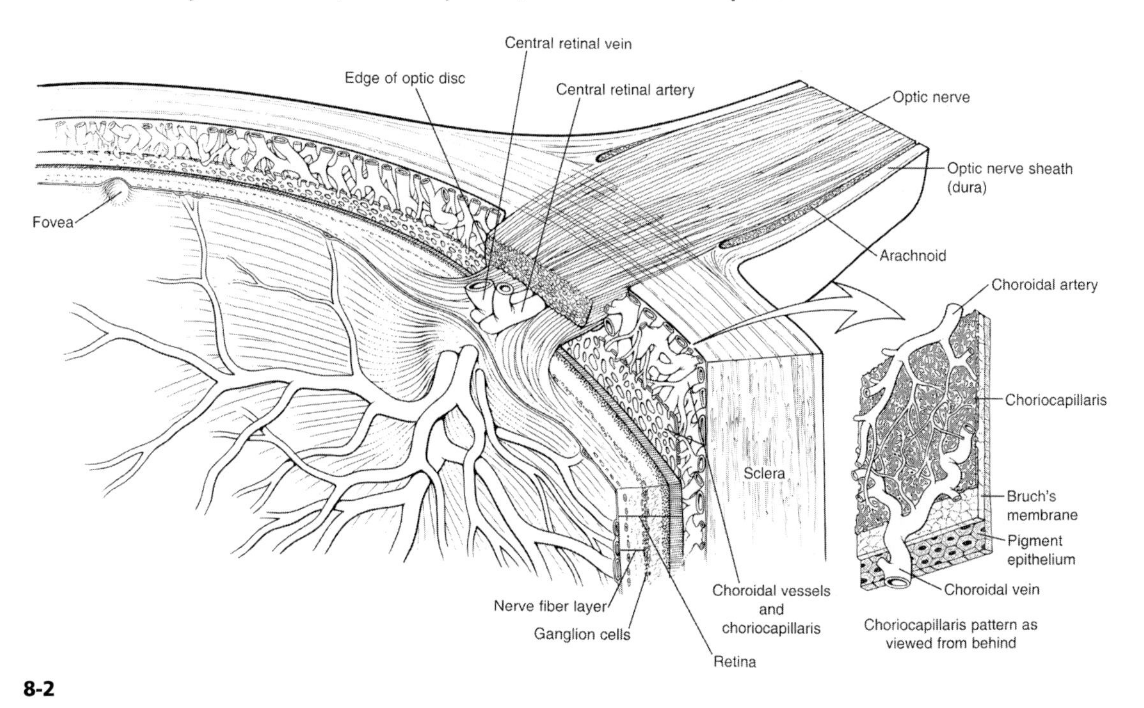

8-2

The choroid, which is very vascular, contains many melanocytes interspersed throughout the vessels. If these melanocytes hypertrophy, nevi are formed. If the melanocytes undergo malignant transformations, melanomas are formed.

Forms of Pigment Seen

Salt and pepper fundus is the term used to describe diffuse pigment granules caused by processes that are rapid in development and affect the retina in a widespread manner.[2] A classic example is seen in congenital syphilis. This pattern can be seen in other retinal/brain abnormalities such as rubella or even retinal degenerations.

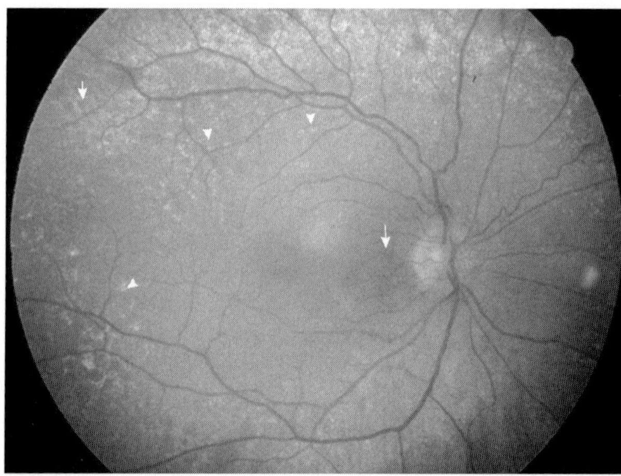

8-3

Figure 8-3. ***Salt and pepper fundus*** **is named for the white dots (salt), which are plentiful (*arrowheads*), and small black dots (pepper, *arrows*), such as in this case of congenital syphilis.**

Pigmented clumps, or *bone spicules*, are caused by conditions that develop more slowly, allowing for pigmented aggregation in the retina and around blood vessels.

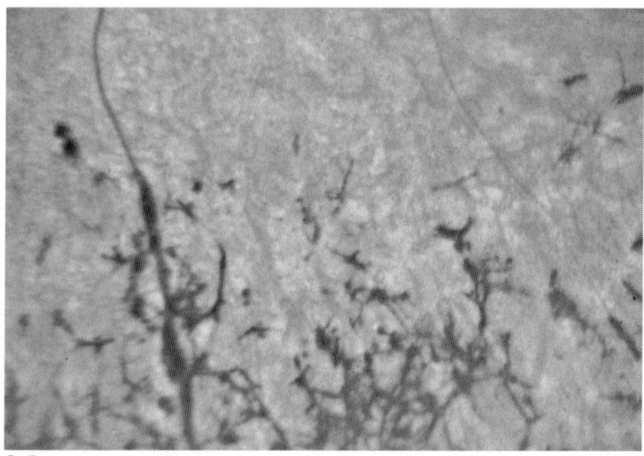

8-4

Figure 8-4. Pigmented clumps of bone spicules are typical in many of the inherited retinal degenerations, such as RP. (Photograph courtesy of W.T. Shults, M.D.)

Plaques of pigment can occur on the disc or in the retina as developmental phenomena.[3] Congenital pigmentation in the retina is fairly common. Plaques of pigment may be grouped and produce a "bear track" appearance to the pigmentation. This is a benign, congenital condition associated with RPE hypertrophy, and retinal function is normal.[4] In addition, pigment also commonly adorns the margins of infectious scars such as toxoplasmosis or presumed ocular histoplasmosis syndrome.

Figure 8-5. A,B. ***Bear tracks*** **are plaques of pigment. The name comes from their appearance. They represent a congenital hypertrophy of the RPE, and retinal function is normal. They can confuse observers into thinking that they are RP. (Photographs courtesy of Paul Zimmerman, M.D.)**

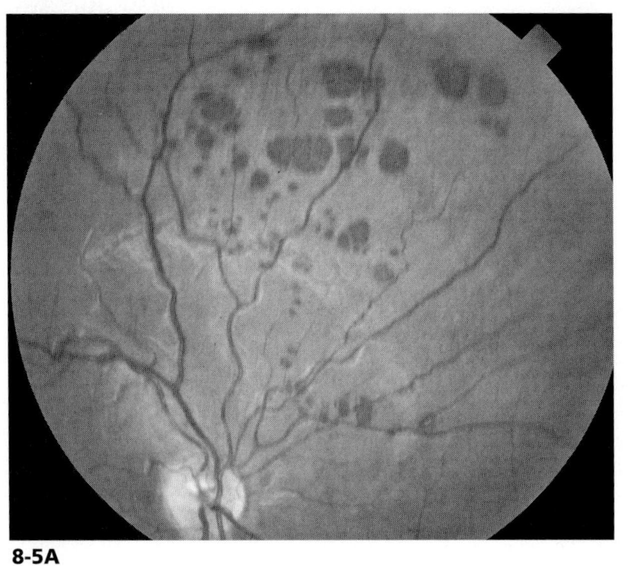

8-5A

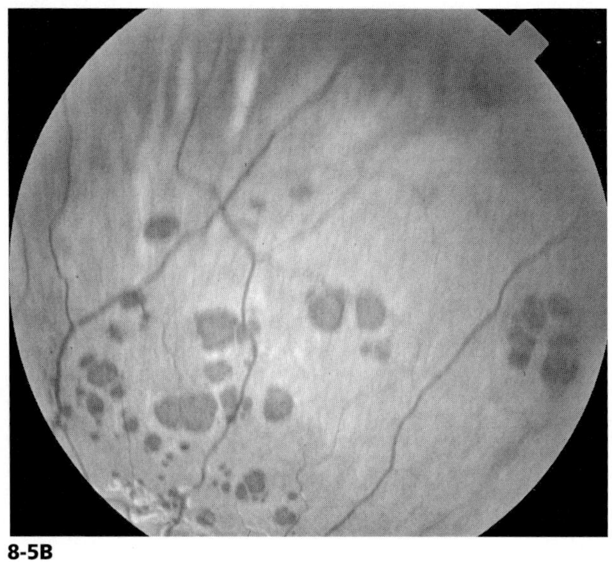

8-5B

NORMAL DISC PIGMENT

First, it is common to see pigmentation around the disc—especially in scleral crescents.

Figure 8-6. This tilted disc has pigmentary changes temporally (*arrow*) typical of pigmentary crescents.

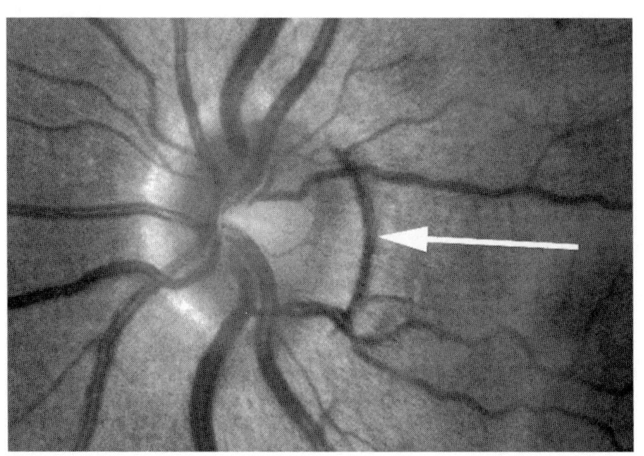

8-6

Figure 8-7. A. **Congenital optic disc pigmentation.** B. **Gray discs can occur in albino retinas. Although gray discs have been reported in normal infants, most cases are related to albinism. (Photographs courtesy of Michael Brodsky, M.D.)**

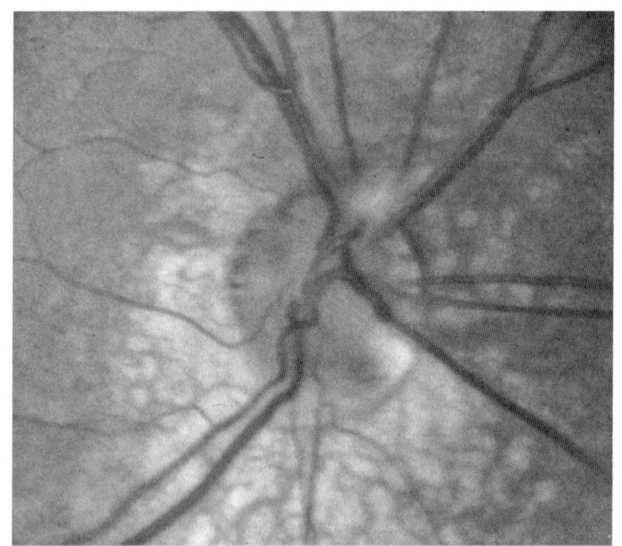

8-7A

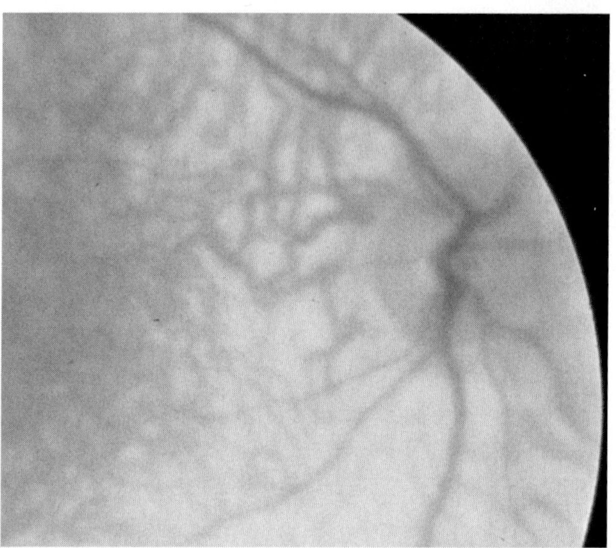

8-7B

The optic nerve may appear gray in otherwise normal infants in whom there is a delay in myelination. According to Pinckers et al., these babies are otherwise normal and do well.[5] In these same cases, many of the babies were albinotic. Pigmented discs have been reported in ocular albinism; why this occurs is a mystery. Some believe that the "gray" disc in this situation is an optical illusion—the disc simply looks gray next to the albinotic retina.

PATHOLOGIC PIGMENTATION—ON THE DISC

Table 8-1. Causes of Pigmented Disc Lesions

Hyperplasia of retinal pigment epithelium or congenital hypertrophy of retinal pigment epithelium
Melanocytoma
Papilla nigra
Optic nerve transection/trauma immediately retrotubular
Peripapillary choroidal nevus
Combined hamartoma of retinal pigment epithelium and sensory retina
Malignant melanoma
Chromosomal abnormalities—chromosome 17[7]
Retinal detachment surgery

Source: Adapted from reference 6.

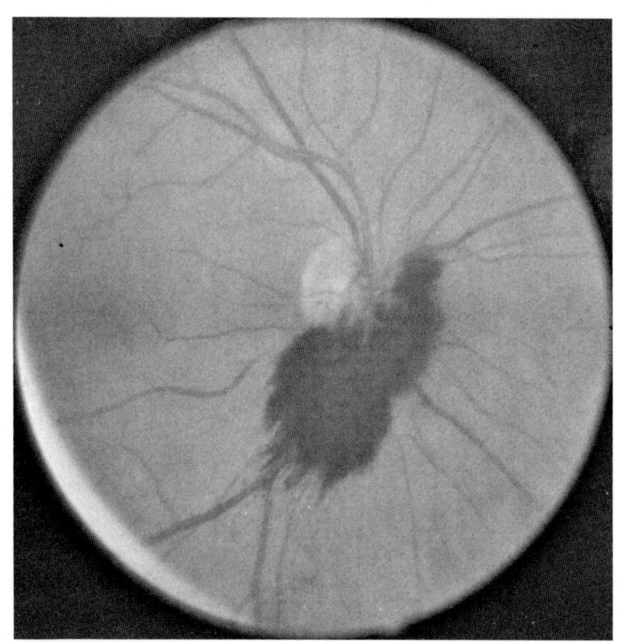

8-8A

Melanocytoma of the optic disc is a usually nonmalignant tumor that arises out of the optic disc from melanocytes in the choroid/uveal system. The disc is elevated, gray to black, and often pigmented eccentrically. Although the tumors can cover the entire disc, they more frequently cover less than one-half of the disc. Melanocytomas are accompanied by disc edema, probably owing to slowed axoplasmic flow, and retinal vessels may be sheathed; they are slightly more common in more heavily pigmented individuals and appear gray to black. In general, melanocytomas do not change. However, malignant transformation can occur,[8] and differentiating these lesions from melanoma of the disc can be a challenge.[9] Close follow-up by an ophthalmologist is necessary. Joffe et al. reported in a study of 27 patients who were followed for 1–19 years that 81% showed no change.[10]

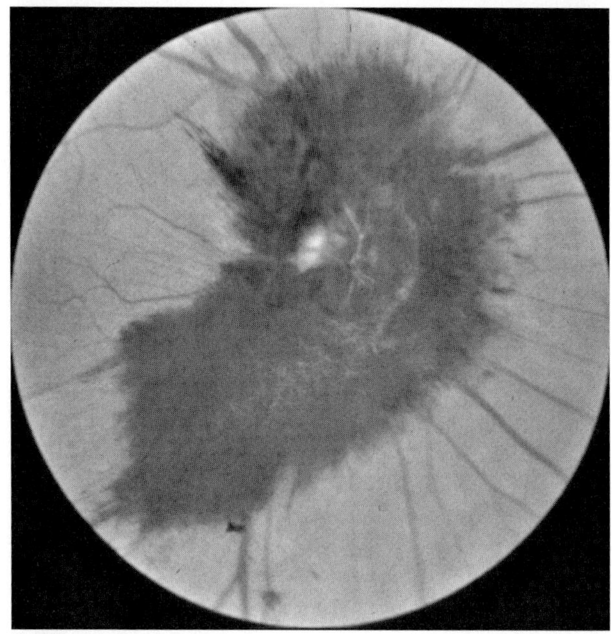

8-8B

Figure 8-8. Melanocytoma is a nonmalignant tumor of the optic disc. A. **The disc when the melanocytoma was discovered.** B. **Four years later, showing tumor enlargement.**

Table 8-2. Differentiating Black Discs

Features	Melanocytoma[11]	Melanoma[9]	Optic nerve transection/trauma
Race	Equal frequency in whites and blacks	Unusual in blacks	Associated with no racial predilection, trauma, or surgical removal of the optic nerve
Visual acuity/ visual field	Normal function	Frequent visual acuity/field loss	Usually no light perception
Source of pigment	Can arise and be contiguous with choroidal nevus	Most arise from peripapillary choroidal melanoma; can arise from melanocytoma (very rarely)	Pigmented cells at the lamina
Appearance	Does not project more than 1 mm into the vitreous; pigment is usually black in optic nerve melanocytoma; disc melanocytomas are variable color; sometimes see a feathery margin	Frequently projects more than 1 mm into the vitreous	Is almost always associated with attenuation of the vessels
Fluorescein features	Blocks fluorescence; may see hyperfluorescence if the disc is swollen	Hypofluorescent[8]	Variable
Evaluation	Usually none; baseline ultrasonography or imaging	Ultrasonography; computed tomography; magnetic resonance characteristics	CT scan with bone window
Treatment	Follow with fundus photography	Enucleation	None; sometimes steroids
Natural history	Benign—81% do not progress	Poor outcome	Related to trauma
Frequency	Rare	Rare	Common

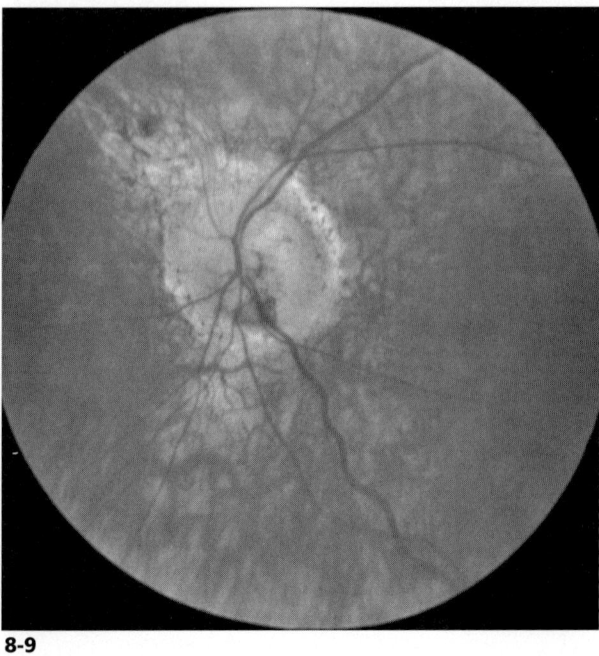

8-9

Figure 8-9. This optic nerve was removed due to an optic nerve glioma. The disc shows pigmentation typical of post-trauma or transection of the optic disc. The pigment is on the disc.

PATHOLOGIC PIGMENTATION—IN THE RETINA

There are many causes of pathologic pigment in the retina, including infection, genetic disorders, toxins, tumors, and trauma. Anything that injures the RPE or stimulates the melanocytes produces pigment.

Pigment is common after acute infections: Acute chorioretinitis is discussed in Chapter 9. However, some chorioretinitis is associated with pigmentary changes, the classic example being congenital syphilis that produces salt and pepper fundus changes.

Congenital and Secondary Syphilis

Appearance of the fundus after acute infections is similar to RP, with pigmentary clumping throughout the retina. However, there are many other retinal findings that are found in addition to syphilitic chorioretinitis, which include arterial occlusion, macular edema, macular star with neuroretinitis, retinal detachment, retinal vein occlusion, and big blind spot syndrome.[12]

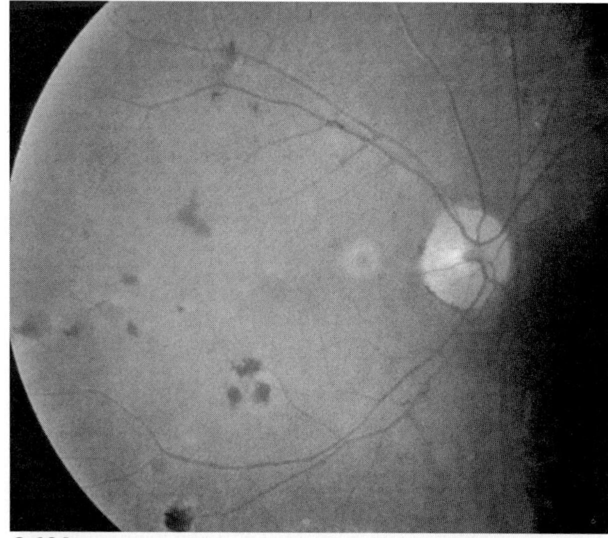

8-10A

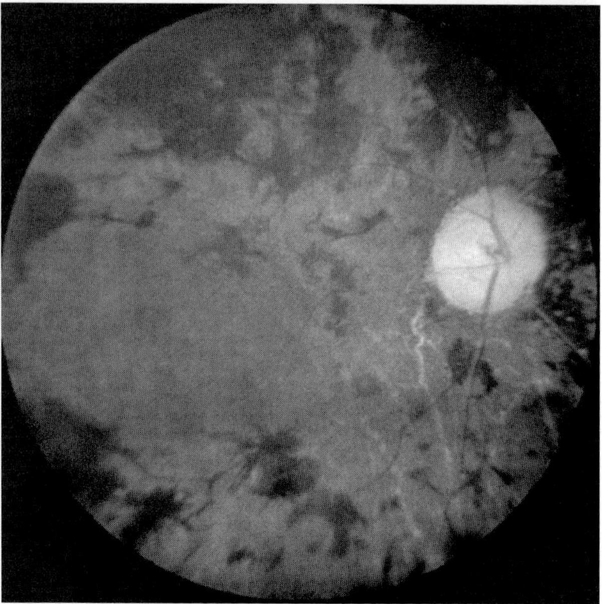

8-10B

Figure 8-10. A. **This individual has chorioretinal changes from congenital syphilis. Although some of the pigment is in dots, there are also small pigment clumps.** B. **This individual had severe syphilitic retinitis, with severe changes in the retina, narrowing of the retinal vasculature, and optic disc pallor. The residue is chorioretinopathy with pigment.**

Histoplasmosis

Figure 8-11. A. **So-called ski-track pigmentary change is typical for histoplasmosis.** B. **Typical peripapillary atrophy (*arrowheads* point to the peripapillary atrophy), lesion at 8 o'clock (*arrow*), and punched-out white lesions (*thicker white arrows*) with pigmentary changes are characteristic of histoplasmosis. (Photographs courtesy of C.J. Chen, M.D.)**

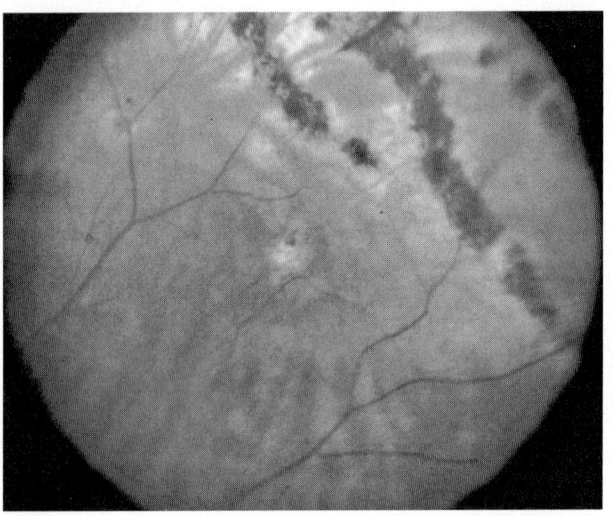

8-11A

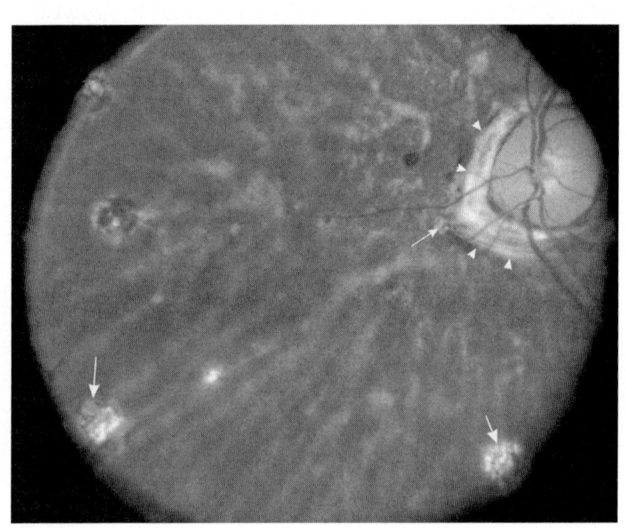

8-11B

Toxoplasmosis

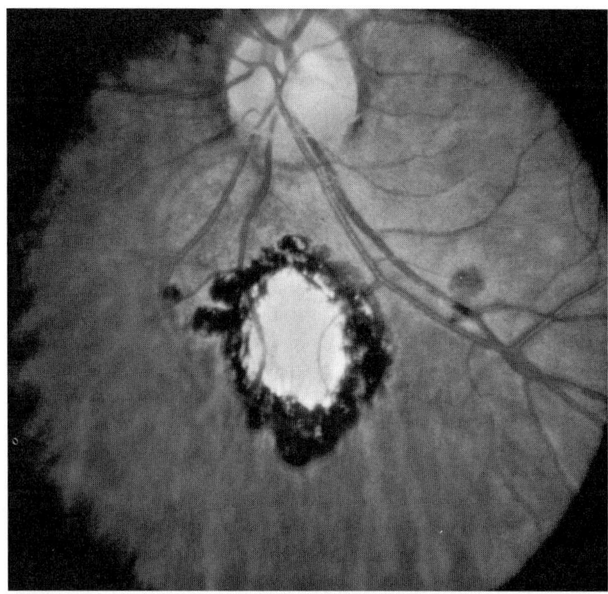

8-12

Figure 8-12. Old toxoplasmosis scars appear as heavily pigmented rings around punched-out areas of the retina, as shown here.

Retinitis Pigmentosa

RP is a retinal/choroidal degeneration caused by various genetic defects. The term *retinitis pigmentosa* is really a misnomer because it is not inflammation of the retina (retinitis) and not a disease of the pigmentary system (pigmentosa), but a disease of the primary visual sensory system, namely, the rods and cones and their cell bodies. The pigmentary changes seen are really secondary to the disease of the rods and cones. The pigment of RP is melanin liberated as the RPE degenerates.

The classic appearance of RP is "bone spicules," which really are perivascular clumps of melanin that are much more apparent in the retinal periphery. Some of the pigmentation can be more granular. Aside from the pigmentation, the arterioles are strikingly narrowed, and early the disc may be slightly swollen. Later, the disc has a classic "waxy" appearance. There may be disc drusen that may be confused with papilledema.

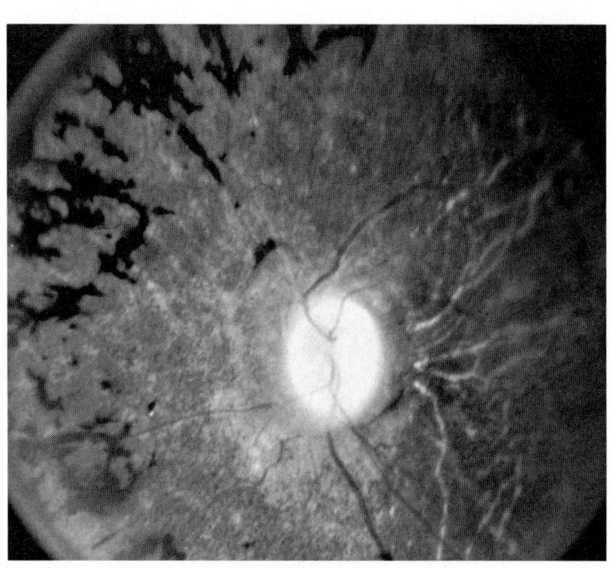

8-13

Figure 8-13. This disc displays the classic fundus findings in RP, including (1) threadlike retinal vessel attenuation, (2) perivascular pigmentary clumping and bone spicule formation, (3) mottling and granularity of the RPE, and (4) waxy appearance of the optic disc.

RP is a large group of conditions that occurs in 1 in 2,000 (Native American) to 1 in 7,000 (in Switzerland).[13] It is usually bilateral, but may present more predominantly in one eye. RP can appear in only one sector or quadrant. Occasionally, RP can appear without pigmentary changes—retinitis pigmentosa *sine pigmento.* Although the symptoms are similar (decreased night vision, etc.), no pigmentary changes are present in the fundus. Sometimes vascular attenuation and disc pallor may provide a clue. An electroretinogram (ERG) and visual field are required because retinal appearance alone would not make the diagnosis.

Figure 8-14. A,B. **This 19-year-old woman was referred for what was believed to be hysterical visual field constriction. Her examination showed disc pallor, narrowing of the arterioles, and no evidence of pigmentary changes of RP (**A, **left eye;** B, **right eye).** C. **Her visual fields were constricted. Because there was a scrap of peripheral visual field in both eyes (*arrow*), it made the diagnosis of functional vision loss less likely. Her ERG was typical for RP, showing a poor scotopic response. This is retinitis pigmentosa *sine pigmento*.**

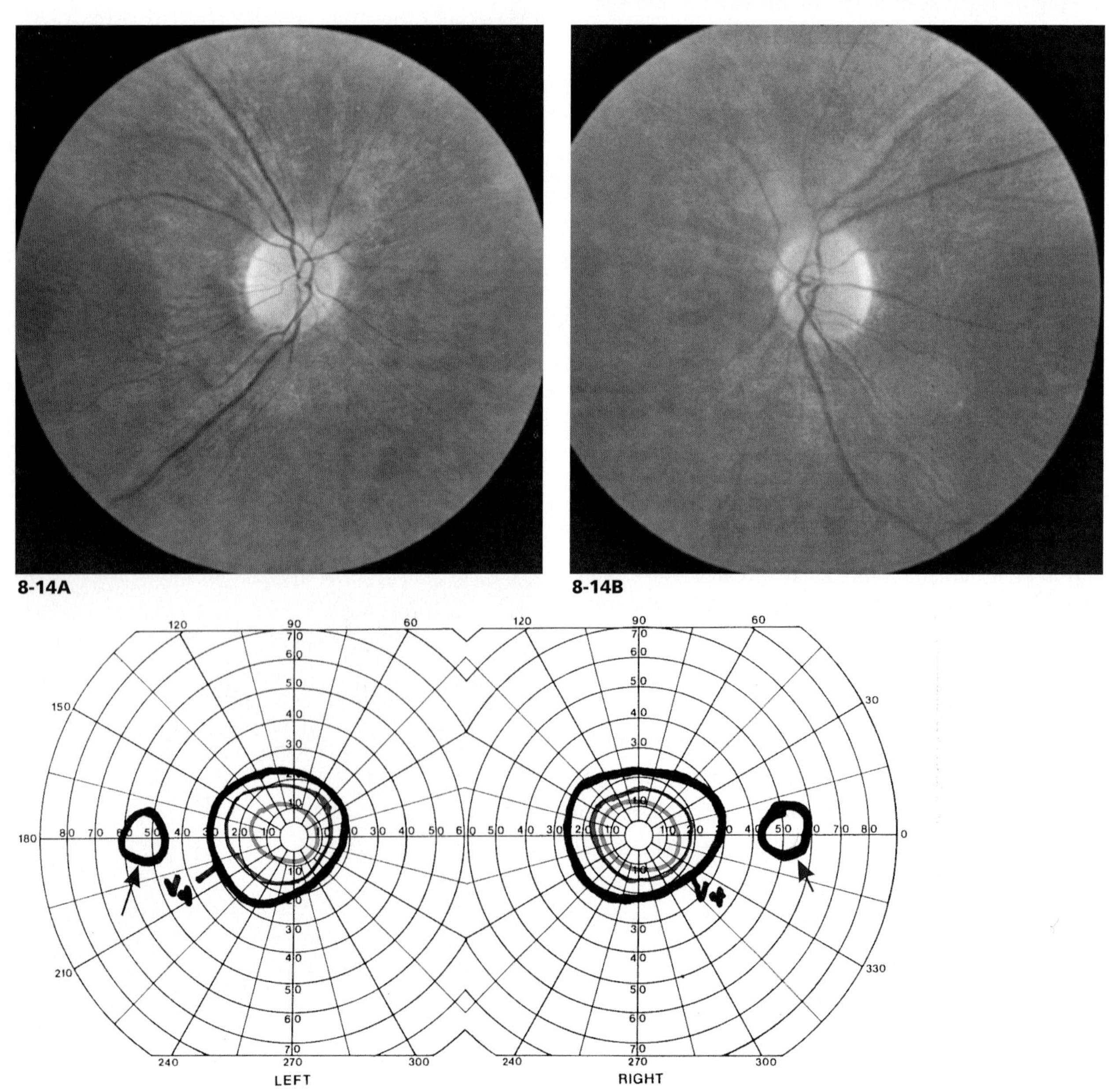

8-14C

Symptoms of all types of RP are classically decreased night vision—"I can't see the stars" (of course, no one in the city can see the stars anyway!)—and photopsias. Ophthalmic examination will show intact acuity and color vision often to the end. Visual field examination early on shows classic ring scotomas that are caused by the degenerative process in the mid-periphery where you see the pigmentary changes. The visual field progressively constricts and finally is extinguished. The central field is the last to disappear; therefore, visual acuity may be preserved until late, but peripheral vision suffers severely.

The most helpful test when you suspect someone has RP is the ERG. The ERG is measured using a contact lens electrode on a patient's cornea. Flashes of light at various frequencies and intensities stimulate the retina. The stimulated retina causes firing of millions of neural cells, which translates into an electrical signal that can be measured at the corneal electrode. The traces we see are the *A-wave*, which is a negative or downward deflection generated by the photoreceptors (cones and rods). The *B-wave* is a positive or upward tracing generated by the bipolar cells, Müller cells (glial cells). The tracings also reflect the lighting conditions: *photopic* means that the condition is a light-adapted state and tests mainly the photoreceptors. The *scotopic* wave is under dark-adapted state and tests mainly the rods (with some contribution from the cones). The scotopic state can be measured after a white light or a dim blue light. The dim blue light tests mainly the rod signal. The third tracing often seen is the *oscillatory potential* (30-Hz flicker), which is measured in the light-adapted state and reflects the cone photoreceptors.

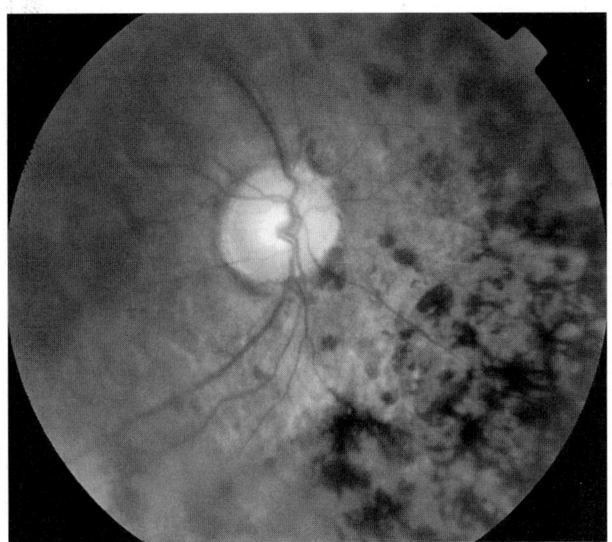

8-15A

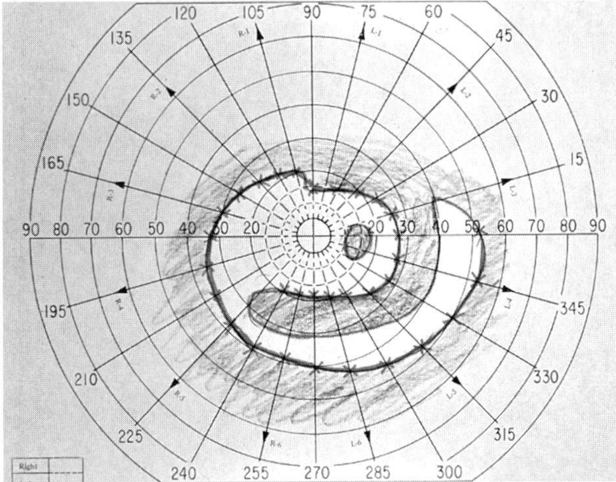

8-15B

Figure 8-15. A. **This individual has poor night vision and slightly decreased visual acuity to 20/30. The funduscopic examination shows typical pigmentation owing to RP.** B. **The visual field shows a mid-peripheral scotoma.**

Figure 8-16. Typical ERG, a part of the ophthalmologic examination, which tests rod and cone function. There are three tracings: normal, RP (a disorder of rod functioning), and cone dystrophy (a disorder of cone function). The top three tracings are scotopic (dark adapted state) to stimulate the rods. The fourth tracing is a 30-Hz flicker or oscillatory potential that is done in the light. The final tracing is the photopic tracing (light state). You will notice that in RP all of the tracings look somewhat abnormal and flat. There is some photopic B-wave and some flicker following, whereas in the cone dystrophy the scotopic tracings look normal but the flicker and photopic tracings are abnormal. (Tracings courtesy of Donnell Creel, Ph.D.)

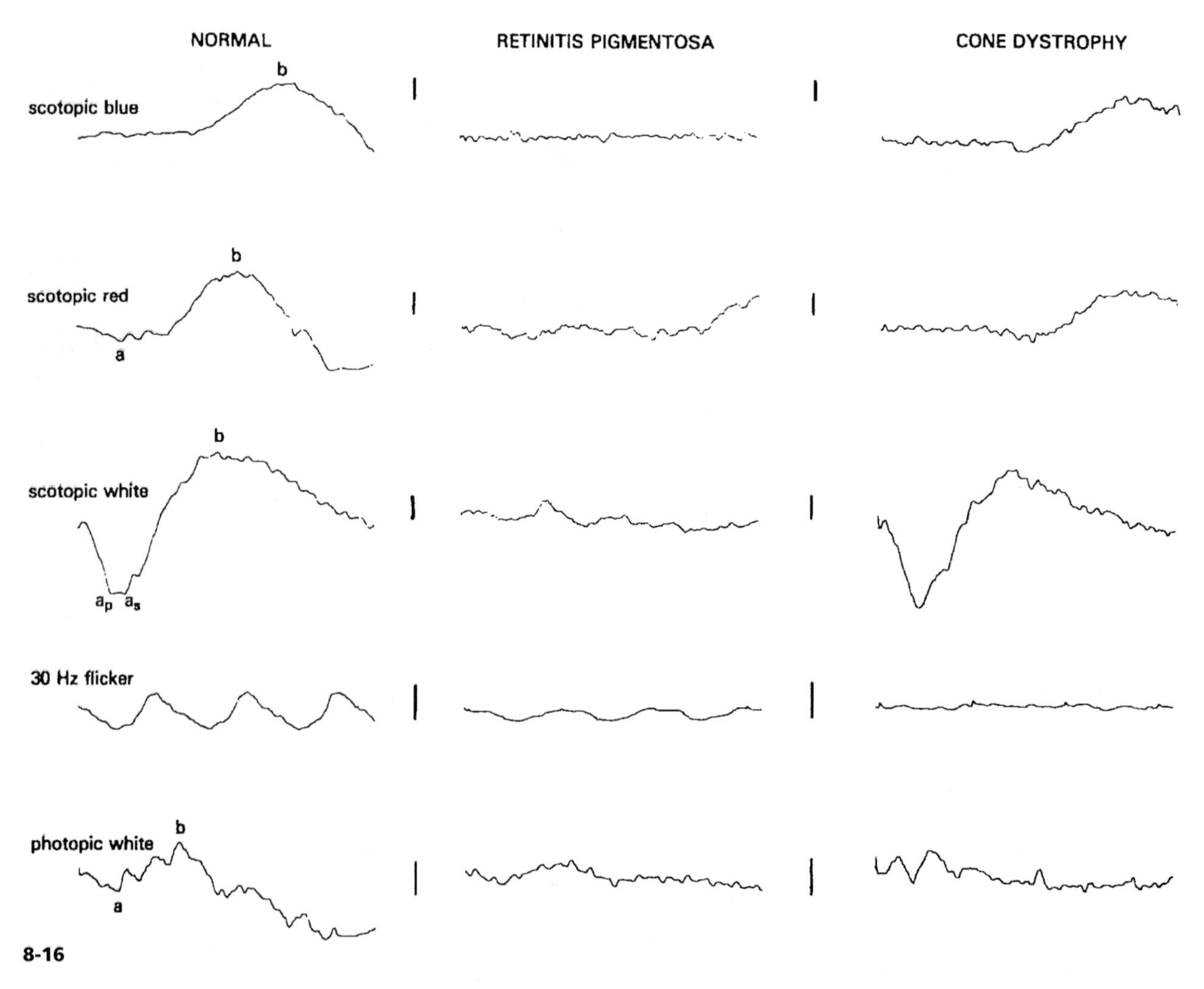

8-16

Table 8-3. Conditions That May Be Mistaken for Retinitis Pigmentosa

Retinal inflammatory disorders
Congenital rubella
Congenital syphilis
Cytomegalovirus
Toxoplasmosis
Congenital herpes infections
Cancer-associated retinopathy/melanoma-associated retinopathy
Autoimmune retinopathy (systemic lupus erythematosus)
Drug toxicity
Thioridazine (Mellaril): the only phenothiazine definitely linked to retinal toxicity
Chloroquine
Chlorpromazine (Thorazine)
Quinine
Trauma
Bear tracking
Congenital hypertrophy of the retinal pigment epithelium (associated with familial polyps)

Source: Adapted from reference 4.

Although most cases of RP have no other associated symptoms or findings, there are many neurological conditions associated with concomitant RP. See Table 8-4 for a list of many of these.

Table 8-4. Neurologic Conditions Associated with Pigmentary Retinopathy

Condition	Symptoms	Neurologic findings	Other features	Genetics	Evaluation/ diagnosis
Kearns-Sayre syndrome	Ptosis, external ophthalmoplegia—first or second decade	Ptosis, ophthalmoparesis; deafness on occasion	Heart block; diabetes, short stature, subnormal intelligence, hearing loss, high CSF protein	Mitochondrial	MR may show T2 signals in basal ganglia; muscle biopsy shows ragged red fibers; electrocardiogram
Chronic progressive external ophthalmoplegia	Progressive ptosis, ophthalmoplegia; adolescence; even older	Ptosis, ophthalmoparesis	Heart block possible	Mitochondrial defect	Muscle biopsy shows ragged red fibers; electrocardiogram
Usher's syndrome (type 1, early onset and severe; type II, variable)[17]	Congenital deafness + retinitis pigmentosa	Deafness; vestibular abnormalities in type 1; associated with multiple sclerosis on occasion[17]	Most common association with retinitis pigmentosa; type 1 is more severe with onset congenital; type 2 milder, onset around puberty	Autosomal recessive	Hearing test
Mitochondrial encephalopathy and lactic acidosis with strokelike episodes (MELAS)	Progressive dementia; strokelike episodes; complicated migraine; reversible neurologic deficits	Ptosis, ophthalmoparesis; with progression neurologic deficits accumulate	—	Mitochondrial[18]	MR abnormal; spectroscopy: elevated lactate; increased serum lactic acid
Myoclonic epilepsy with ragged red fibers (MERRF)	Myoclonic epilepsy; ataxia, dysarthria	Spasticity; ataxia; optic atrophy; dementia	—	Mitochondrial	Muscle biopsy shows ragged red fibers
Neuropathy, ataxia,[19] retinitis pigmentosa (NARP)	Sensory neuropathy and ataxia	Developmental delay, seizure	—	Mitochondrial	Mitochondrial testing of muscle
Friedreich's ataxia	Trouble walking; young age	Ataxia, hyporeflexia, dysarthria, pes cavus deformity; deafness	Optic atrophy is more common than retinitis pigmentosa	Autosomal dominant	Vitamin E therapy

Abetalipoproteinemia (Bassen-Kornzweig disease)	Malabsorption syndrome with hypovitaminosis A/E	Neuropathy and cerebellar dysfunction; see eye movement abnormalities like internuclear ophthalmoplegia; angioid streaks	Absent beta-lipoproteins; acanthocytosis; low cholesterol	Autosomal recessive	Blood smear; serum lipoproteins; cholesterol profile; see ERG changes; supplement with vitamins A, E
Alström disease	Severe vision loss within the first 10 years, cataract	Deafness	Diabetes, obesity, renal failure, acanthocytosis nigricans, hypogonadism, baldness	French Acadians	—
Arteriohepatic dysplasia (Alagille syndrome)	Axenfeld's anomaly; corectopia, esotropia; disc has horizontal elongation; also can see pseudopapilledema	Abnormal vertebrae; absent stretch reflexes	Neonatal jaundice owing to decreased number of biliary ducts; pulmonic stenosis, abnormal face	Autosomal dominant; variably expressed	High serum porphyrins; liver biopsy
Bardet-Biedl syndrome	Macular atrophy	Mental retardation; Laurence-Moon-Biedl form has spastic diplegia, deafness	Obesity, polydactyly, interstitial nephritis; hypogenitalism	Autosomal recessive	—
Cockayne's syndrome	Severe vision loss by age 30 years owing to optic atrophy; band keratopathy (owing to dry eyes), cataracts; pigmentary retinopathy	Deafness; mental deterioration, cerebellar dysfunction with motor deterioration; intracranial calcifications	Growth failure; rapid facial aging; photosensitive dermatitis; joint contractures	Autosomal recessive	CT scan shows basal ganglia and dentate calcification; MR shows delayed myelination
Cystinosis	Corneal deposits with erosion; photophobia; flecked retinopathy	Growth retardation; confusion and memory loss	Renal failure owing to crystal nephropathy	Autosomal recessive	—

Continued

Table 8-4. *Continued*

Condition	Symptoms	Neurologic findings	Other features	Genetics	Evaluation/ diagnosis
Flynn-Aird syndrome	Myopia, cataracts	Deafness, ataxia, peripheral neuropathy, epilepsy, dementia; cataracts, myopia; hearing loss	Dental caries, chronic skin ulcers, baldness	Autosomal dominant	—
Neuroaxonal dystrophy (Hallervorden-Spatz)	Blepharospasm, apraxia of eye lid opening; some have optic atrophy; 25% bull's eye maculopathy	Choreoathetosis, dysarthria, gait impairment, severe rigidity; dementia; epilepsy	Death within 15 years of onset	Autosomal recessive	T2 image on MR shows decreased signal intensity in the globus pallidus and substantia nigra—iron deposition
Refsum's disease (phytanic acid storage disease)	Macular degeneration; clumped pigmentary change, not bone spicules; optic atrophy	Deafness, hypotonia, peripheral neuropathy (painful); anosmia; cerebellar ataxia; mental retardation	Hepatomegaly; cardiac conduction defect	Autosomal recessive	Elevated phytanic acid; increased protein in cerebrospinal fluid; treatable with low phytanic acid diet
Jeune's syndrome (thoracic-pelvic phalangeal dystrophy)	Poor visual acuity (myopia), strabismus; photophobia	Nystagmus; ataxia	Dwarfism, polydactyly, long thorax, short ribs; respiratory insufficiency, renal failure, liver abnormal	Autosomal recessive	Kidney biopsy
Mucopolysaccharidoses (accumulations of glycosaminoglycans) (Scheie's, San Filippos, Hunter's syndrome)	Corneal clouding; optic atrophy; pseudopapilledema	Mental retardation; hearing loss	Hepatosplenomegaly; coarse facial features; skeletal abnormality—claw hand	Autosomal recessive	Urine for dermatan sulfate and heparan sulfate; sulfate assays in white blood cell count, fibroblasts

Neuronal ceroid lipofuscinosis—Batten's disease; Haltia-Santavuori (infantile) disease; Jansky-Bielschowsky (late infantile) disease; Batten's disease (juvenile); Kufs' disease (adult onset)	Severe visual abnormality; retinal hypopigmentation; macula brown; bull's eye maculopathy	Ataxia, hypotonia, microcephaly; intellectual and motor deterioration; seizures, absent visual evoked potential; cataracts	—	Autosomal recessive	Conjunctival biopsy shows granular inclusions; MR shows severe white and gray atrophy
Familial juvenile nephronophthisis (Senior syndrome; renal–retinal dysplasia)	Congenital blindness; sector (mild) retinitis pigmentosa	Rarely mental retardation	Anemia; interstitial nephritis; hepatic fibrosis	Autosomal recessive	Kidney biopsy
Cerebrohepatorenal syndrome (Zellweger's syndrome)	Corneal clouding	Hypotonia, seizures,	Hepatomegaly, renal failure—cysts	Autosomal recessive	Elevated very long chain fatty acids
Spinocerebellar degenerations olivopontocerebellar atrophy (OPCA)	Retinitis pigmentosa; maculopathy	Progressive ataxia; SCA type 1 and type 2	—	Autosomal dominant	—
Hereditary motor and sensory neuropathy	Retinitis pigmentosa	Progressive ataxia; peripheral neuropathy; sometimes deafness	Related to Refsum's disease	Variable	—

MR = magnetic resonance.
Source: Adapted in part from references 13–16 and CA Grant, EC Berson. Treatable forms of retinitis pigmentosa associated with systemic neurological disorders. Int Ophthalmol Clin 2001;41:103–110.

Figure 8-17. This 53 year old had seizures, encephalopathy, and lactic acidosis typical of mitochondrial encephalopathy, lactic acidosis, and stroke-like symptoms (MELAS). A. His ophthalmoscopic examination showed granularity and some mild pigmentary changes in the retina. The pigmentary change was subtle and easy to overlook. The abnormal ERG was helpful in making the diagnosis. The arrows point to small pigment clumps. B. The left eye showed similar changes. C. His ERG showed abnormalities in scotopic waveforms. The top line shows slightly reduced but present oscillatory potentials. The next line shows reduced scotopic white waveform, but the blue scotopic light shows no A-wave and marked diminished B-wave. All of these ERG responses are consistent with rod dysfunction typically seen in RP.

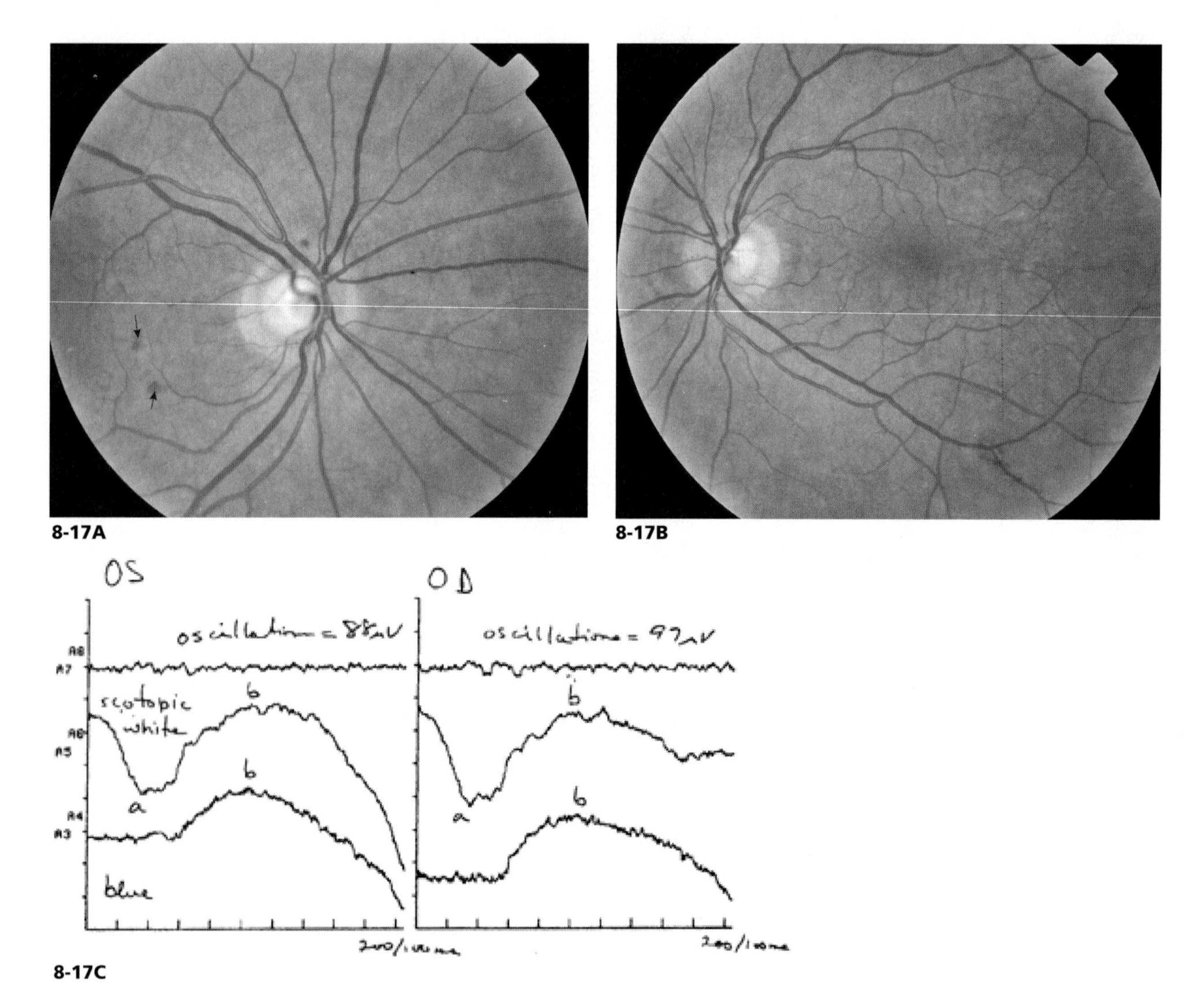

8-17A

8-17B

8-17C

Toxins/Drugs That Induce Pigmentary Changes

Table 8-5. Toxins Producing Pigmentary Changes

Toxin	Use	Features	Associated findings	Evaluation/ treatment
Chloroquine	Antimalarial; treats lupus; lower risk if less than 250 mg/day	Pigment in periphery like retinitis pigmentosa; pigmentary changes around the macula; see bull's eye macula; ring scotoma (see Chapter 10)	Hearing loss	Dose-related defect—watch Amsler's grid; stop drug
Thioridazine (Mellaril)[22]	Antipsychotic	Diffuse, granular (salt and pepper) pigmentary changes	Blurred vision, poor night vision; electroretinogram shows diffusely reduced photopic and scotopic state	Stop drug—appearance may not change, but the progressive retinal changes stabilize
Chlorpromazine (Thorazine)	Antipsychotic	Pigmentary changes if high dose for long time	Has been associated with poor dark adaptation on electroretinogram and delayed visual evoked potential	Stop drug and retinopathy improves
Quinine	Antimalarial	Pigment not prominent; change in optic nerve, vessels	Usually a very large dose	Stop drug; some recovery
Deferoxamine[21]	Iron chelator	Decreased vision, retinal pigment epithelium changes; leads to pigmentation—especially in macula	Usually at high dosages	Stop drug; recovery

Source: Adapted from references 13,20.

Phenothiazines, especially thioridazine (Mellaril), can produce pigmentary changes that are similar to the pigmentary granularity of some forms of RP. This occurs because the phenothiazine accumulates in the melanin of the RPE; it occurs usually in doses of more than 1,000 mg per day and rarely in doses of less than 700 mg per day.[20] Recommendations are to follow the retinal examination in anyone who is taking more than 800 mg per day for signs of retinal toxicity. The pigmentary changes are most frequently in the posterior pole and typically spare the macular region. Frequently, the changes are salt and pepper pigmentary changes.[22] There is no "bull's eye" change, such as is seen in chloroquine maculopathy. Symptoms are similar to RP—night blindness, but blurred vision, drop in visual acuity, and changes in color vision can also be seen. Ophthalmologic examination may show decreased visual acuity. Stopping the drug may improve vision, although in some the pigmentary changes do not reverse themselves.

Recently, anticonvulsants have been reported to cause visual symptoms, visual field constriction, and ERG changes. Although no discrete retinal pigmentary disturbance has been reported, the ERG is useful in following patients who take drugs that may have an affect on retinal function.[23]

Nevi and Melanomas

Choroidal nevi are common incidental findings on examination. Occasionally there is malignant transformation. The appearance of a choroidal nevus is usually a round, flat, pigmented area. Because it is in the choroid, the retinal vessels are easily seen overlying it. Furthermore, there is no disruption of the retina above.

Figure 8-18. A. **A congenital nevus. (Photograph courtesy of Paul Zimmerman, M.D.)** B. **A congenital nevus is a pigmented, usually flat-appearing lesion deep to the retina (hence, you see blood vessels on top of the lesion). The congenital nevus can be photographed and followed.**

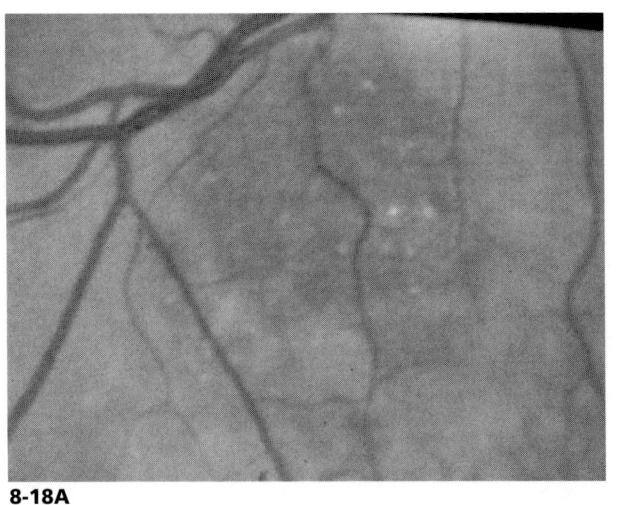

8-18A

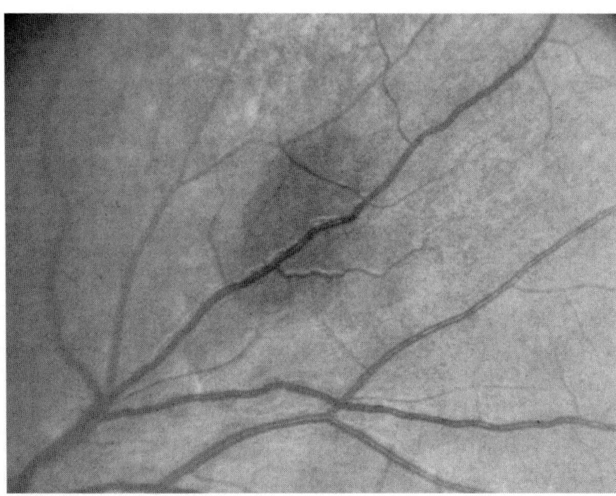

8-18B

Malignant melanoma is the most common malignant, intraocular tumor. Melanomas arise from melanocytes in the choroid and uveal system. Therefore, they can be seen in the iris and inside the eye. Appearance of a malignant melanoma is that of a variably pigmented mass arising from the choroid, protruding into the vitreous. Approximately 70% are pigmented, and 30% are not. Most choroidal melanomas are detected on routine fundus examinations because few patients have symptoms.[24] The fluorescein angiogram shows hyperfluorescence in the early venous phase, and late leakage of the vessels and a multifocal punctate appearance of the late fluorescence.[25]

Figure 8-19. A. **A malignant melanoma showing pigmentary changes not far from the disc. The arrows outline the extent of the melanoma.** B. **Some melanomas are not pigmented, but look elevated and white. The arrows outline the limit of the melanoma. Again, you know that it is beneath the retina because you see the retinal vessels overlying the melanoma.**

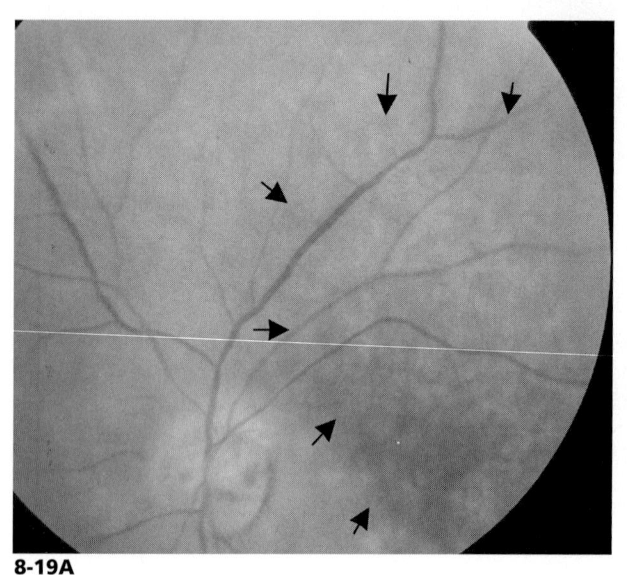

8-19A

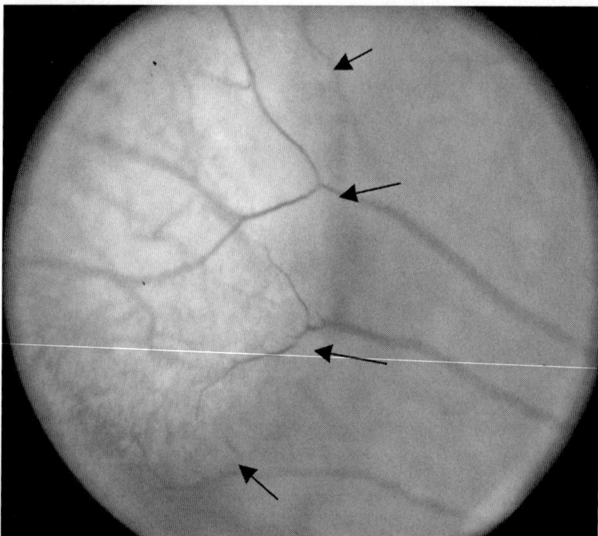

8-19B

Table 8-6. Differential Diagnosis of Choroidal Melanoma

Choroidal nevus
Metastatic carcinoma
Choroidal osteoma
Choroidal hemangioma
Hypertrophy of the retinal pigment epithelium
Intraocular hemorrhages of the choroid

Source: Adapted from reference 25.

The importance of recognizing malignant melanoma is that patients die from this tumor if not treated.

Practical Viewing Essentials

1. Sometimes indirect illumination makes the black spot more visible.
2. Notice the relationship of pigment to blood vessels. Is the pigment clumped around the vessels, or does the pigment lie under the vessel?
3. Sometimes to see pigment you have to look in the periphery.
4. If you think there is RP, look for other neurologic findings.

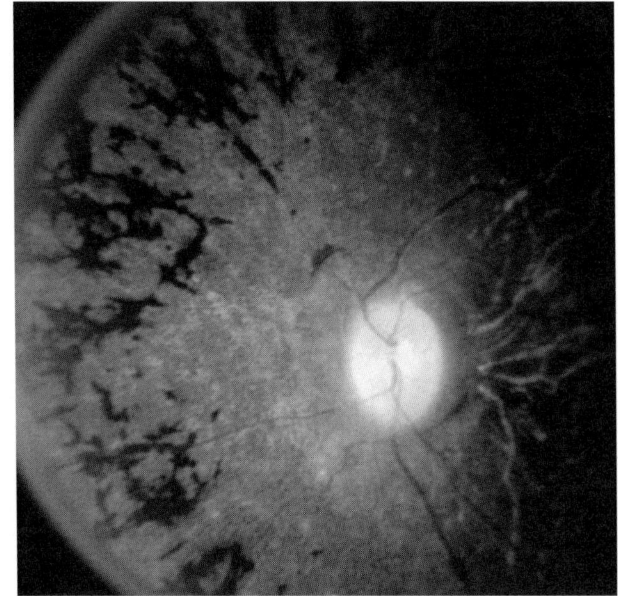

8-20

References

1. Gowers W. A Manual and Atlas of Medical Ophthalmoscopy. London: J & A Churchill, 1879:111–112.
2. Cogan D. The Neurology of the Visual System. Springfield, IL: Thomas, 1967.
3. Mann I. Developmental Abnormalities of the Eye. London: British Medical Association, 1957.
4. Weleber RG, Gregory-Evans K. Retinitis pigmentosa and allied disorders. In Ryan SJ (ed), Retina. St. Louis: Mosby, 2001;362–460.
5. Pinckers A, Cruysberg JRM, Renier WO. Delayed myelination of the optic nerve and pseudo optic atrophy of Beauvieux. Neuroophthalmol 1993;13:165–170.
6. Apple DJ, Rabb MF, Walsh PM. Congenital anomalies of the optic disc. Surv Ophthalmol 1982;27:3–41.
7. Brodsky MC, Buckley EG, McConkie-Rosell A. The case of the gray optic disc! Surv Ophthalmol 1989;33:367–372.
8. DePotter P, Shields CL, Eagle RC, et al. Malignant melanoma of the optic nerve. Arch Ophthalmol 1996;114:608–612.
9. Erzurum SA, Jampol LM, Territo C, O'Grady R. Primary malignant melanoma of the optic nerve simulating a melanocytoma. Arch Ophthalmol 1992;110: 684–686.
10. Joffe L, Shields JA, Osher RH, Gass JD. Clinical and follow-up studies of melanocytomas of the optic disc. Ophthalmology 1979;86(6):1067–1083.
11. Brown GC, Shields JA. Tumors of the optic nerve head. Surv Ophthalmol 1985;29(4):239–264.
12. Margo CE, Hamed LM. Ocular syphilis. Surv Ophthalmol 1992;37:203–220.
13. Weleber RG. In SJ Ryan (ed), Retina (2nd ed). St. Louis: Mosby, 1994;335–466.
14. Pagon R. Retinitis pigmentosa. Surv Ophthalmol 1988;33:137–177.
15. Drack AV, Traboulsi EI. Systemic associations of pigmentary retinopathy. Int Ophthalmol Clin 1991;31: 35–59.
16. Kelly J, Maumenee IH. Hereditary macular diseases. Int Ophthalmol Clin 1999;39(4):83–115.
17. Lynch SG, Digre K, Rose JW. Usher's syndrome and multiple sclerosis. Review of an individual with Usher's syndrome with a multiple sclerosis-like illness. J Neuroophthalmol 1994;14(1):34–37.
18. Dimauro S, Moraes CT. Mitochondrial encephalomyopathies. Arch Neurol 1993;50:1197–1208.
19. Kerrison JB, Biousse V, Newman NJ. Retinopathy of NARP syndrome. Arch Ophthalmol 2000;118:298–299.
20. Grant WM. Toxicology of the Eye. Springfield, IL: Thomas, 1974;1005–1006.
21. Mehta AM, Engstrom RE, Kreiger AE. Deferoxamine-associated retinopathy after subcutaneous injection. Am J Ophthalmol 1994;118:260–261.
22. Shah G, Auerbach DB, Augsburger JJ, Savino PJ. Acute thioridazine retinopathy. Arch Ophthalmol 1998;116:826–827.
23. Miller NR. Using the electroretinogram to detect and monitor retinal toxicity of anticonvulsants. Neurology 2000;55:333–334.
24. Grin JM, Grant-Kels JM, Grin CM, et al. Ocular melanomas and melanocytic lesions of the eye. J Am Acad Dermatol 1998;38:716–730.
25. Reinke MH, Gragoudas ES. Unusual hemorrhagic lesions masquerading as choroidal melanoma. Int Ophthalmol Clin 1997;37:135–147.

9 What Is That in the Retina?

Apart from the vessels and the optic disc, the changes in the retina . . . are those which are special to certain general diseases. . . . The only common feature which these morbid states possess, is the development in the retina of haemorrhages and white spots and patches.

William Gowers[1]

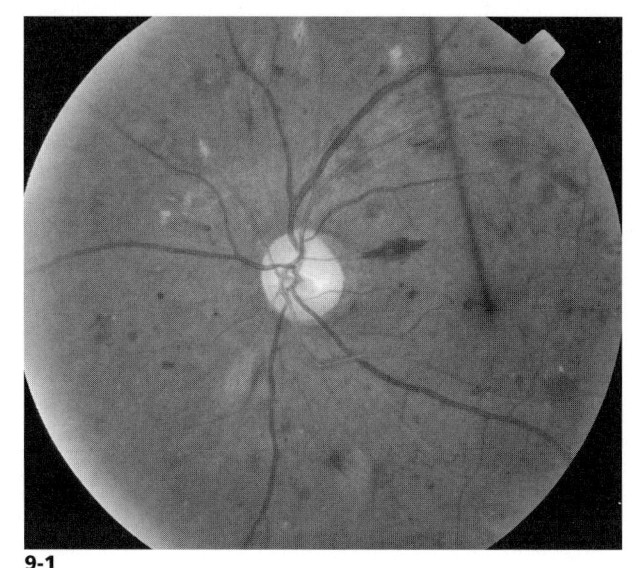
9-1

Figure 9-1. The retina has only a few ways to respond to insults—white spots, hemorrhage, pigmentary changes, neovascularization, and edema. Here is typical diabetic retinopathy.

There is no other place in the human body where the overall health of the arteries and veins can be observed more easily than the posterior pole of the eye. Not only have we seen that viewing the optic nerve can tell us a lot about the neurologic condition of a person, but we see in this chapter that viewing the retina is essential to the examination of the general vascular status of a person. Nowhere else in the body can we be as close to viewing small arterioles and capillaries. Aside from the changes seen in the fundus with two very common conditions, diabetes and hypertension, there are changes in the fundus that can help make the diagnosis of infections, genetic disorders, and autoimmune diseases. The retina has only a few ways to respond to insults that are vascular, infectious, degenerative, or genetic; armed with this knowledge, we can guide our viewing to look for patterns of hemorrhage (Chapter 7), white spots (Chapter 6), pigment changes (Chapter 8), neovascularization, and edema. In this chapter we explore common forms of retinal disease related to metabolic conditions (diabetes), vascular disease (hypertension), infections, inflammations, and toxin to the retina.

Remember that when we view the fundus with the direct ophthalmoscope we see only small areas of the retina. For a comprehensive view of the retina, the indirect method of ophthalmoscopy must be performed. General neurologists, internists, family practitioners, obstetricians, and otolaryngologists do not have access to this equipment or the skills to perform the examination. Therefore, there are certain things we can look for in the retina with the direct ophthalmoscope, but if we suspect retinal changes due to systemic disease, a full evaluation including an indirect ophthalmoscopic examination and slit-lamp biomicroscopy by an ophthalmologist or optometrist are suggested.

How the Retina Responds to Injury

The responses of the retina to injury are white spots, hemorrhages, neovascularization, and edema (cloudy swelling). The retina's response to *ischemia* from any cause includes infarcts, cotton-wool spots, hemorrhage, and angiogenesis or neovascularization. The stimulus for angiogenesis can come from ischemia, inflammation, or tumor. Neovascularization is not a unique retinal process, but because of the eye's vascularity and easy accessibility for viewing, it has been well studied. The steps for angiogenesis and the growth factors in the eye have been outlined in detail.[2] A classic example of angiogenesis is seen in proliferative diabetic retinopathy. However, other vascular, inflammatory, and infectious causes have been associated with "proliferation" of new blood vessels. These blood vessels are often weak, fragile, and bleed easily. The bleeding sets up further ischemic changes, and this cycle can end in blindness. The most common causes of retinal neovascularization are diabetes, macular degeneration, retinopathy of prematurity, central and branch retinal vein occlusion, and sickle cell disease.[3]

Figure 9-2. Typical neovascularization from proliferation of blood vessels: Look for it around the disc (A) **and distal to the disc** (B)**. Any process that causes ischemia to the retina can result in neovascularization.**

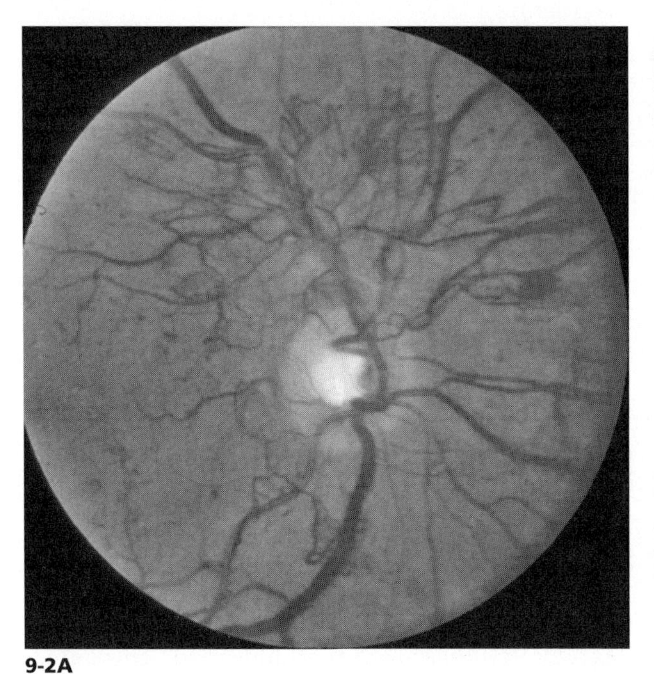

9-2A

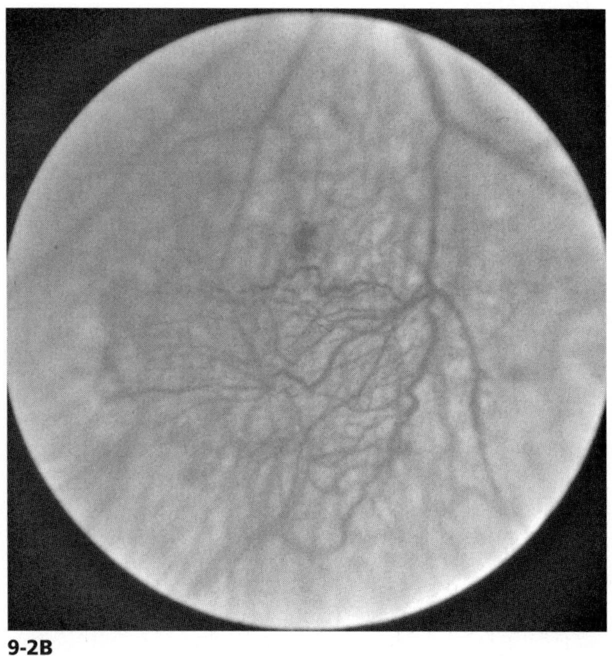

9-2B

What conditions should you be able to recognize in the retina? The two most important systemic conditions that we should recognize when viewing the retina are changes associated with diabetes and hypertension.

Table 9-1. Diseases Associated with Proliferation of Blood Vessels/Angiogenesis/Neovascularization of the Retina

Ischemia	Ocular disease	Inflammatory	Infectious	Genetic
Sickle cell hemoglobinopathy	Macular degeneration	Sarcoid	Toxoplasmosis	Incontinentia pigmenti
Eales' disease	Retinal detachment	Retinal vasculitis; systemic lupus erythematosus	Syphilis	Retinitis pigmentosa
Diabetes		Uveitis	Cytomegalovirus	Inherited retinal venous beading
Branch retinal vein occlusion		Birdshot retinopathy	Epstein-Barr virus	Retinoschisis
Branch retinal artery occlusion		Acute retinal necrosis	Herpes viruses	
Retinal embolization		Cocaine abuse	Lyme disease	
Retinopathy of prematurity		Eales' disease		
Hyperviscosity syndromes		Multiple sclerosis		
Ocular ischemic syndrome from any cause (carotid insufficiency, arteritis, aortic arch syndrome)		Tumors		
Carotid cavernous fistula				
Buckling operation for retinal detachment				
Takayasu's disease				

Source: Adapted from references 2,3.

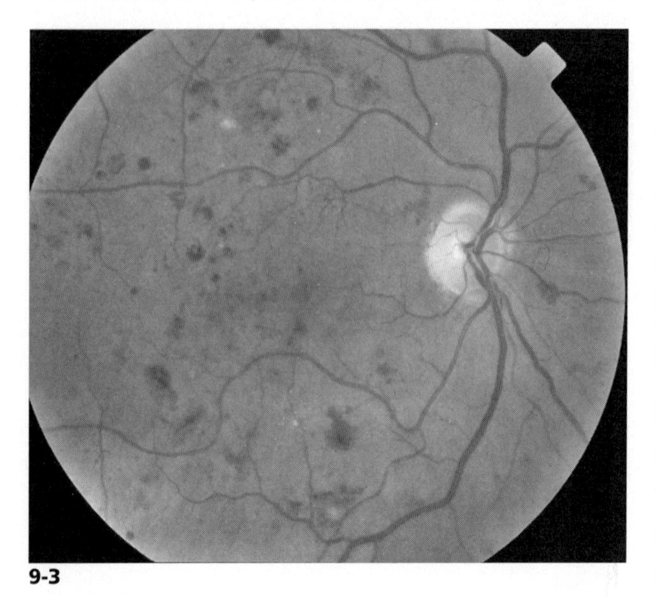

9-3

Metabolic Retinopathies

DIABETIC RETINOPATHY

Figure 9-3. Diabetic retinopathy is the most common treatable retinopathy that all physicians encounter. Most of the pathology is out of the viewing of the normal fundus examination without dilation of the pupil. Dilate the patient with diabetes to view changes of diabetic retinopathy.

Sixteen million people are known to have diabetes mellitus in the United States; however, an additional 5 million people who have the condition go undiagnosed. Diabetes is the fifth leading cause of death in developed countries of the world. The prevalence is expected to almost double in the world in the next 10 years.[4] Diabetic retinopathy causes approximately 85% of the blindness associated with diabetes, and diabetic retinopathy is the leading cause of blindness in the United States in people younger than age 60.[5] Therefore, early recognition and treatment are essential for successful therapy of diabetic retinopathy.

Retinopathy is seen in approximately 50% of patients with type I diabetes within 10 years and 75% within 20 years. Approximately one-fourth of patients with type I diabetes develop the proliferative form.[5] In an ophthalmologist's practice, most of the patients have type II diabetes because it is so much more common.

Because diabetic retinopathy is a treatable condition, screening for the disease is very important. Sussman showed that 9% of ophthalmologists, 33% of diabetologists, and 52% of internists missed the diagnosis of proliferative diabetic retinopathy.[6] The American Academy of Ophthalmology has endorsed that individuals 10–30 years of age who have had the diagnosis of diabetes for more than 5 years should have a baseline dilated ophthalmoscopic examination. Individuals older than 30 years diagnosed with diabetes should have a baseline dilated examination at the time of diagnosis. Those individuals older than 30 years are probably type II diabetics, and may have had the disease for a prolonged period of time before diagnosis was made. Thereafter, all groups should be evaluated with a dilated examination once each year.[7]

What causes the changes in the retina? The answers are hypoxia, changes in the blood vessels, and changes in the blood itself. *Hypoxia* develops by way of many factors, including increased levels of hemoglobin A1C. Normally, hemoglobin A1C is only 3–6% of the total hemoglobin. In diabetes, the concentration of hemoglobin A1C increases to 10–25%. Higher levels of hemoglobin A1C block the oxygen-releasing capacity of 2,3-diphosphoglycerate. When this happens, oxygen release is impaired and retinal hypoxia occurs. Initially, the retina may autoregulate and increase blood flow; later, this regulatory function is lost. Further hypoxia occurs when cellular glucose is converted to sorbitol (a polyol) within the cell. This leads to increased osmotic pressure and cellular edema. The edema leads to poor oxygen diffusion and retinal hypoxia. Sorbitol, as well as hyperglycemia, increases free radicals and weakens capillary wall integrity, which leads to hemorrhages, edema, and hard exudates. With time, diabetes also affects the basement membrane of the capillaries, causing thickening and narrowing of the blood vessels, which then decreases blood flow and further contributes to hypoxia. Because the arterial side is affected first, microaneurysms develop in capillaries near the underperfused areas of retina. In addition, the retina's response to hypoxia is to secrete angiogenic growth factors,[8] which stimulate new vessel growth and lead to more microaneurysms and venous-arterial shunts. Also, pericyte death may lead to endothelial proliferation and neovascularization. The shunts are makeshift vessels with no true underlying laminated vascular wall structure. Thus, they are weak and bleed frequently. Finally, the blood itself in diabetic patients is somewhat hypercoagulable, with increased fibrinogen, thromboxane A2, and other proteins, leading to aggregation of red cells and platelets. Occlusion of already damaged small vessels leads to cotton-wool spots, arteriolar occlusion, and further hypoxic damage to the retina.

Diabetic retinopathy, therefore, has many clinical features. *Microaneurysms* are dilations in the capillaries and appear as small, smooth, sharp red dots. The number of microaneurysms is important to diabetic retinal specialists. We compared microaneurysms with hemorrhages in Chapter 7, Figure 7-3. Aneurysms occur near areas of hypoperfusion and are best detected by fluorescein angiography.

Figure 9-4. Diabetic retinopathy typically has microaneurysms, hemorrhages, and cotton-wool spots. A. **Here you see aneurysms (*arrows*) that are large enough to be seen easily.** B. **The corresponding fluorescein angiogram shows the "pin-points" of fluorescence (*arrows*), which characterize aneurysms. You can appreciate that there are many, many points of light present on the fluorescein that you cannot see in the fundus photograph** (A). **This is very typical of aneurysms and shows the value and importance of fluorescein angiography in looking at patients with diabetic retinopathy.**

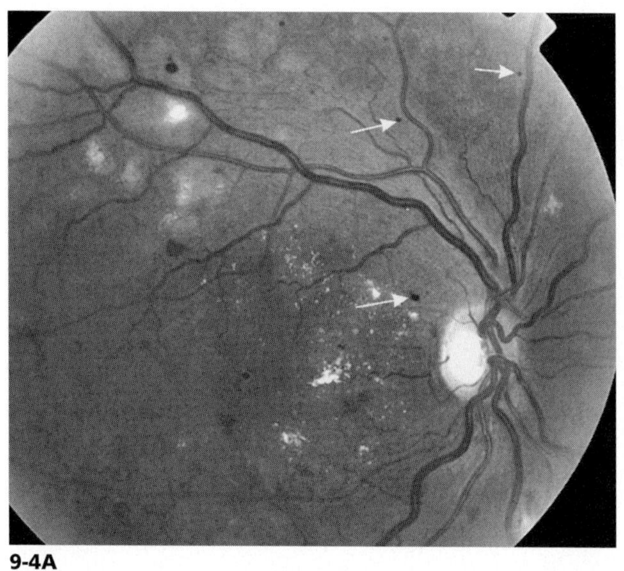

9-4A

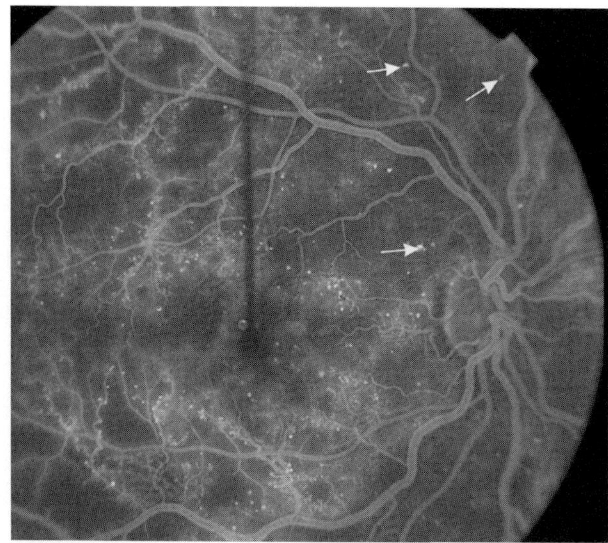

9-4B

Hemorrhages in diabetes are *dot and blot* in the middle retinal layers and *flame-shaped* in the nerve fiber layer. A large hemorrhage from rupture of new fragile vessels—preretinal or into the vitreous—automatically suggests neovascularization and is more severe.

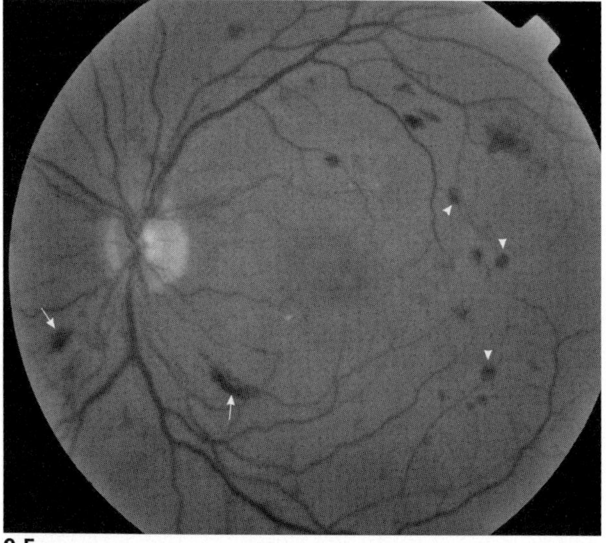

9-5

Figure 9-5. Typical hemorrhages with diabetes, including flame-shaped nerve fiber layer hemorrhages (*arrows*) and dot-and-blot type (*arrowheads*).

Retinal edema is caused by fluid accumulation from leaky vessels in the retina. The edema appears as a gray-white color when viewed with the direct ophthalmoscope. However, subtle edema may not be apparent with this method, and more sophisticated techniques are required to see macular edema. Intraretinal edema usually resolves, but when it remains for a prolonged period, a hard exudate (lipoprotein deposit) may appear.

Figure 9-6. A. **Retinal edema is severe in the macula. Around the retina are lipoproteinaceous deposits.** B. **Macular edema alone commonly occurs with diabetic retinopathy and is associated with decreased vision. Visual acuity loss is the rule in patients with these kinds of changes in the macula. (Photograph courtesy of Paul Zimmerman, M.D.)**

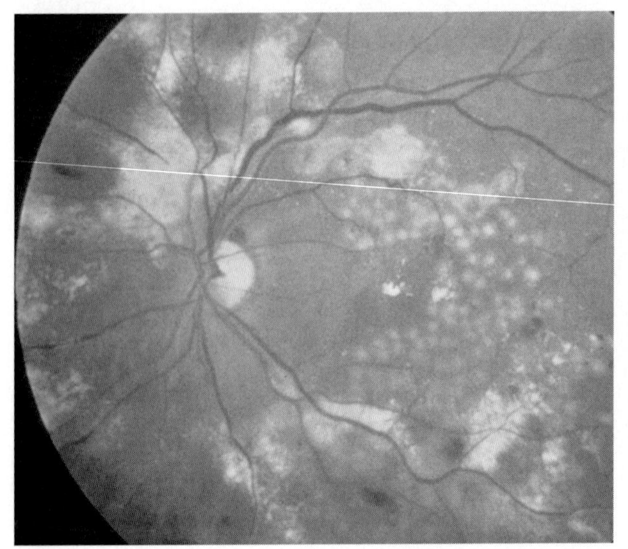

9-6A

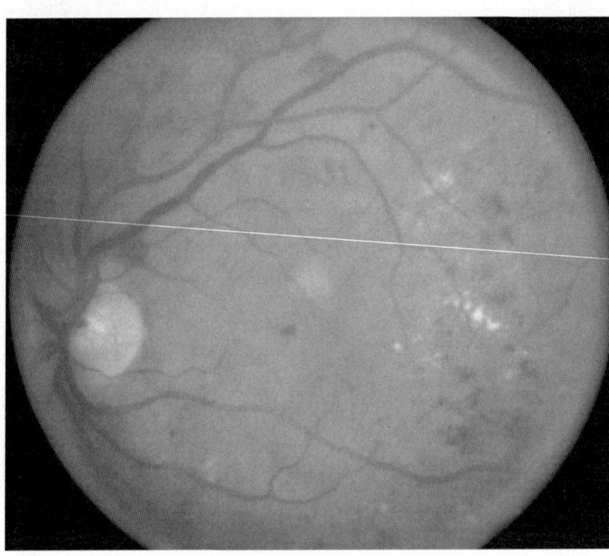

9-6B

Hard exudates , which are lipoprotein deposits in the outer plexiform layer, appear as whitish-yellow spots with definite borders. These persist for months or years and seem to occur after edema. The amount of retina covered by hard exudates is important to specialists.

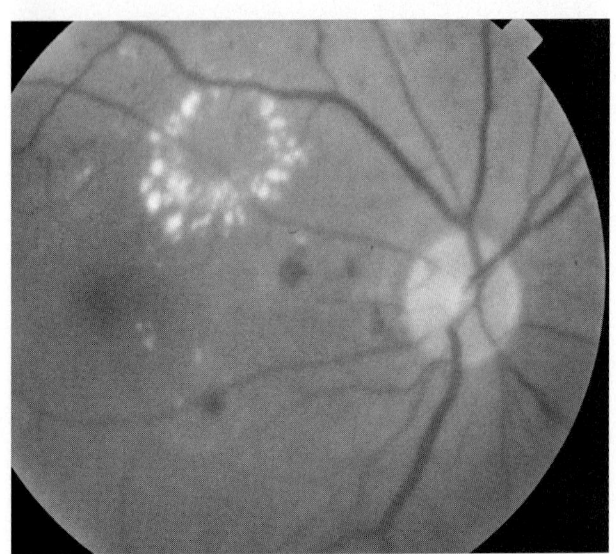

9-7

Figure 9-7. This hard exudate developed after retinal edema. The borders are distinct. (Photograph courtesy of Marie Acierno, M.D.)

Soft exudates, or *cotton-wool spots*, are larger than hard exudates. Although dramatic, cotton-wool spots are the least significant predictors of progression to proliferative diabetic retinopathy.[9]

Figure 9-8. Cotton-wool spots (*arrows*) are frequently present in diabetic retinopathy. In this photograph, not only do you see cotton-wool spots, but there are also new vessels forming on the disc.

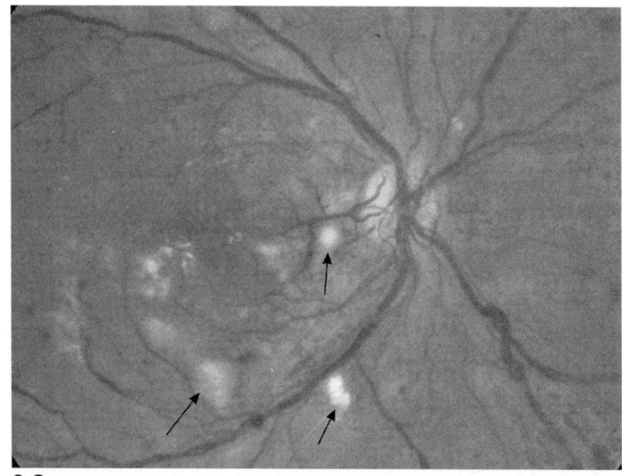

9-8

Arterial narrowing, sheathing of arterial vessels, and *arterial occlusion*, which may appear as thin white threads where the arteries should be, are important signs; frequently occlusion is not seen unless a fluorescein angiogram is performed.

Venous dilation and beading are caused by increased retinal blood flow. Dilated veins are an early but variable sign of diabetic retinopathy. As the disease progresses, veins become more tortuous, with constricted areas followed by dilated areas, hence the term *beading*. Venous beading is thought to be the most significant predictor of retinopathy progressing to the proliferative stage.[9] Often, large venous loops are seen within areas of capillary nonperfusion. Venous sheathing, perivenous exudates, and narrowing may also be seen.[10]

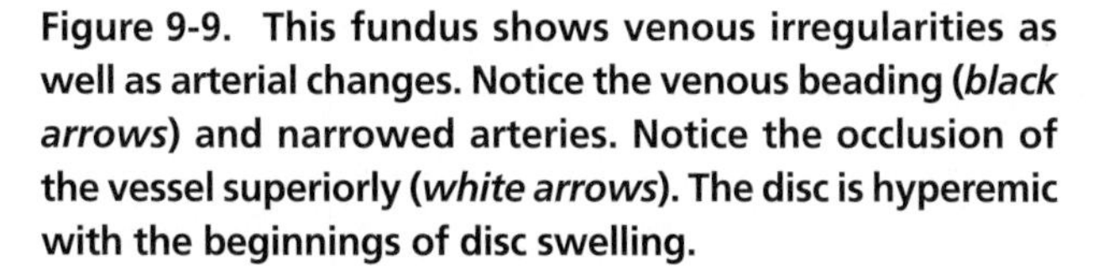

Figure 9-9. This fundus shows venous irregularities as well as arterial changes. Notice the venous beading (*black arrows*) and narrowed arteries. Notice the occlusion of the vessel superiorly (*white arrows*). The disc is hyperemic with the beginnings of disc swelling.

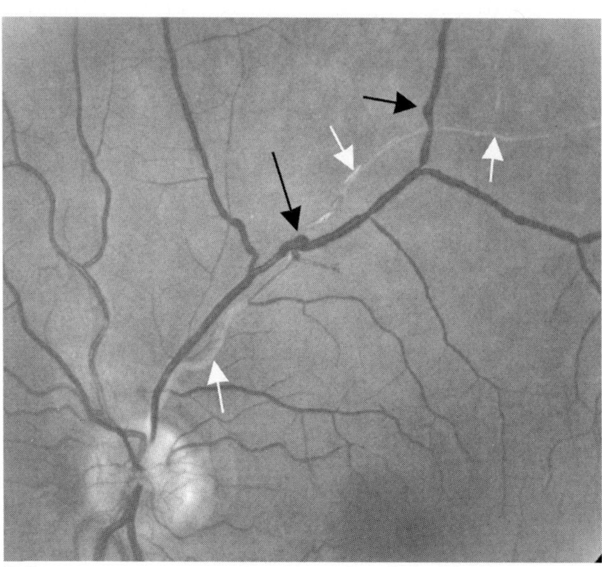

9-9

Intraretinal microvascular abnormalities (IRMA) is a term used to describe areas of capillary nonperfusion next to areas of capillary dilation. These are areas of tortuous intraretinal vasculature. The term is meant to encompass dilated capillaries and neovascularization, because sometimes you cannot tell them apart.[11] These used to be interpreted as "shunt" vessels, dilated capillaries, or intraretinal neovascularization. The term *IRMA* was chosen at the Airlie House Classification Congress.[10] IRMA is the closure of the capillaries, leading to ischemic changes. The amount of area with IRMA is important because it is the amount of IRMA that frequently determines the severity of diabetic retinopathy. These areas are associated with cotton-wool spots. Sometimes it is difficult to distinguish IRMA from neovascularization.

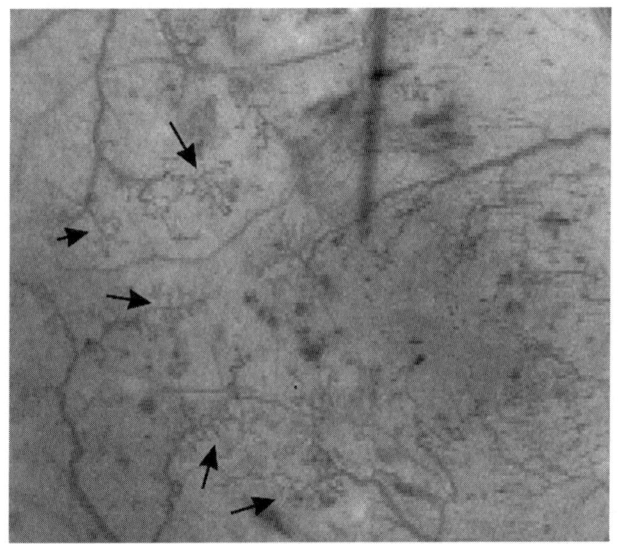

9-10A

Figure 9-10. Dilated, tortuous small blood vessels make up IRMA. Sometimes it is difficult to distinguish IRMA from neovascularization. IRMA does not include neovascularization on the surface of the retina—it has to be intraretinal. The amount of the retina that has IRMA is what is important. A. **Intraretinal microvascular abnormalities: IRMA. These look like dilated capillaries or neovascularization (*arrows*). Can you identify more areas of IRMA on this photograph?** B. **The arrows point to areas of IRMA. The amount of IRMA seen in the retina is one indicator of the severity of the retinopathy.** C. **The black arrow points to IRMA and the white arrows point to dot hemorrhages. The IRMA areas appear to be more filigree work.**

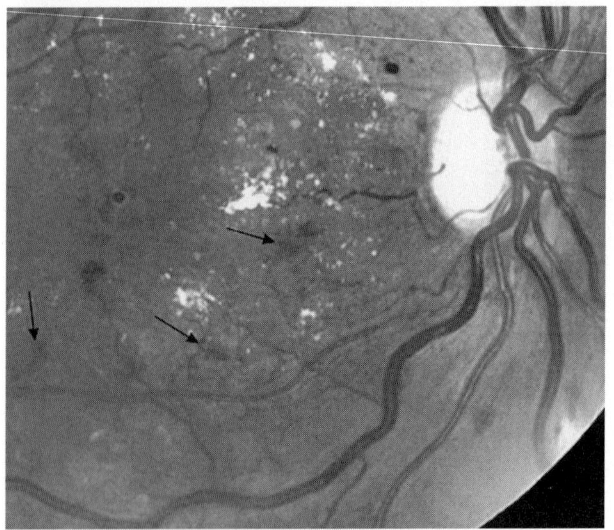

9-10B

9-10C

Neovascularization and *fibrous proliferation* are the hallmarks of proliferative diabetic retinopathy. This really is a process in which the vasogenic factors respond to hypoxia, leading to new vessel development. The new vessels are structurally defective and therefore leak fluid (edema, a true exudate) and red cells (hemorrhages). This in turn stimulates connective tissue growth. Retinal experts have labeled two types of neovascularization: NVD (new vessels on the disc) and NVE (new vessels elsewhere in the retina). What is the difference? The importance of knowing NVD and NVE is that it guides your viewing—look at the disc, look at the retina. If you see neovascularization, these patients need immediate attention by a retinal specialist.

Figure 9-11. Neovascular fronds can be present around the disc and distally in the retina: here we see neovascularization elsewhere (A) **and neovascularization of the disc** (B).

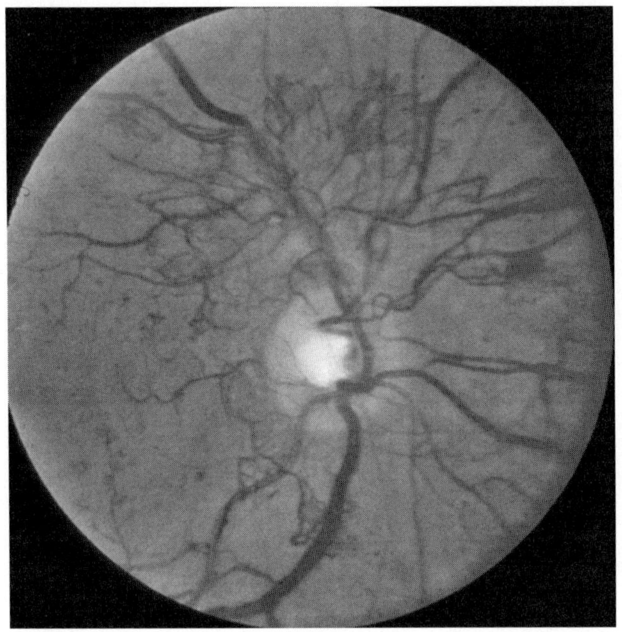

9-11A

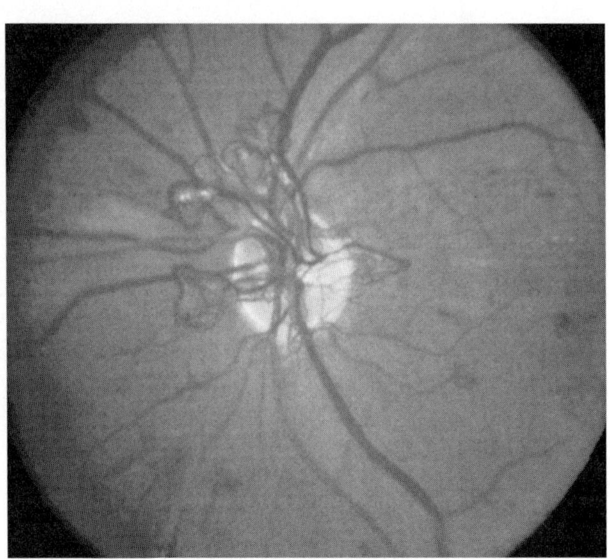

9-11B

Figure 9-12. A. **New vessels on the disc.** B. **New vessels elsewhere. (Photograph courtesy of Marie Acierno, M.D.)**

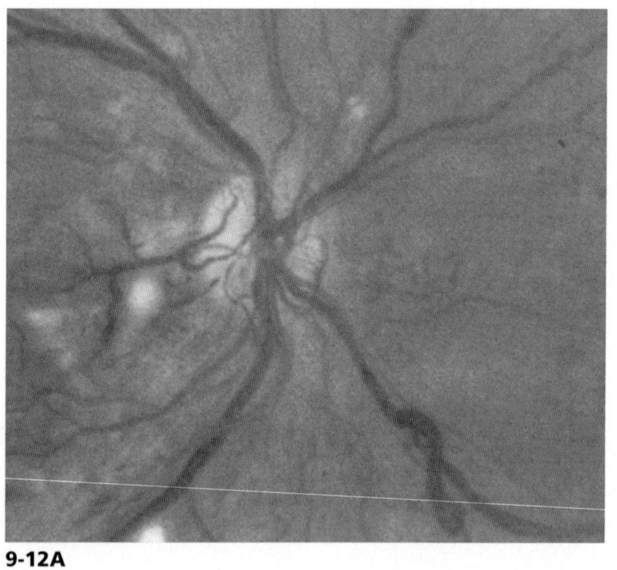

9-12A

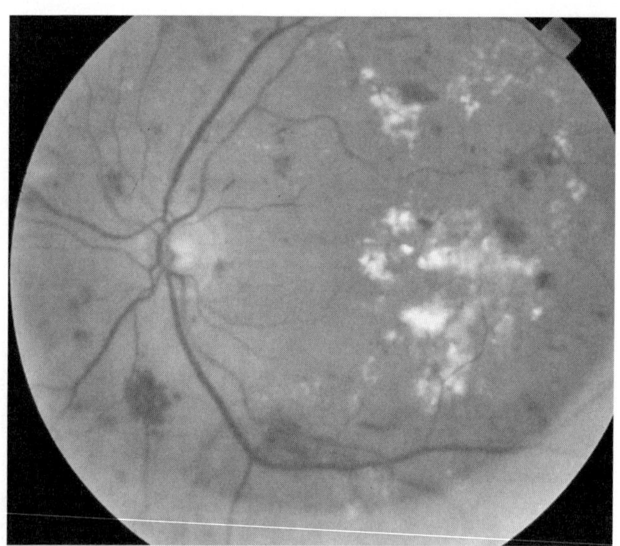

9-12B

Table 9-2. Distinguishing Neovascularization of the Disc from Neovascularization Elsewhere

Characteristic	Neovascularization of the disc (NVD) (see Figure 9-12A)	Neovascularization elsewhere (NVE) (see Figure 9-12B)
Location	Within 1 disc diameter of the disc	The rest of the retina—not around the disc
Arterial system affected	Peripapillary artery system	Arterioles from the retinal arteries
Site of neovascularization	Vessels grow from front of retina or disc into the vitreous	Vessels grow at the proximal end of a non-perfused area
Fluorescein angiography	Large areas of nonperfusion around the disc	Areas of nonperfusion around the neovascularization

Retinal detachment is the end result of neovascularization followed by fibrous proliferation, which creates traction on the retina. This process is frequently accompanied by recurrent hemorrhages in the vitreous.

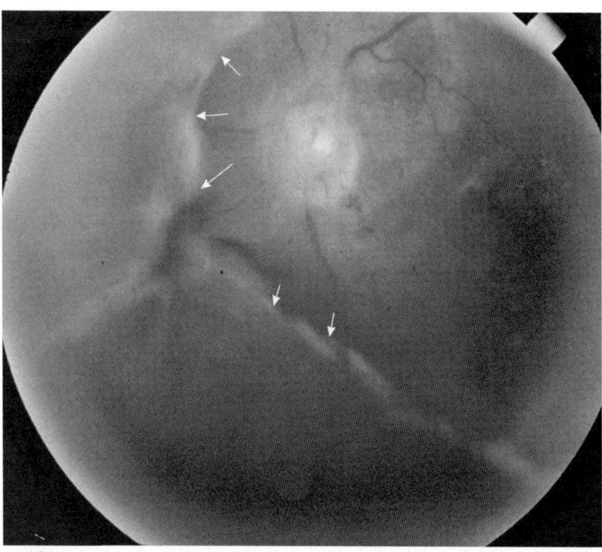

9-13

Figure 9-13. We try to avoid retinal detachment because profound vision loss usually accompanies this late proliferate stage. The arrows mark out the areas of detachment. (Photograph courtesy of Marie Acierno, M.D.)

Disc swelling is also important to consider in looking at diabetic retinopathy. This may involve ischemic changes of the disc.

Retinal specialists have also divided background diabetic retinopathy into two types: nonproliferative and proliferative. The reason for the division has to do with the prognosis and treatment of the proliferative type and the significance of this stage. Nonproliferative retinopathy has been divided into three stages: mild, moderate, and severe.

The classification most often used in studies on diabetic retinopathy is based on the Airlie House classification set up in 1968 during a consensus conference at Airlie House in Warrenton, Virginia.[12] This classification has been modified somewhat by the Early Treatment Diabetic Retinopathy Study (ETDRS).[10] The Airlie House and ETDRS classifications set up specified viewing fields around the disc, around the macula, temporal to the macula, and above and below the disc.

The ETDRS and Airlie House classifications then provide photographic definitions of what constitutes each characteristic evaluated within each field (e.g., microaneurysms, hard exudates, venous abnormalities, neovascularization, hemorrhage). For study purposes, they grade how many of each there are in each field to assess the effect of various treatments. Furthermore, they use photographic fields—the original Airlie House photographs and new photographs—to define each stage. Frequently, retinal specialists further subdivide patients into even finer classifications, such as microaneurysms only and subdivisions of moderate and severe based on photographs.[13,14] What most clinicians need to know is that we can recognize some of these findings, and if we see any of them, the patient should be referred for a dilated examination by a specialist.

Figure 9.14. A. Mild nonproliferative diabetic retinopathy: microaneurysms, hemorrhages, occasional soft/hard exudates. B. Moderate nonproliferative diabetic retinopathy: microaneurysms, hemorrhages, soft exudates, and early IRMA. C. Many microaneurysms, hemorrhages, large IRMA, arteriole occlusion, venous beading, and beginning areas of nonperfusion on fluorescein. D. Proliferative diabetic retinopathy shows neovascularization of the disc, macula, or both; hemorrhages into the vitreous; and, when severe, retinal detachment. (Photograph courtesy of Marie Acierno, M.D.)

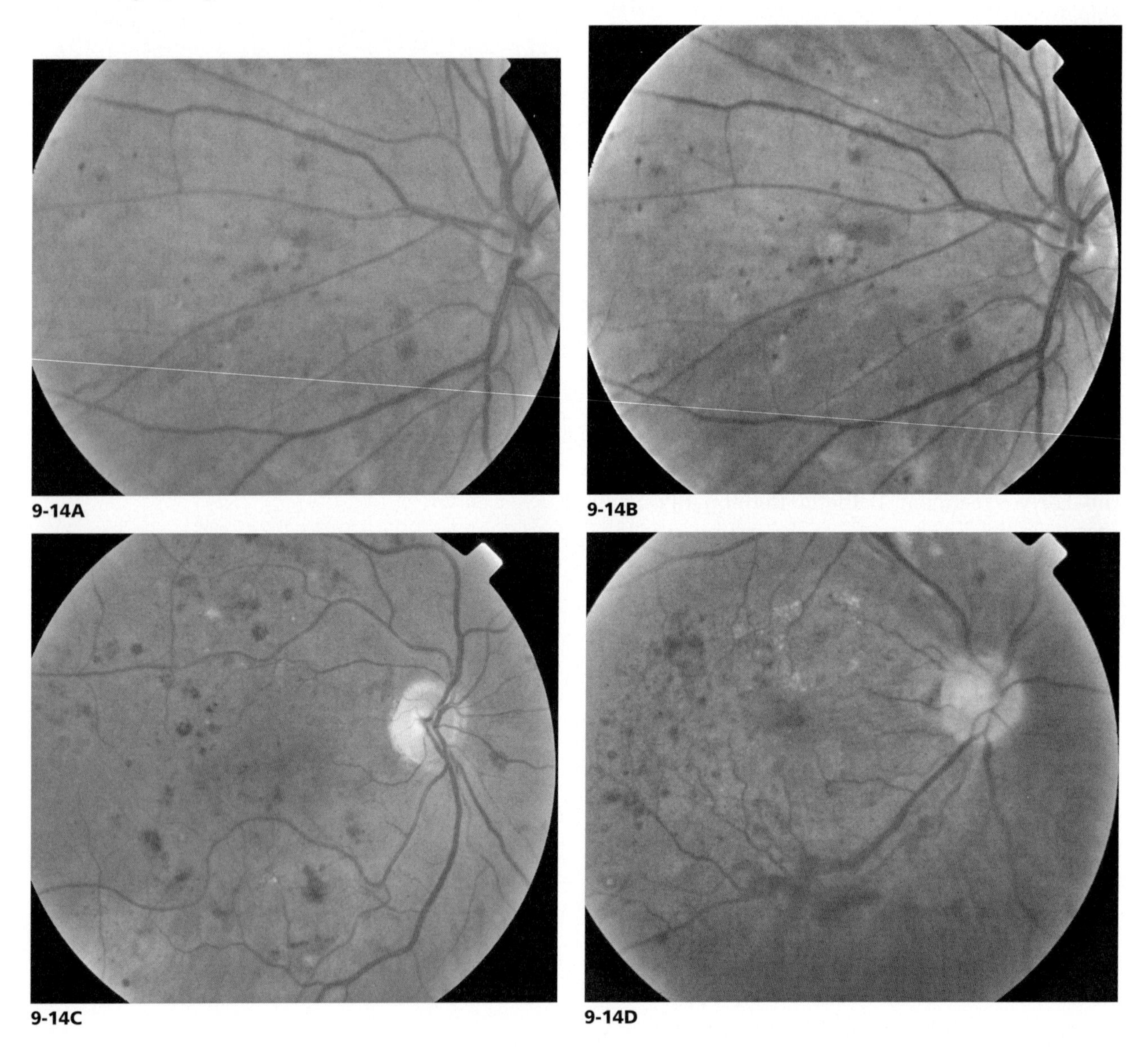

Table 9-3. Nonproliferative Background Retinopathy Classification and Findings*

Mild	Severe
Microaneurysms	Many microaneurysms, hemorrhages
Hemorrhages	Large IRMA
Occasional (rare) soft/hard exudates	Arteriole occlusion
Moderate	Venous beading
Microaneurysms	Areas of nonperfusion on fluorescein
Hemorrhages	Proliferative diabetic retinopathy
Soft exudates	Neovascularization of the disc, macula, or both; hemorrhage into the vitreous; retinal detachment
Early IRMA	

IRMA = intraretinal microvascular abnormalities.
*As classified by the Early Treatment Diabetic Retinopathy Study, and based also on the Airlie House Classification.
Source: Adapted from reference 5.

Table 9-4. Stages of Nonproliferative Background Diabetic Retinopathy

Severity	Microaneurysm	Hemorrhage	Soft/hard exudate	Intraretinal microvascular abnormalities	Arteriolar occlusion	Venous beading	Nonperfusion
Mild	X	X	X	—	—	—	—
Moderate	XX	XX	XX	X	—	—	—
Severe	XXX	XXX	XXX	XXX	XX	XX	XX

X = present; XX = more frequent; XXX = very frequent.
Source: Adapted from reference 15.

The Diabetic Retinopathy Study looked at what clinical features are seen that predict severe vision loss with diabetes.

Table 9-5. Risk Factors for Vision Loss with Diabetic Retinopathy (from Diabetic Retinopathy Study)

New blood vessels on the optic nerve or within 1-disc diameter (NVD)—strongest predictor
Presence of microaneurysms and hemorrhage
Presence of vitreous or preretinal hemorrhage
Any neovascularization (e.g., intraretinal microvascular abnormalities)—especially severe

Source: Adapted from reference 16.

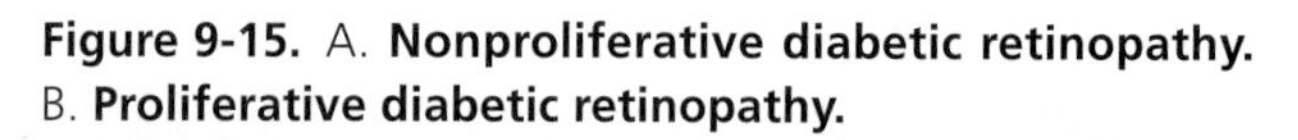

Figure 9-15. A. **Nonproliferative diabetic retinopathy.** B. **Proliferative diabetic retinopathy.**

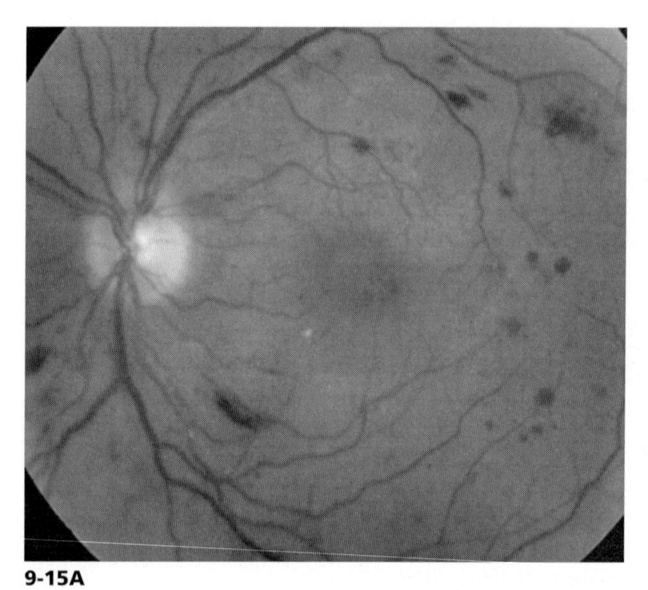

9-15A

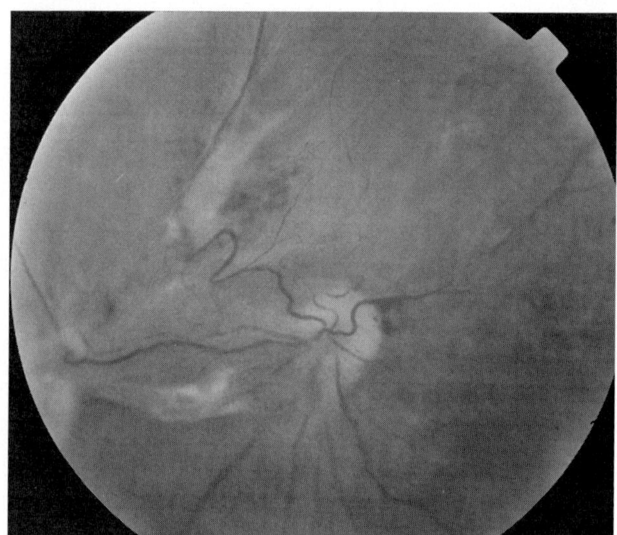

9-15B

Table 9-6. Differences between Nonproliferative and Proliferative Diabetic Retinopathy

Characteristics	Nonproliferative (see Figure 9-15A)	Proliferative (see Figure 9-15B)
Age and years of diabetes	Virtually all have some type of retinopathy by 15 yrs of onset of the disease	Diabetes present for at least 10 yrs; usually longer duration
Type of diabetes	Type I and type II	Occurs in 25–50% of type I diabetes patients after 15–20 yrs (more common in type I than II); occurs in type II patients who are insulin dependent rather than diet
Features seen	Hemorrhages, microaneurysms, cotton-wool spots, hard exudates, capillary dilation, intraretinal microvascular abnormalities	All the features of nonproliferative diabetes + neovascularization, macular edema, vaso-occlusion, fibrous tissue growth
Visual acuity	Fine unless there is macular edema	Decreased by macular edema and vitreal hemorrhages
Fluorescein angiogram	Areas of nonperfusion; no new vessels	Large areas of nonperfusion; new vessels leaking, staining
Treatment	Tight control of diabetes; early laser treatment of moderate to severe; watch blood pressure	Tight control of diabetes; laser coagulation; watch blood pressure
Prognosis	<3% blind at 5 yrs	NVE better than NVD; poor prognosis if untreated
Complications	Proliferative retinopathy	Neovascular glaucoma
		Retinal detachment

If a person had four risk factors, prognosis was very poor; with three risk factors, the patient was still at serious risk of severe vision loss. Interestingly, the presence of urine protein was the best systemic predictor of vision loss.[17]

Macular edema can occur in nonproliferative or proliferative diabetic retinopathy. The incidence is approximately 20% in those with younger onset.[18] Macular edema is caused by fluid collecting under the macula. The patient complains of decreased vision. It may be slight (not clinically significant) or severe (clinically significant). An examiner may see thick, cloudy, or grayish color in the macula, which would correspond to edema. *Cystoid macular edema* refers to a "petal" or "pebble" shape in the macula. Subtle forms of edema can only be seen with slit-lamp biomicroscopy and a contact lens. Fluorescein angiography may also detect the edema.

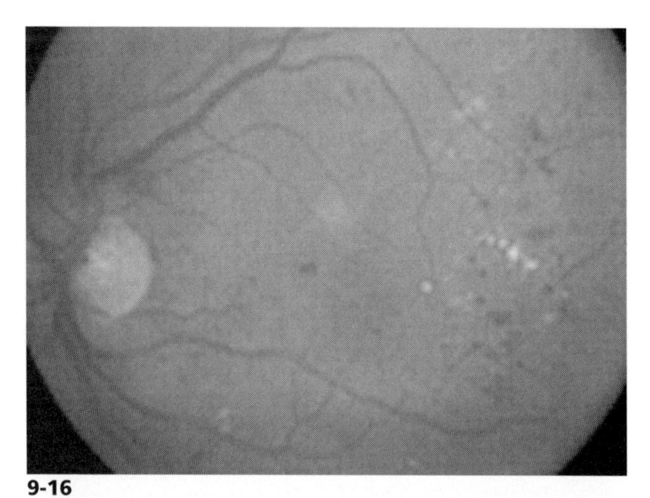

9-16

Figure 9-16. Macular edema causes decreased visual acuity. To detect macular edema, you must dilate the pupil. You will see that the bright "floating" foveal reflex is gone, and the macula has a grayish color.

The use of laser photocoagulation has reduced the vision morbidity associated with diabetic retinopathy. The indications for laser treatment include proliferative retinopathy, clinically significant macular edema, and severe nonproliferative retinopathy.

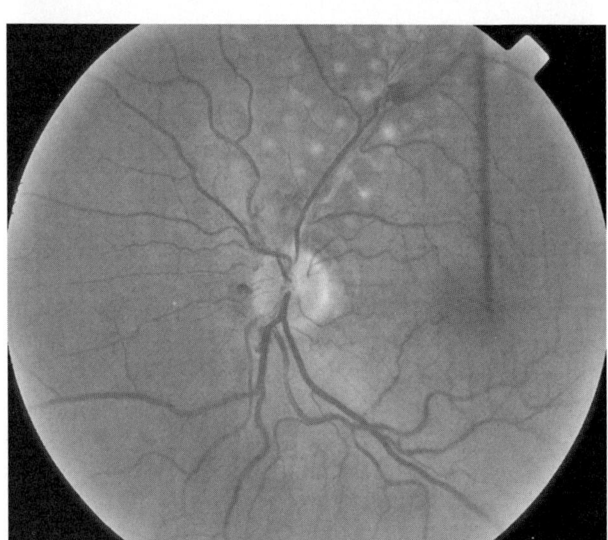

9-17A

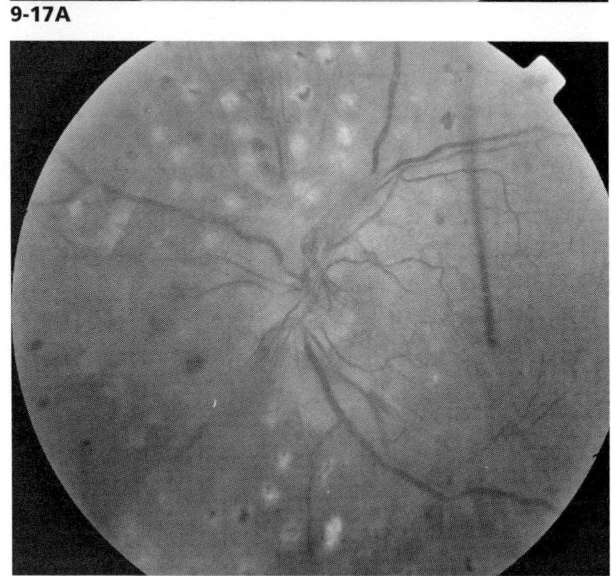

9-17B

Figure 9-17. A,B. **The goal of laser treatment is to destroy hypoxic retina so as to reduce the amount of the vasogenic factor production. Many techniques have been developed: "Local photocoagulation"** (A) **is used for patches of neovascularization. "Focal photocoagulation" is used in treatment of macular edema. In** A **you see small, regular, round, white spots along the superior temporal arcade to prevent neovascularization.** B. **"Full scatter panretinal photocoagulation" is treatment of the entire retina. Here you can appreciate the numerous small round spots across the entire background. Some of the older spots have pigmentary changes.**

Complications of photocoagulation include: decreased vision, constricted visual field, decreased accommodation, choroidal effusion, decreased night vision, and diminished contrast sensitivity and color vision. The pupil can have a reduced reaction to light after photocoagulation.

Hypertensive Retinopathy

Hypertension affects 50 million people in the United States (24–31% of the population), with individuals on anti-hypertensive medication for blood pressure elevation greater than 140 mm Hg systolic or 90 mm Hg diastolic.[19] A large percentage of the world suffers from hypertension as well. Hypertension is a significant risk factor for myocardial infarction, stroke, congestive heart failure, renal disease, and peripheral vascular disease.

For more than 100 years we have known that hypertension affects blood vessels in the eyes. The early classification of these changes was first made when patients presented with long-standing, uncontrolled hypertension. Now patients are routinely screened for hypertension, making the severe retinal changes much less common. However, examination of the fundus for changes in vasculature related to hypertension is still important.[20]

Table 9-7. Blood Pressure Classification from the Joint National Committee (JNC-V)

Category	Systolic blood pressure (mm Hg)	Diastolic blood pressure (mm Hg)
Normal	<130	<85
High normal	130–139	85–89
Hypertension		
Stage 1 mild	140–159	90–99
Stage 2 moderate	160–179	100–109
Stage 3 severe	>180	>110

Source: Adapted from references 21,22.

Figure 9-18. A,B. **Acute hypertensive retinopathy including disc swelling, splinter disc hemorrhages, and exudates. (Photographs courtesy of William T. Shults, M.D.)** C. **Diffuse arterial narrowing from long-standing hypertension. There are also scattered hemorrhages.**

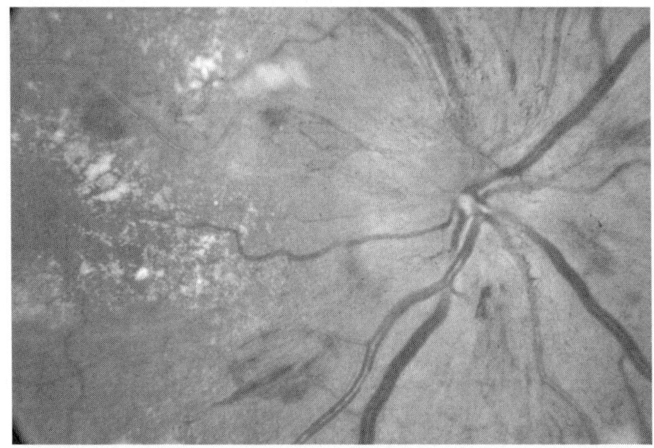

9-18A

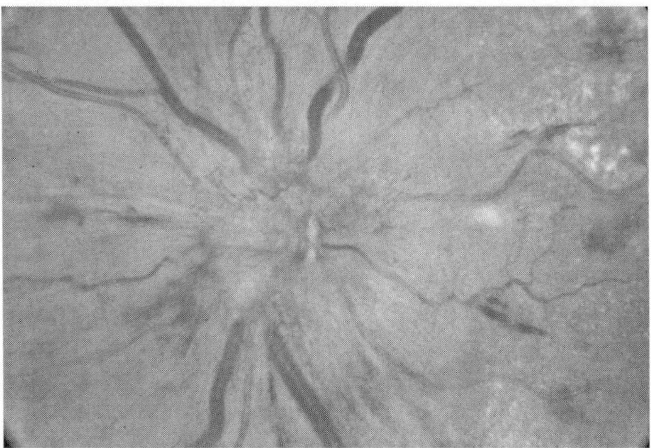

9-18B

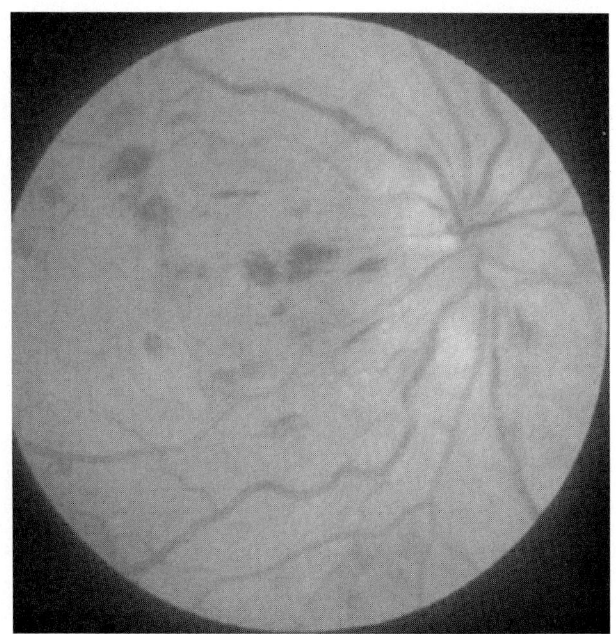

9-18C

Typical hypertensive changes in the retina include the following elements.

Arteriolar narrowing is the hallmark sign in the retina of hypertension. By itself, it is not pathognomonic, but when compared with a person without hypertension, narrowing does occur. In the Beaver Dam, Wisconsin, population study, arteriolar narrowing was present in 13.5% of patients with hypertension (582 of 1,479).[23]

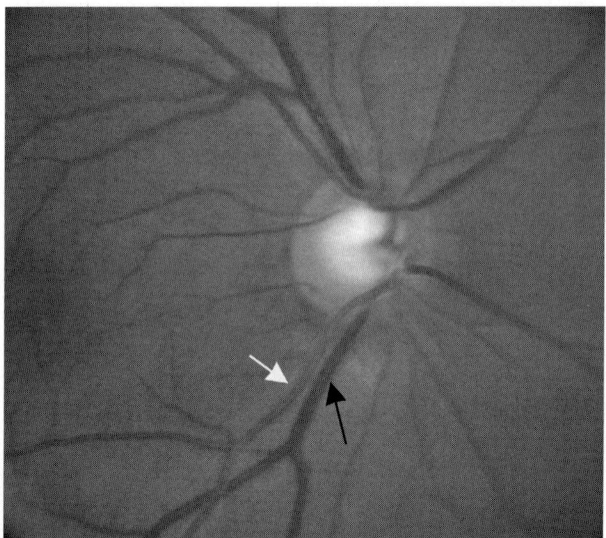

9-19A

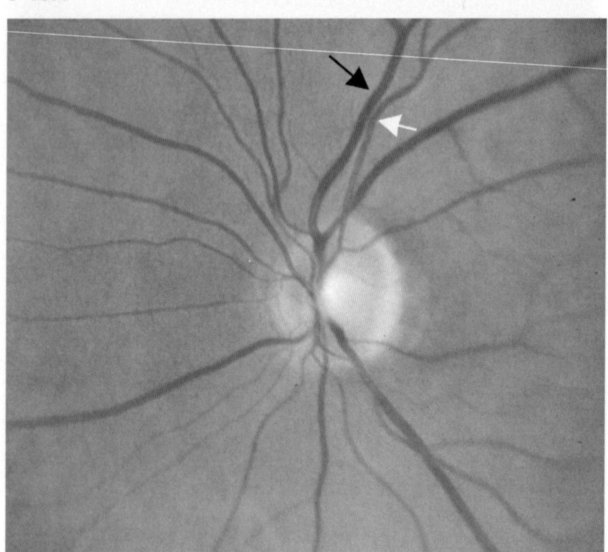

9-19B

Figure 9-19. A. **The normal A-V ratio is approximately 2:3 (i.e., the artery is approximately two-thirds of the size of the vein, or better). The black arrow points to the vein and the white arrow points to the artery.** B. **The narrowed arteries here make the A-V ratio smaller—no more than 1:2 in this case. The black arrow points to the vein and the white arrow points to the artery.**

Comparison of arterial and venous sizes is another way to look at the effect of hypertension on vessel size. Stanton et al. found that as the diastolic blood pressure increased, the diameter of the arterioles decreased and the diameter of the venules increased, leading to a decreasing arteriovenous (A-V) ratio with an increase in blood pressure.[20] The normal A-V ratio is approximately 2:3. The change in the ratio occurs when the arteries get smaller and the veins stay the same or enlarge slightly. Most of the change in the A-V ratio in hypertension is owing to the arteriolar narrowing.

Vessel coloring. "Copper-wiring" is really an increase in the light reflex caused by thickening of the vessel wall. The vessel wall normally is transparent, and what we actually see is the blood column; however, if the wall thickens, the color of the oxygenated blood carried in the vessel appears less red and more copper-orange. If this process continues, "silver wiring," or a white-appearing artery, ensues, meaning the vessel is further narrowed. Thickening of the vessel wall is owing to the increase in the intimal components in the vessel wall induced by hypertension. This process is called *arteriolosclerosis* (as opposed to *atherosclerosis*, which is atheromatous and lipid deposit in the intima of large vessels). Copper and silver wiring changes are very uncommon in treated hypertension.

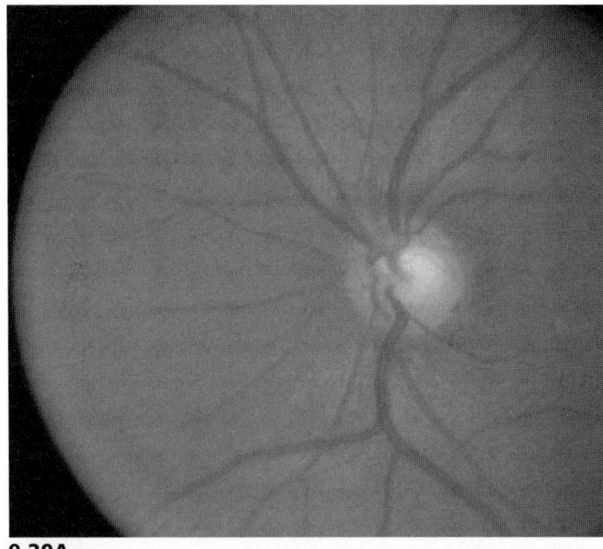

9-20A

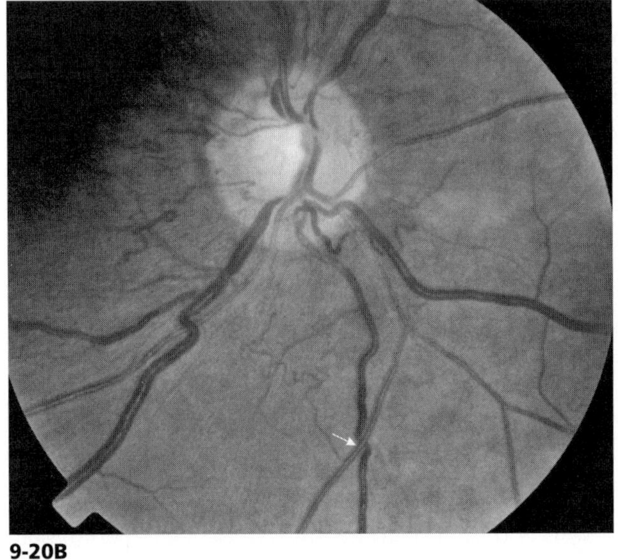

9-20B

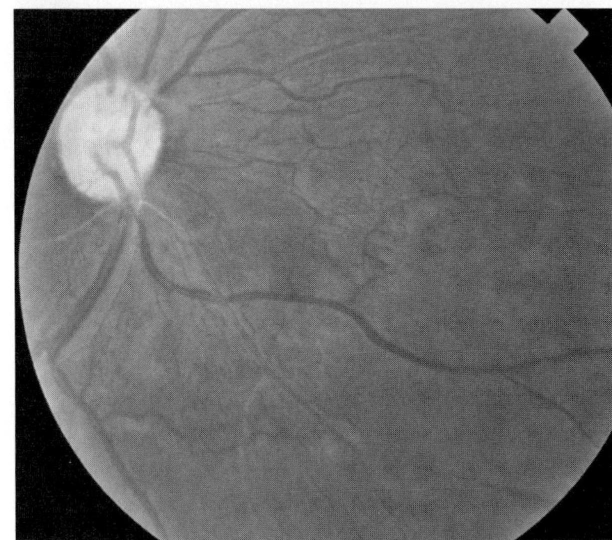

9-20C

Figure 9-20. A. **The normal color of the vessels is red, because the wall is transparent and what we see is the blood column.** B. **Copper wiring: The increased thickening of the vessel wall causes the blood column/the light reflex on the vessel wall to look less red, and more of a copper color. See the color photograph on the accompanying CD-Rom. Also, notice nicking changes (*arrow*).** C. **Silver wiring: As the hypertensive process continues, the vessel looks more white and narrow owing to the arteriolosclerotic process that thickens of the vessel wall. (Photographs in** B **and** C **courtesy of Marie Acierno, M.D.)**

Arteriovenous nicking. As the vessel wall thickens owing to arteriolosclerosis, the vein is displaced. Remember that the artery usually, but not always, crosses over the vein; if the vein is compressed, it looks "nicked." The vein may also, less commonly, hump up over the artery. In the Beaver Dam study, 95 of 1,479 (2.2%) hypertensive patients had A-V nicking changes.[23] Early on, only vessel displacement would be seen. As the arteriolar thickening continues, the venule appears tapered and constricted on

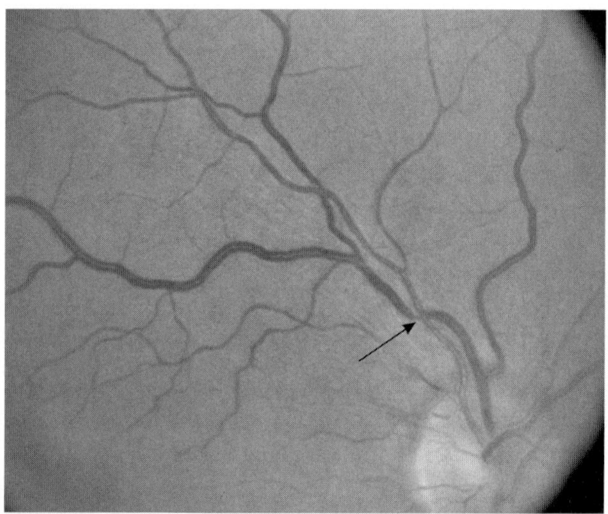

9-21A

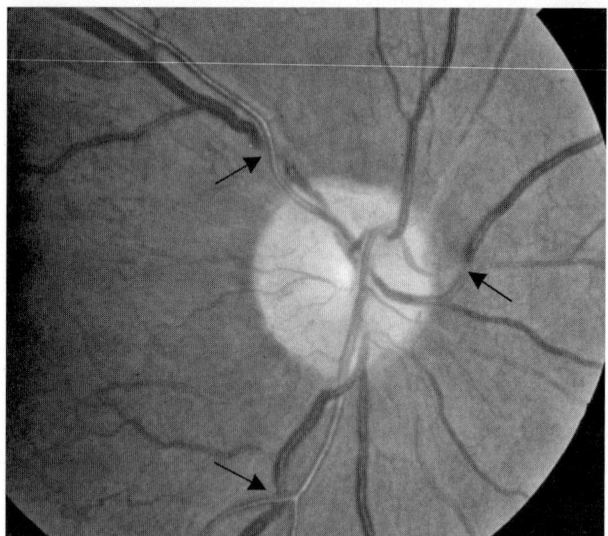

9-21B

either side of the crossing arteriole. At its worst, the vein can appear to disappear on either side of the arteriole, or if the vein crosses above the arteriole, it may hump over the arteriole like a little Japanese bridge.

Figure 9-21. A. **The artery goes over the vein in this case (*arrow*), and the vein appears to be "nicked."** B. **A-V nicking can be seen in multiple sites (*arrows*). Notice the caliber of vein passing under the arteriole at 11 o'clock. Distally the vessel is fat and tortuous, and proximally the vein is narrowed. This is a precursor to branch retinal vein occlusion. (Photograph courtesy of Marie Acierno, M.D.)**

Other findings include microaneurysms, cotton-wool spots, and capillary nonperfusion, which can only be appreciated on fluorescein angiography.

Hypertensive retinopathy follows when the arteriolar thickening progresses to produce ischemic changes in the retina. The Beaver Dam Population Study showed that 336 of 1,479 patients with hypertension (7.8%) had hypertensive retinopathy.[23]

Although the choroid is often forgotten in hypertensive retinopathy, a hypertensive "choroidopathy" can also occur simultaneously. This is difficult to appreciate with the direct ophthalmoscope; fluorescein angiography is more helpful. There may be a yellow change in color over the retinal pigment epithelium (RPE) and fluorescein leaks. These have been called *Elschnig's spots*.[24] If this is severe enough, a serous retinal detachment can be seen. See hypertensive choroidal changes in eclampsia (see Chapter 13, Figure 13-11).

The optic disc may also show swelling. Although the cause of the swelling is controversial, with some thinking it is owing to increased intracranial pressure, most agree that there is probably some ischemic change causing axoplasmic stasis and disc "edema."

Hypertensive retinopathy consists of a number of stages. Most today do not bother to stage hypertensive changes because they are fairly arbitrary, but at least the staging gives one an idea of progression. The two classifications are the Keith-Wagener-Barker classification (refined by Wagener),[25] which relied heavily on arteriolar constriction, and the Scheie classification. Scheie attempted to delineate the classification from normal to most severe.[26] The Scheie classification is most often referred to today.[24]

Classification of Hypertensive Retinopathy—Modified Scheie Classification

Stage 0: The patient has hypertension, but there are no retinal changes.

Figure 9-22. A. **Stage 1: Early changes include focal and diffuse narrowing of the arteries. No A-V crossing changes. If the hypertension is acute, such as in eclampsia, these changes may reverse themselves when blood pressure normalizes. With long-standing hypertension, the narrowing persists.** B. **Stage 2 consists of arterial narrowing, copper/silver wiring, and A-V nicking (*arrows*). Focal areas of arteriolar constriction. (Photograph courtesy of Marie Acierno, M.D.)** ***Continued***

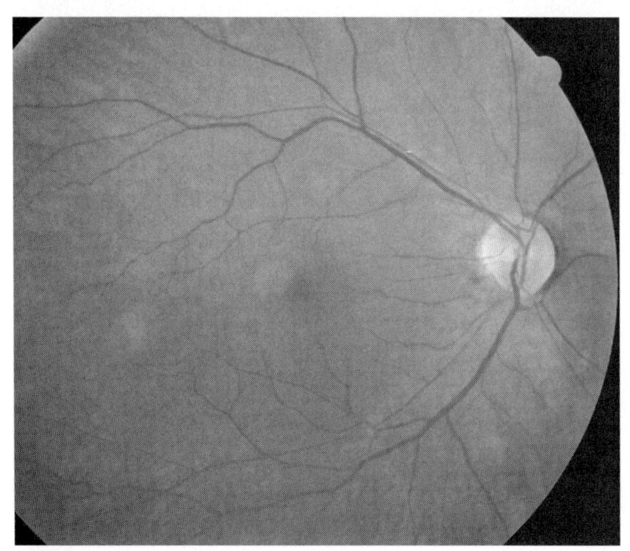

9-22A

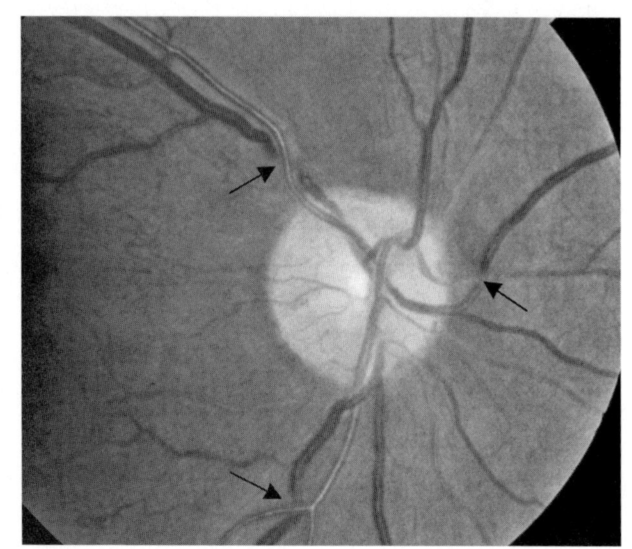

9-22B

Figure 9-22. *Continued.* C. Stage 3 consists of arterial narrowing, copper/silver wiring, retinal hemorrhages, and cotton-wool exudates (*arrowheads*). The hemorrhages are typically nerve-fiber-layer flame-shaped. With acute accelerated hypertension, such as with renal failure, there are more cotton-wool exudates. You can also appreciate a hemimacular star (*arrow*). (Photograph courtesy of Marie Acierno, M.D.) D. Stage 4 is all of the aforementioned changes plus retinal edema, hard exudates, and disc swelling. Hard exudates (*arrows*) occurring in the macular region form a "star" (see Macular Star, Chapter 10, Figure 10-18). Disc leakage on fluorescein angiography indicates a breakdown of the blood retinal barrier and dilation of precapillary arterioles,[27] although similar changes occur with swelling caused by increased intracranial pressure. The disc swelling has frequently been attributed to papilledema associated with increased intracranial pressure, but is more likely caused by microangiopathy of the optic nerve head—an ischemic optic neuropathy.

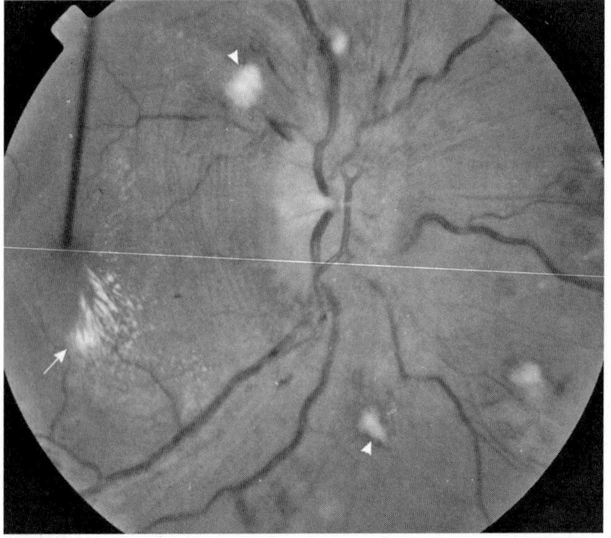

9-22C

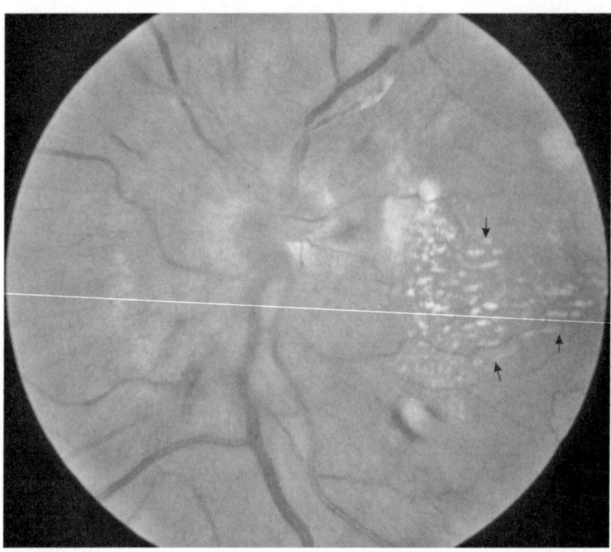

9-22D

Figure 9-23. A,B. **This woman has stage 4 hypertensive retinopathy owing to severe pre-eclampsia in pregnancy (see Chapter 13). (Photographs courtesy of Paul Zimmerman, M.D.)**

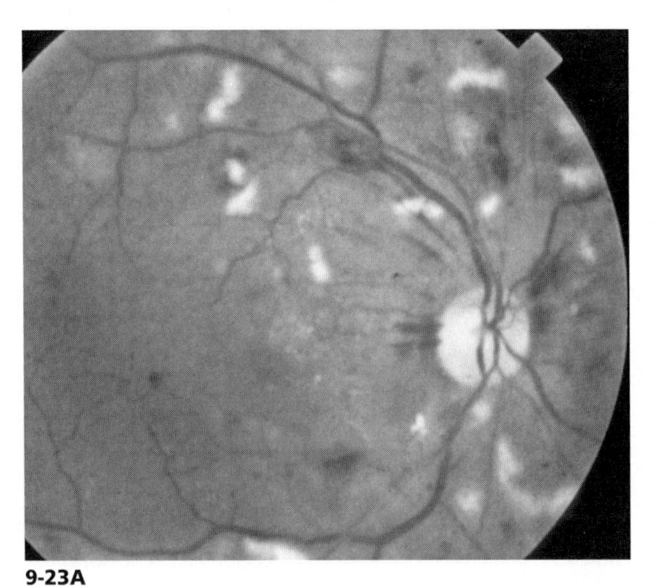

9-23A

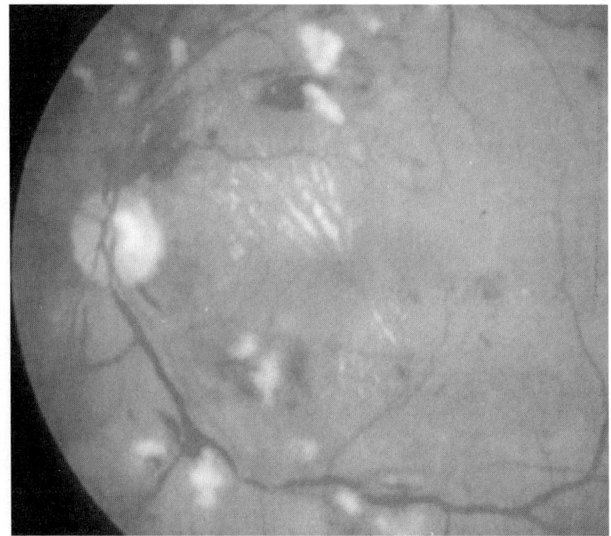

9-23B

Hypertension also affects the choroid. In fact, the choroid is one of the most commonly affected blood vasculatures in hypertension. Frequently, it is difficult to appreciate injury to the choroid. Typical changes include choroidal infarctions leaving Elschnig's spots. Later, these spots may actually become pigmented. If the ischemic injury is severe enough, a serous retinal detachment may occur. Fluorescein angiography is frequently helpful.

Figure 9-24. A. **Elschnig's spots (*arrows*). The way that you know it is a choroidal location is that the retinal vessels overlie the spot (*top arrow*). With the direct ophthalmoscope you have to look closely to see this relationship.** ***Continued***

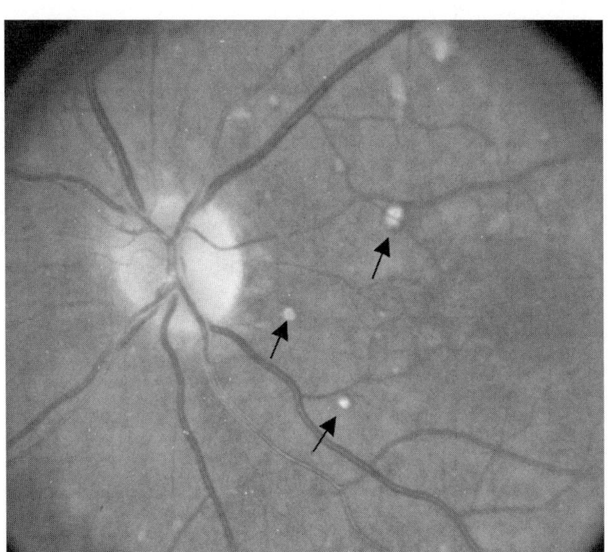

9-24A

Figure 9-24. ***Continued.*** B. **Old Elschnig's spots cause pigmentary changes (*arrows*).** C. **If choroidal ischemia is severe enough, serous retinal detachments occur (*arrows* outline the detachment).** D. **An Elschnig's spot in the choroid is sometimes hard to see.** E. **The fluorescein angiogram can sometimes elucidate the area of injury (*arrow*).**

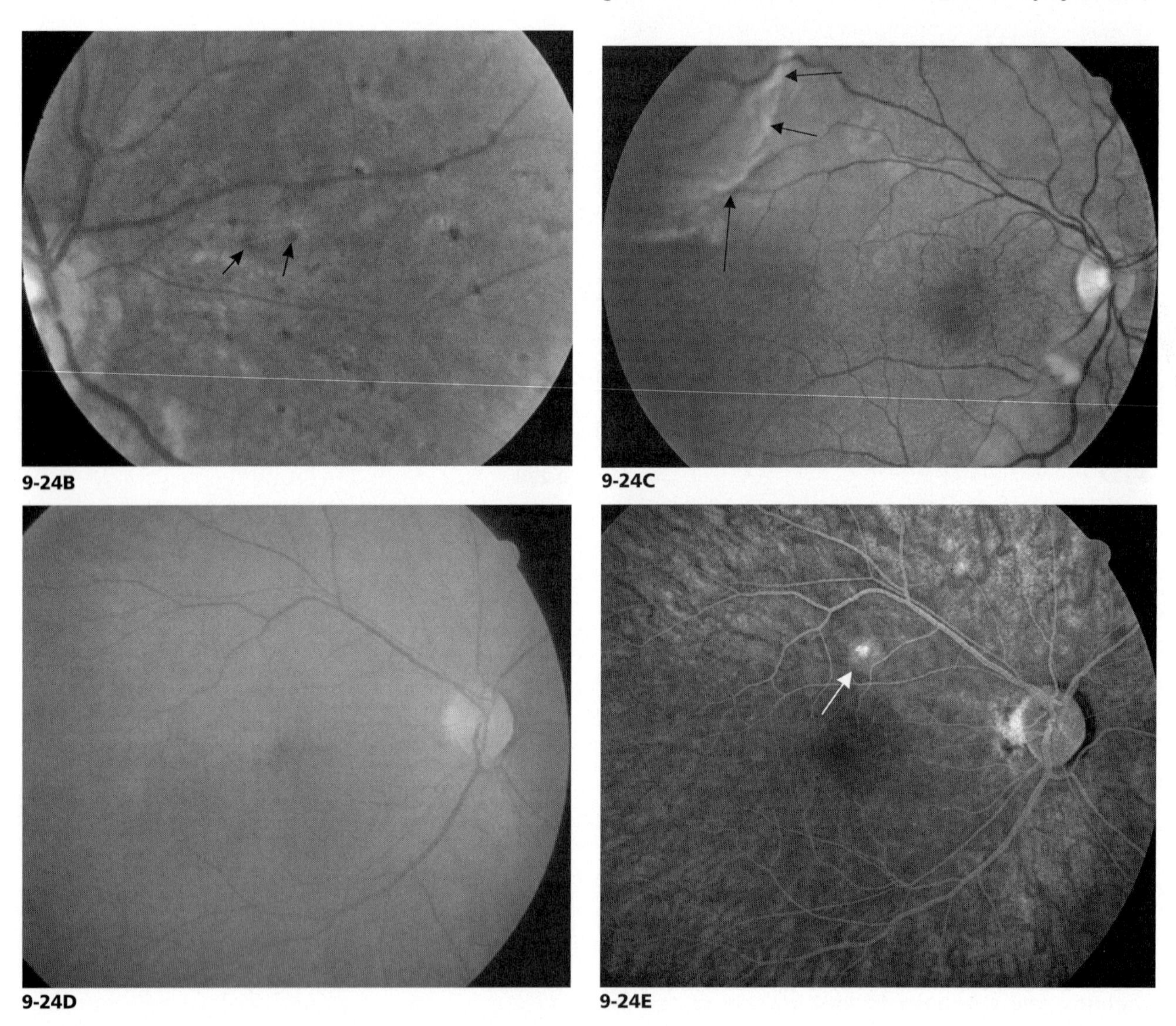

Asymmetry of hypertensive retinopathy, in which one eye is slightly affected and the other is seriously affected, suggests a lower blood pressure (carotid stenosis or occlusion) on the less severely affected side.

Importantly, finding retinopathy, arteriolar narrowing, or A-V nicking is *not* pathognomonic for systemic hypertension; blood pressure measurement remains the best way to diagnose hypertension.[23]

Radiation Retinopathy

Whenever there is a history that a patient has received radiation, especially of the orbit or the brain, radiation changes in the retina should be considered. Vision loss, commonly stepwise, is the complaint. Radiation damages the blood vessels first. Later, the neural elements, cones, rods, nerve fibers, and optic nerve are affected. Focal, whole-brain, proton-beam, and gamma-knife radiation, especially applied around the eyes, can produce radiation retinopathy, optic neuropathy, or both. The major damage in radiation is to the blood vessels of the eye. Usually, changes in small vessels do not occur until approximately 6 months after treatment (7–36 months or longer, with a mean of 19 months). The dose of radiation that can cause retinopathy is as low as 1,500 cGy (15 Gy), but more frequently it occurs with doses of 3,000 cGy (30 Gy).[28] Lower doses of radiation are obviously much less likely to cause retinopathy.

The development of radiation retinopathy is stepwise and depends on the total dose of radiation received, the size of the fraction, whether chemotherapy is given concomitantly, and pre-existing vascular conditions.[29] What do you see in radiation retinopathy? First, there is the dropout of retinal capillaries, and then cotton-wool spots appear, followed by capillary nonperfusion. These changes may be extremely subtle on ophthalmoscopy, but the patient will be symptomatic, and, at times, changes will not be appreciated without the aid of fluorescein angiography. When larger retinal vessels become thickened, neovascularization can be seen.[28] The course is similar to diabetic retinopathy. Neovascularization of the iris and subsequent glaucoma may occur. An animal model study by Irvine and Wood systematically studied monkeys who were treated with 30 Gy to the eye. They found that changes characteristically occurred 12–24 months after treatment. Table 9-8 lists the stepwise changes they saw.[30] Interestingly, the photoreceptors and ganglion cells seem to be resistant to radiation. Rods are more sensitive than cones, in that even a single dose of 20 Gy can damage the rods, whereas cone damage occurs in radiation doses of 100 Gy.[31]

Table 9-8. Stepwise Progression of Radiation Damage to the Retina Showing up 12–24 Months after Treatment

Loss of pericytes and capillary endothelial cells in blood vessels
Cotton-wool spots (nerve fiber layer infarcts)
Retinal capillary nonperfusion
Microaneurysms
Choriocapillaris occlusion—less pronounced
Retinal pigment epithelium atrophy and "salt and pepper" appearance to retina
Intraretinal neovascularization
Hemorrhages—vitreal
Retinal detachment
Late (3 yrs) neovascularization of the iris and neovascular glaucoma

Source: Adapted from references 30,31.

Table 9-9. Retinopathy Findings in Patients with Local and External Beam Irradiation

Finding	Focal (n = 20 eyes) (%)	External beam (n = 16 eyes) (%)
Microaneurysms	75*	81*
Intraretinal hemorrhage—dot-blot	65*	88*
Telangiectases	35	38
Hard exudates	85*	38
Cotton-wool spots	30	38
Vascular sheathing	20	25
Neovascularization of the disc/retina	—	31.25
Fluorescein findings		
Capillary dropout	100	100
Macular edema—leakage	65	58

*Most prominent findings.
Source: Adapted from reference 32.

Additionally, Brown and others have found that chemotherapy or underlying diabetes makes a person more susceptible to severe retinal damage.[32] One feature that can help distinguish radiation retinopathy from diabetic retinopathy is atrophy of the RPE, which can accompany radiation retinopathy, but not diabetic retinopathy.[29]

Figure 9-25. A. **This woman had radiation for progressive vision loss owing to a left sphenoid ridge meningioma. Early on, she had cotton-wool spots (*arrows*) in the retina of her right eye.** B. **Later, there was capillary dropout, narrowing of the blood vessels, small dot hemorrhages, and areas of early neovascularization (*arrows*).** C. **The left eye was more severely affected. She also received focal photocoagulation therapy (*arrow*) for severe neovascularization in the left eye, creating the small round spots between the disc and the macula.**

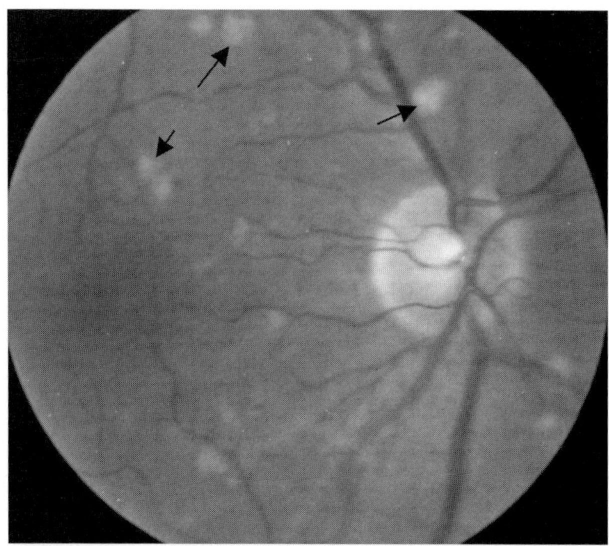

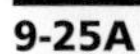

9-25A

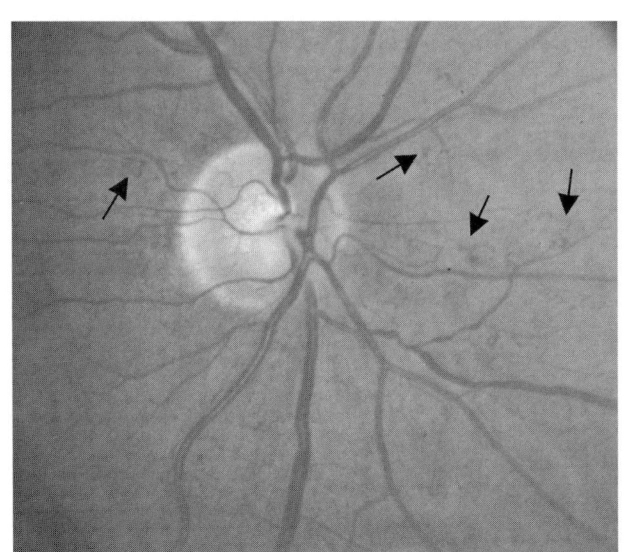

9-25B

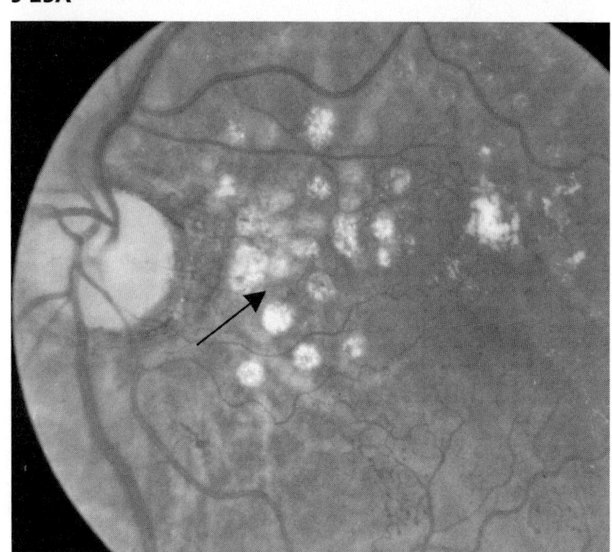

9-25C

Radiation Optic Neuropathy

Radiation damage to the optic nerve(s), chiasm, or tract can occur after radiation to the orbit, frontal lobe, pituitary gland, or middle fossa for tumors. Depending on the radiation portal used, the optic neuropathy may be unilateral or bilateral and characterized by acute vision loss, radiation retinopathy with or without disc swelling, and progressive optic atrophy. The incidence of optic neuropathy after radiation is variable, from less than 0.5% to 25.0%. The peak incidence seems to be 1–1 $1/2$ years, but usually within 3 years. Of patients with adenomas, those receiving concurrent chemotherapy are at greater risk to develop radiation-induced optic neuropathy. The diagnosis can be made by magnetic resonance imaging, which shows swelling and radiation necrosis of the chiasm or adjacent frontal and temporal lobes. The amount of radiation needed to produce radiation optic neuropathy is 4,200–5,000 rad,[33] which produces optic neuropathy in 1% of such patients. "Safe" dosages have been stated to be less than 7,000 rad, delivered at a rate of less than 200 rad per day.[33] Pathological evaluation of the optic nerves shows changes of demyelination and obliterative endarteritis.[34] High-dose steroids, hyperbaric oxygen therapy, and heparin rarely halt the progression of blindness.[34,35]

Bone Marrow Transplant Retinopathy

Bone marrow transplant has become an increasingly important treatment for leukemia, aplastic anemia, and other malignant conditions. Not only is the patient exposed to high doses of chemotherapeutic agents, which destroy bone marrow, but also bone marrow reintroduced from self or from a human leukocyte antigen–compatible donor. Donor bone marrow transplants predispose the patient to develop graft-versus-host disease. Furthermore, in some protocols, radiation is also added.[36]

Table 9-10. Retinal Complications with Bone Marrow Transplant (n = 397)

Intraretinal, vitreous hemorrhage (3.5%)
Cotton-wool spots (4.3%)
Disc edema (2.8%), with most owing to cyclosporin
Serous retinal detachments (0.5%)
Infectious retinitis (2%) (fungal, toxoplasmosis, varicella-zoster, cytomegalovirus)

Source: Adapted from reference 36.

CANCER-ASSOCIATED RETINOPATHY/ MELANOMA-ASSOCIATED RETINOPATHY/PARANEOPLASTIC RETINOPATHY

These retinopathies are recently described and rare, characterized by degeneration of many retinal layers caused by an immune mechanism. The diagnosis is difficult to make by appearance alone. The history and ancillary findings become important. In fact, the triad of photosensitivity, ring scotomas on the visual field, and retinal arteriole attenuation should alert one to this diagnosis.[37] Symptoms include light-induced glare, photosensitivity, reduced vision, and bizarre transient entoptic phenomena (e.g., spots and dots of light over the entire visual field). Although a history of cancer may be present (small cell cancer of the lung is most frequent), sometimes the retinopathy can be the presenting feature of a malignancy. Other cancers associated with this syndrome include melanoma, ovarian cancer, oat cell carcinoma of the lung, non–small cell cancer of the lung, cancer of the cervix, and ductal breast cancer.[38]

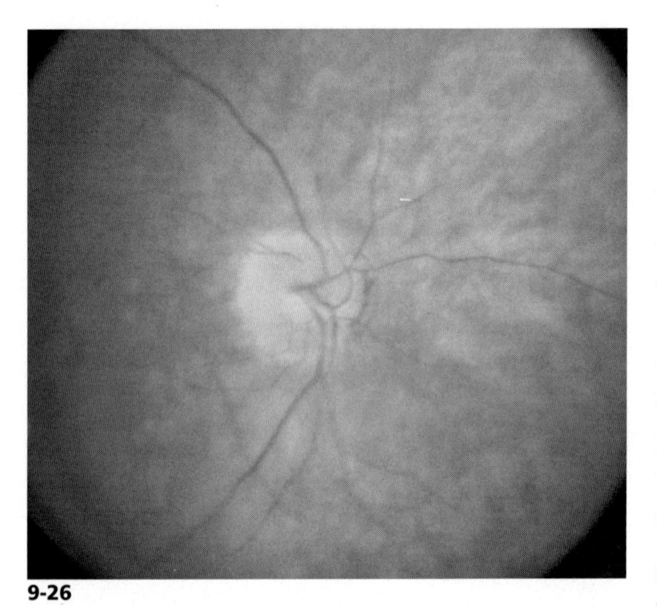
9-26

Ophthalmologic examination shows variable visual acuity and decreased color vision. The visual field shows peripheral and ring scotoma, like a picture of retinitis pigmentosa. Further blood may be sent for testing for antiretinal antibodies—the cancer-associated retinopathy and melanoma-associated retinopathy antigens.

Appearance of paraneoplastic retinopathy is variable. Sometimes the retina may appear normal. Late in cancer-associated retinopathy, a salt and pepper pigmentary change may occur. Findings in the retina that suggest a paraneoplastic retinopathy include retinal artery attenuation.

Figure 9-26. Typical findings of vascular attenuation with cancer-associated retinopathy. Otherwise, there are few clues to the cause of vision loss. (Photograph courtesy of Daniel Jacobson, M.D.)

Inherited Retinopathy

SICKLE CELL HEMOGLOBINOPATHY

Blacks are at risk for sickle cell trait (8.5%); the incidence is 0.4% sickle cell anemia, 0.2% sickle cell hemoglobin C, and 0.03% thalassemia.[9,39] Sickle cell retinopathy is rare; like diabetic retinopathy, it is nonproliferative or proliferative. There are characteristic hemorrhages and retinal changes associated with sickle cell nonproliferative retinopathy (background retinopathy).

A *salmon-patch hemorrhage* is a round hemorrhage, approximately the size of the disc or smaller, located within the retina. Although it is initially red, within days the color is more orange or salmonlike. If the hemorrhage produces a cavity, an *iridescent spot* is left behind that looks yellow or orange-yellow and signifies that there are macrophages with hemosiderin. The *black sunburst* is a pigmented chorioretinal scar that develops in the retina after a hemorrhage.

"Sea fans," which are neovascular tissue growing onto the vitreous, are a sign of proliferative disease. Other signs include arteriolar occlusions, vitreous hemorrhage, retinal detachment,[3] and angioid streaks that become clearly visible as patients age.[40] (See angioid streaks, Figure 9-47, later in this chapter.)

Figure 9-27. A. **A salmon patch (*arrow*) is a round hemorrhage in the retina; it is named for its more orangelike color. Although initially red, within days the color is more orange or salmonlike.** B. **Once the hemorrhage produces a cavity, an iridescent spot (*arrows*) is left behind that is yellow or orange-yellow and signifies macrophages laden with hemosiderin.** C. **A black sunburst (*arrows*) is really a chorioretinal scar that occurs after the hemorrhage has been resorbed. Neovascularization can occur. (Photographs in** A–C **courtesy of C.J. Chen, M.D.)** D. **A close-up of a black sunburst.**

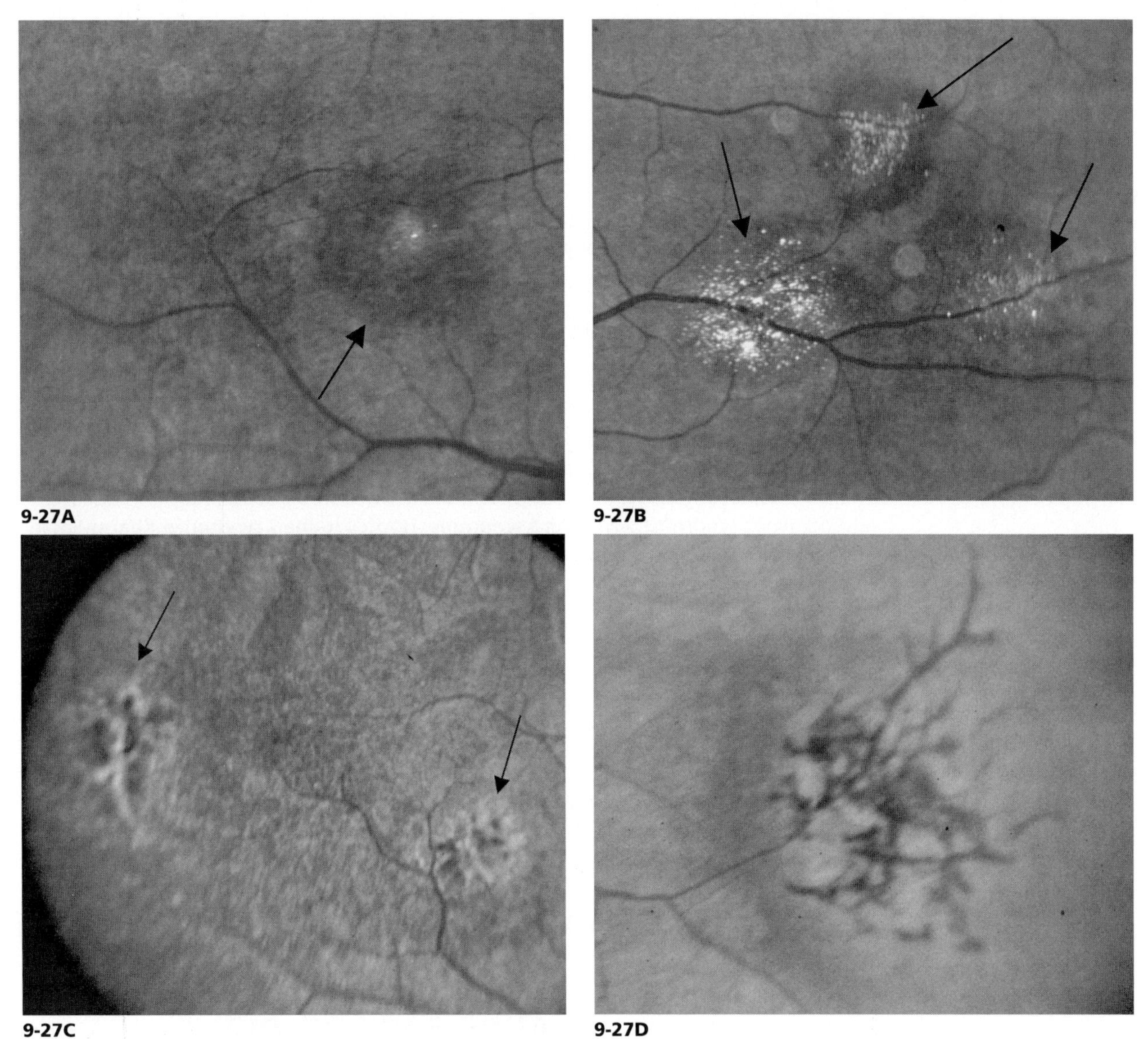

RETINAL CHANGES WITH INHERITED DEGENERATIVE NEUROLOGIC DISEASES

Although the most frequent retinal change with neurologic disease is retinitis pigmentosa, other changes in the retina can accompany progressive, degenerative neurologic disease. Certainly, degenerative conditions can cause changes in the retina, especially pigmentary changes. See Chapter 8 on pigment—retinitis pigmentosa. In addition, there can be other degenerative/hereditary conditions diagnosed in children (see Chapter 11).

Table 9-11. Retinal Changes with Degenerative Neurologic Disease

Retinal appearance	Diseases
Gray fovea	Metachromatic leukodystrophy; Farber's lipogranulomatosis
Vascular tortuosity	Fabry's disease
Brown macula and hypopigmentation of retina	Neuronal ceroid lipofuscinosis
White spots	Gaucher's disease
Pigmentary changes	Gaucher's disease, gangliosidoses, type 2, mucolipidosis, neuronal ceroid lipofuscinosis, mucopolysaccharidoses, abetalipoproteinemia, apoceruloplasmin deficiency, cystinuria, homocarnosinosis, hyperpipecolatemia, McArdle's disease, Refsum's disease, Cockayne's syndrome, Flynn-Aird syndrome, Hooft's Joubert syndrome, Kearns-Sayre syndrome, Laurence-Moon-Bardet-Biedl syndrome, Letterer-Siwe disease, Marinesco-Sjögren syndrome, Pelizaeus Merzbacher disease, Rud's syndrome, Senior's syndrome, Sjögren-Larsson syndrome, Tuck-McLeod syndrome, Usher's syndrome, Zellweger's syndrome, Friedreich's ataxia, Hallervorden-Spatz syndrome, Leber's congenital amaurosis, Lytico-Bodig, spinocerebellar degeneration
Cherry-red spot	Tay-Sachs disease, Sandhoff's gangliosides, type 2, Niemann-Pick disease, sialidoses, Farber's lipogranulomatosis, metachromatic leukodystrophy
Gyrate atrophy	Hyperornithemia

Source: Adapted in part from reference 41.

Infections/Inflammation/ Infiltrations of the Retina and Choroid

Uveitis is inflammation of the pigment-bearing portions of the eye. Uveitis can be anterior or posterior.

In anterior uveitis, there is reddening of the eye, cells, and protein in the anterior chamber leading to hypopyon (layered cells or whitening in the anterior chamber). Posterior uveitis is really an inflammation of the choroid. *Vitreitis* is an inflammation within the eye, which inflames the vitreous—one sees cells in the vitreous. Cells in the vitreous obscure the view of the fundus when using a direct ophthalmoscope. *Choroiditis* is an inflammation primarily in the choroid—see the section on white spots in Chapter 6. Choroiditis appears as white-yellow patches. *Retinitis* is an inflammation primarily in the retina. *Chorioretinitis* is an inflammation mainly of the choroid but involves the retina. *Retinochoroiditis* is inflammation of the retina that also involves the choroid.

The effect of all of these inflammatory reactions is to make the fundus difficult to see because of vitreous cells.

Toxoplasmosis owing to the parasite *Toxoplasma gondii* is the most common cause of chorioretinitis in the United States. The parasite, often carried by cats, infiltrates and encrypts in the retina, causing an immune inflammatory response and a threat to vision. Retinal pigmentary scars are seen as evidence of a prior infection by toxoplasmosis in 1–8% of the adult population.[42] The acute systemic infection in adults or children exposed to cats can be almost asymptomatic or can be accompanied by fever and lymphadenopathy. Ocular manifestations generally are of two types: old toxoplasmosis scar as a result of congenital toxoplasmosis, or reactivation of recent infection. Reactivation and acute toxoplasmosis pose the most trouble. Because the organism has an affinity for neural tissue, the lesions begin in the superficial retina and cause inflammation. If it is severe and continuous, involvement of the deep retina and choroid ensues. Because there is significant inflammation, cells are plentiful in the vitreous. The patient may complain that everything looks like a "headlight in the fog."[43] Patients also lose vision if the infection involves the macula.

Figure 9-28. Retinitis.

Figure 9-29. Choroiditis.

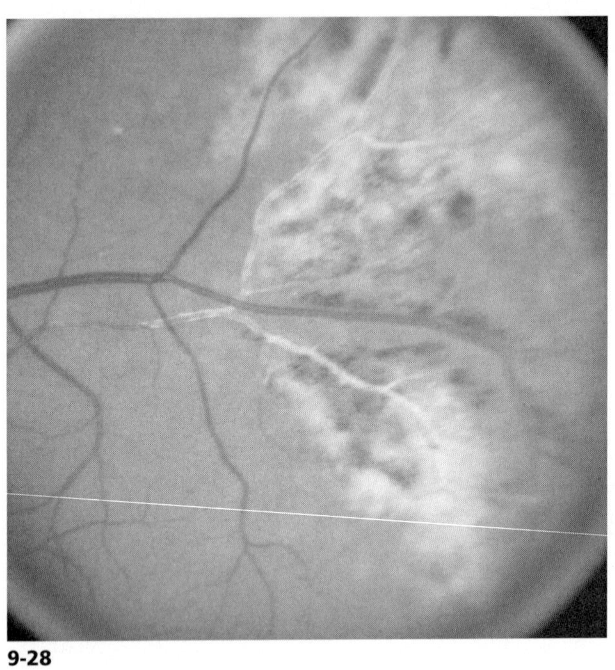

9-28

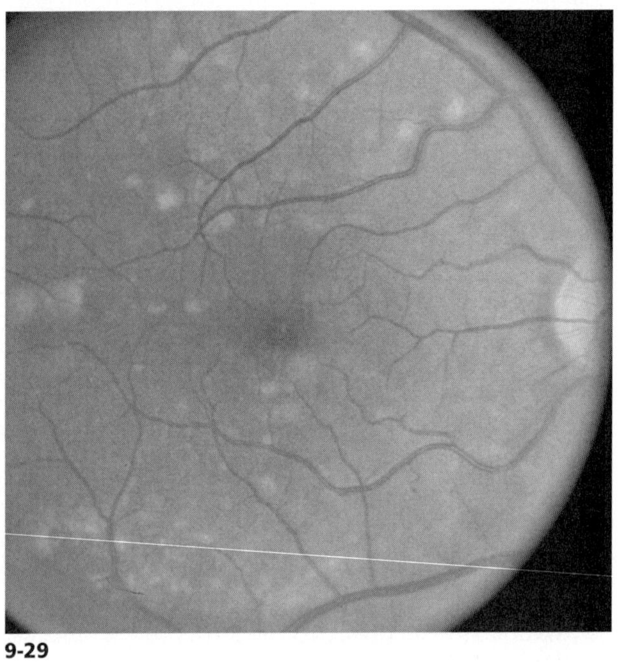

9-29

Table 9-12. Differentiating Choroiditis and Retinitis

	Retinitis (see Figure 9-28)	**Choroiditis (see Figure 9-29)**	**Chorioretinitis (see Figure 9-30)**
Fundus features	Hemorrhage, exudates, cotton-wool spots, edema; late pigmentary changes	White spots deep to the retina; usually no edema or hemorrhage; late pigmentary changes	See features of retinitis and choroiditis
Optic disc	Possible	Possible	Possible
Macula	Macular star; macular edema	Possible macular edema	Variable macular findings
Vasculature	Sheathing of the blood vessels	Usually normal or narrowed	Variable blood vessels
Cells in the vitreous	Significant	May be present, but not severe	Variable cells
Vision loss	Usually severe	Mild to moderate	Variable
Treatment	Often treatable	Sometimes treatable	Variably treatable
Examples	Cytomegalovirus retinitis, *Candida* retinitis; toxoplasmosis (acute), fungal retinitis, tubercular retinitis, syphilis	Sarcoid, white dot syndromes; multifocal choroidopathy	Infectious causes: *Toxoplasma*, syphilis, histoplasmosis, cytomegalovirus, fungal infections
			Inflammatory causes: systemic lupus erythematosus

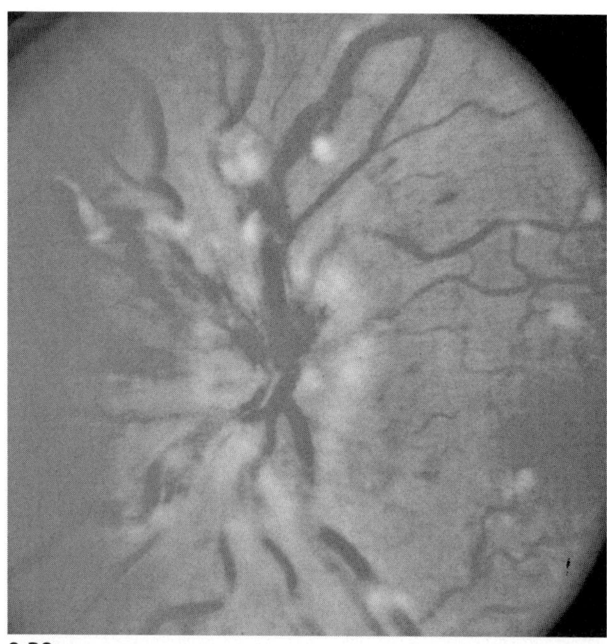
9-30

Figure 9-30. Chorioretinitis.

Rarely, the presentation may be of papillitis. Congenital toxoplasmosis, the second most common congenital infection (after cytomegalovirus), can occur in the first trimester of pregnancy, causing severe ocular and cerebral complications. If it is acquired in the third trimester, there is less morbidity. The importance of recognizing toxoplasmosis is that it is treatable with antibiotics.

Figure 9-31. A. **Appearance of early acute toxoplasmosis in the retina shows yellow/white in the retina with an inflammatory reaction in the vitreous. In this case, the disc is almost obscured by the inflammatory reaction and white infiltrates.** B. **As the lesion heals, a chorioretinal scar forms that is surrounded by pigmentation. In congenital toxoplasmosis, pigmented chorioretinal scars are normally seen. The finding of pigmentation related to toxoplasmosis is more common than seeing acute toxoplasmosis. (Photographs courtesy of Hussein Wafapoor, M.D.)**

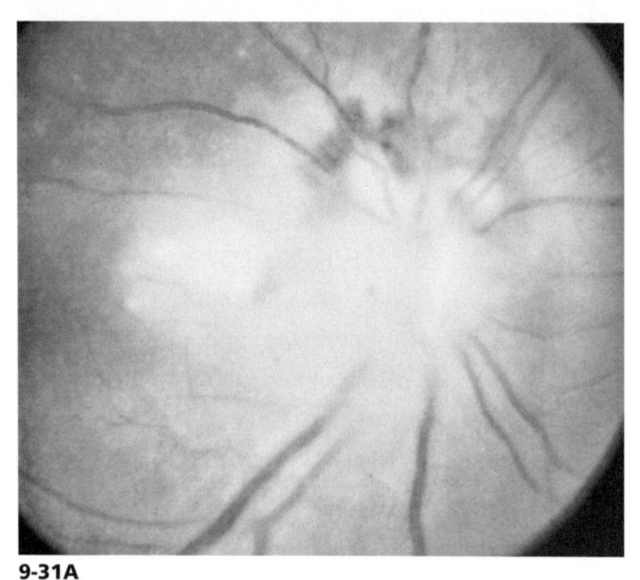

9-31A

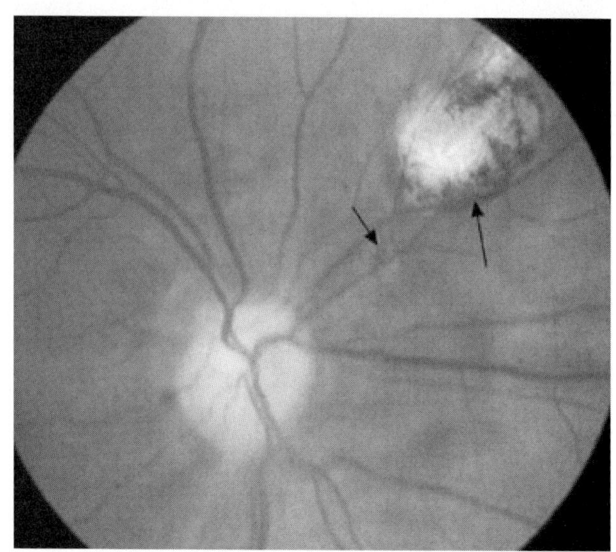
9-31B

Another common infection is *presumed ocular histoplasmosis syndrome*. The organism is seen especially in the Mississippi Valley area of the United States, and it occurs in 1.6–4.6% of the people in that area.[44] It is "presumed" because the organism has never been identified or cultured from a lesion. Although commonly benign and often asymptomatic, a spot in the retina can confuse the examiner. See Chapter 6, Figure 6-22.

Figure 9-32. A. **Appearance of histoplasmosis is characteristically scarring in the peripapillary area (*arrowheads*), with focal areas of scarring at 5 o'clock and 6 o'clock (*black arrows*), accompanied by small chorioretinal scars in the periphery (*white arrows*). Macular lesions are common, as illustrated by this case (*top white arrow*).** B. **Sometimes histoplasmosis can cause neovascularization and hemorrhage (*arrows*). In this case, the hemorrhage is by the macula (*top black arrow*). The white arrow points to the disc. (Photograph courtesy of C.J. Chen, M.D.)**

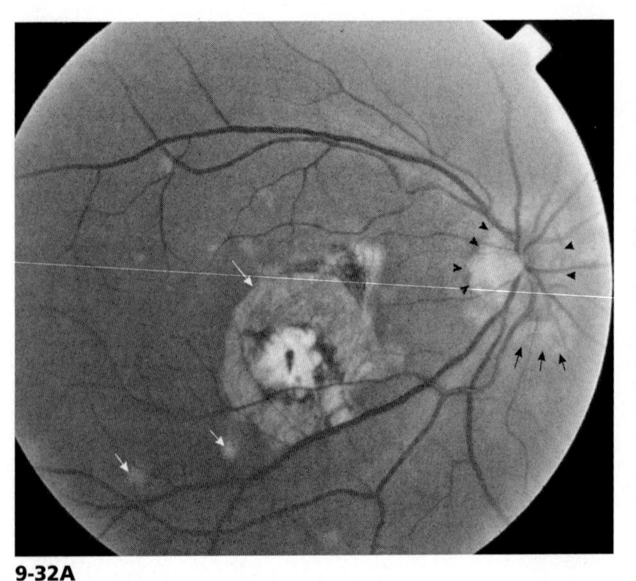

9-32A

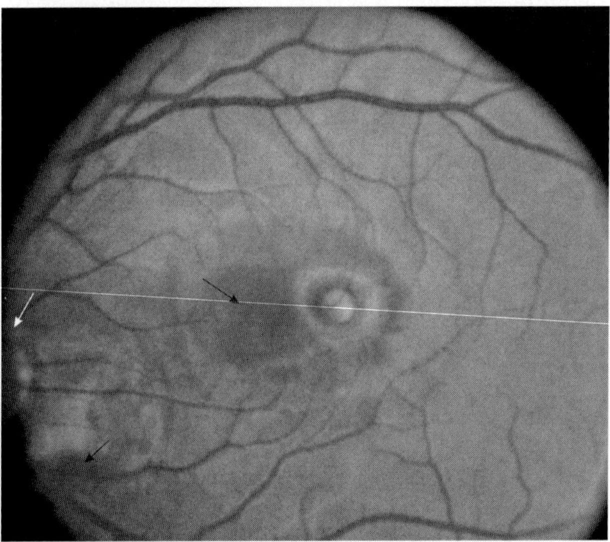

9-32B

Cytomegalovirus (CMV) retinitis is caused by a herpes (DNA) virus in immune-compromised individuals, including patients undergoing immunosuppression for bone marrow or organ transplant; patients with cancer, lymphoma, or leukemia; or patients with acquired immunodeficiency syndrome (AIDS). It is the single most common congenital infection. Active infections in this group present with retinitis, pneumonitis, hepatitis, colitis, sialadenitis, and nephritis. Patients with CMV retinitis are usually asymptomatic or may have only slight visual complaints.[45] CMV retinitis is rare in immune-competent subjects, but CMV has widespread exposure, with 50–70% of adults in Western countries having antibodies to the organism. It is important to recognize CMV retinitis because it is treatable with ganciclovir.[46]

Figure 9-33. A. Acute CMV infection, with a classic brush fire appearance. B. Appearance of CMV retinitis early on consists of white dots at the level of the RPE, vessel sheathing focally, and hemorrhages. Later, more diffuse changes with the retinitis, especially severe hemorrhages, ensue. Vessels are white and atrophic. The classic "brush fire" or "pizza pie" appearance is typical of CMV infection. The virus damages the retina. Retinal detachments are possible. Eventually, the retina becomes scarred and atrophic.[45] C. Retinitis with disc swelling can also occur. Although the disc appearance may be mistaken for papilledema, there is usually severe vision loss and commonly only one disc is swollen. (Photographs courtesy of Paul Zimmerman, M.D.)

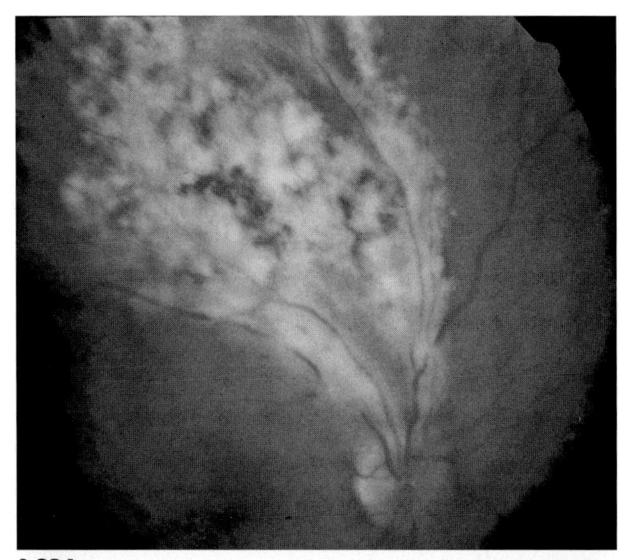

9-33A

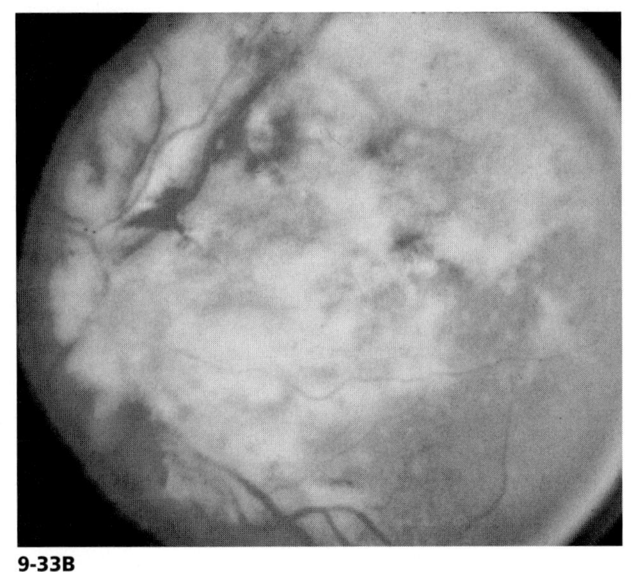

9-33B

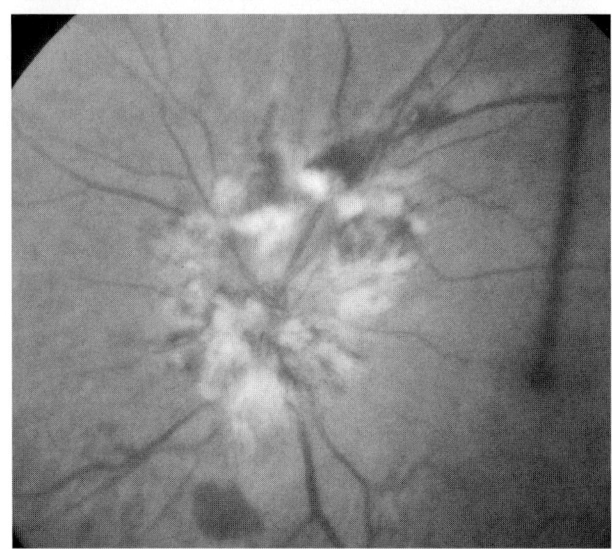

9-33C

Human immunodeficiency virus (HIV) can cause retinopathy, with cotton-wool spots, intraretinal hemorrhage, and capillary changes. Retinopathy is the most common retinal manifestation of HIV infection and may not be related to direct infection of the retina but is caused by viral antigens and antibodies, creating a noninfectious retinopathy. Retinopathy occurs to some degree in approximately one-half of patients with AIDS.[47] Cotton-wool spots are seen in 25–92% of patients with AIDS.[47] In addition, patients are at risk for CMV retinitis, which is the most common infectious retinitis in

HIV patients.[45] AIDS patients with vision complaints should be examined by an ophthalmologist.

Table 9-13. Acquired Immunodeficiency Syndrome–Associated Retinopathies

Type of retinitis/choroiditis with AIDS	Major retinal finding	Other
HIV retinopathy	Cotton-wool spots and hemorrhages	—
CMV retinitis	"Brush fire" or "pizza pie" hemorrhagic appearance	Polymerase chain reaction to diagnose on any fluid; treat with ganciclovir
Acute retinal necrosis	Peripheral retinal vascular occlusion with white retina; may also see vascular occlusion and cherry-red spot	Caused by herpes simplex and varicella-zoster
Syphilis	Neuroretinitis (with macular star); chorioretinitis	Optic nerve—optic neuritis
Tuberculosis (mycobacteria)	Yellow-white choroidal infiltrates; low-grade vitreitis	—
Toxoplasmosis	Focus of chorioretinitis with vitreitis	—
Pneumocystis carinii	Multifocal white-yellow, raised choroidal lesions—little inflammation	—
Cryptococcal disease	Chorioretinitis	Usually severe papillitis
Candida	"Fluff ball" vitreitis	—
Ocular histoplasmosis	Chorioretinitis—little inflammation	—
Lymphoma	Yellow-white infiltrates, perivascular sheathing	—

Source: Data from references 47,48.

Inflammatory Conditions of the Retina

See also retinal vasculitis (Chapter 5, Amaurosis Fugax).

Systemic lupus erythematosus is an autoimmune condition with multisystem involvement. The retina is the second most frequently involved structure in the eye, next to the lacrimal gland (which causes dry and red eyes). The classic finding is multiple cotton-wool spots with or without hemorrhage. There can also be intraretinal edema. Renal involvement and systemic hypertension can be seen. The vessels in the retina may also be occluded, and vasculitis can be present.[49] Occlusive vasculitis may also occur.[50] Fluorescein angiography is helpful in making the diagnosis of retinal vasculitis and can assist in making the diagnosis of primary central nervous system vasculitis (see Chapter 6, Figure 6-20). In addition, retinal vein occlusion, retinal artery occlusions, and ischemic optic neuropathy can occur with systemic lupus erythematosus. Choroidopathy has also been reported with serous retinal detachments.[51,52]

Table 9-14. Rheumatologic/Vasculitides with Retinal Findings

Condition	Retinal finding	Other
Rheumatoid arthritis, ankylosing spondylitis, Reiter's syndrome	Rare	Scleritis
Systemic lupus erythematosus	Cotton-wool spots with or without hemorrhages; rarely choroidopathy	Severe vaso-occlusive disease associated with central nervous system lupus; rare autoimmune retinopathy, such as cancer-associated retinopathy
Scleroderma	Cotton-wool spots, hemorrhage, disc edema associated with hypertension	Skin findings prominent
Sjögren's syndrome	Rare	Rare anterior ischemic optic neuritis
Relapsing polychondritis	Posterior scleritis with exudative detachment	—
Goodpasture's syndrome	Hemorrhages, exudates, retinal detachment; associated with hypertension	Pulmonary hemorrhages and glomerulonephritis
Inflammatory bowel disease—ulcerative colitis and Crohn's disease	Posterior uveitis, retinitis, vitreitis, posterior scleritis	Papillitis
Vasculitis	Cotton-wool spots, hemorrhage; see vessel sheathing; fluorescein abnormal	—
Polyarteritis nodosa	Vasculitis; hypertensive retinopathy owing to renal involvement	Scleritis
Wegener's granulomatosis	Vasculitis; cotton-wool spots, hemorrhage; branch retinal artery occlusion	Optic nerve—anterior ischemic optic neuritis, disc vasculitis
Giant cell arteritis	Cotton-wool spots	Anterior ischemic optic neuritis; choroidal dropout
Behçet's disease	Retinal vasculitis—veins and arteries; arterial occlusion; neovascularization; retinal detachment	Optic neuropathy
Other: sarcoid	Retinal vasculitis—sheathing of veins; retinal occlusions	May see optic neuropathy, papilledema, disc swelling, uveitis, chorioretinitis

Source: Data from reference 52.

MALIGNANCIES AND THE RETINA

Leukemia causes changes in the retina by directly infiltrating the retina and choroid. Indirect retinal involvement occurs with anemia, thrombocytopenia, and hyperviscosity, causing retinal changes. Other malignancies, like lymphoma and metastatic disease, may also affect the retina.[53]

Figure 9-34. A. **Leukemia can cause changes in the retina—hemorrhages as well as leukemic infiltrates can be present. Leukemic infiltrates can be present in white-centered hemorrhages (*arrows*).** B. **After treatment, the hemorrhages are resolving. (Photographs courtesy of Paula Morris, CRA.)**

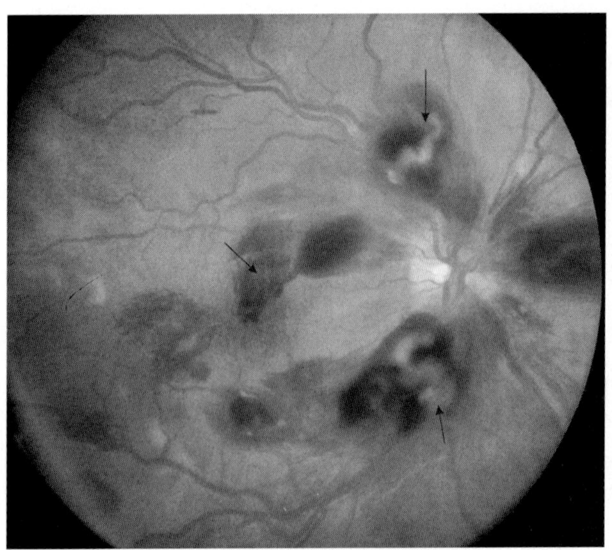

9-34A

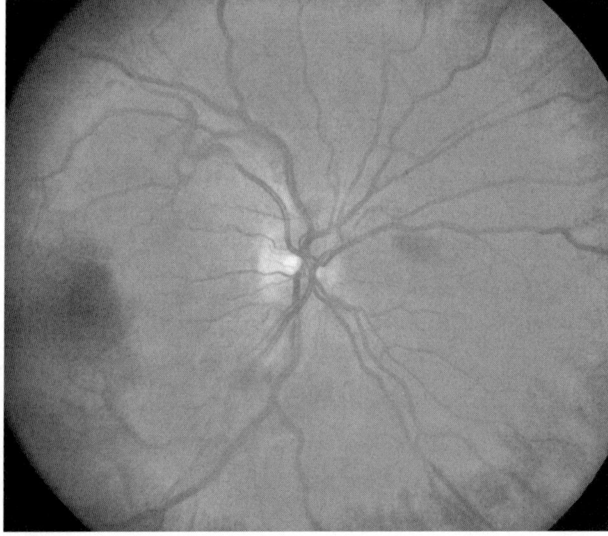

9-34B

Table 9-15. Retinal Changes Associated with Malignancy

Type of malignancy	Retinal change	Other
Leukemia with leukemic retinopathy	Hemorrhages in one-third to one-half; Roth's spots (white-centered hemorrhages) in many—the white center may be leukemic infiltrate; macular hemorrhage; retinal detachments possible; choroid most frequently involved	Retinopathy worse with associated anemia and thrombocytopenia; retinitis infiltrated in 31% of autopsied cases of leukemia; more frequent involvement with acute leukemia; intraretinal hemorrhage a poor prognosis in leukemia[56]
Multiple myeloma	In one-third: hemorrhages; some Roth's spots; microaneurysms	—
Lymphoma	Vitreitis; posterior uveitis; see choroidal infiltrates	Central nervous system involvement common, but retinal findings may antedate brain lesion by mos
Metastatic disease	Yellow, elevated lesions in the choroid	Breast and lung most common; gastrointestinal, testes, prostate, cutaneous melanoma

Source: Adapted from references 53–56.

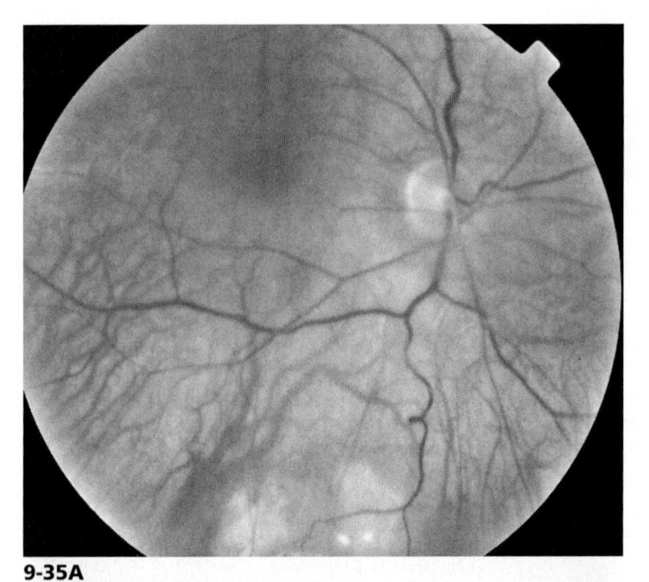

9-35A

Figure 9-35. Primary ocular tumors include retinoblastoma, melanoma, and vascular tumors. A. **Here is a "burned-out" retinoblastoma without progression.** B. **This shows what is left of the tumor.** C. **A computed tomographic scan shows the calcified mass in the left orbit. Most retinoblastomas are discovered in childhood and the eye is enucleated. Metastatic tumors to the eye can occur from breast, lung, and gastrointestinal cancers, renal carcinoma, and cutaneous melanoma. The appearance of choroidal metastasis is usually a yellow, elevated lesion deep to the retina. There may be secondary detachments.**

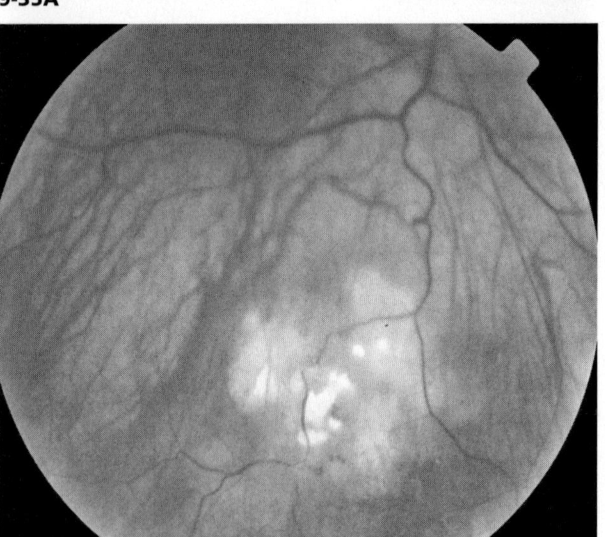

9-35B

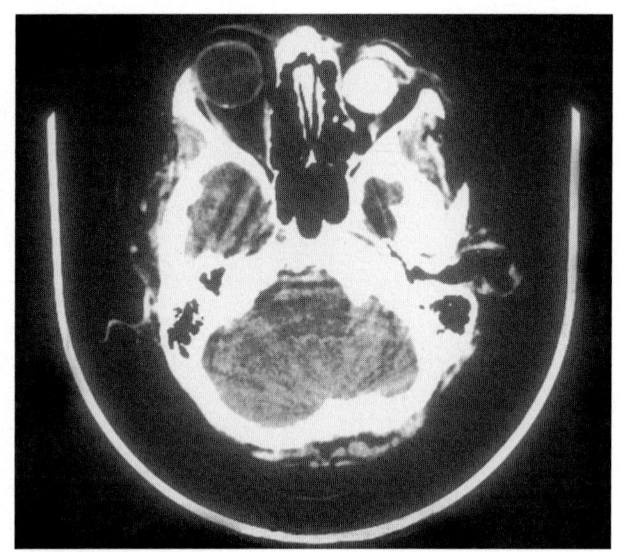

9-35C

CHANGES IN THE RETINA RELATED TO DRUGS AND TOXINS

You may be able to view the effects of drugs in the retina. In general, when the RPE is affected by medications or toxins, the retinal appearance can be pigment clumping, like salt and pepper changes. Some toxins affect the retinal elements (rods and cones) as well as the ganglion cells and axons (see Chapter 4, Table 4-19, Figures 4-48 and 4-49 for toxic optic neuropathy). Certainly, many drugs can cause a pigmentary change (see Chapter 8, Table 8-5 on pigment). Furthermore, some drugs affect the macula specifically (see Chapter 10, Table 10-10 and Figure 10-26 on viewing the macula). Other drugs are considered in the following section.

Table 9-16. Drug and Toxin Effects on the Retina

Drug or toxin	Use	Symptoms	Findings
Digitalis	Heart arrhythmias	Yellow vision (this complaint may be related to cortical effects)	Usually no obvious clinical changes; electroretinogram may show decreased cone amplitudes
Quinine	Malaria; leg cramps	Decreased vision	Normal fundus early; later electroretinogram B-wave decline, venous distention, retinal opacification; bone spicules
Tamoxifen	Antiestrogen used for breast cancer treatment	Few symptoms	Crystalline retinopathy—small white flecks throughout the retina, in the perifoveal region
Canthaxanthine	Oral carotenoid used for tanning	See tamoxifen	See tamoxifen
Methoxyflurane	Methoxyflurane anesthetic	See tamoxifen	See tamoxifen
Clofazimine	Leprosy, mycobacterium, psoriasis	Few	Macular pigmentary changes; peripheral retinal atrophy
Intraarterial chemotherapy (cisplatin, bischloroethylnitrosourea, others)	Central nervous system malignancy	Vision loss	Changes in macula; severe pigmentary retinopathy
Interferon-alpha	Hepatitis, chronic active infections	Blurred vision	Cotton-wool spots and hemorrhages
Chloroquine	Treatment of autoimmune disorders	Blurred vision; decreased vision	Retinal pigment epithelium toxicity in the macula; bull's eye maculopathy (see Figure 10-27)
Talc retinopathy	Comes from intravenous drug abuse (i.e., injection of substances like heroin, methylphenidate—fillers in these preparations)	Sometimes asymptomatic	Glistening yellow crystals in the arterioles–often perifoveal

Source: Adapted from references 57–59.

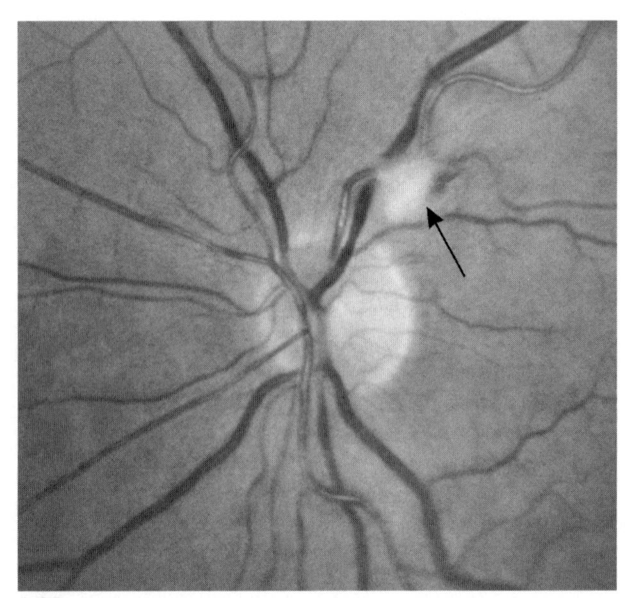

9-36

See Chapter 8 for other drugs that cause pigmentary changes in the retina.

Figure 9-36. This woman was treated with interferon alpha for her hepatitis C infection. She presented with visual blurring. Cotton-wool spots were seen (*arrow*).

Phakomatoses

The *phakomatoses* are a group of inherited diseases with distinct lesions that affect the skin and eye. For a review of the major features of these, see Shields et al.[60]

von Hippel-Lindau disease (angiomatosis retinae) (VHL) is a dominantly inherited condition on chromosome 3p (VHL gene locus) associated with tumors in the retina, brain, and other organs. Technically, when only the eye is affected, the disorder is called *von Hippel's disease*, and when other systemic findings are present, it is called *von Hippel-Lindau disease*. A German ophthalmologist, Eugen von Hippel, described the retinal angiomas in 1904, and a Swedish pathologist, Arvid Lindau, recognized the association between the retinal angiomas and tumors and cysts of the cerebellum in 1927.[61] The hemangioblastoma of the retina may be the earliest, and is the single most reliable manifestation. The retinal angioma is the first manifestation of the disease in just under one-half of the patients. Retinal angiomas continue to appear with greater frequency as the patient ages, so that the chance of having an angioma by age 80 years is 80%.[62] More than one-fourth to two-thirds of patients with VHL have cerebellar, brainstem, or spinal cord hemangioblastomas, which commonly present with headache, possibly papilledema, ataxia, and spastic paraparesis.

Figure 9-37. A. **The retinal tumors in VHL are hamartomas of the blood vessels—artery, vein, and capillaries. Therefore, the appearance is a tumor with dilated vessels seen in the posterior pole, sometimes near the disc and sometimes in the mid-periphery. Approximately 50% of the time they are bilateral. Here you can appreciate the vascular retinal mass (reddish color) with a dilated feeder artery going from the disc to the tumor and a draining vein going back to the disc (*arrow*). (Photograph courtesy of Judith E.A. Warner, M.D.)** B. **Here is a close-up of the tumor with a feeding artery.** C. **Pathologically, you can see the hemangioblastoma of the disc (*arrow*) arising from retinal architecture with a nearby large vessel.**

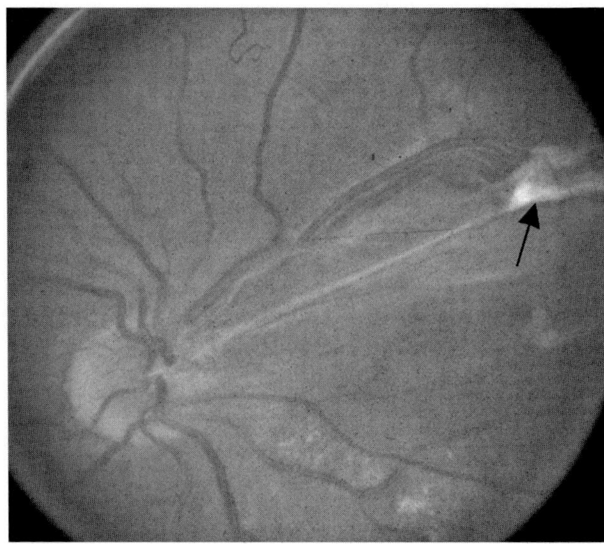

9-37A

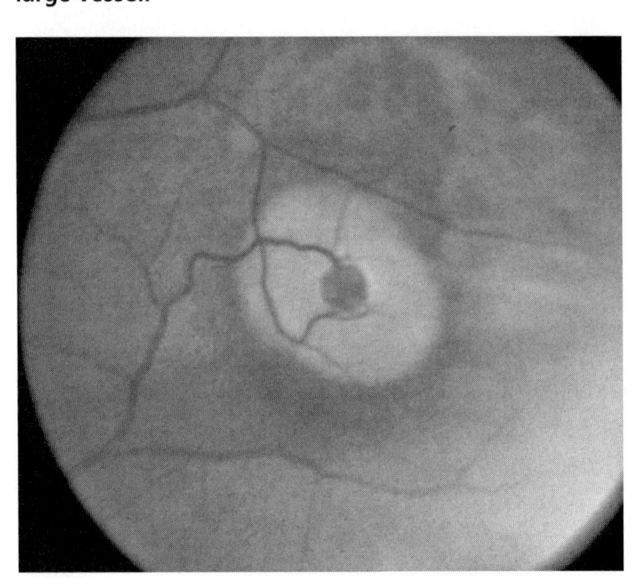

9-37B

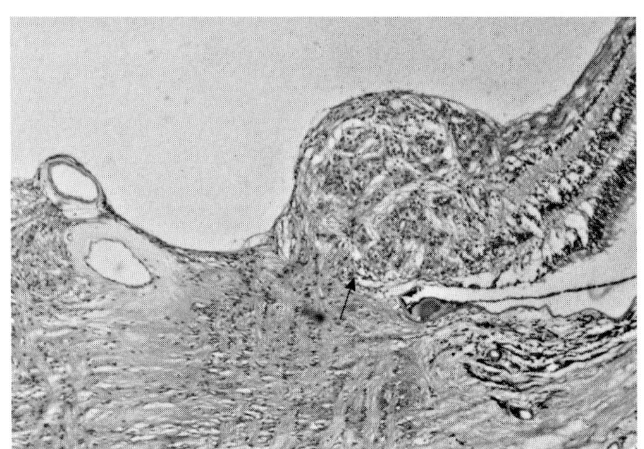

9-37C

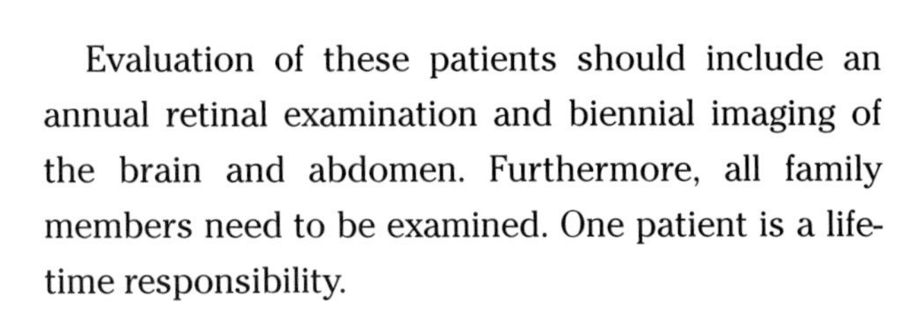

Evaluation of these patients should include an annual retinal examination and biennial imaging of the brain and abdomen. Furthermore, all family members need to be examined. One patient is a lifetime responsibility.

Figure 9-38. This individual with a family history of VHL presented with headache and ataxia. A large cerebellar hemangioblastoma was demonstrated on computed tomographic scan with contrast. There is also mild hydrocephalus on the far right scan owing to obstruction of the fourth ventricle.

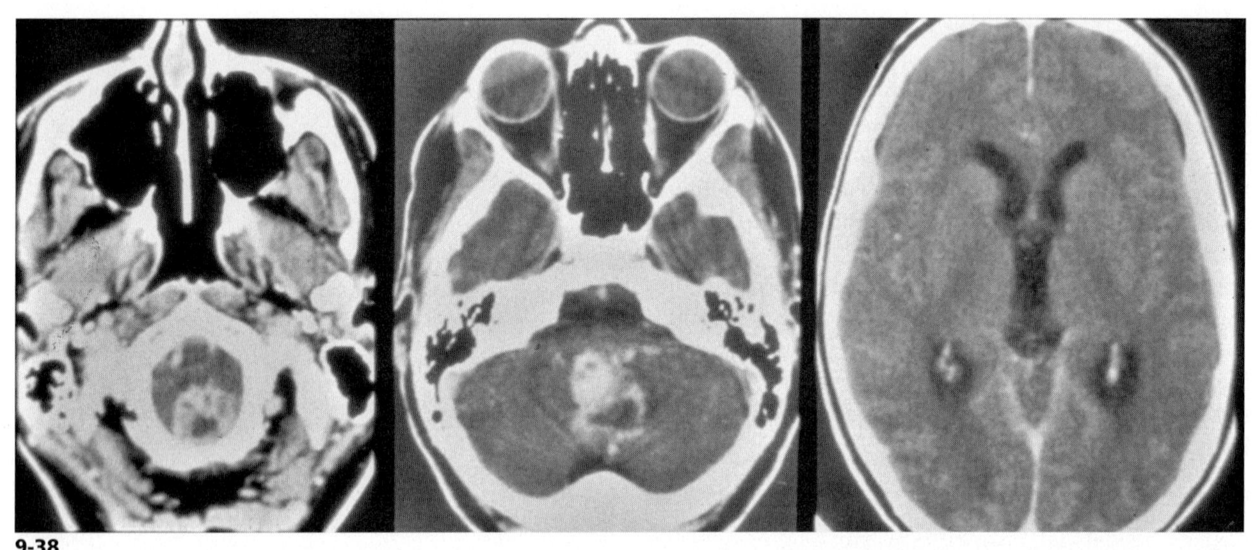

9-38

Screening of children of parents with VHL should begin at the age of approximately 5 years. VHL is an autosomal dominant defect in a tumor-suppressor gene, which causes tumors in many organs, including the eye. The tumor in the eye is similar to the cerebellar hemangioblastoma—a combination of capillaries and glial cells. Treatment of the eye tumors has included laser coagulation, but even with treatment, retinal tumors continue to appear de novo.

Figure 9-39. (opposite page) A. **Angiomas can also occur on the disc. When this occurs, one sees a reddish-orange elevated lesion that presents with vision loss from macular edema. (Photograph courtesy of Judith E.A. Warner, M.D.)** B–F. **Illustrated here is a typical hemangioma with feeder vessel and draining vein.** B. **These tumors can occur in the mid-peripheral retina.** C. **Fluorescein angiography shows a peripheral tumor with early filling.** D. **Early staining of the mass.** E. **Filling of the venous drainage system.** F. **Late leaking and staining of dye of the mass.**

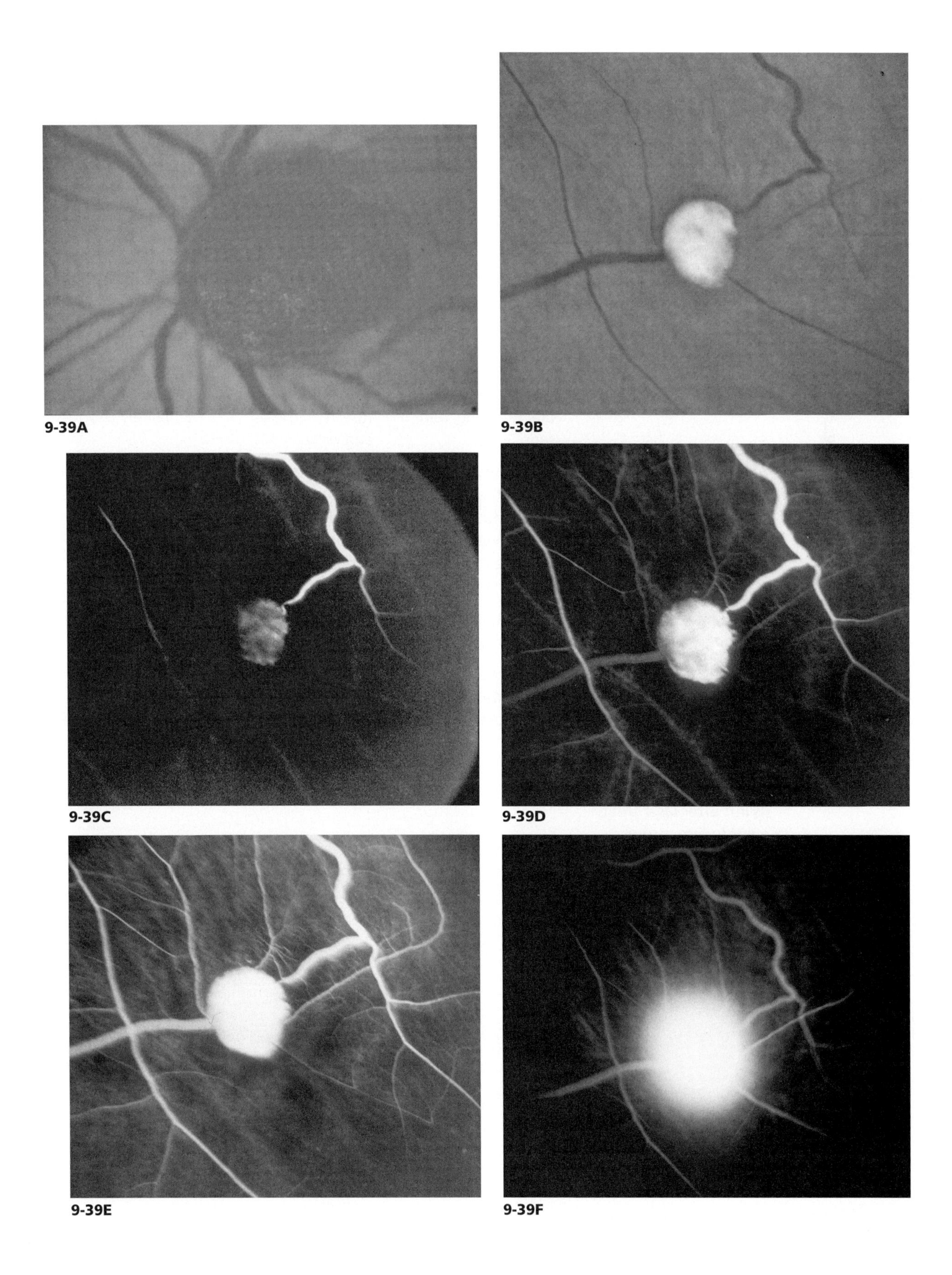
9-39A
9-39B
9-39C
9-39D
9-39E
9-39F

Finally, papilledema or optic atrophy may occur independent of VHL hemangioblastomas because obstructive hydrocephalus can occur with the cerebellar tumors.

Table 9-17. Stages of Retinal Angiomas in von Hippel-Lindau Disease

Characteristic stage	Figure	Ophthalmoscopic features	Fluorescein features	Risk of hemorrhage or complication
Stage 1	9-40A	Small gray or pink spot	No perfusion of the spot	None
Stage 2	9-40B	Elevated, red nodule; draining vein seen	See leaking and perfusion of the angioma	No hemorrhage, but will likely progress
Stage 3	9-40C	Elevated red nodule with arterial and venous feeder vessels; may see exudates	See severe leakage, dropout of surrounding capillaries; prolonged hyperfluorescence	Hemorrhage is likely; begin treatment at this stage, otherwise progression is certain
Stage 4	9-40D—The disc is in the center field, but you can see detachment superiorly	See all of the above plus exudate detachment	—	Severe consequence; progress to stage 5
Stage 5	9-40E—This tumor has been treated with laser, but is still growing; you can appreciate the pigmentary deposits left after laser treatment (*white arrow*) and the feeding arteriole (*black arrows*)	Total exudative detachment	—	Terminal stage: glaucoma, uveitis, cataract leads to globe removal

Note: (A) is not exactly only a pink spot, because there are technically exudates present; nevertheless, it is early on in the disease.
Source: Adapted from reference 61.

Figure 9-40. The stages of VHL: Stage 1 (A), Stage 2 (B), Stage 3 (C), Stage 4 (D), and Stage 5 (E). The two black arrows point to the narrow feeding arteriole (right) and the fat tortuous draining vein (left). The hemangioblastoma is below.

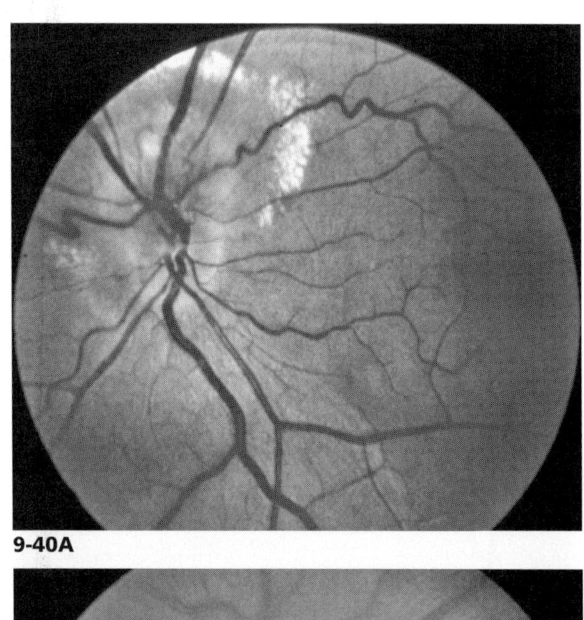

9-40A

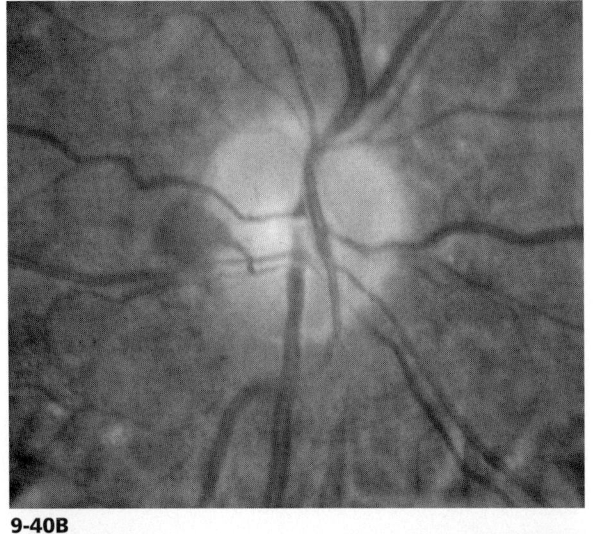

9-40B

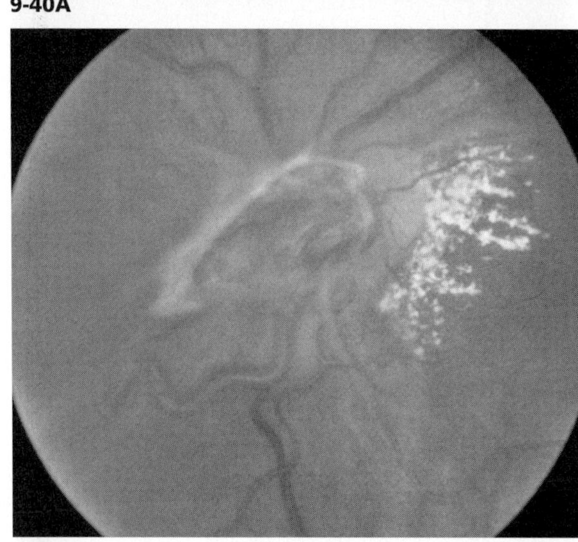

9-40C

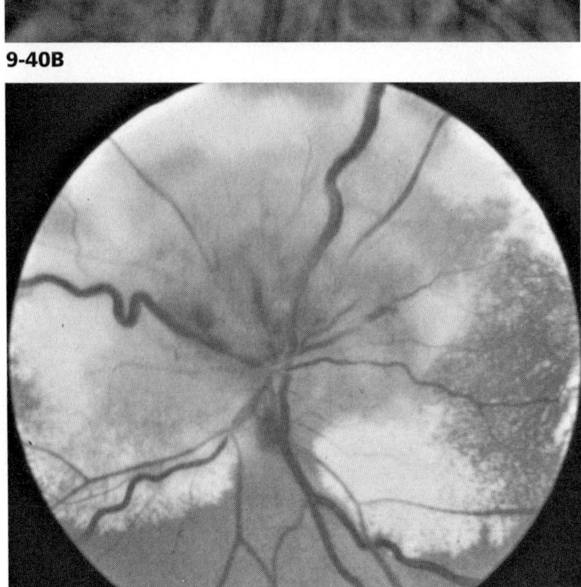

9-40D

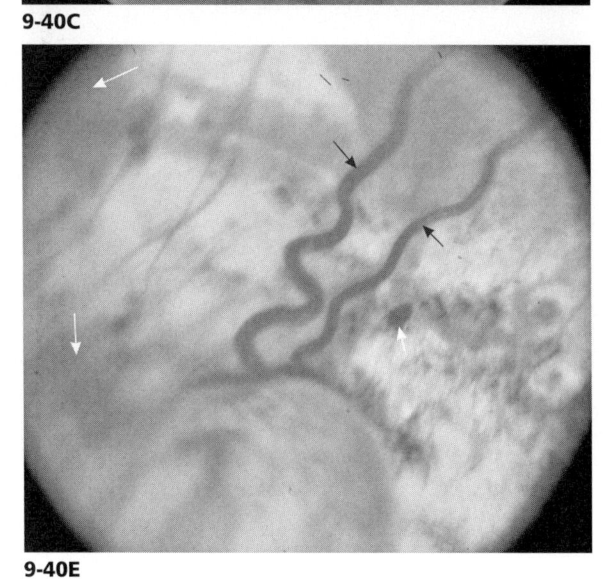

9-40E

Tuberous sclerosis is an autosomal dominant disorder (chromosome 9, TSC1 gene, and chromosome 16 TSC2 gene) that produces hamartomas (i.e., tumors of embryological tissue from the organ in which it grows). The classic triad of seizures, mental retardation, and adenoma sebaceum is not seen in all affected individuals. Tuberous sclerosis occurs in 1/10,000–50,000 people. Patients may have only seizures or be sent for evaluation of mental retardation.[62] There are frequently no visual symptoms. Systematic examination is very helpful. First, look for facial adenoma sebaceum—groups of soft, fleshy, elevated spots on the malar and perialar aspect of the face. Furthermore, one may find subungual fibromas in the skin around fingernails, and also ash-leaf spots. In the retina, look for hamartomas.

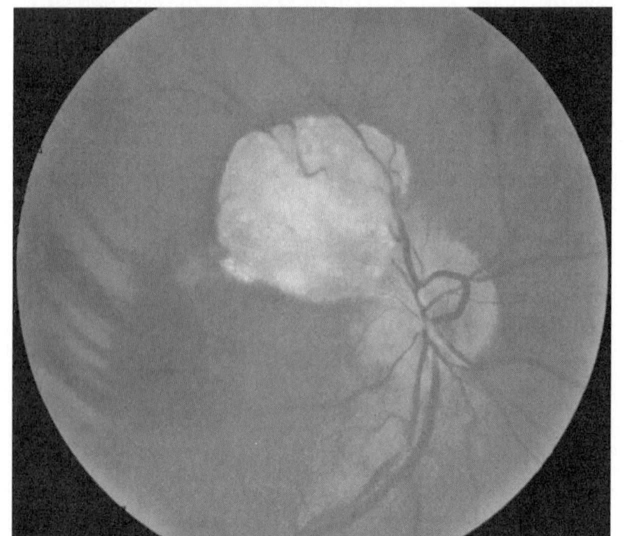

9-41A

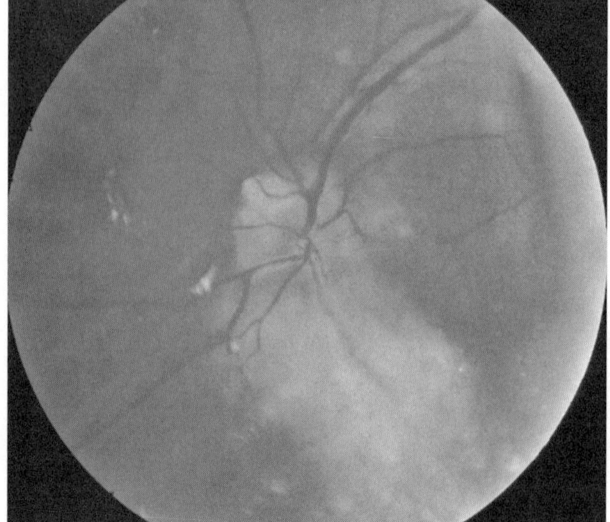

9-41B

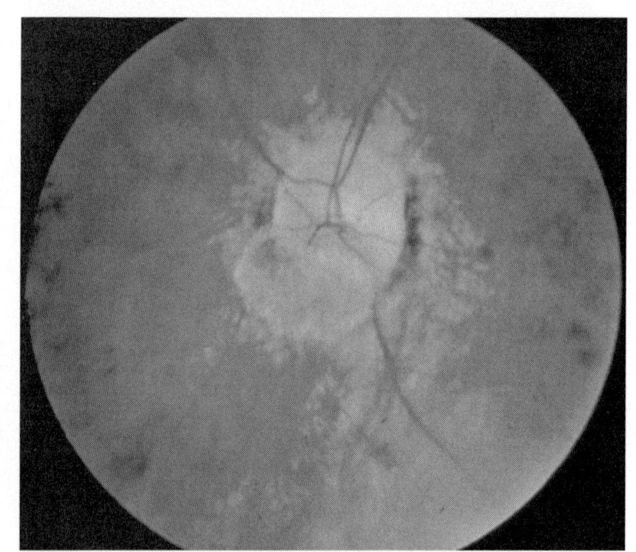

9-41C

Figure 9-41. A. **Retinal hamartomas consist of smooth, round, calcific, gliotic elevations. They have been called "mulberries" because of their lumpy-bumpy appearance.** B. **Others have called them "giant drusen," like disc drusen, because of their almost geodelike appearance.**[62] C. **They often appear around the disc and occasionally may need to be differentiated from a tumor, like a retinoblastoma in a child.** ***Continued***

Figure 9-41. ***Continued.*** D,E. **Other typical hamartomas of tuberous sclerosis occur in the retina.**

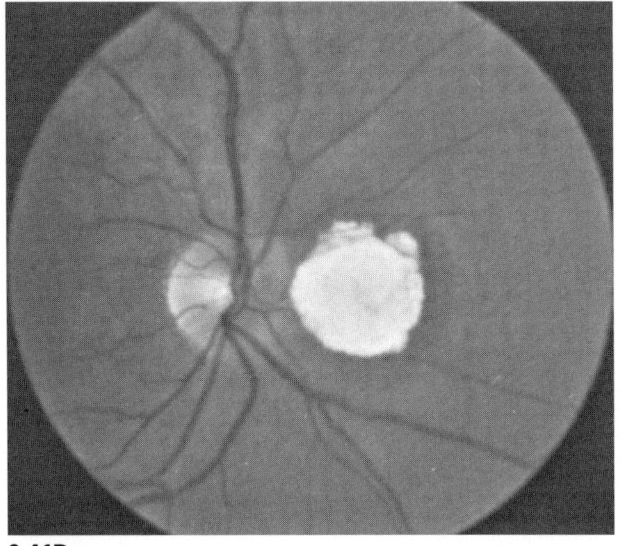

9-41D

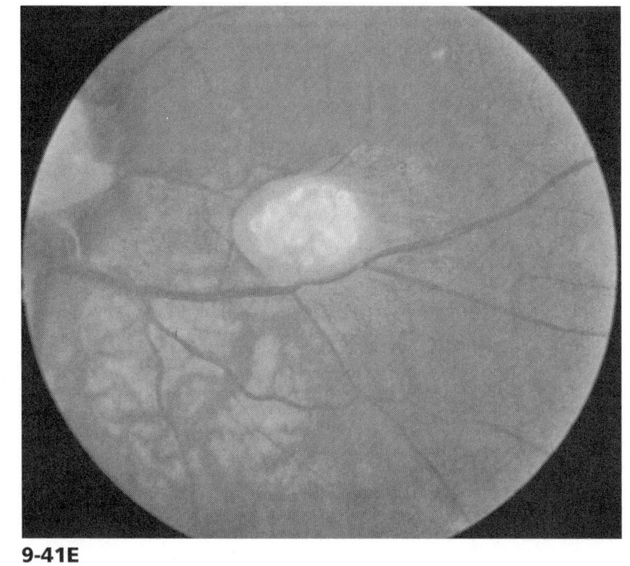

9-41E

Figure 9-42. A. **Soft, fleshy, elevated spots on the malar aspect of the face are characteristic of adenoma sebaceum.** B. **The skin may also show hypopigmented spots called "ash-leaf spots" (best viewed with an ultraviolet Wood's lamp) and hyperpigmented spots (so-called café-au-lait spots).** C. **Subungual hamartomas are common in the finger- and toenails (*arrow*). Hamartomas also may affect the kidneys (horseshoe kidney) and heart (leiomyoma).**

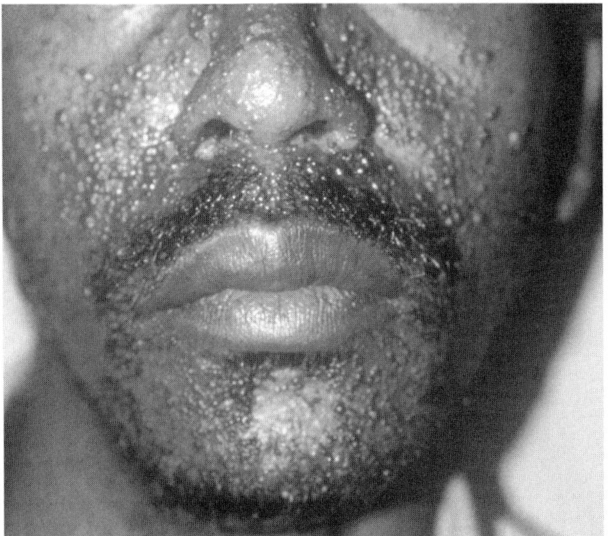

9-42A

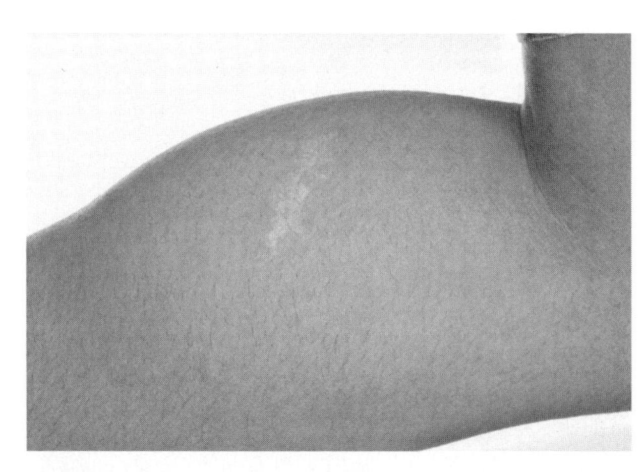

9-42B

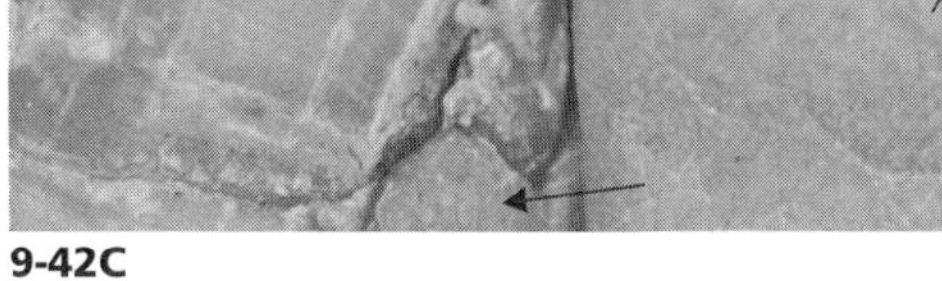

9-42C

Neurofibromatosis is another autosomal dominant phakomatosis that affects the skin, nervous system, and eyes; it is discussed in Chapter 4, Figure 4-21. There are no characteristic retinal changes.

Sturge-Weber disease (also called *encephalotrigeminal angiomatosis*) is characterized by a large port wine stain on the face in the territory of the first division of the trigeminal nerve, first division and an accompanying venous malformation of the frontal meninges, and choroidal angioma with associated abnormal veins and possible glaucoma. Retinal detachment with Sturge-Weber disease is uncommon. Ophthalmoscopically, choroidal angiomas appear as an area of very red hue. Fluorescein angiography shows a spotted appearance.[63] Aside from the angioma, the disc may display findings associated with glaucoma ipsilateral to the port wine stain.

Wyburn-Mason syndrome is a syndrome characterized by A-V anastomoses in the retina and midbrain. Although these were recognized before they were described by Dr. R. Wyburn-Mason, his name is affixed to the condition.[64] The retinal vascular lesion consists of small to large anastomoses between the artery and vein. These vascular anomalies, unlike those of von Hippel-Lindau, do not cause exudation and retinal detachment. Larger vascular anomalies in the retina are more likely to have central nervous system vascular anomalies.[64]

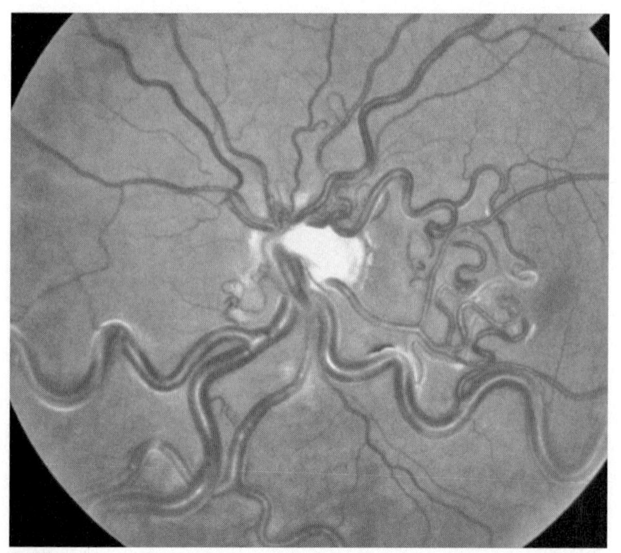

9-43

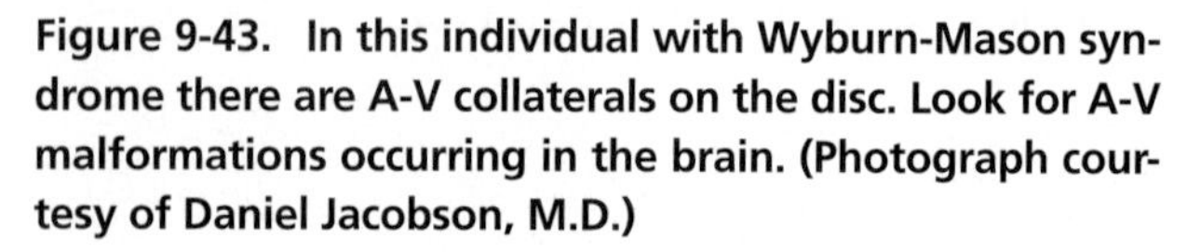

Figure 9-43. In this individual with Wyburn-Mason syndrome there are A-V collaterals on the disc. Look for A-V malformations occurring in the brain. (Photograph courtesy of Daniel Jacobson, M.D.)

What Else Should You Look for in the Retina?

CHOROIDAL FOLDS

Choroidal folds occur whenever there is alteration of the choroid by edema or pressure by a mass that causes the RPE and choroid to be put into folds or parallel grooves, which are alternating dark and light lines. The lines are usually in a horizontal direction. Many conditions cause chorioretinal folds, including tumors pressing on the back of the globe, Graves' orbitopathy, hypotony, and acquired hyperopia; they may also be idiopathic. When you see unilateral chorioretinal folds, think of an orbital mass and look for proptosis. When the folds are bilateral, consider hyperopia, hypotony, scleritis, papilledema, and thyroid eye disease. Symptoms include metamorphopsia (distorted vision) and sometimes acquired hyperopia.[65] Look for evidence of orbital tumors and Graves' disease by observing for proptosis, reduced ability to retropulse the globe, or signs of optic neuropathy. Imaging can be very helpful, showing not only orbital processes like masses or enlarged muscles, but also flattening of the posterior globe seen in idiopathic choroidal folds. If imaging does not reveal a cause of choroidal folds, a lumbar puncture can be helpful to show increased intracranial pressure.[66]

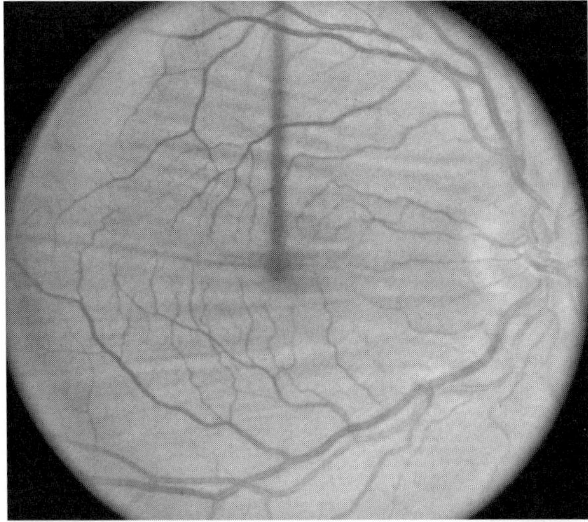

9-44A

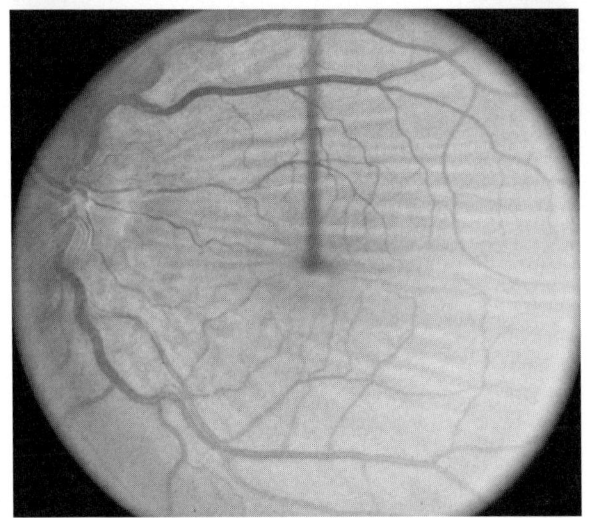

9-44B

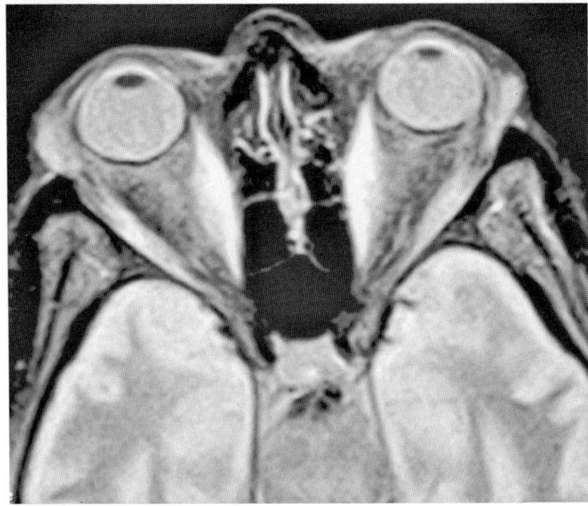

9-44C

Figure 9-44. A. **Choroidal folds commonly appear as horizontal lines in the posterior pole in this woman with Graves' disease.** B. **The folds are often seen through the macula as alternating yellow and darkish streaks. The vertical line in the center of the photograph is a fixation device used at the time of the photograph and does not represent the pathology.** C. **In this case, the cause was markedly enlarged muscles from Graves' disease documented on magnetic resonance imaging.**

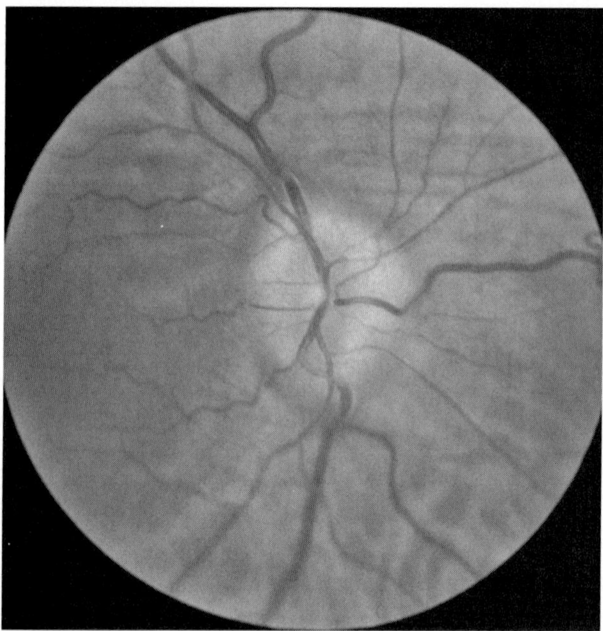

9-45A

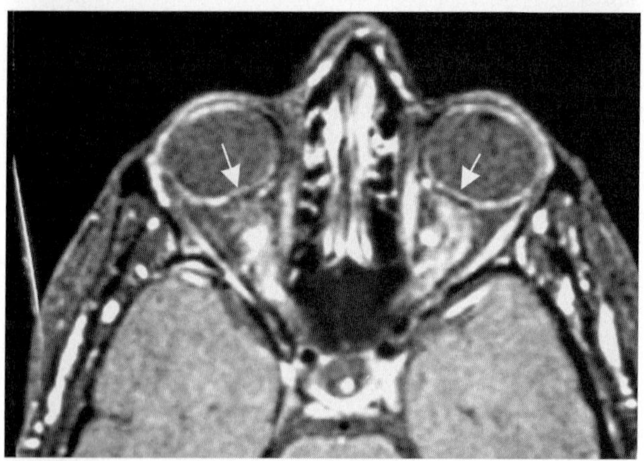

9-45B

Table 9-18. Etiologies of Choroidal Folds

Idiopathic
Hyperopia
Hypotony
Scleritis
Uveitis
Choroiditis
Orbital tumor
Choroidal tumor
Pseudotumor of the orbit
Frontoethmoidal mucoceles[67]
Papilledema
Graves' ophthalmopathy
Postsurgical procedures

Source: Adapted from references 65,66.

Figure 9-45. A. **This woman presented with visual obscuration and acquired hyperopia. Choroidal folds and disc swelling were found on examination. Notice the tessellated fundus in this patient.** B. **Magnetic resonance imaging showed flattening of the posterior globe (*arrows*) by an optic nerve sheath meningioma. In cases of choroidal folds, look for the flattening of the globe and for the process causing that flattening on an imaging study.**

RETINAL STRIAE

Retinal striae are very subtle wrinkles in the internal limiting membrane (similar to cellophane wrinkling) of the retina. These cannot be seen without a dilated pupil and a careful examination.

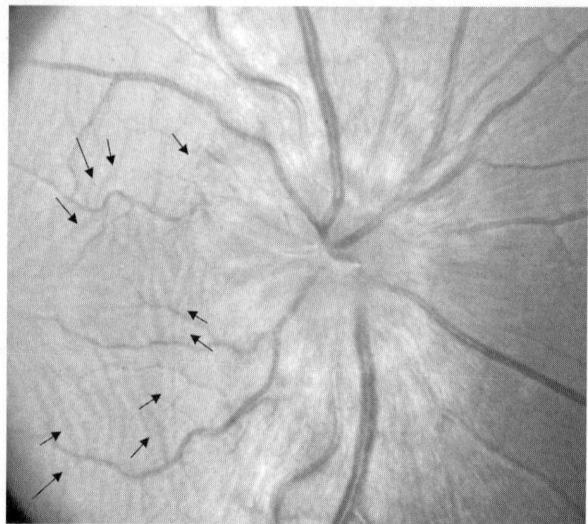

9-46

Figure 9-46. Retinal striae (*arrows*) are around the macula owing to disc swelling associated with Vogt-Koyanagi-Harada disease. (Photograph courtesy of Paul Zimmerman, M.D.)

ANGIOID STREAKS

Angioid streaks are not very common, but can be seen in systemic conditions like pseudoxanthoma elasticum, Ehlers-Danlos syndrome, Paget's disease, and sickle cell anemia (see also Figure 1-31A). Angioid streaks are caused by breaks in Bruch's membrane (see also Figure 6-16). Angioid streaks are asymptomatic unless the break in the membrane is near the macula, in which case there may be visual blurring and vision loss. Furthermore, if there is vascular proliferation or neovascularization under the retina, hemorrhage can occur.

Figure 9-47. In this woman with documented Marfan's syndrome and pseudoxanthoma elasticum, angioid streaks were present. A. **At first blush, angioid streaks may appear to be a blood vessel with a white spot. As they develop, pigment forms because of damage to the RPE.** B. **In this case, 2 years later, more pigment is seen. Angioid streaks are seen around the disc, in the macula, and anywhere in the retina.** C. **A fluorescein angiogram demonstrates these breaks dramatically. Notice that the breaks typically radiate from the disc. The black spots on fluorescein are pigmentary changes.** ***Continued***

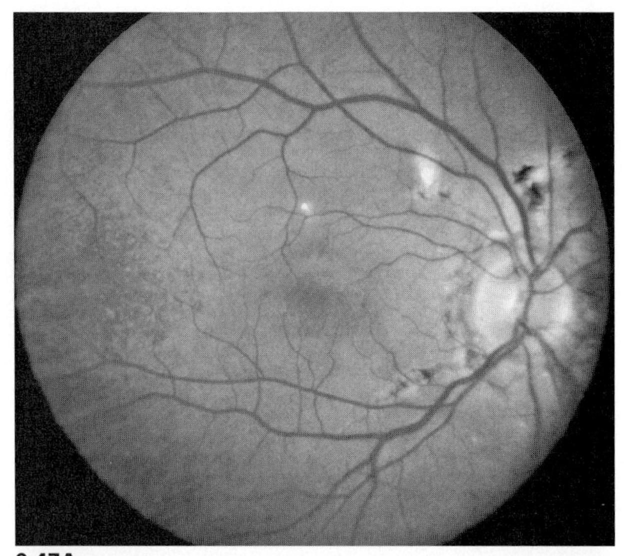

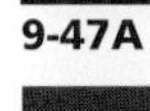

9-47A

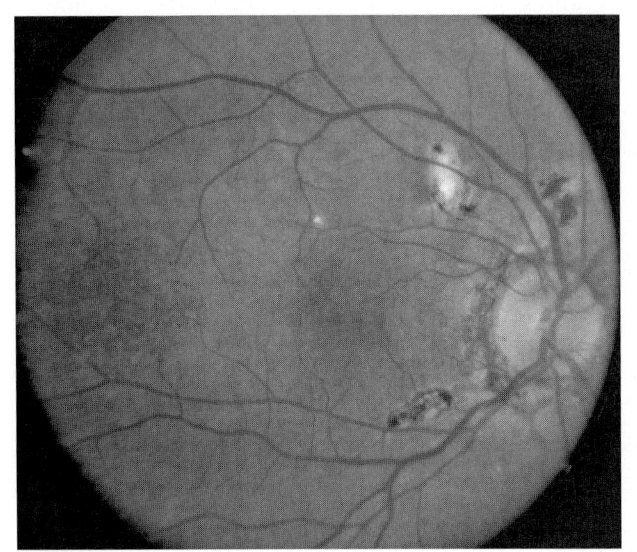

9-47B

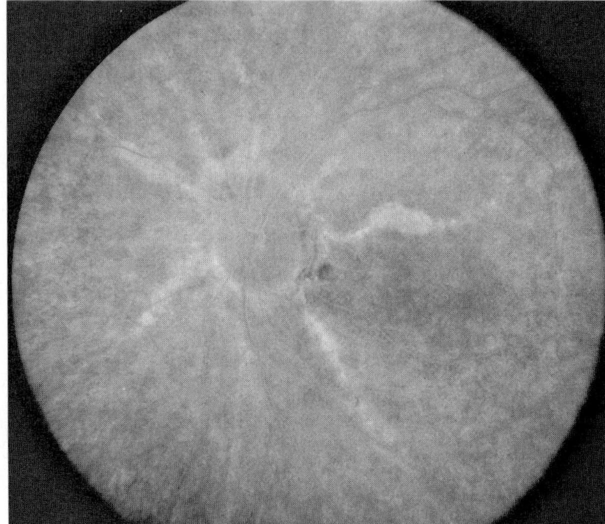

9-47C

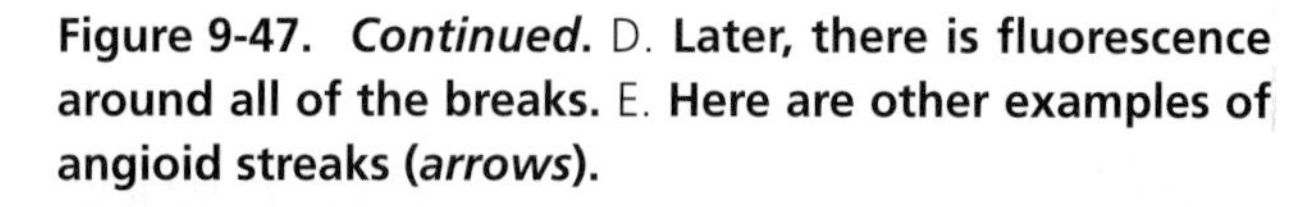

Figure 9-47. *Continued.* D. **Later, there is fluorescence around all of the breaks.** E. **Here are other examples of angioid streaks (*arrows*).**

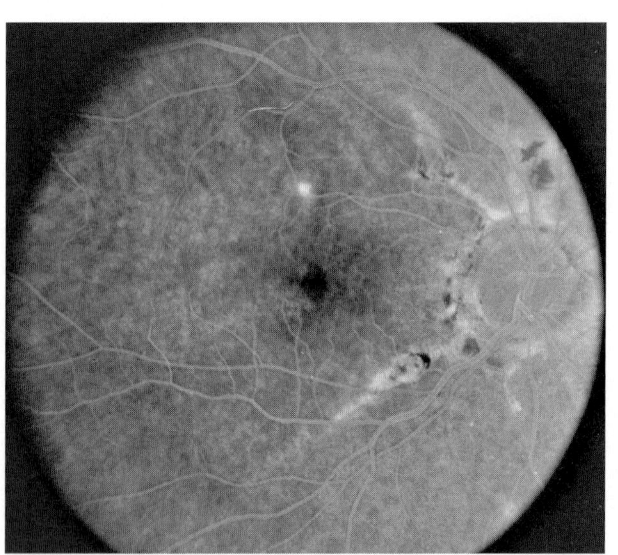

9-47D

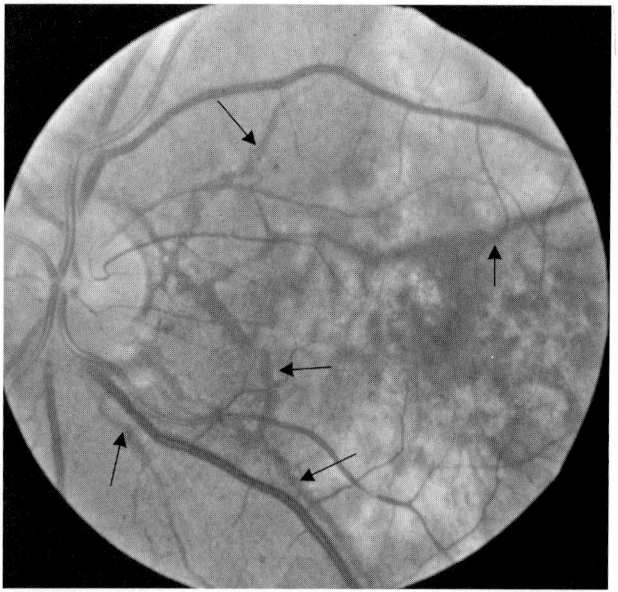

9-47E

RETINAL DETACHMENT

Retinal detachment is an ominous event, which often requires quick attention by not only an ophthalmologist, but also a retinal specialist. The symptoms include a sudden shower of floaters and sparkles, and perhaps blurring of vision. Myopic individuals are at higher risk for a retinal detachment. Frequently, the detachment is difficult to see because it is further in the periphery than the posterior pole, which is accessible by direct ophthalmoscopy. If you suspect someone has had a retinal detachment he or she should be referred immediately, that same day, for a dilated examination by an ophthalmologist. Sometimes you may be able to view the detachment with your direct ophthalmoscope.

Figure 9-48. A. This man presented with an increased number of floaters and decreased vision in his left eye. Follow the vessels out temporally from the disc to the periphery (the *arrow* marks the superior temporal vessel at a bifurcation). B. A retinal detachment is visible. The arrowheads outline the detachment, whereas the arrow points to the same temporal vessel bifurcation that you see in A. C. The visual field revealed a defect where the detachment was. Repair of the detachment returned his vision and visual field to normal.

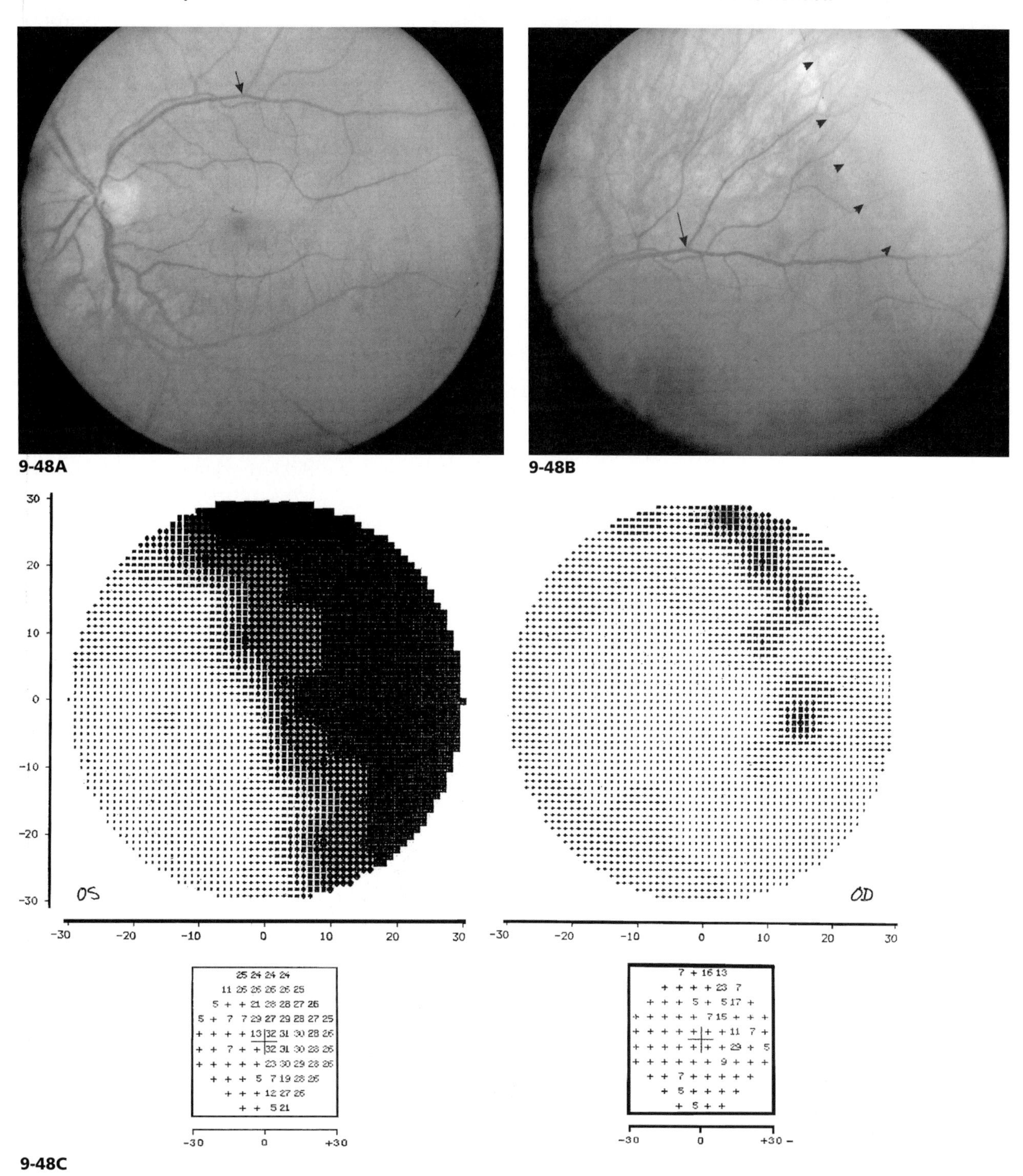

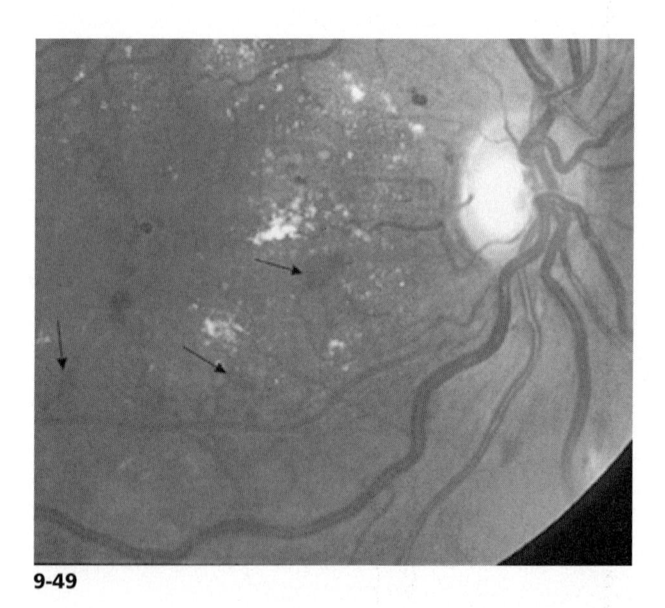

9-49

Practical Viewing Essentials

1. When viewing the retina, be sure to look not only with the regular white light, but also the red-free (green) light.
2. Dilate the pupils—you won't see much of the retina without having done so.
3. Although an indirect examination of the retina gives a bigger picture, your direct ophthalmoscope gives a satisfactory look at the retina.
4. Look for hemorrhages, white spots, and pigment. What is the pattern?
5. Neovascularization has many causes.
6. When you see retinal disease, look for systemic clues that may be helpful, including the skin, blood, and blood pressure.
7. If you see abnormalities in the retina, the patient needs a dilated examination by an ophthalmologist.

References

1. Gowers W. A Manual and Atlas of Medical Ophthalmoscopy. London: J & A Churchill, 1879.
2. Jampol LM, Ebroon DA, Goldbaum MH. Peripheral proliferative retinopathies: an update on angiogenesis etiologies and management. Surv Ophthalmol 1994;38:519–540.
3. Lee P, Wang CC, Adamis AP. Ocular neovascularization: an epidemiological review. Surv Ophthalmol 1998;43:245–269.
4. Amos AF, McCarty DJ, Zimmet P. The rising global burden of diabetes and its complications: estimates and projections to the year 2010. Diabet Med 1997;14(Suppl 5):S1–S85.
5. Neely KA, Quillen DA, Schachat AP, et al. Diabetic retinopathy. Med Clin North Am 1998;82:847–876.
6. Sussman EJ, Tsiaras WG, Soper KA. Diagnosis of diabetic eye disease. JAMA 1982;247:3231–3234.
7. Singer DE, Nathan DM, Fogel HA, Schachat AP. Screening for diabetic retinopathy. Ann Intern Med 1992;116:660–671.
8. Wiedemann P. Growth factors in retinal diseases: proliferative vitreoretinopathy, proliferative diabetic retinopathy and retinal degeneration. Surv Ophthalmol 1992;36:373–384.
9. Federman JL, Gouras P, Schubert H, et al. Textbook of Ophthalmology, Vol 9. St. Louis: Mosby, 1994.
10. Grading diabetic retinopathy from stereoscopic color fundus photographs–an extension of the modified Airlie House classification. ETDRS report number 10. Early Treatment Diabetic Retinopathy Study Research Group. Ophthalmology 1991;98(5 Suppl):786–806.
11. Chew EY, Ferris FL. Nonproliferative Diabetic Retinopathy. In SJ Ryan, AP Schachat, RP Murphy (eds), Retina. St. Louis: Mosby, 2001;1295–1308.
12. Goldberg MF, Fine SL. Symposium on the Treatment of Diabetic Retinopathy. Arlington, VA: U.S. Department of Health, Education, and Welfare (Publication No 1890), 1969.
13. Klein R, Klein BE, Magli YL, et al. An alternative method of grading diabetic retinopathy. Ophthalmology 1986;93:1183–1187.
14. Klein BE, Davis MD, Segal P, et al. Diabetic retinopathy. Assessment of severity and progression. Ophthalmology 1984;91:10–17.
15. Garcia CA, Ruiz RS. Ocular complications of diabetes. Clin Symp 1992;44:2–32.
16. Rand LI, Prud'homme GJ, Ederer F, Canner PL. Factors influencing the development of visual loss in advanced diabetic retinopathy. Diabetic Retinopathy Study (DRS) Report No. 10. Invest Ophthalmol Vis Sci 1985;26(7):983–991.
17. Arango J, Pavan PR. Diabetic retinopathy treatment trials: a review. Int Ophthalmol Clin 1998;38(2):123–154.
18. Klein R, Klein BE, Moss Se, Cruickshank KJ. The Wisconsin Epidemiologic Study of Diabetic Retinopathy, XV. The long-term incidence of macular edema. Ophthalmology 1995;102:7–16.
19. Hyman BN, Moser M. Hypertension update. Surv Ophthalmol 1996;41:79–89.
20. Stanton AV, Mullaney P, Mee F, et al. A method of quantifying retinal microvascular alterations associated with blood pressure and age. J Hypertens 1995;13:41–48.
21. Pogue VA, Ellis C, Michel J, Francis CK. New staging system of the fifth Joint National Committee report on the detection, evaluation, and treatment of high blood pressure (JNC-V) alters assessment of the severity and treatment of hypertension. Hypertension 1996;28(5):713–718.
22. National high blood pressure education program. The Sixth Report of the Joint National Committee on Prevention, Detection, Evaluation, and treatment of High Blood Pressure. Bethesda, MD: U.S. Department of Health and Human Services, Public Health Service, National Institutes of Health, National Heart, Lung, and Blood Institute, 1997; NIH Publication No. 98-4080.
23. Klein R, Klein BE, Moss SE, Wang Q. Hypertension and retinopathy, arteriolar narrowing, and arteriovenous nicking in a population. Arch Ophthalmol 1994;112:92–98.
24. Murphy RP, Chew EY. Hypertension. In SJ Ryan, AP Schachat, RB Murphy (eds), Retina. St. Louis: Mosby, 2001;1404–1409.
25. Wagener HP, Clay GE, Gipner JF. Classification of retinal lesions. Trans Am Ophthalmol Soc 1947;45: 57–73.
26. Scheie HG. Evaluation of ophthalmoscopic changes of hypertension and arteriolar sclerosis. Arch Ophthalmol 1953;49.
27. Hayreh SS, Servais GE, Virdi PS. Fundus lesion in malignant hypertension. V. Hypertensive optic neuropathy. Ophthalmology 1986;93:74–87.
28. Boozalis GT, Schachat AP, Green WR. Subretinal neovascularization from the retina in radiation retinopathy. Retina 1987;7:156–161.
29. Zamber RW, Kinyoun JL. Radiation retinopathy. West J Med 1992;157:530–533.
30. Irvine AR, Wood IS. Radiation retinopathy as an experimental model for ischemic proliferative retinopathy and rubeosis irides. Am J Ophthalmol 1987;103:790–797.
31. Maguire AM, Schachat AP. Radiation retinopathy. In

SJ Ryan, AP Schachat, RP Murphy (eds), Retina. St. Louis: Mosby, 2001;1509–1515.
32. Brown GC, Shields JA, Sanborn G, et al. Radiation retinopathy. Ophthalmology 1982;89:1494–1501.
33. Kline LB, Kim JY, Ceballos R. Radiation optic neuropathy. Ophthalmology 1985;92:1118–1126.
34. Guy J, Schatz NJ. Hyperbaric oxygen in the treatment of radiation-induced optic neuropathy. Ophthalmology 1986;93:1083–1088.
35. Borruat FX, Schatz NJ, Glaser JS, et al. Visual recovery from radiation-induced optic neuropathy. The role of hyperbaric oxygen therapy. J Clin Neuroophthalmol 1993;13(2):98–101.
36. Coskuncan NM, Jabs DA, Dunn JP, et al. The eye in bone marrow transplantation. VI. Retinal complications. Arch Ophthalmol 1994;112:372–379.
37. Jacobson DM, Thirkhill CE, Tipping SJ. A clinical triad to diagnose paraneoplastic retinopathy. Ann Neurol 1990;28:162–167.
38. Dhaliwal RS, Schachat AP. Remote effects of cancer on the retina. In SJ Ryan, AP Schachat, RP Murphy (eds), Retina. St. Louis: Mosby, 2001;617–624.
39. Cohen SB, Van Houten PA. Hemoglobinopathies. In SJ Ryan, AP Schachat, RP Murphy (eds), Retina. St. Louis: Mosby, 1994;1465–1472.
40. Cohen SB, Godber MF, Fletcher ME, Jednock NJ. Diagnosis and management of ocular complications of sickle hemoglobinopathies: Part II. Ophthalmol Surg 1986;17:110–116.
41. Rizzo JF. Neuro-ophthalmologic disease of the retina. In DM Albert, FA Jakobiec (eds), Principles and Practice of Ophthalmology. Philadelphia: Saunders, 1994;2507–2529.
42. Holland GN. Reconsidering the pathogenesis of ocular toxoplasmosis. Am J Ophthalmol 1999;128:502–505.
43. Sherman MD, Nozik RA. Other infections of the choroid and retina. Toxoplasmosis, histoplasmosis, Lyme disease, syphilis, tuberculosis, ocular toxocariasis. Infect Dis Clin North Am 1992;6:893–906.
44. Hawkins BS, Alexander J, Schachat AP. Ocular histoplasmosis. In SJ Ryan, AP Schachat, RP Murphy (eds), Retina. St. Louis: Mosby, 2001;1687–1701.
45. Hennis HL, Scott AA, Apple DJ. Cytomegalovirus retinitis. Surv Ophthalmol 1989;34:193–203.
46. Nussenblatt RB, Palestine AG. Uveitis Fundamentals and Clinical Practice. Chicago: Year Book, 1989.
47. Graham K, Pinnolis M. AIDS and the posterior segment. Int Ophthalmol Clin 1998;38(1):265–280.
48. DeSmet MD. Differential diagnosis of retinitis and choroiditis in patients with acquired immunodeficiency syndrome. Am J Med 1992;92(Suppl 2A):S17–S21.
49. Stafford-Brady FJ, Urowitz MB, Gladman DD, Easterbrook M. Lupus retinopathy. Arthritis Rheum 1988;31:1105–1110.
50. Read RW, Chong LP, Rao NA. Occlusive retinal vasculitis associated with systemic lupus erythematosus. Arch Ophthalmol 2000;118:388–389.
51. Jabs DA, Hanneken AM, Schachat AP, Fine SL. Choroidopathy in systemic lupus erythematosus. Arch Ophthalmol 1988;106:230–234.
52. Jabs DA. Rheumatic diseases. In SJ Ryan, AP Schachat, RP Murphy (eds), Retina. St. Louis: Mosby, 2001;1410–1433.
53. Holt JM, Gordon-Smith EC. Retinal abnormalities in disease of the blood. Br J Ophthalmol 1969;53:145–159.
54. Rennie IG. Ocular manifestations of malignant disease. Br J Hosp Med 1992;47:185–189.
55. Allen RA, Straatsma BR. Ocular involvement in leukemia and allied disorders. Arch Ophthalmol 1961;66:490–508.
56. Reddy SC, Quah SH, Low HC, Jackson N. Prognostic significance of retinopathy at presentation in adult acute leukemia. Ann Hematol 1998;76:15–18.
57. Swartz M. Other Diseases: Drug toxicity and metabolic and nutritional conditions. In SJ Ryan, AP Schachat, RP Murphy (eds), Retina. St. Louis: Mosby, 1994;1755–1766.
58. Kempen JH. Drug-induced maculopathy. Int Ophthalmol Clin 1999;39(4):67–82.
59. McLane NJ, Carroll DM. Ocular manifestations of drug abuse. Surv Ophthalmol 1988;30:298–313.
60. Shields JA, Shields CL. Systemic hamartomoses (phacomatoses). In Shields JA, Shields CL (eds), Intraocular Tumors. A Text and Atlas. Philadelphia: WB Saunders, 1992;513–539.
61. Wittebol-Post D, Hes FJ, Lips CJM. The eye in von Hippel-Lindau disease. Long-term follow-up of screening and treatment: recommendations. J Int Med 1998;243:555–561.
62. Sharma S, Cruess AF. Tuberous sclerosis and the eye. In SJ Ryan, AP Schachat, RP Murphy (eds), Retina. St. Louis: Mosby, 2001;588–595.
63. Ferry AP. Other phakomatoses. In SJ Ryan, AP Schachat, RP Murphy (eds), Retina. St. Louis: Mosby, 2001;596–597.
64. Wyburn-Mason R. Arteriovenous aneurysm of midbrain and retina, facial naevi and mental changes. Brain 1943;66:163–203.
65. Jacobson DM. Intracranial hypertension and the syndrome of acquired hyperopia with choroidal folds. J Neuroophthalmol 1995;15:178–185.
66. Griebel SR, Kosmorsky GS. Choroidal folds associated with increased intracranial pressure. Am J Ophthalmol 2000;129:513–516.
67. Leventer DB, Linberg JV, Ellis B. Frontoethmoidal mucoceles causing bilateral chorioretinal folds. Arch Ophthalmol 2001;119:922–923.

10 What Is That in the Macula?

The macula lutea (yellow spot) is an ill-defined area at the posterior pole of the eye having approximately the same dimensions as the optic disc. The yellow color is not ordinarily visible during life against the orange background of the choroid but stands out in death or whenever the retina becomes opaque. The yellow color increases with age and corresponds to the 'pigment' granules in the ganglion cells seen by electron microscopy.

David Cogan[1]

The macula serves the highest visual acuity and the structure of the macula promotes this function. The macula area lies temporal to the disc, approximately 2 disc diameters away. In real life, this is really a short distance—only 3–4 mm. The macula appears darker than the rest of the retina. When viewing the macula, it is important to first remember the structure of this part of the retina. First, anatomically, the macula consists of the foveola umbo, fovea, parafovea, and perifovea.

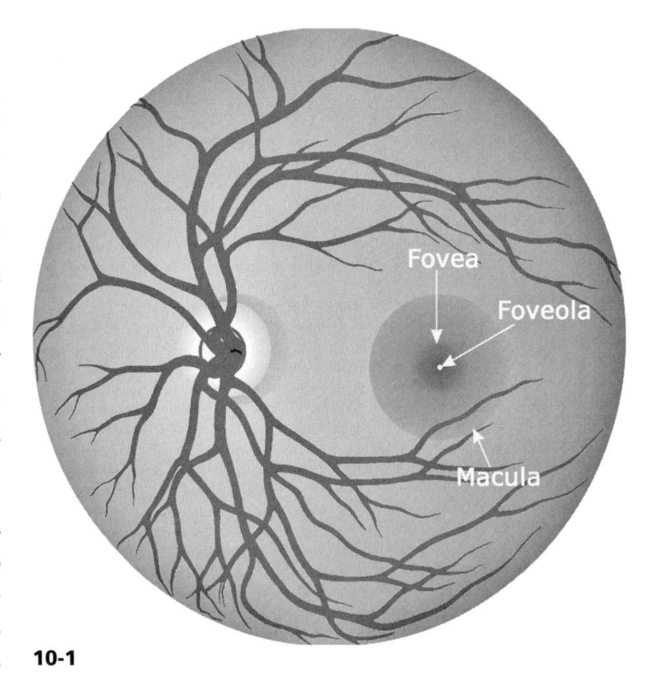

Figure 10-1. The macula is temporal and slightly inferior to the disc. The center spot is called the *foveola*. The *fovea* is the area just around the foveola, and the *macula* is the entire structure. The fovea has only cone cells, and corresponding ganglion cells are radially displaced. **10-1**

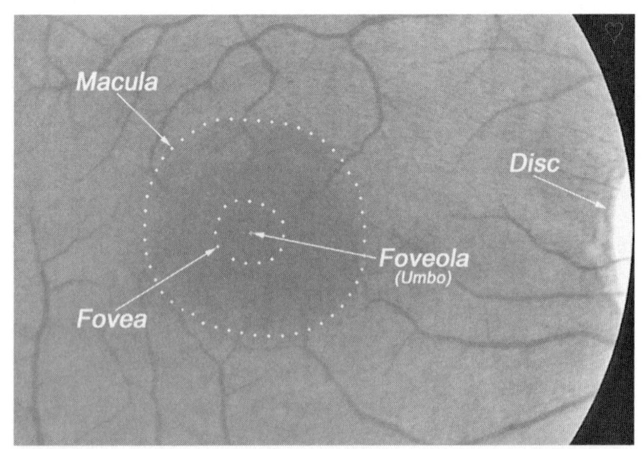

10-2A

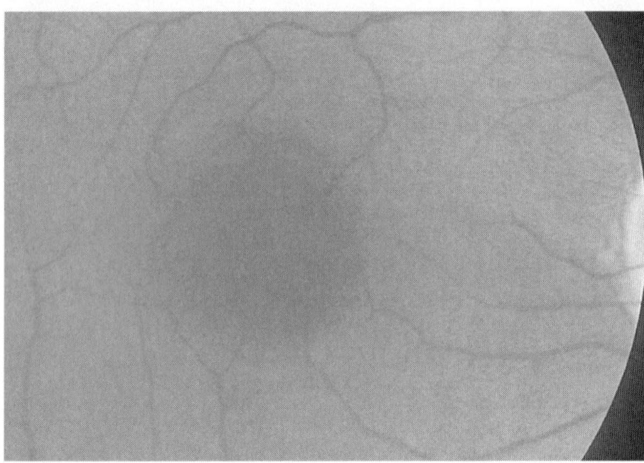

10-2B

Figure 10-2. A. **This labeled photograph of the macula demonstrates the macula, fovea, and foveola.** B. **Now can you find the foveola, fovea, para fovea, peri fovea, and macula?**

We can actually see the foveola (the umbo is simply the microscopic center of the foveola), in which there are only cones and Müller's cells from the inner nuclear layer. Notice the yellow dot of the foveola. The yellow dot is a xanthopigment—lutein and zeaxanthin that act as an optical filter and antioxidant.[2] Look at the macula with the red-free light (green)—it may accentuate the yellow dot. Around the foveola is the fovea. This is a space that on microscopic sections encompasses the area in which there are still no rods and no blood vessels (the foveal avascular zone). Finally, surrounding the fovea are the parafoveal area (the area around the fovea) and the perifoveal area (which makes it almost to the disc).

There are also light aberrations around the macula, with lines of watery glistening around the area. This is light reflecting off of the internal limiting membrane as it drapes over vessels (see Figure 10-3).

The macula has only cones. There are no rods and no blood vessels from the retinal circulation to obscure vision, and the macula relies on blood supply from the choroidal circulation. Unlike the rest of the retina, the macula continues to differentiate after birth until approximately 4 months of age.[3]

The nerve fiber layer is peculiar in the macular region. First, there are no ganglion or bipolar cells in the macula. The axons of the cone cells in the outer nerve fiber layer, called *Henle's layer*, radiate obliquely, not vertically. Henle's layer is quite thin in the center. Polyak noted that "Its fibers are swept aside as if pulled by centrifugal force."[4] The rest of the nerve fiber layer from the retina goes superior and inferior to the macula, producing an arching arrangement of nerve fibers around the fovea (review Figure 2-23).[1] If you view the macula with the red-free light, you may be able to see the macular nerve fibers going above and below the fovea. These fibers form the papillomacular bundle.

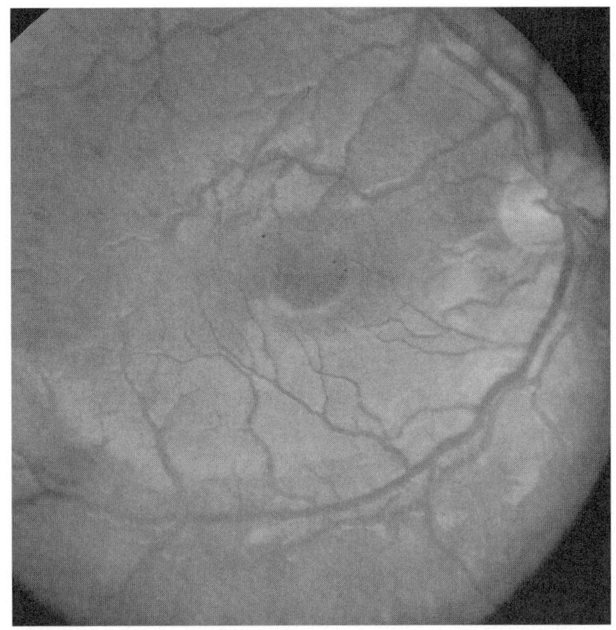
10-3

Figure 10-3. The internal limiting membrane makes reflections occur around the macula. These reflections are very prominent in younger individuals, and, as a person ages, the reflections lessen.

Viewing the macula routinely takes practice. First, it is extremely uncomfortable for the patient, because the bright light maximally stimulates the cones. Second, in an undilated eye, the bright light causes extreme pupillary constriction. Third, most of us do not make it a habit to look at the macula—the optic nerve is what we usually want to see.

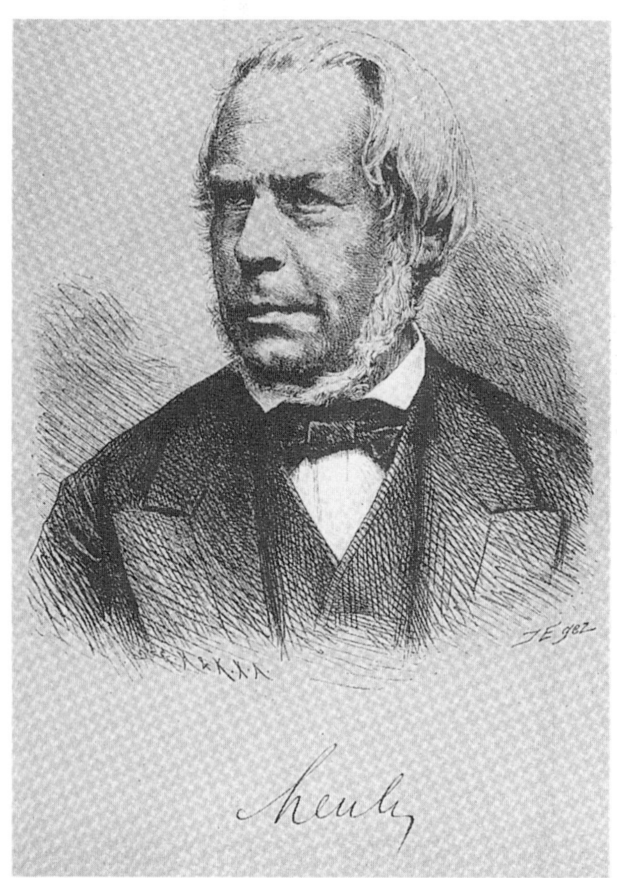

10-4A

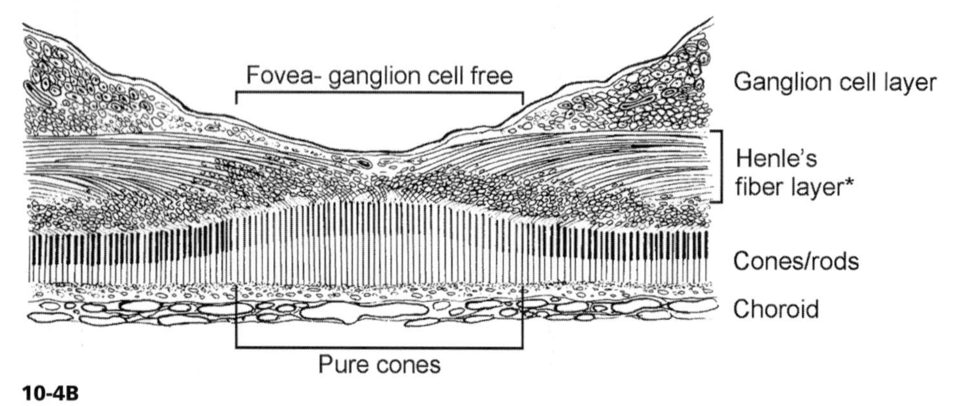

10-4B

Figure 10-4. A. **Jakob Henle (1809–1885) was a professor of anatomy in Zürich, Heidelberg, and Göttingen. He first described the outer fiber layer of the retina, hence the name *Henle's layer* (photograph from reference 4, with permission).** B. **Pick out Henle's layer from this diagram and notice that the fovea has cones only. (* = Lipoproteinaceous deposits in Henle's layer produce a characteristic "macular star.")**

There are good clinical reasons to know how to look at the macula. Loss of visual acuity is the first complaint in macular disorders, and patients notice it immediately. Any change in visual acuity should alert the physician to include a look at the macula. Furthermore, changes can be seen on macular examination that can make a diagnosis: For example, a macular star seen with disc swelling gives the diagnosis of neuroretinitis. Finally, there can be changes in the macula that can be confusing to the examiner—what does the change really mean?

Testing Macular Function—How Do You Know If the Macula Is Functioning Normally?

First, look at visual acuity and color perception. Visual acuity is one of the best tests of macular function. If the macula is diseased, acuity falls. Another clue to a macular disorder is that the patient may not be able to see the center letter, but can see the letters on the side. This is because of the central scotoma on visual fields seen with macular disease. Testing color vision is also a good "macular test" because color is sensed in the cones.

Another useful test to determine whether macular function is normal is the macular or photo stress test. In this test, the patient first reads the eye chart as far down as possible—get him or her to read the smallest print. Then, the patient stares at a bright light (e.g., your ophthalmoscope light) for 10 seconds. The examiner times how long it takes to see one line above the best line on the hand-held Snellen chart read by the patient. Normally, an eye recovers vision in less than 50 seconds. An eye with a macular problem recovers in 120–480 seconds.[5] You can also notice whether both macular stress times are equal; when not approximately the same, then consider a unilateral macular disorder.

The macular stress test separates vision loss owing to primarily optic nerve disease from macular disease. If the patient's vision loss is owing to optic nerve disease, the macular stress test will not be too long. If, however, the macula is at fault, then the patient will not see anything for a very long time.

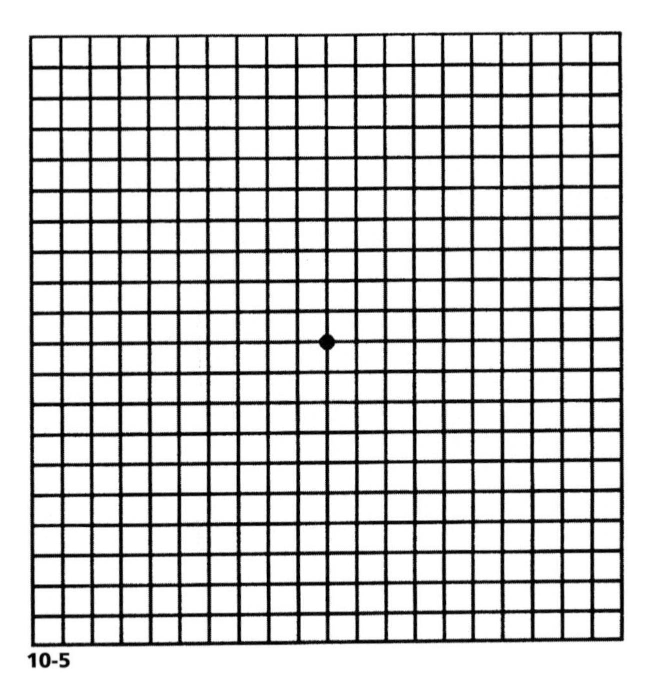

10-5

Still another test of macular function uses Amsler's grid (named for Dr. Marc Amsler, who first developed it).[6] It tests the central 10 degrees of vision. The patient wearing reading glasses focuses on a central point on a grid, with one eye approximately 14 in. (or 0.33 m) from the grid, and reports the following: (1) if the dot is present, (2) if lines or corners are present or absent (scotomas), and (3) if the lines (horizontal and vertical) are straight. It is another sensitive test of macular function. When the lines are curved or not straight, metamorphopsia can be present, indicating macular dysfunction.

Figure 10-5. This is the black and white grid used to test macular function. Each eye is tested separately wearing best reading correction. Amsler's grid can be used to detect subtle loss of central visual field.

Visual field testing with static perimetry (e.g., Humphrey visual field analyzer) can be customized for the central field. Some static perimetry programs test only the central 10 degrees of field. The foveal threshold value correlates well with visual acuity.

Electrophysiology is also useful for testing macular function. An electroretinogram (ERG) measures the electrical response of the retina after a brief light flash. There are two types of ERG. The full-field ERG sums the response of the retina as a whole, including all cone function (mainly macula) and all rod function. The focal and multifocal ERG specifically tests the macula. So, although the ERG is abnormal in patients with retinitis pigmentosa, the central visual acuity is normal. On the other hand, if the patient has severe macular degeneration with poor visual acuity (i.e., worse than 20/400), the full-field ERG can be normal. This is because although the macula has many cones, the macula has only 10% of the total number of cones in the retina.[7] The focal or multifocal ERG shows an abnormality if there is a macular dystrophy or macular abnormality.

Electrooculography usually tests the difference in electrical potential between the front and back of the globe, and reflects retinal pigment epithelium integrity. Although it usually gives similar responses as the ERG, sometimes a retinal condition can have a normal ERG and an abnormal electrooculogram, an example of which is Best's disease.

Visual evoked potentials (VEPs), frequently used to detect optic neuropathy, can be used to detect macular dysfunction. A maculopathy reducing visual acuity to 20/40 or greater would be expected to show a loss of visual evoked potential amplitude and perhaps a slight prolongation of the P100 latency.

Fluorescein angiography is helpful in evaluating macular disease. After the injection of fluorescein dye, any disruption of the blood retinal barrier in the macula demonstrates leakage of the dye around the macula.

Maculopathy is a general term for macular disease. Like optic neuropathy, it does not tell what is causing the problem, but rather that the source of the decrease in vision is in the macula. The range of appearance in maculopathy includes everything from simple macular edema to white/yellow infiltrates in the macula, suggesting infection. The most common form of maculopathy is age-related macular degeneration (ARMD). *Macular dystrophy* refers to inherited forms of maculopathy.

Common Macular Findings

Retinal drusen (not the same as drusen of the disc) are extracellular deposits that are probably derived from the retinal pigment epithelium. They are found between the retinal pigment epithelium and Bruch's membrane.[8] Drusen of the retina seem to be of at least two types. *Hard drusen* , which are small, yellow, well-demarcated deposits, can be found in individuals as early as their 20s–30s; these drusen do not signify ARMD. On the other hand, *soft drusen* are slightly larger, have indistinct borders, and occur after age 55 years. Soft drusen form the basis for the beginning of ARMD.[8] Almost everyone older than 50 years has small drusen, but large drusen suggest macular degeneration.[9]

Figure 10-6. Retinal drusen are found between the retinal pigment epithelium and Bruch's membrane. They are deep in the retina and can be a precursor to macular degeneration.

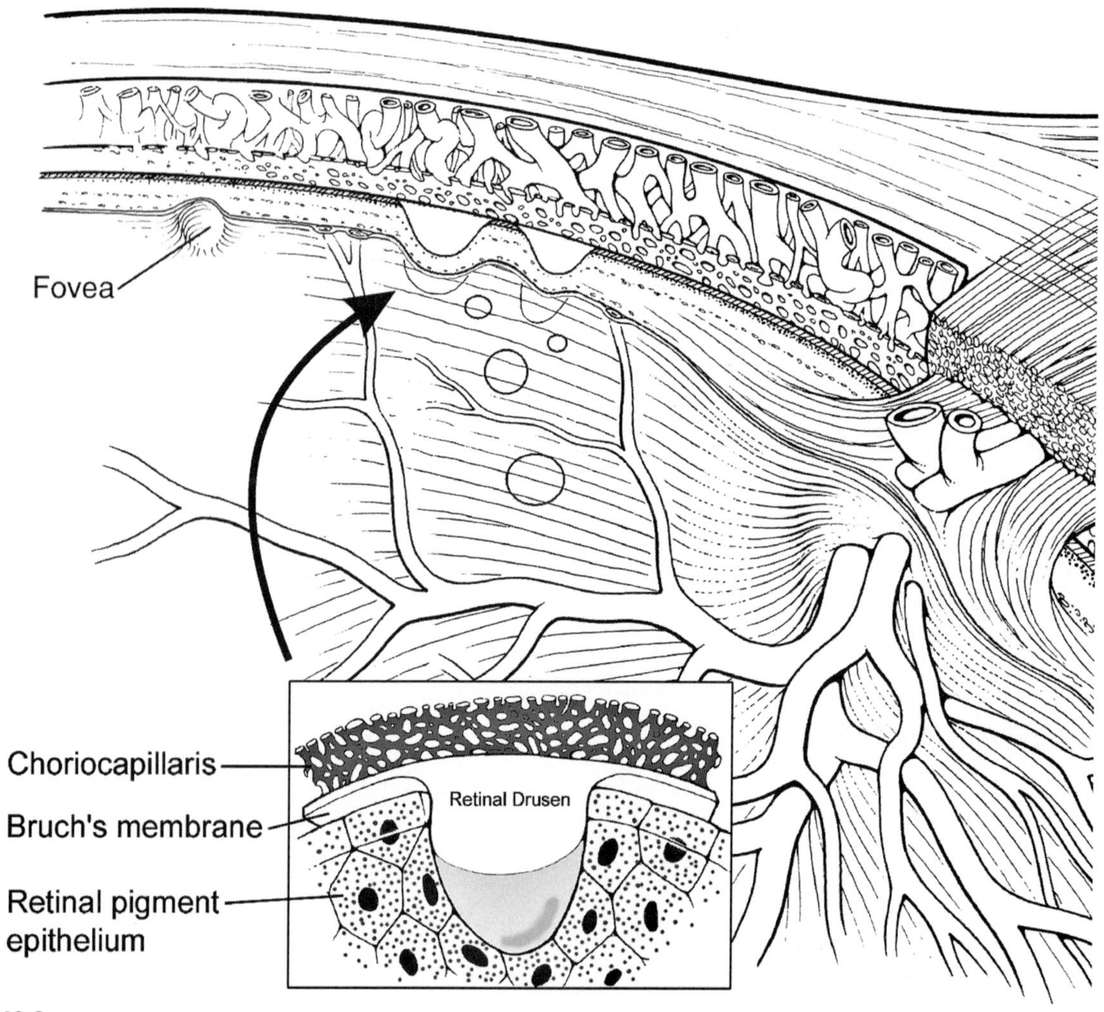

Figure 10-7. A. **Hard drusen are deposits between the retinal pigment epithelium and Bruch's membrane. By themselves, they do not signify macular degeneration and can be seen in many normal individuals.** B. **Soft drusen are larger and have more indistinct borders.**

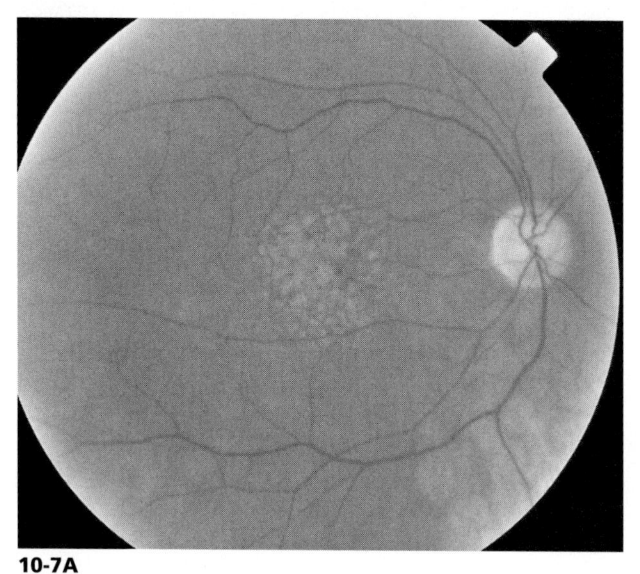

10-7A

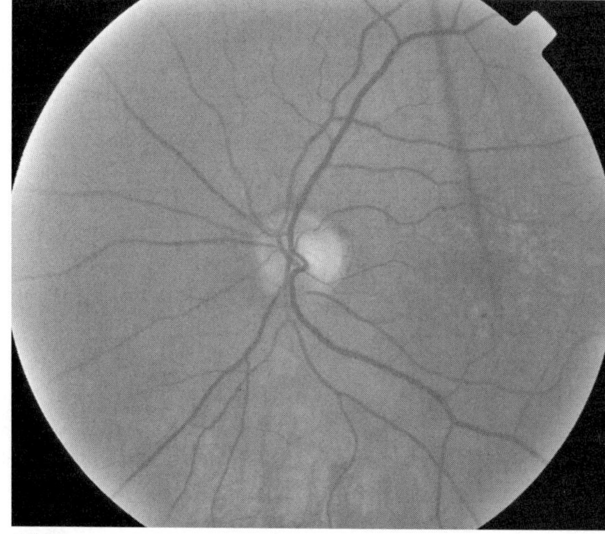

10-7B

AGE-RELATED MACULAR DEGENERATION (ARMD)

ARMD is the most common maculopathy, affecting 6.5% of the population older than 65 years and 20% of people older than 75 years. It is the most common cause of blindness in the Western world.[10] The condition is slowly progressive, causing first pigmentary changes in the macula with loss of the foveolar reflex, and loss of the usual pigmentation, centrally leaving the orange color of the choroid visible. The most striking finding is that the macular appearance precedes visual symptoms and loss of visual acuity. Vision loss appears in all forms of ARMD. In the nonatrophic form, the vision may be good (i.e., better than 20/40), but patients can have complaints of problems with night vision or reading under low illumination.[9]

Figure 10-8. This older gentleman has 20/25 visual acuity; however, on examination of the macula, the observer sees atrophy of the macula with hard drusen in the retina (*arrows*). Notice, on the accompanying CD-Rom, how the macula has a bright-orange appearance. On this black and white photograph, the arrows mark out the area of atrophy.

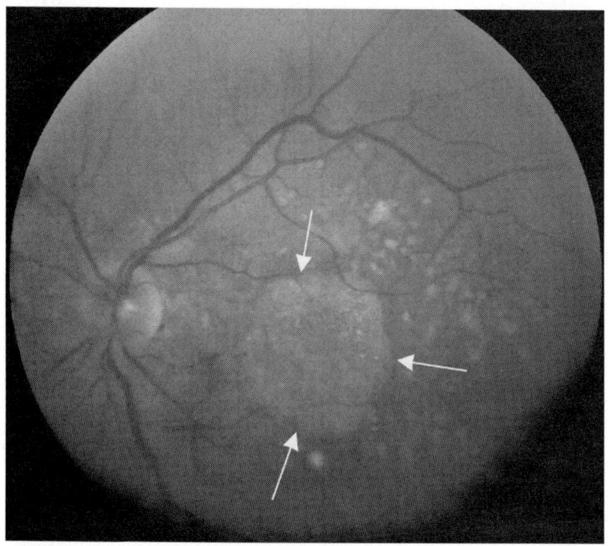

10-8

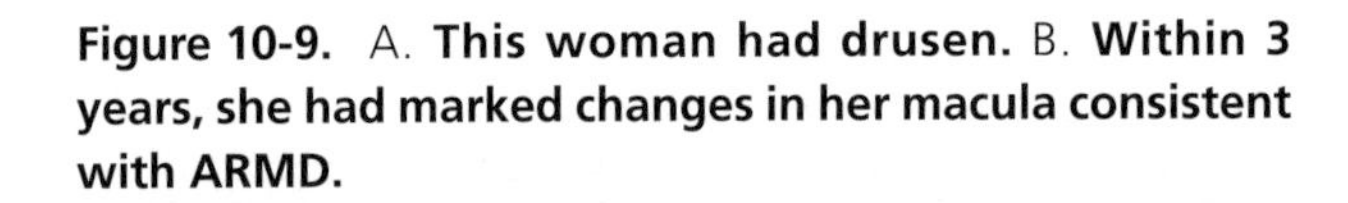

Figure 10-9. A. **This woman had drusen.** B. **Within 3 years, she had marked changes in her macula consistent with ARMD.**

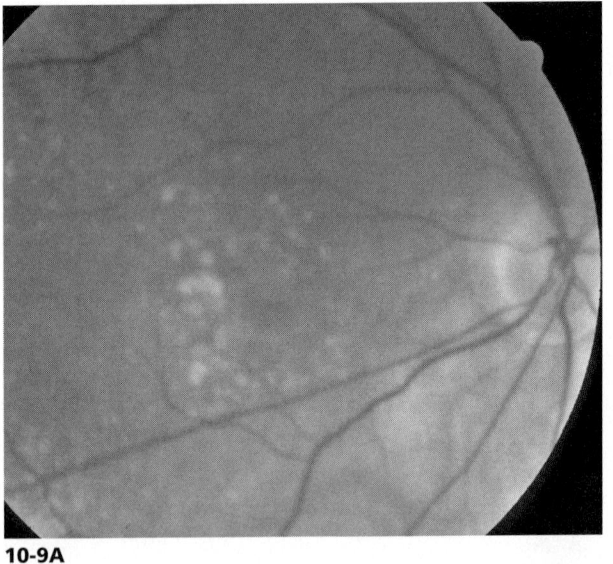

10-9A

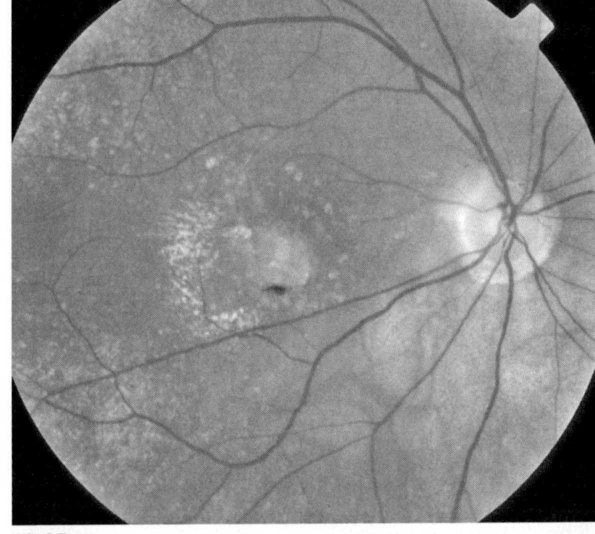

10-9B

There are two types of ARMD. The first is atrophic, nondisciform (dry-type) atrophy, in which there is a progressive change in the retinal pigment epithelium, choriocapillaris, and rods and cones to the point at which the macula is atrophied as well as the choriocapillaris. Vision is slightly reduced, but patients complain of trouble with reading, seeing in reduced illumination, and night vision.[9] There is no blood vessel involvement.

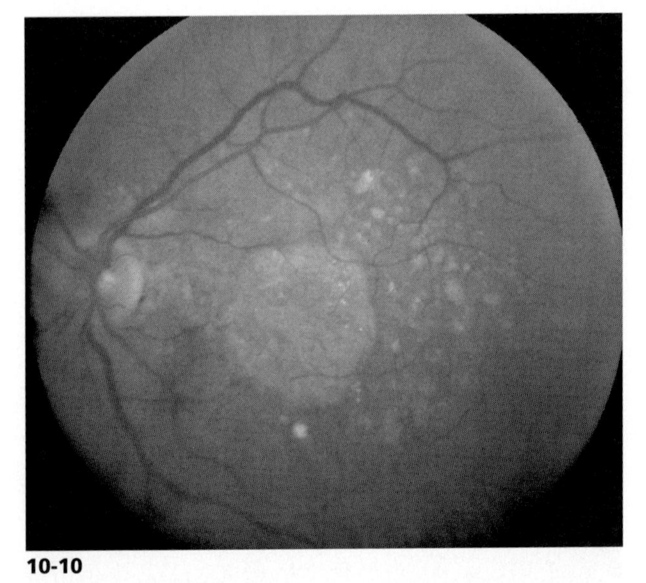

10-10

Figure 10-10. Photograph of geographic atrophy or dry macular degeneration. The visual acuity is relatively spaced.

The other form of macular degeneration is the neovascular, "exudative," disciform (wet-type) form. This type is rarer, but it is also the cause of the most severe forms of blindness. In this form there is a submacular proliferation of blood vessels, which makes the macula more prone to hemorrhage and visual loss. *This form requires prompt treatment before hemorrhage occurs*. Scarring and permanent vision loss ensue. This form is caused by choroidal neovascularization. The risk factors for developing this form include more than five drusen, very large drusen, pigment clumping, and hypertension.[9] These patients have severe vision loss centrally. Even with the worst central visual acuity, patients with macular degeneration tend to maintain peripheral vision useful in ambulation.

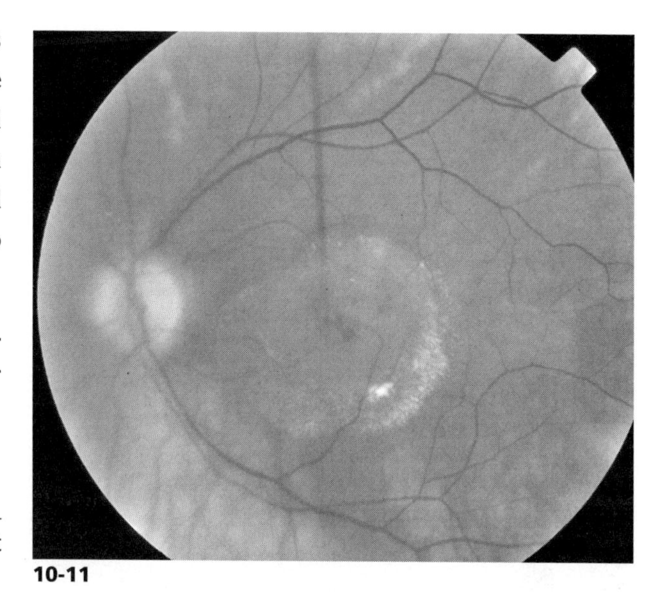
10-11

Figure 10-11. Photograph of exudative macular degeneration. The visual acuity is decreased and visual prognosis is poor.

Table 10-1. Risk Factors for ARMD

Age—the older you are, the more likely you are to have it
Women (although women tend to live longer)
Hereditary (most have a family history)
Systemic disease: cardiovascular disease
Smoking
Light exposure
Nutritional factors—lack of antioxidants and zinc

Source: Adapted from reference 9.

See Chapter 12 on viewing the disc in the elderly.

MACULAR EDEMA

Macular edema can be caused by a large number of processes. Normally, there is no fluid present in the macula because there are tight junctions in the endothelium of retinal vessels around the macula and tight junctions of the retinal pigment epithelium. When these break down, plasma proteins and water enter the macular space owing to disease processes, and macular edema results. Fluid generally accumulates between the outer plexiform and inner nuclear layers. The fluid causes a thickening of the normally thinner macular area.[11]

To view macular edema with the direct ophthalmoscope takes practice and knowledge about what is normal. Because the view is not stereo (i.e., you won't be able to see elevation), detecting elevation is more difficult. Focus the slit illumination at the edge of the macula—this side illumination provides better viewing of elevation and a clearer view of the fluid-filled spaces.

Fluorescein angiography is also essential in diagnosing macular edema. Normally, there is no leakage of fluid if there is no edema. When fluid is present, however, the fluid leaks.

Figure 10-12. A. **This fundus shows drusen all around the macula. In the center of the macula, you can see the discoloration associated with edema. If you use slit illumination on the edema, you may be able to detect elevation.** B. **Here the macular edema is well seen (*arrows*).** ***Continued***

10-12A

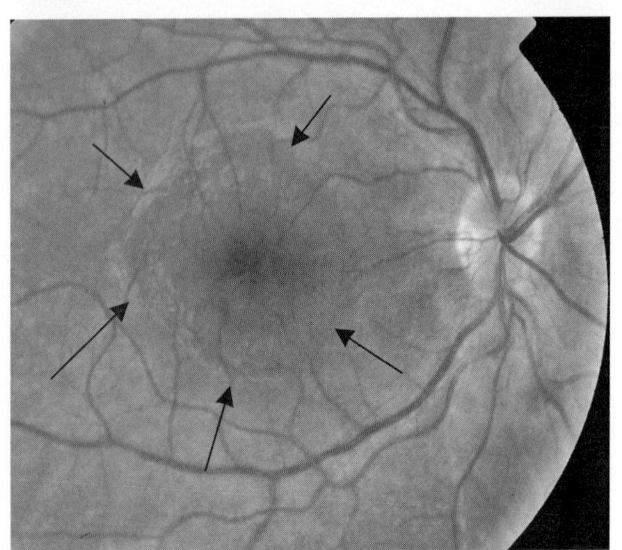

10-12B

Figure 10-12. ***Continued.*** C. ***Cystoid macular edema***, **so named because of its petaloid appearance, is barely perceptible in this photograph (*arrows*).** D. **The fluorescein angiogram beautifully demonstrates the petaloid appearance of cystoid macular edema (*arrow*).** E. **Diabetic macular edema may be diffuse and poorly appreciated. The arrow points to the macular fluid.** F. **The fluorescein angiogram shows active leaking from the nearby incompetent vessels. In the macula, however, you can also see a faint leakage centrally where the edema is (*arrows*). The fluorescein findings take several minutes to appear—in this case, more than 8 minutes (see the time on the far right of the picture).**

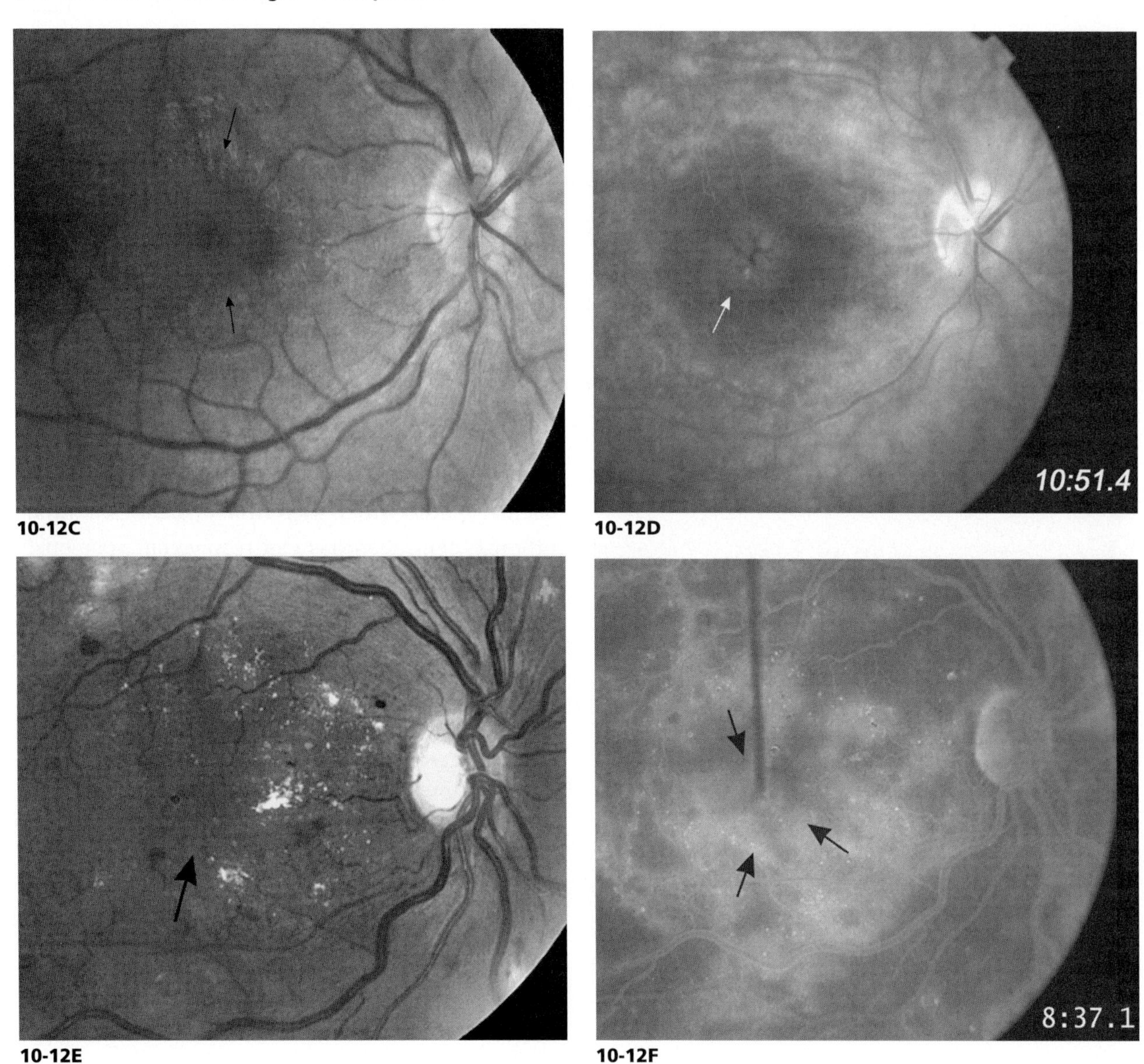

10-12C **10-12D**

10-12E **10-12F**

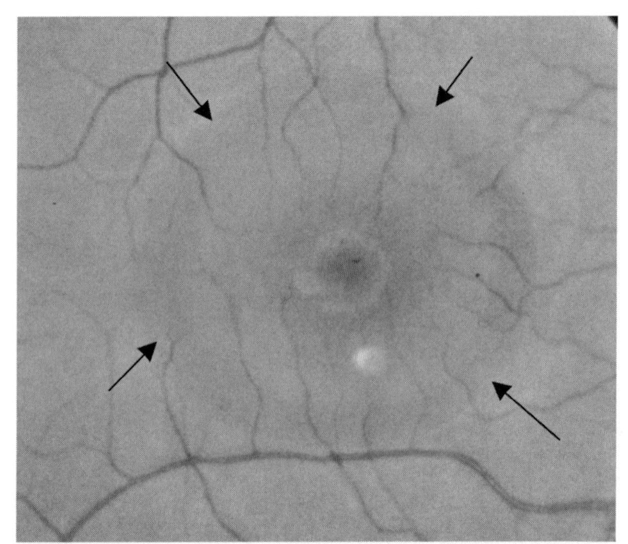

10-13A

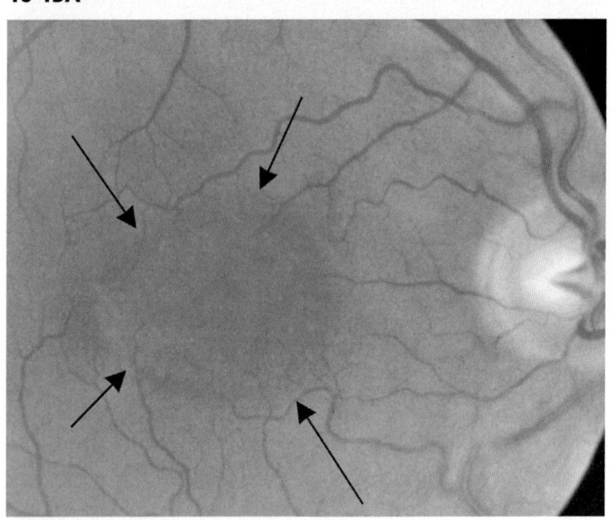

10-13B

Causes of macular edema include metabolic disturbances such as diabetes; hereditary diseases like retinitis pigmentosa; ischemic diseases of the choroid, such as hypertension; collagen-vascular disease; retinal vein occlusions (branch and central); low intraocular pressure; vitreoretinal traction from membranes; inflammation associated with uveitis; pars planitis; radiation damage to the retina; von Hippel-Lindau disease; and drugs such as epinephrine and latanoprost (a synthetic prostaglandin which is supposed to increase anterior chamber outflow in high intraocular pressure).[11,12]

Cystoid macular edema can be caused by many of the aforementioned causes but can also develop after cataract surgery, and anyone with decreased vision after cataract surgery should be checked for cystoid macular edema.

A specific type of macular edema, confused with optic neuritis, is *central serous maculopathy.* This condition is seen in young, healthy adults (men more than women) who present with decreased vision in one eye. When there is no afferent pupillary defect to go along with the decrease in vision, think of this condition and check the macula carefully. A macular photo stress test will also be abnormal. Although central serous can resolve spontaneously in weeks without treatment, on occasion patients are left with permanent vision loss.

Figure 10-13. A,B. **These two young men presented with blurring of vision in the right eye. There was no afferent pupillary defect. A macular stress test was prolonged. A careful examination of the macula revealed slight elevation owing to serous fluid under the macula. Arrows mark the sides of the elevation. Notice in** A **that the vessels curve up over the fluid. (Photographs courtesy of Christopher Blodi, M.D.)**

Table 10-2. Differentiating among Macular Edemas

	Macular edema (see Figure 10-12E,F)	Cystoid macular edema (see Figure 10-12C,D)	Central serous macular edema (see Figure 10-13A,B)
Clinical appearance	Retinal thickening within two disc diameters of the center of the macula	Thickening around the macula; loss of the macular light reflex	Loss of the normal macular light reflex; may see a halo of light around the darker-colored macula; very slight elevation of the macula
Fluorescein appearance	Diffuse leakage in the area of the macula	Petaloid appearance of leakage in the macula	See accumulation of fluorescein in the macula; the fluorescein stains and leaks; the foveal area typically does not; look at the disc for staining owing to optic pit
Level involved	Intraretinal	Outer plexiform, inner nuclear layer	Between the retinal pigment epithelium and the retina; inner nuclear layer
Outcome	Variable	Variable	Variable, but can be reversible
Examples and risk factors for development	Diabetes; branch and central vein occlusion; hypertensive retinopathy	Postcataract surgery; diabetes; retinal vein occlusion; retinal vascular malformation; radiation retinopathy; retinitis pigmentosa; infections	Seen usually in young men; optic pits; increased incidence in type A personality; pregnancy; steroid use

Source: Adapted from references 12–15.

MACULAR HOLE

A *macular hole* is a macular lesion that is visible with a direct ophthalmoscope. Most macular holes occur in the elderly; they are 2.5 times more common in women than in men.[16] Macular holes are thought to be caused by traction of the vitreous on the fovea.

Holes can occur after long-standing macular edema and many occur spontaneously. Symptoms are decreased vision or distortion of vision. Ophthalmologic examination shows a variable visual acuity—20/25 to 20/200. A central scotoma may be present on Amsler's grid or on visual field testing. Furthermore, place the slit illumination on the fovea and ask the patient if there is a break in the beam of light. If there is a break, there could be a macular hole. This has been labeled the *Watzke*

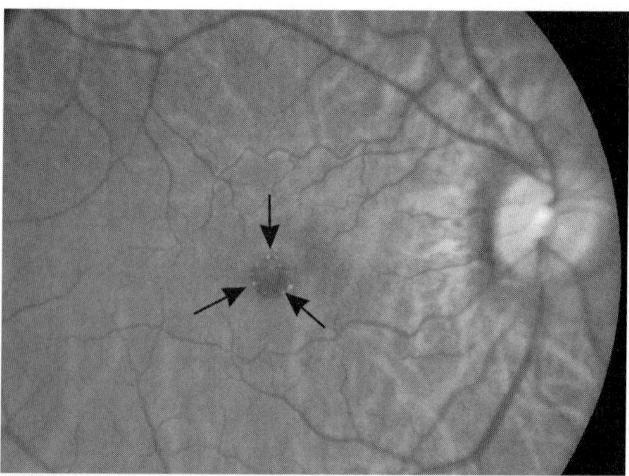

10-14A

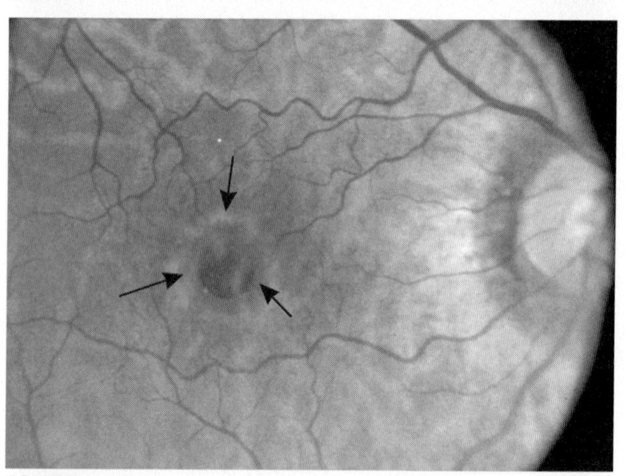

10-14B

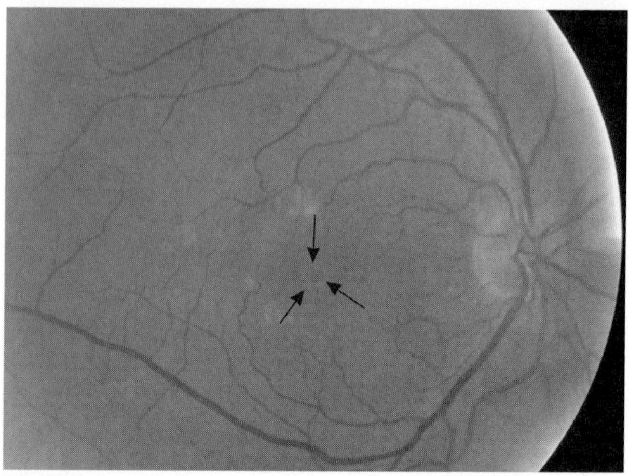

10-14C

sign.[17] Recognition of this disorder is important, because it is now treatable.

Table 10-3. Causes of Macular Holes

Trauma
Severe retinopathies (diabetic, hypertensive)
Myopic degeneration
Macular disease: macular dystrophy (Best's, macular degeneration)
Vitrectomy
Lightning
Welding

Source: Adapted from references 16,17.

Figure 10-14. A. **The macula looks like a red, round, punched-out spot. This woman had the beginnings of her macular hole more than 10 years ago.** B. **Follow-up 10 years later shows the hole is slightly larger. The arrows show the punched-out spot.** C. **Can you see the small macular hole in this macula (*arrows*)?**

Solar maculopathy is a common cause of small macular holes. This maculopathy occurs frequently in military populations, sun eclipse watchers, solar telescope observers, and drug abusers. Patients report blurred vision, continuous after-image, scotomas, and reddening of the vision (erythropsia). What is viewed in the macula of solar maculopathy is a yellow-white foveolar spot acutely, which then becomes a small macular hole.[18]

Figure 10-15. A. **This individual watched a sunrise and presented with vision of 20/200. (Photograph courtesy of Christopher Blodi, M.D.)** B,C. **This welder experienced an electrical explosion in front of his face. His visual acuity was reduced to 20/60 in both eyes. Both his right** (B) **and left** (C) **macula showed typical "solar" injury.** D,E. **The visual fields show bilateral central scotomas. (Photographs in** B,C **and visual fields** D,E **courtesy of W.T. Shults, M.D.)**

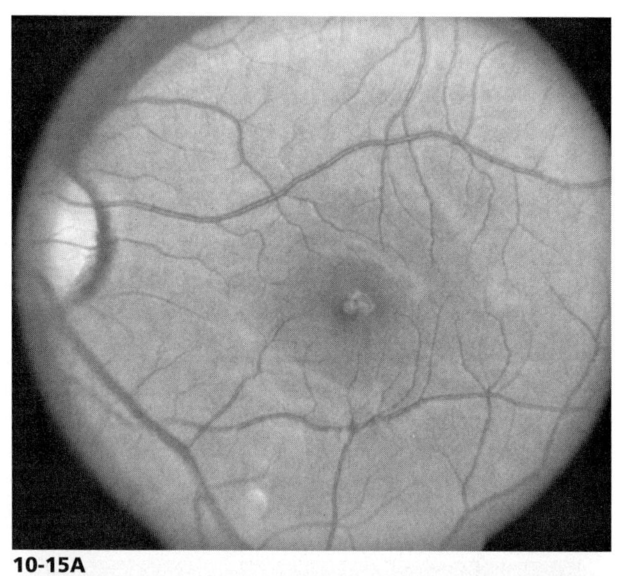

10-15A

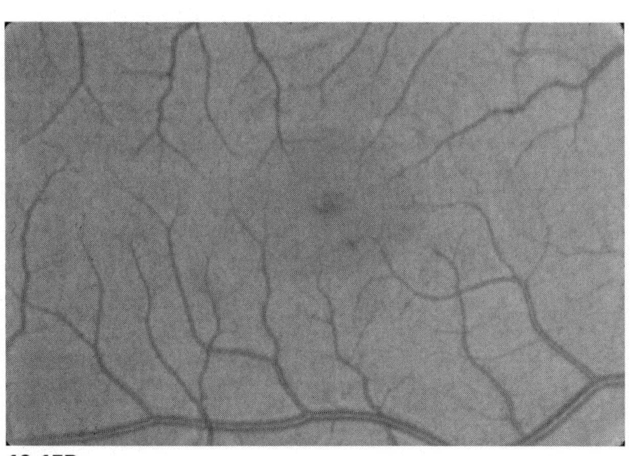

10-15B

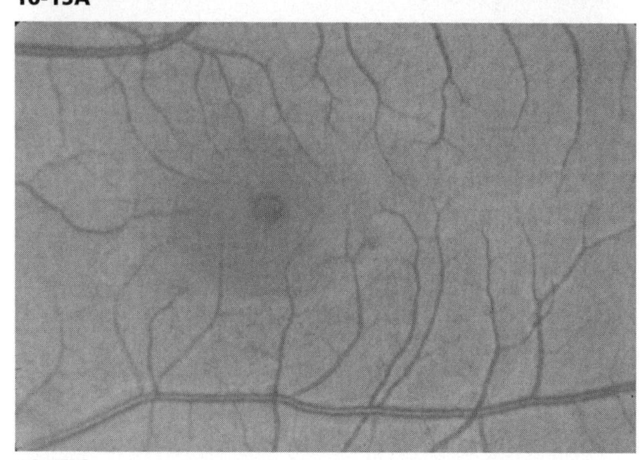

10-15C

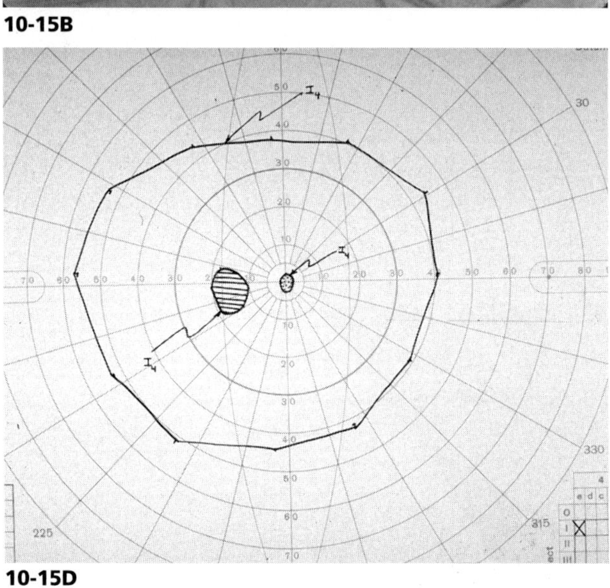

10-15D

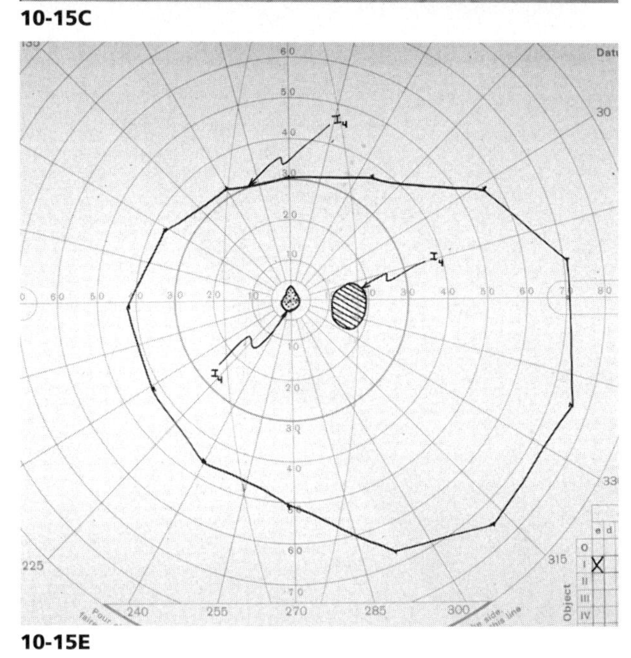

10-15E

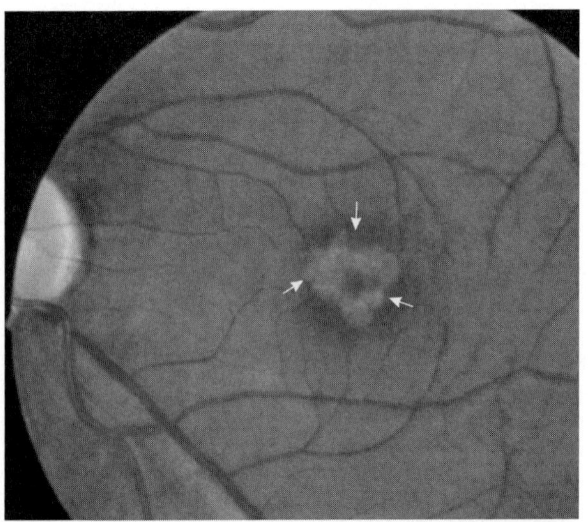

10-16A

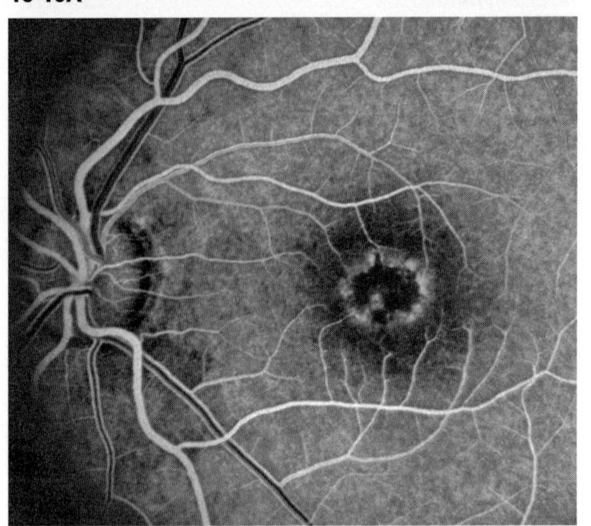

10-16B

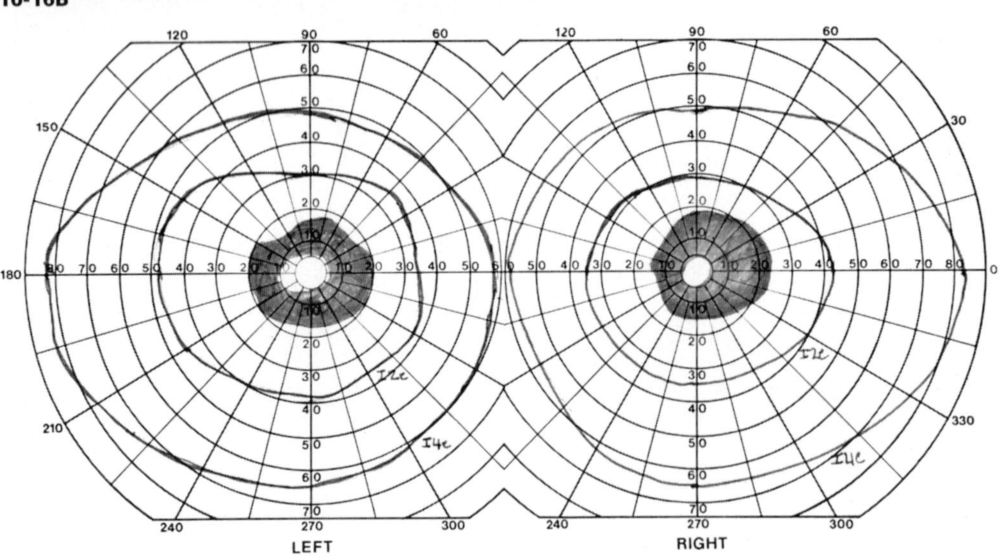

10-16C

VIRAL MACULOPATHY

Viralmaculopathy or*macularneuroretinopathy* may occur abruptly during or after a viral illness, with decreased vision unilaterally or bilaterally. There may be little to be seen other than some browning or darkish dots in the macula. In some, wedge-shaped or teardrop-shaped defects are present. Visual acuity is often normal. Visual field defects are common. The fluorescein is also frequently normal. This disorder may be related to acute (posterior) multifocal placoid pigment epitheliopathy (see Chapter 6).[19]

Figure 10-16. A. **This young woman presented with bilaterally decreased vision after a viral illness. Her macula shows pigmentary changes (*arrows*). She had a viral cerebellitis and proven adenovirus.** B. **The fluorescein angiogram shows leakage around the macula.** C. **The visual fields show a small ring scotoma around the central portion of the visual field.**

MACULAR STAR

Macular star is another manifestation of systemic infections that can involve the macula. Henle's layer has a peculiar axonal radiating pattern toward the center of the fovea. Hard exudates accumulate in this layer in this region, and a "star" lesion is produced.

Figure 10-17. Lipid deposits form in Henle's layer, and because of its configuration, a star is formed. (* = Lipoproteinaceous deposits in Henle's layer produce a characteristic "macular star.")

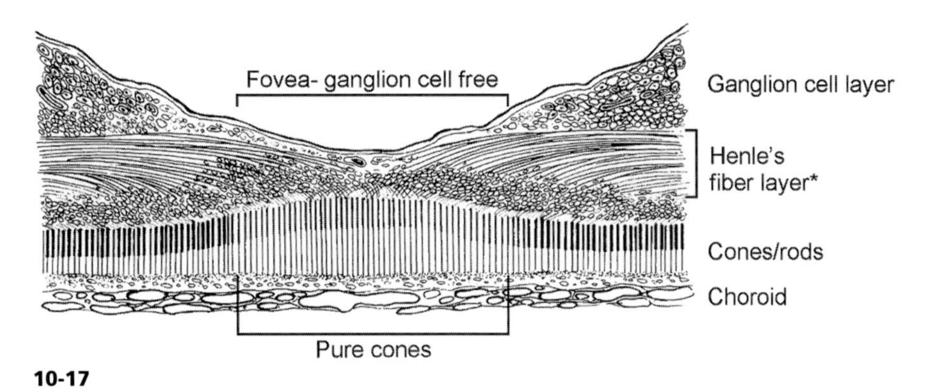

10-17

Figure 10-18. A. **Bilateral macular stars owing to cat-scratch fever (*Bartonella henselae* infection). Look also for peripapillary serous retinal detachment.[23]** B. **Here is a complete macular star in another patient with cat-scratch fever. Notice the delicate radiations in all directions. (Photographs courtesy of Marie Acierno, M.D.)**

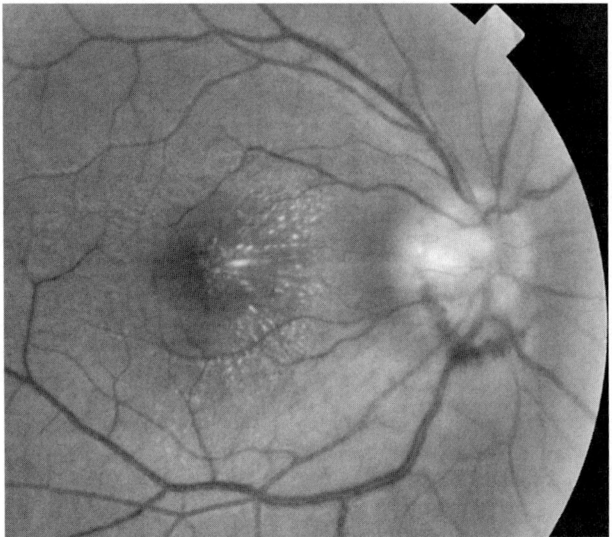

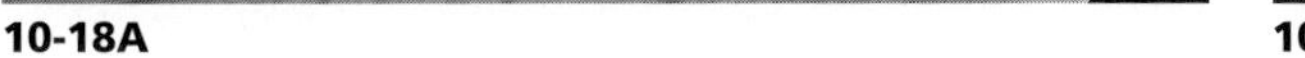

10-18A

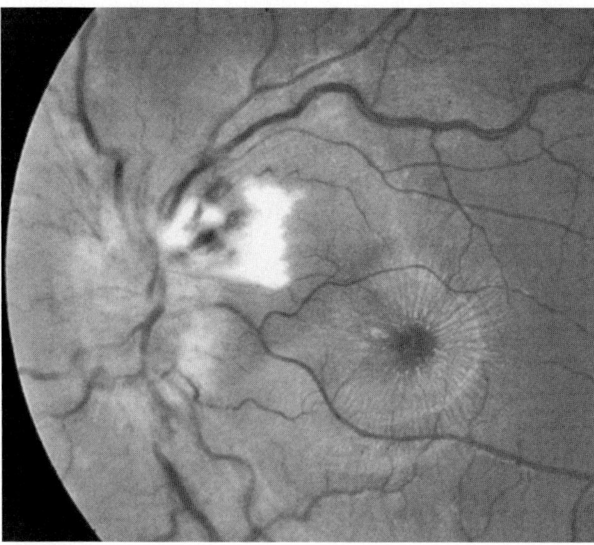

10-18B

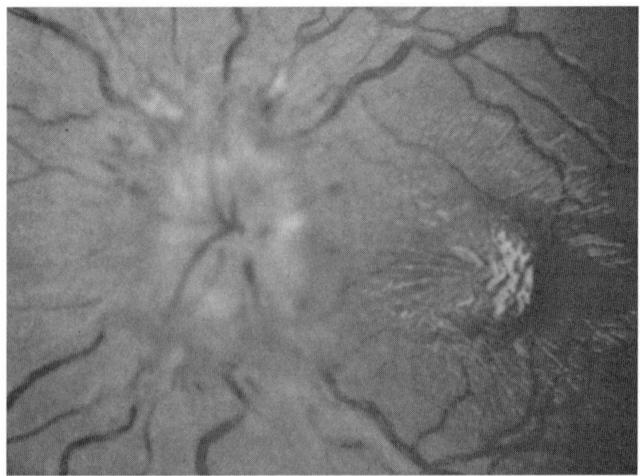

10-19A

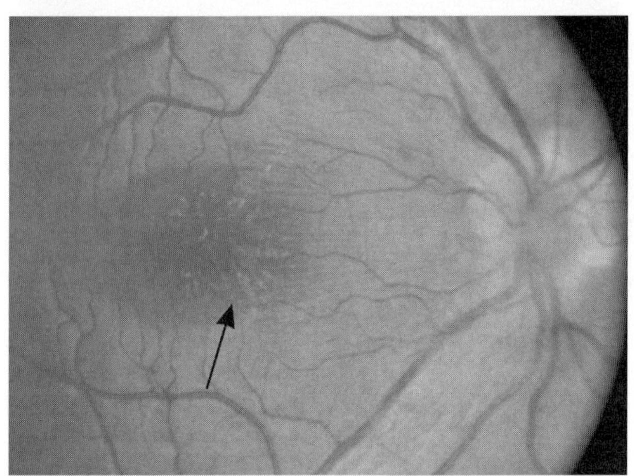

10-19B

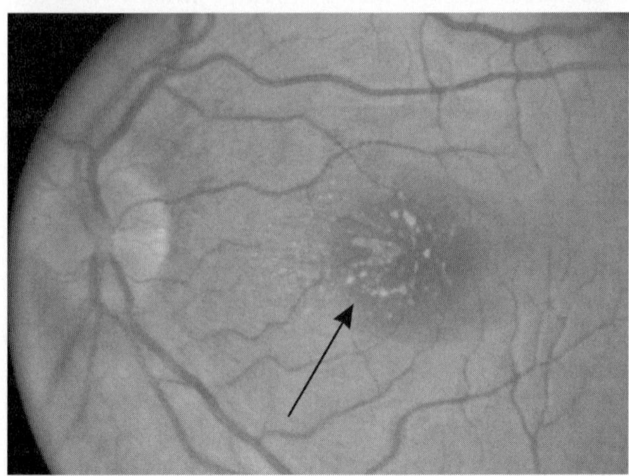

10-19C

Figure 10-19. A,B. **Bilateral macular stars (*arrow*, B) owing to idiopathic intracranial hypertension, seen acutely.** C. **Although the disc swelling has gone, the macular stars are still present (*arrow*).**

Table 10-4. Causes of Macular Star

Idiopathic stellate neuroretinitis
Infectious forms of neuroretinitis
Bartonella henselae (cat-scratch disease)
Mumps
Borrelia burgdorferi (Lyme disease)
Toxocara
Tuberculosis
Syphilis
Leptospirosis
Infectious mononucleosis (Epstein-Barr virus)
Toxoplasmosis neuroretinitis
Influenza
Poliomyelitis
Coxsackie virus
Psittacosis
Papilledema
Posterior scleritis
Diffuse unilateral subacute neuroretinitis
Diabetic papillitis
Anterior ischemic optic neuropathy
Papillophlebitis
Acute hypertensive optic neuropathy

Source: Adapted from references 20,21, and MC Brodsky, RS Burke, LM Hamel. Pediatric Neuro-Ophthalmology. New York: Springer-Verlag, 1996.

Table 10-5. Differential Diagnosis of Disc Swelling with a Macular Star

Condition	Associated symptoms	Associated findings	Risk factors	Evaluation
Idiopathic	Visual loss—usually unilateral	—	Febrile illness	Search for infectious cause
Infectious				
Bartonella henselae (cat-scratch disease)[22]	Fever, lymphadenopathy	Hepatosplenomegaly; skin rash; lymphadenopathy	Scratch or bite from full-grown cat/kitten	Serology
Borrelia burgdorferi (Lyme disease)	Rash	Erythema migrans, carditis, arthritis, cranial nerve VII palsy	Tick bites; northeastern and midwestern United States	Serology
Toxoplasmosis	Fever, flulike illness	Lymphadenopathy, myalgias	Congenital; cats	Serology
Toxocara	Fever, splenomegaly, rash	Splenomegaly, pneumonitis	Cats and dogs	Toxocara enzyme-linked immunosorbent assay
Epstein-Barr	Fatigue, fever	Lymphadenopathy, organomegaly	Ubiquitous	Serology
Leptospirosis	Headache, fatigue, myalgias	Encephalitis, meningitis, renal disease	Contaminated water, animals	Serology
Papilledema	Headache, transient monocular blindness	Papilledema	Multiple etiologies	Magnetic resonance imaging and lumbar puncture
Posterior scleritis	Eye pain, red eye, diplopia	Also see retinal and choroidal striae; look for retinal detachment	Collagen-vascular disease	Ultrasonography, computed tomography shows thickened posterior sclera
Diffuse unilateral subacute neuroretinitis	Blurred vision	See white and yellow spots in deep layers of retina and retinal pigment epithelium	Nematodes	Toxocara enzyme-linked immunosorbent assay
Diabetic papillitis	May be none; decreased vision	Peripheral neuropathy	Family history	Glucose; hemoglobin A1C
Hypertension	None or decreased vision	Elevated blood pressure	Family history	Renal function

Uncommon Macular Findings

CHERRY-RED SPOT

Although a cherry-red spot can be seen with a central retinal artery occlusion, in which case a pale retina is seen all around (see also Chapter 5, Figure 5-5), a cherry-red spot is a finding associated with a degenerative neurologic disorder; Tay-Sachs disease and Sandhoff's disease are examples, as well as older children with Niemann-Pick disease (see Chapter 11). The appearance is a red-appearing spot at the macula. The reason for the appearance is that the ganglion cells of the retina have become opaque owing to the presence of storage material—glycolipids or swelling. Because ganglion cells are not present in the macula, the choroidal vasculature and the single layer of pigment make the spot look very red.

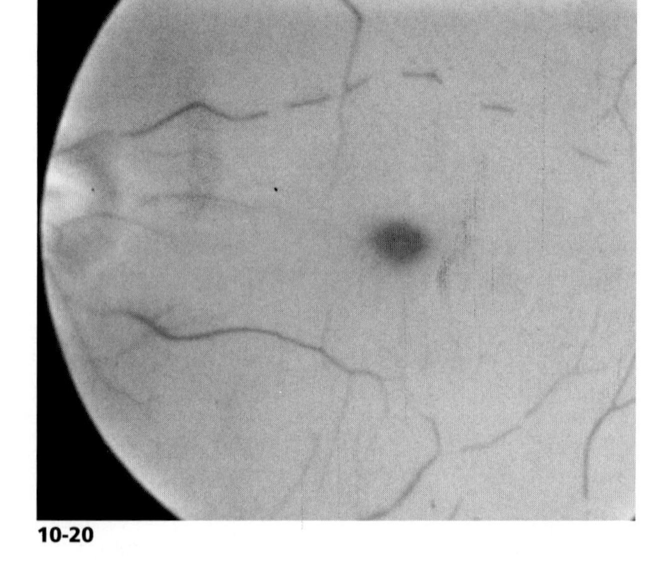

10-20

Figure 10-20. This woman had a sudden onset of blindness owing to a central retinal artery occlusion. The cherry-red spot is owing to the pale retina surrounding the normal pigmentation of the choroidal vessel-fed macular elements.

Figure 10-21. A,B. **A cherry-red spot (*arrow,* A) in Tay-Sachs disease is owing to glycolipid deposits in ganglion cells everywhere except in the macula (where there are no ganglion cells).**

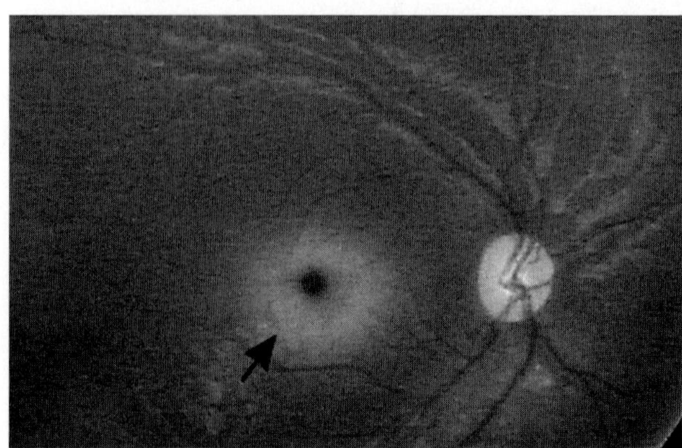

10-21A

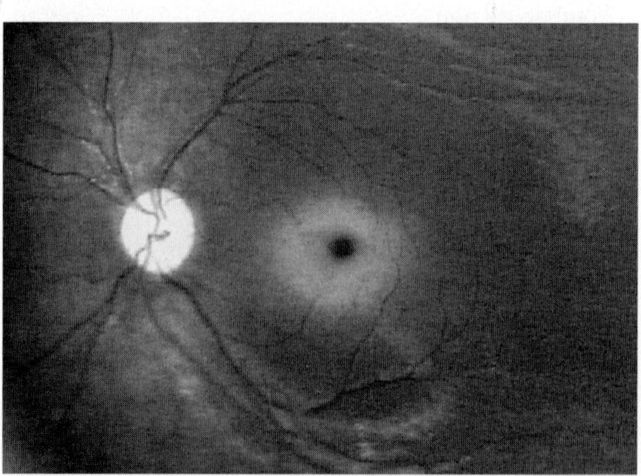

10-21B

Table 10-6. Causes of a Cherry-Red Spot

Central retinal artery occlusion
Retinal edema after trauma
Quinine toxicity
Inherited disorders
Tay-Sachs disease
Sandhoff's disease
Gangliosidoses, type 1
Niemann-Pick disease
Rarer causes
Sialidoses
Farber's lipogranulomatosis
Metachromatic leukodystrophy
Goldberg's syndrome
Krabbe's disease
Nephrosialidosis

Source: Adapted from references 24–26.

The macula can also be involved in degenerative neurologic and inherited problems.

Table 10-7. Other Inherited Macular Changes Associated with Neurologic Disease

Inherited condition	Features	Macular finding
Metachromatic leukodystrophy	Peripheral neuropathy; fatal encephalopathy	Gray opacification of fovea; cherry-red spot acutely
Niemann-Pick type A	Motor and cognitive dysfunction	Cherry-red spot
Niemann-Pick type B	Organomegaly, intact neurologically	Halo of white around macula
Neuronal ceroid lipofuscinosis	Motor dysfunction	Brownish macula; hypopigmented retina
Gaucher's disease	Organomegaly with supranuclear gaze palsy, seizures	White spots; cherry-red spot
Cerebellar ataxia	Progressive ataxia	Bull's eye maculopathy; beaten metal
Fucosidosis	Coarse external features with growth retardation	Bull's eye maculopathy

Source: Adapted from references 24–27.

See also Tables 8-4 and 9-11 for a discussion on retinal degenerations.

INHERITABLE MACULAR DISEASE

Cogan described the maculopathy of Stargardt's disease in this way:

Some forms of macular degeneration fall into the category of hereditary degeneration of the outer retinal layers. They are the reverse of retinitis pigmentosa in that the central areas are preferentially involved and they do not customarily extend to the periphery; they are sometimes called retinitis pigmentosa inversa (or Stargardt's disease) . . . [1]

Stargardt's disease is an inherited maculopathy that frequently presents with a loss of central vision. Dr. Karl Stargardt first described this familial condition in 1909.[28] Most people reserve the term for a macular dystrophy with yellow flecks. Some people also talk about a "beaten-metal appearance" to the macula and perimacular areas. Early on there may be few clues, and the young person may be misdiagnosed as malingering. Stargardt's disease should be on the list of causes of unexplained vision loss in the young adult. Examination should include a fluorescein angiogram because there may be defects in the foveal region on fluorescein; there may also be choroidal nonperfusion or choroidal silence. Furthermore, an ERG may be normal early on, but a multifocal ERG of the macular region can be diagnostic.

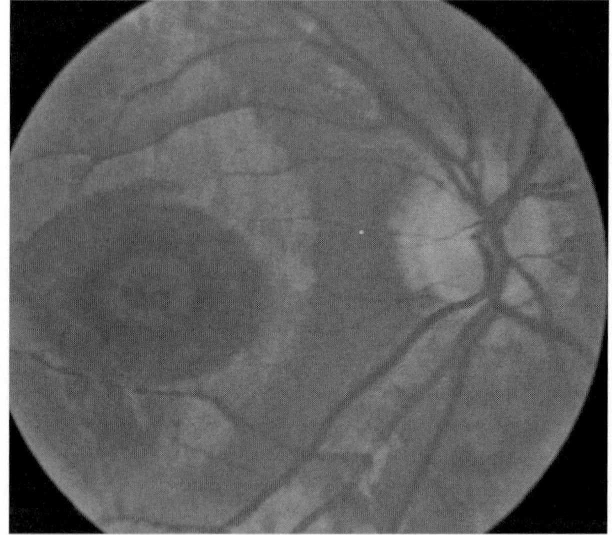

10-22A

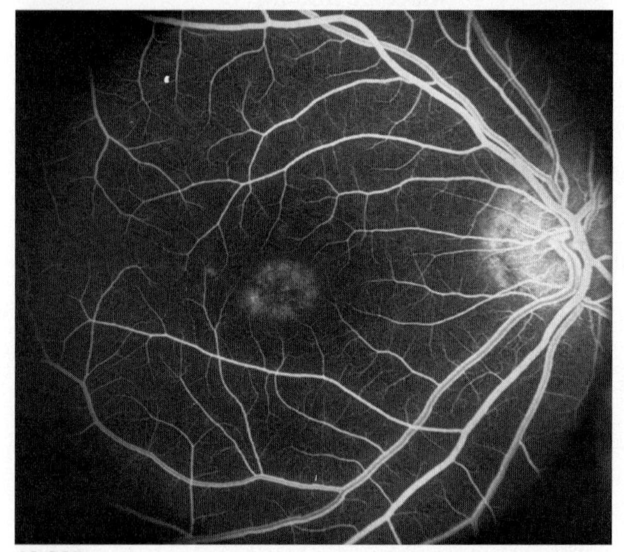

10-22B

Figure 10-22. A. **This young man was referred for possibly nonorganic vision loss. His macula had a slightly granular appearance. The focal ERG was flat.** B. **A fluorescein angiogram showed lack of normal choroidal fluorescence, which is typical of Stargardt's disease.**

Another inherited maculopathy is *cone dystrophy*. Like Stargardt's disease, patients present with decreased central acuity with few initial findings in the macula. Cone dystrophy is an inherited degeneration that presents between 10 and 30 years of age. Patients complain of decreased visual acuity, poor color vision, and sometimes light sensitivity. Like Stargardt's patients, they may be misinterpreted as being malingerers with complaints of decreased vision without obvious findings. An ERG (i.e., full photopic field and especially focal ERG) is helpful in making the diagnosis. Later, typical changes in the macula include a bull's eye maculopathy, so-called because of rings of hypertrophy of the retinal pigment epithelium followed by atrophy in the macula, giving it a "bull's eye" appearance.

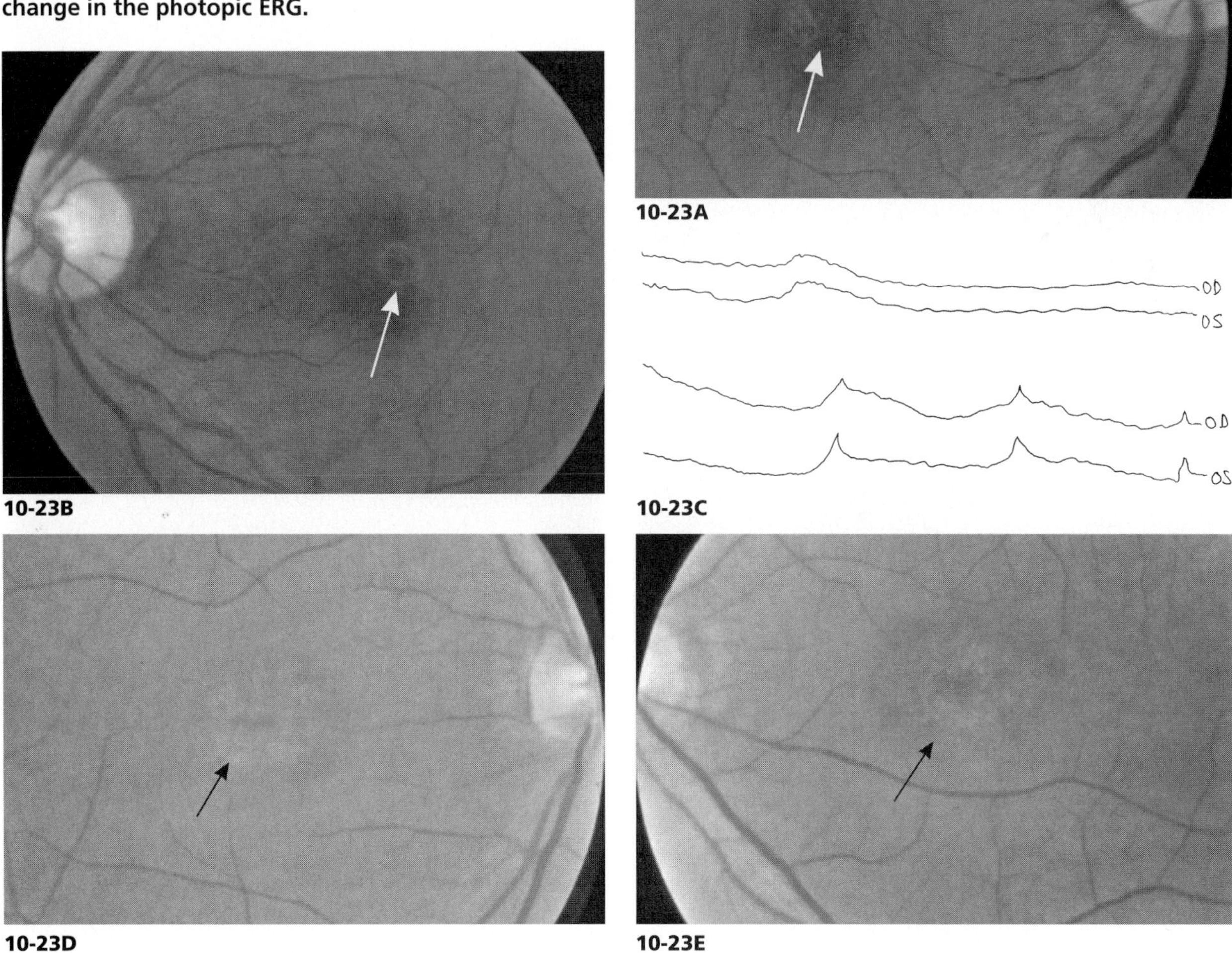

Figure 10-23. This woman was diagnosed as being a malingerer with unexplained decreased vision. A,B. **Her maculas had a somewhat unusual pattern, with mild granularity (*arrows*).** C. **An ERG was diagnostic, showing little cone functioning.** D,E. **Another individual referred for unexplained vision loss. Decreased visual acuity was found on examination. There were subtle changes in the macula (*arrows*) associated with a change in the photopic ERG.**

A specific maculopathy is seen with the spinocerebellar degeneration SCA-7. This autosomal dominant degenerative condition begins with progressive cerebellar ataxia. SCA-7 has a prominent maculopathy that presents subtly with decreased color vision and, later, loss of central acuity and abnormalities on focal ERG.

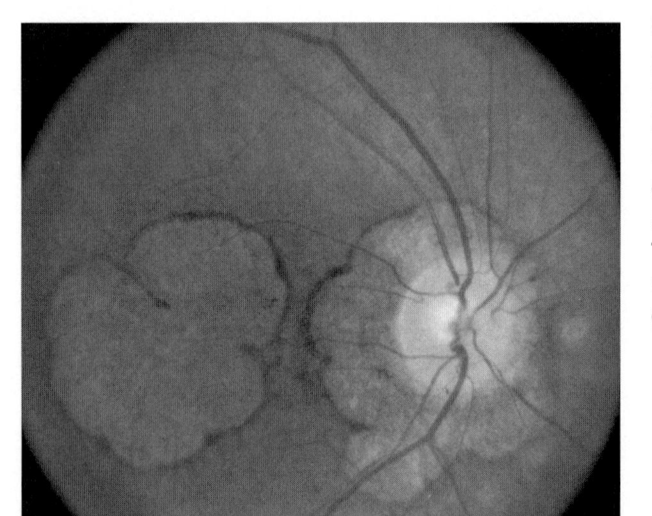

10-24A

Figure 10-24. A. **This 28-year-old woman was completely disabled by ataxia, dysarthria, dysphagia, and poor vision, all related to familial ataxia: SCA-7. She had poor vision in both eyes and large central scotomas. (See full report in LG Gouw, KB Digre, CP Harris, et al. Autosomal dominant cerebellar ataxia with retinal degeneration. Neurology 1994;44:1441–1447.)** B,C. **This woman is a cousin to the first patient; she had much milder involvement of the macula. Notice the granularity of the macula.**

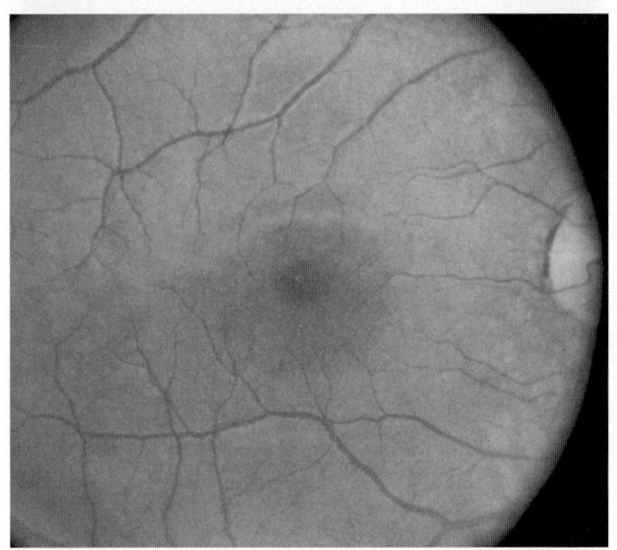

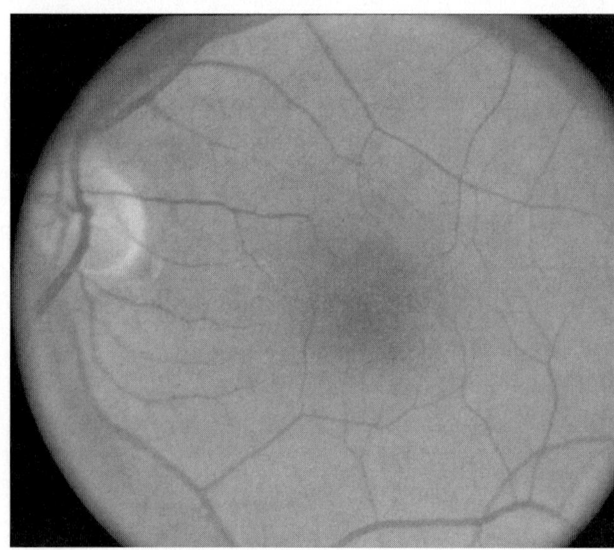

10-24B

10-24C

Other Maculopathies/Cone Dystrophies

In general, all of the macular dystrophies are inherited and present with decreased visual acuity. Early complaints are considered with suspicion, because there is often no obvious change in the macula, and these patients are often referred for functional visual loss or malingering. Often the visual fields are normal early, aside from a reduced foveal threshold. Color vision is almost invariably affected. A Farnsworth D-15 or Farnsworth-Munsell 100-hue color test may reveal a tritan axis (blue-yellow) defect. Although the full-field ERG may be normal, photopic ERG may be low. Focal ERG (testing only the macular function) is diagnostic.[29] Fluorescein angiography is helpful in that it may reveal the diagnosis (i.e., choroidal silence, as in Stargardt's, or bull's eye maculopathy). In general, there is no treatment for the macular dystrophies at this time.

Table 10-8. Macular Dystrophies

Maculopathy	Clinical	Appearance	Other
Vitelliform maculopathy (Best's)	Slowly decreasing vision in a child; few symptoms; autosomal dominant	Fried egg appearance (also "peach half")	Atrophy of the retinal pigment epithelium
Cone dystrophy (there are several forms)	Variable genetics: autosomal dominant; see better at dusk; prefer sunglasses	See bull's eye appearance also on fluorescein angiogram; pigment stippling; sometimes very subtle	See loss of cones
Stargardt's disease	Autosomal recessive; vision loss	Initially no findings; fluorescein angiogram may show earliest change; later yellowish, perifoveal flecks	Fluorescein: choroidal silence; atrophy of cones, retinal pigment epithelium
Achromatopsia	Autosomal recessive; poor visual acuity, absence of color perception, photophobia; stationary—doesn't progress	See associated nystagmus and blepharospasm; early on no obvious macular change; later may see bull's eye maculopathy	ERG makes the diagnosis; cones are abnormal

Source: Adapted from references 26,30,31.

Table 10-9. Causes of Bull's Eye Maculopathy

Chloroquine
Cone dystrophies
Achromatopsias
Hallervorden-Spatz syndrome
Spinocerebellar atrophy
Fucosidosis

Figure 10-25. A,B. **This 14-year-old girl presented with decreased vision, headaches, and central scotomas. She was found to have bilateral papilledema related to idiopathic intracranial hypertension and also Best's vitelliform maculopathy. The maculas are commonly described as having a "fried egg" sunny-side-up appearance (*arrows*).**

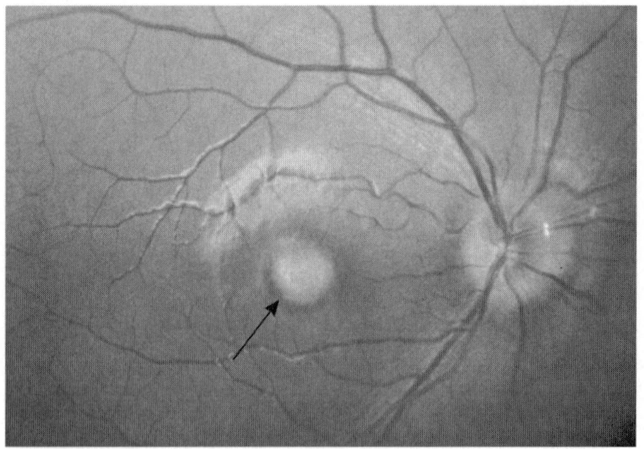

10-25A

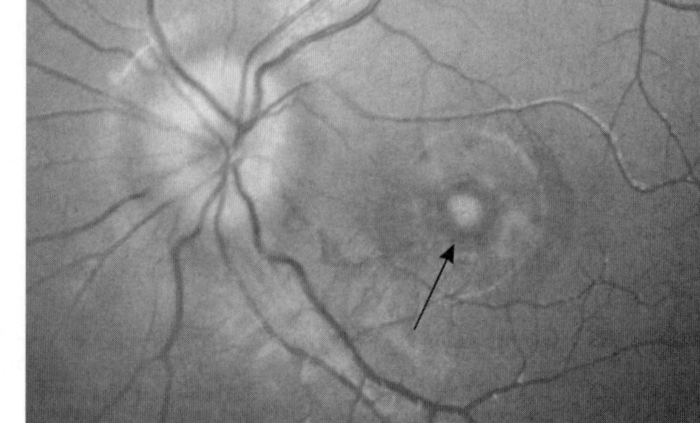

10-25B

Figure 10-26. A,B. Chloroquine maculopathy, as well as other toxic maculopathies, can produce a "bull's eye" pattern of depigmentation. The outer ring (*black arrows*) outlines the outermost abnormal area, whereas the inner circle (*white arrowheads*) is the "bull's eye." C,D. The fluorescein angiogram shows a central nonfluorescent spot surrounded by hyperfluorescence. Sometimes cone dystrophies can have this appearance as well. See Chapter 4 (toxins associated with optic nerve disorders) and Chapter 9 (toxins associated with retinal disorders).

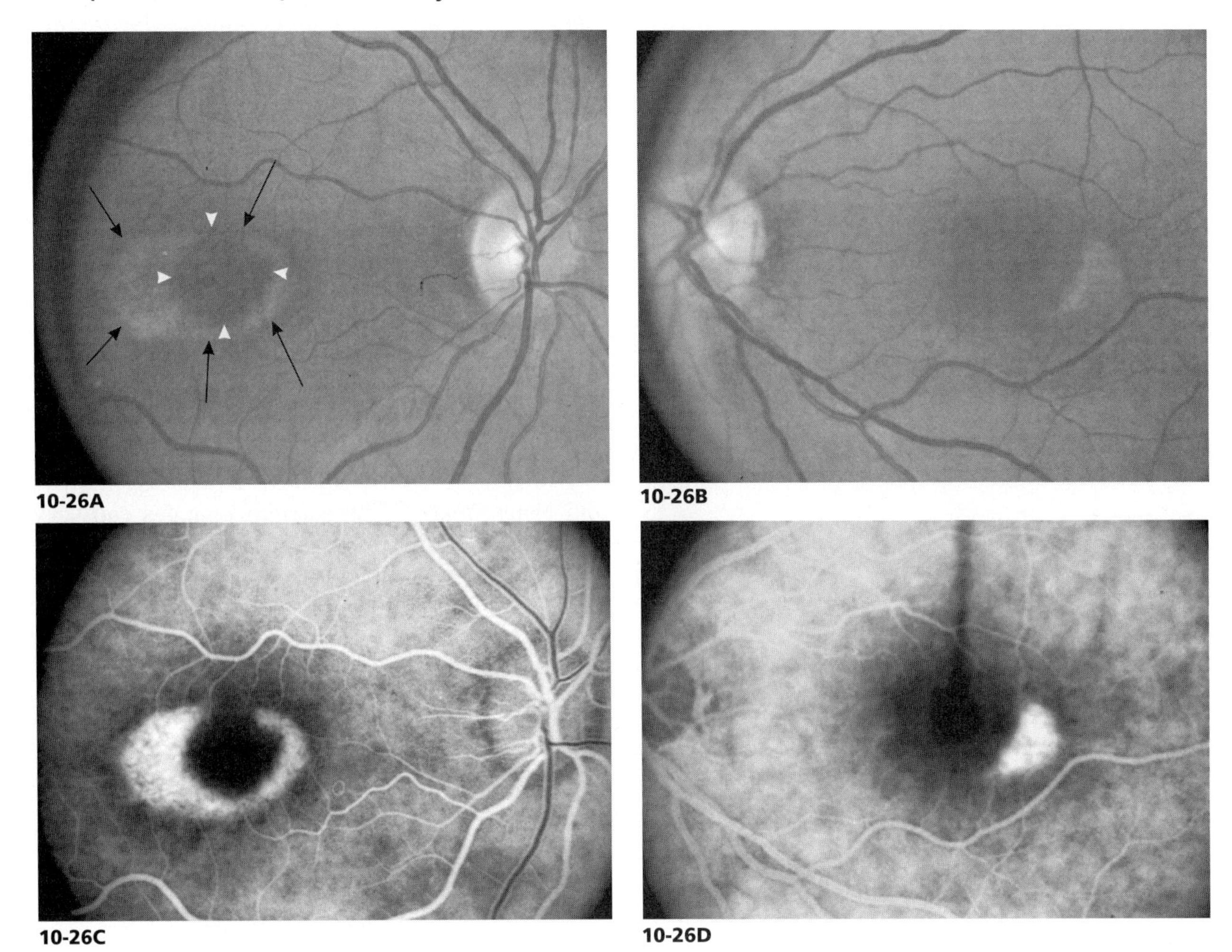

Changes in the Macula Owing to Toxins and Drugs

Many drugs and toxins affect the macular function. One of the more common drugs used includes hydroxychloroquine (Plaquenil) for the treatment of malaria and collagen-vascular diseases. It is the prototype of macular toxicity from a medication.

There appears to be little risk of retinopathy in patients on maintenance doses of less than 6.5 mg per kg per day, particularly if the treatment lasts less than 10 years in duration and renal insufficiency is not present. Patients should have color vision testing, visual field tests (usually the Humphrey 10-2, macular program), an Amsler's grid check monthly by the patient, and examinations approximately every 6 months after the baseline and then annually. If a patient is on more than 6.5 mg per kg per day, examinations should be more frequent. On examination, the cornea may show deposition but is not symptomatic.[32] The definition of hydroxychloroquine retinopathy (maculopathy) is the "presence of bilateral, reproducible, positive field defects that can be demonstrated by two different tests of the visual field" (e.g., Amsler's grid and visual field).[33] The macular changes can very closely mimic macular degeneration and the appearance of the macula per se is not the best way to follow patients.[33]

Table 10-10. Drugs and Toxins Affecting the Macula

Drug or toxin	Use	Symptoms	Clinical findings
Chloroquine/hydroxy-chloroquine	Malaria and collagen-vascular disease	Few; later visual acuity loss	Bull's eye maculopathy (late)
Clofazimine	Leprosy, mycobacterium, psoriasis	Few	Macular pigmentary changes; peripheral retinal atrophy
Deferoxamine	Iron toxicity	Blurred vision	Pigmentary change in the macula
Tamoxifen	Breast cancer	Blurred vision	Macular edema; crystalline retinopathy—see small refractile spots in the macula
Canthaxanthin	Carotenoid used as artificial tanning agent	Usually none	See small deposits in the macula
Epinephrine	Allergic reactions; many uses	Decreased vision	Cystoid macular edema
Niacin (nicotinic acid)	Hypercholesterolemia	Usually none	Yellow foveola with possible cystoid macular edema

Source: Adapted from references 13,34,35.

What Diseases Could Mimic Macular Diseases?

Optic neuropathies with central scotomas may mimic disease of the macula. An afferent pupillary defect is present in unilateral optic neuropathies. Optic pits may be accompanied by serous macular detachment, and although the macula is involved in this case, the primary problem is the optic pit.

Table 10-11. Conditions That Mimic Macular Disease

Optic neuropathy
Optic pit
Optic nerve drusen with serous retinal detachment
Neuroretinitis (primarily optic nerve with macular star)

Practical Viewing Essentials

Figure 10-27.

1. Signs of macular involvement include decreased visual acuity, reduced color vision, and changes on an Amsler's grid.
2. To view the macula, you have to dilate the pupil and use the dimmest light possible on the ophthalmoscope so that the patient can tolerate the examination and you can see the macula.
3. Investigation of macular disease requires a sensitivity to changes in the appearance of the macula over time.
4. The macula may be entirely normal in appearance, and yet be the seat of dysfunction, such as is seen in Stargardt's disease and cone dystrophy.
5. Fluorescein angiogram and an ERG (especially multi-focal ERG) are essential tools in the evaluation of a patient with suspected macular disease.
6. Macular disease should be seen by an ophthalmologist.

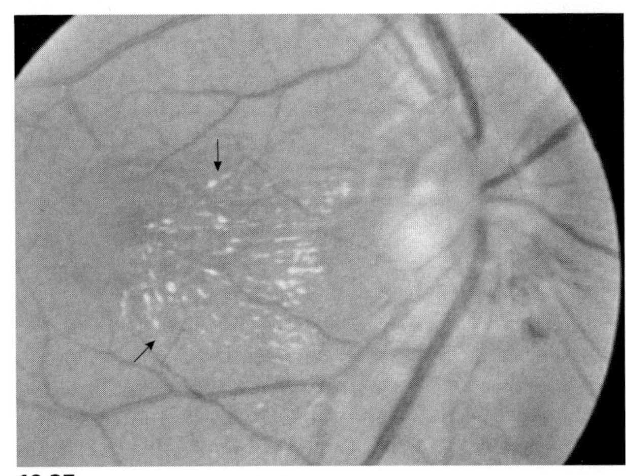

10-27

References

1. Cogan DG. Neurology of the Visual System. Springfield, IL: Thomas, 1966.
2. Rapp LM, Maple SS, Choi JH. Lutein and zeaxanthin concentrations in rod outer segment membranes from perifoveal and peripheral human retina. Invest Ophthalmol Vis Sci 2000;41:1200–1209.
3. Walsh FB, Hoyt WF. Clinical Neuro-ophthalmology. Baltimore: Williams & Wilkins, 1969;10–11.
4. Polyak S. The Vertebrate Visual System. Chicago: University of Chicago Press, 1957;272.
5. Glaser JS, Savino PJ, Sumers KD, et al. The photostress recovery test in the clinical assessment of visual functions. Am J Ophthalmol 1977;83(2):255–260.
6. Amsler M. Quantitative and qualitative vision. Trans Ophthalmol Soc UK 1949;69:397–410.
7. Sunness J. Evaluating macular function. Int Ophthalmol Clin 1999;39(4):19–31.
8. Abdelsalam A, Priore LD, Zarbin MA. Drusen in age-related macular degeneration: pathogenesis, natural course, and laser photocoagulation-induced regression. Surv Ophthalmol 1999;44:1–29.
9. Fine SL, Berger JW, Maguire MG, Ho AC. Age-related macular degeneration. N Engl J Med 2000;342:483–492.
10. Sarks SH, Sarks JP. Age-related maculopathy: neovascular age-related macular degeneration and the evolution of geographic atrophy. In SJ Ryan, AP Schachat (eds), Retina (3rd ed). St. Louis: Mosby, 2001;1064–1099.
11. Dick JS, Jampol LM. Macular edema. In SJ Ryan, AP Schachat (eds), Retina (3rd ed). St. Louis: Mosby, 2001;967–981.
12. Dick JS. Macular edema. Int Ophthalmol Clin 1999;39:1–18.
13. Kempen JH. Drug-induced maculopathy. Int Ophthalmol Clin 1999;39(4):67–82.
14. Aiello LM. Diagnosis, management, and treatment of non-proliferative diabetic retinopathy and macular edema. In DM Albert, FA Jakobiec (eds), Principles and Practice of Ophthalmology. Philadelphia: Saunders, 1994;747–760.
15. Gass JD. Stereoscopic Atlas of Macular Diseases. St. Louis: Mosby, 1987.
16. Pearlman J, Pieramici D. Diagnosis and management of macular holes. Int Ophthalmol Clin 1999;39:175–189.
17. Ho AC, Guyer DR, Fine SL. Macular hole. Surv Ophthalmol 1998;42:393–416.
18. Mainster MA, Khan JA. Photic retinal injury. In SJ Ryan, AP Schachat, RP Murphy (eds), Retina (2nd ed). St. Louis: Mosby, 1994;1767–1781.
19. Rush JA. Acute macular neuroretinopathy. Am J Ophthalmol 1977;83:490–494.
20. Leavitt JA, Pruthi S, Morgenstern BZ. Hypertensive retinopathy mimicking neuroretinitis in a twelve-year-old girl. Surv Ophthalmol 1997;41:477–480.
21. Dreyer RF, Hopen G, Gass DM, Smith JL. Leber's idiopathic stellate neuroretinitis. Arch Ophthalmol 1984;102:1140–1145.
22. Cunningham ET, Koehler JE. Ocular bartonellosis. Am J Ophthalmol 2000;130:340–349.
23. Wade NK, Levi L, Jones MR, et al. Optic disk edema associated with peripapillary serous retinal detachment: an early sign of systemic *Bartonella hensleae* infection. Am J Ophthalmol 2000;130:327–334.
24. Rizzo JF. Neuroophthalmologic disease of the retina. In DM Albert, FA Jakobiec (eds), Principles and Practice of Ophthalmology. Philadelphia: Saunders, 1994;2507–2529.
25. Kivlin JD, Sanborn GE, Myers GG. The cherry-red spot in Tay-Sachs and other storage diseases. Ann Neurol 1983;17:356–360.
26. Kelly J, Maumenee IH. Hereditary macular diseases. Int Ophthalmol Clin 1999;39(4):83–115.
27. Rosenberg RN, Prusiner SB, Di Mauro S, Barchi RL. The Molecular and Genetic Basis of Neurological Disease. Boston: Butterworth–Heinemann, 1998.
28. Stargardt K. Ueber familiare progressive degeneration in der Maculagegend des Auges. Albrecht Von Graefes Arch Ophthalmol 1909;71:534–550.
29. Piao CH, Kondo M, Tanikawa A, et al. Multifocal electroretinogram in occult macular dystrophy. Invest Ophthalmol Vis Sci 2000;41:513–517.
30. Deutman AF. Macular dystrophies. In SJ Ryan, AP Schachat, RP Murphy (eds), Retina (2nd ed). St. Louis: Mosby, 1994;1186–1240.
31. Simunovic MP, Moore AT. The cone dystrophies. Eye 1998;12:553–565.
32. Easterbrook M. The ocular safety of hydroxychloroquine. Semin Arthritis Rheum 1993;23:62–67.
33. Easterbrook M. Detection and prevention of maculopathy associated with antimalarial agents. Int Ophthalmol Clin 1979;39:49–57.
34. Swartz M. Other diseases: drug toxicity and metabolic and nutritional conditions. In SJ Ryan, AP Schachat, RP Murphy (eds), Retina (2nd ed). St. Louis: Mosby, 1994;1755–1766.
35. Grant WM. Toxicology of the Eye. Springfield, IL: Thomas, 1974.

11 Practical Viewing in Children

It is equally important that [the examiner] should be familiar with those congenital changes in the eye which are of no significance. Many of these will be alluded to in describing the morbid appearance which they are most liable to be confounded.

William Gowers[1]

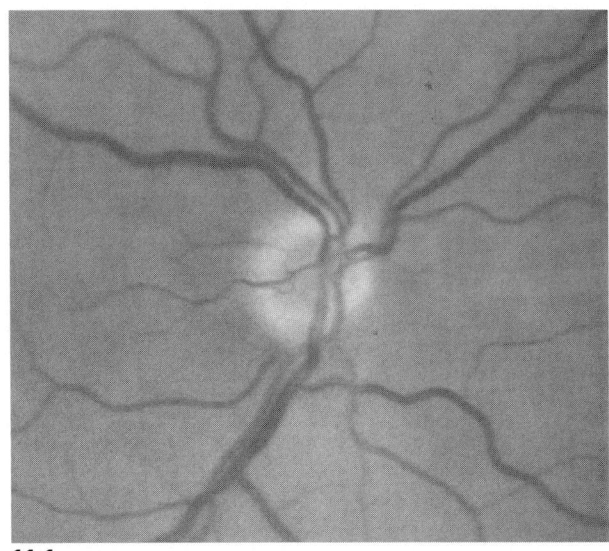

11-1

Figure 11-1. A hypoplastic disc is important to recognize in childhood.

Children represent a special challenge in viewing the optic disc. First, infants and small children may not be able to give a history. We rely totally on the parent or caregiver's observations. Second, infants and small children are uncooperative with our usual examination techniques—we do not have a lot of time to see, and have to be prepared to *look* to see quickly. Third, viewing the optic fundus may provide valuable information about the problem the child has, whether a diagnosis of a genetic syndrome or a visual problem attributable to delayed development—namely, viewing the optic fundus may be an important way to narrow down possible diagnoses.

Here, the history is very important.

Table 11-1. Historical Data to Evaluate in Children

History of the pregnancy
Mother's health
Prenatal care
Time of birth—preterm by how many weeks or term
Complications at delivery (vaginal or cesarean): Apgar scores
Peri/postnatal complications
Neonatal hypoglycemia
Neonatal jaundice
Hypothyroidism
Development to date; development curves
Past history: trauma, illnesses (chronic ear infections)
Family history: Any related vision or eye condition

Which children are at higher risk for visual abnormalities? Children born prematurely (i.e., before 32 weeks of development) are at higher risk not only for acquired disorders such as retinopathy of prematurity (ROP), but also are more frequently associated with genetic disorders, meaning those that could affect the appearance of the optic disc and/or fundus. Children with neurologic disorders, including mental disorders as well as genetic and hearing disorders, should be examined by an ophthalmologist. Children who have a family history of a vision-threatening condition may be at risk for a similar process and should also be seen.

Symptoms reported by the parents, such as that the child does not follow or does not appear to see, should be taken seriously. The most common time for a child to present with vision loss is after failing a school screening examination. Unilateral vision loss before school tests may be hard to detect because neither the child nor the parent notices it. A second common complaint is an eye turning out or in strabismus. This can be owing to vision loss or misalignment, as well as ocular motor problems.

What examination is necessary? First, an assessment of visual acuity is helpful. If the child is too young for the E game, note whether the child fixates on your face or follows your face when you move.

Table 11-2. Normal Visual Development

Age	Normal acuity	What the child should see
Newborn	20/400	Light/dark and contrast
2 Weeks		Regards mother's face
6 Weeks		Steady fixation
3 Months		Fixes and follows an object; smiles at faces
2 Years	20/40	Fixes and follows; can pick up small objects; begin picture chart
Verbal—3 years	20/40	Picture chart
4 Years	20/40	E game
6 Years	20/20	Snellen acuity chart

Source: Adapted from reference 2.

Visual acuity can be slightly decreased in young children, perhaps because of a refractive error or because of not understanding the acuity test directions. Even though decreased vision may be owing to refractive error, prompt referral for refraction can be made. If the visual acuity is asymmetric, refer to an ophthalmologist or optometrist.

School screenings of visual acuity are undertaken in almost all schools in the United States to assure that children are seeing properly out of both eyes. Any abnormality picked up at these screenings is referred to a physician for further evaluation.

With the penlight, notice that the light strikes the cornea at about the same place on each eye. Seeing this assures the examiner that ocular alignment is grossly normal.

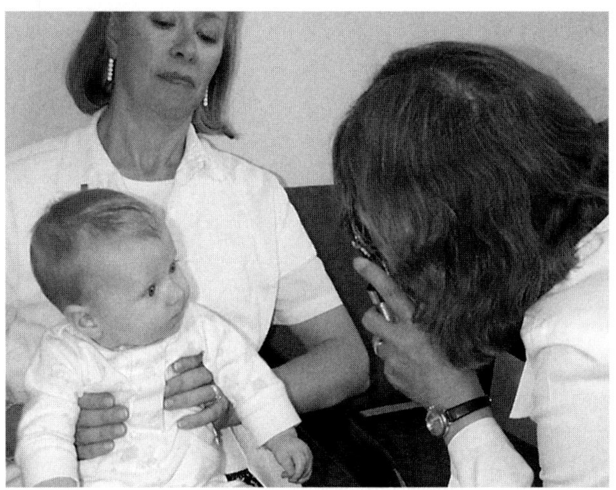

11-2

Figure 11-2. Examining a baby is challenging. Begin by being sure that the ophthalmoscopic light strikes the cornea in approximately the same place. Then look for the red reflex through the ophthalmoscope.

Next, check the pupillary light reflex in both eyes and perform the swinging flashlight test while having the child look in the distance, to see if there is an afferent pupillary defect that may indicate an optic neuropathy.

Examine the pupil in room light—do you see the red reflex, or is the pupil white? A white pupil, leukocoria, should prompt an immediate referral to an ophthalmologist.

Table 11-3. Causes of Leukocoria

Causes of Leukocoria
Cataract
Corneal opacity
Retinoblastoma
Persistent hyperplastic primary vitreous
Retinopathy of prematurity
Vitreous hemorrhage
Other: Coats' disease, Norrie's disease, toxocariasis

Pediatricians and primary care physicians have used the red reflex to examine whether or not there is a gross abnormality in the eye. This reflex usually detects cataracts or gross abnormalities such as retinoblastoma.

The red reflex examination can be performed in any doctor's office. The lights are turned off and the ophthalmoscope lens setting is +2. Shine the light from approximately 2 feet away toward the infant or child. Use a lower-powered light and increase the intensity to the brightest the child can stand without wincing. The examiner looks to be sure that the red reflex is present and complete. You will also see a white light reflex shining off of the cornea; this has been called the *corneal reflex* and should be in the center of the cornea. You can view the red reflex and the corneal reflex simultaneously. *Any abnormality in the red reflex demands an ophthalmologic evaluation.* The red reflex examination can be done with the child's pupil dilated, which increases the sensitivity of detecting retinoblastoma.

Table 11-4. Red Reflex Examination

Condition	Age	Presentation	Finding on red reflex examination	Further workup
Cataract	Infant	Leukocoria	See black irregular object in the red reflex; may see reflected light—white reflex	Glucose, calcium, TORCH battery, consider other metabolic and genetic disorders; refer to ophthalmologist
Retinoblastoma	12–21 mos; unusual after 2 yrs	Leukocoria—more than one-half; strabismus 20%; red eye; poor vision, orbital cellulitis	Red reflex shows a black object obscuring the red reflex	Refer immediately for evaluation; computed tomography scan and ultrasonography
Anisometropia	Infant, child	No particular presentation; early strabismus	See unequal red reflex, with one eye brighter than other	Needs refraction—refer
Strabismus	Infant, child	Eye turning in or out	See red reflex, but corneal reflex is not centered	Refer for evaluation
Persistent hyperplastic primary vitreous	Infant, child	Leukocoria	Red reflex shows changes in the posterior part of the lens	Refer for evaluation
Norrie's disease	Infant, child	Leukocoria	Red reflex is altered owing to cataract, retinal detachment, masses—vitreoretinopathy	Further evaluation with ophthalmologist
Corneal disease—microcornea (e.g., rubella; fetal alcohol syndrome; trisomy 13, 15; Ehlers-Danlos), megalocornea, Peter's anomaly, Marfan's, Sturge-Weber, cloudy cornea (e.g., metabolic disease, corneal dystrophy)	Any child	May present with parents noting the clouding	Red reflex is absent in cloudy cornea; the size of the cornea should be assessed	Refer to ophthalmologist; check pressure—glaucoma associated with megalocornea

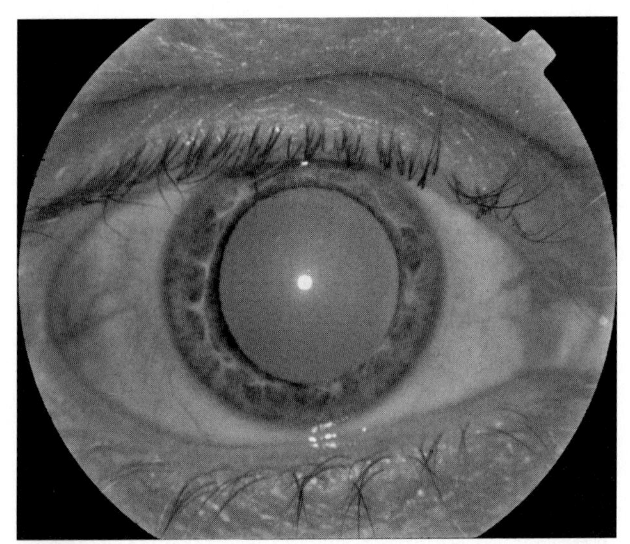

11-3A

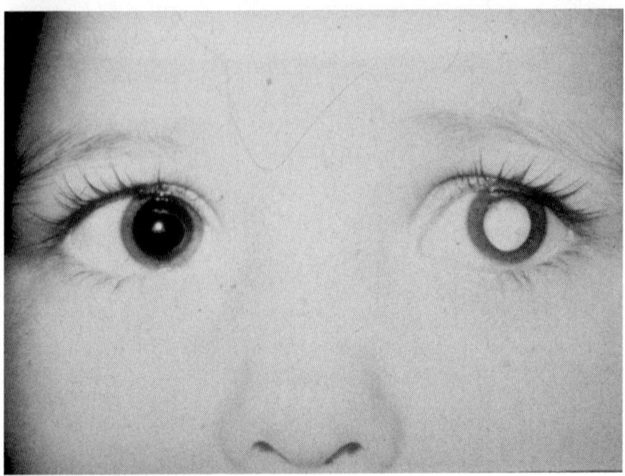

11-3B

Figure 11-3. A. **The normal red reflex.** B. **If the pupil looks white, leukocoria is present. In this case, the leukocoria is owing to a tumor (retinoblastoma). (Photograph courtesy of Nick Mammalis, M.D.)**

What about looking at the disc itself? First, getting a good view requires pupillary dilation. Dilating drops to use in children include phenylephrine 1.0%–2.5% or tropicamide 1% for most routine dilations. If there is a concern about getting a good refraction, ophthalmologists use a cycloplegic agent like cyclopentolate 0.2%–1.0% (Cyclogyl). We avoid atropine.

Even with the pupil dilated, direct ophthalmoscopy may be difficult. In many cases, an indirect examination (with the 20-diopter lens) by an ophthalmologist is necessary. Sometimes, to keep the eyes open in infants, lid specula are used.

On occasion, an examination is performed under anesthesia to adequately view the disc and retina. How does one perform this examination? General anesthesia with an anesthesiologist in attendance, using a sleeping agent like chloral hydrate, is necessary. This should be performed by an ophthalmologist who is experienced in direct and indirect techniques.

Table 11-5. Indications for an Examination under Anesthesia

Suspected glaucoma
Enlarged cornea
Corneal opacification
Cupping
Gonioscopy to evaluate the angle
Suspected peripheral retinal disease
Suspected optic nerve disease
Intraocular tumor
Cataract surgery planning
Retarded or uncooperative child
Unexplained vision loss

Once you are able to view the optic disc, you are looking for features as outlined in Chapter 2—the normal disc and normal variants. However, the anomalous disc is a problem for the pediatrician and family physician, who frequently see the child first. The *anomalous disc* is usually discovered during childhood. Bilaterally anomalous discs usually cause decreased vision at birth, and the child's vision does not develop normally. Unilateral anomalous discs associated with vision loss are often not detected until the school eye exam.

What Should You Think of When Seeing an Anomalous Disc?

We think that the general concepts of Brodsky et al. for evaluating and viewing children with disc anomalies are very important.[3] These include

1. Bilateral optic disc anomalies present in infancy with poor vision and nystagmus.
2. Unilateral optic disc anomalies present during their preschool years with strabismus (esotropia).
3. Malformed discs frequently have associated central nervous system malformations.
4. Anomalous discs have better color vision than discs with an acquired optic neuropathy.
5. Congenital anomalies have a treatable form of vision loss (amblyopia).

All children with anomalous discs and vision loss, especially if there is evidence of neurodevelopmental abnormalities, should have a neuroimaging procedure.

When trying to analyze why the disc does not appear normal, you may wish to divide the anomalous disc into these categories: size, shape, cavitary anomalies, and elevated anomalies.

Table 11-6. Disc Anomalies and Their Associated Defects

Disc anomalies	What to consider
Small discs	
Optic nerve hypoplasia	Midline defects such as absent septum pellucidum; endocrinologic dysfunction and developmental delay
Hyperopic discs	Notice the refraction
Little red discs	Confused with papilledema
Normal-sized discs	
Large cup	Prematurity; look for periventricular leukoencephalopathy
Abnormal vasculature—tortuosity; lack of branch points[4]	Prematurity, fetal alcohol syndrome
Large discs	
Megalopapilla	Usually normal variant
Colobomas	Associated with endocrinologic and midline defects
Morning glory discs	Basal encephaloceles
Staphyloma	Related to myopia
Gray discs	Delayed development; Pelizaeus Merzbacher; albinism

Is the Disc Too Small?

Although some have tried to quantify what is "small," no uniform definition exists. You may want to try the estimating-the-disc-size technique outlined in Chapter 2 with the small aperture of the ophthalmoscope. Is the disc remarkably smaller than that? Otherwise, remember the Supreme Court Justice quote about pornography: "I can't define it, but I know it when I see it."

Hyperopia alone can make the disc appear small. Sometimes these discs are actually slightly smaller than normal and have no cup. The disc is commonly more hyperemic and congested-appearing, hence, "the little red disc" (which we discussed in Chapter 2). Hyperopic discs are frequently mistaken for early disc swelling (see Chapter 2, Figure 2-4 and Chapter 3, Figure 3-1).

OPTIC NERVE HYPOPLASIA

In *optic nerve hypoplasia*, the nerve is small—less than one-half to two-thirds of the normal size. If the mean disc area is approximately 2.89 mm^2, a hypoplastic disc is approximately 1.4 mm^2.[5] Optic nerve hypoplasia is one of the most common optic nerve anomalies. Although there is no great definition of hypoplasia, we agree with the definition of hypoplasia as a small optic disc associated either with decreased vision or changes in the visual field that correspond to nerve fiber layer defects, or both.[5] The cause of hypoplastic discs is still being debated. Some argue that the fibers reach an abnormal chiasm or abnormal midline that prevents normal growth to the opposite optic tract, causing the fibers to then undergo retrograde degeneration. Others think that there was defective differentiation of the retinal ganglion cells to begin with or secondary degeneration of these cells. In most series, the majority of the cases are bilateral with a slight male predominance.[5–7] More recently, Deiner et al. have reported that certain proteins, such as Netrin 1, actually guide the retinal ganglion cell axon through the disc. When these proteins are absent, the axons do not exit into the optic nerve, and optic nerve hypoplasia results.[8]

Optic disc hypoplasia appears to occur anytime between 6 and 16 weeks' gestation, but may occur even later when one considers segmental hypoplasia, which can occur after cerebral hemispheric damage. Bilateral optic nerve hypoplasia has more associated developmental and endocrinologic abnormalities. Patients with good vision and either unilateral or bilateral optic nerve hypoplasia are reported to have less frequent nonvisual problems.[8]

Figure 11-4. A. Hypoplastic discs are usually tiny and pale (the disc is outlined) or slightly gray-appearing with a ring of slightly paler area (*arrows*)—the "double ring" sign.[9] Notice that there is usually combined arterial and venous tortuosity, another sign of hypoplastic discs. The hypoplasia also may be segmental, leading to altitudinal or wedge visual field defects as well. Does the retinal vasculature look tortuous? The black outline is the actual disc. The arrows point to the ring of pallor. B. Now pick out the actual disc and the pale "double ring." C. Another hypoplastic disc—pick out the disc and outline the ring of pallor. D. This optic disc shows the characteristic tortuous blood vessels coming out of the center of the disc. Find the disc and the ring of pallor.

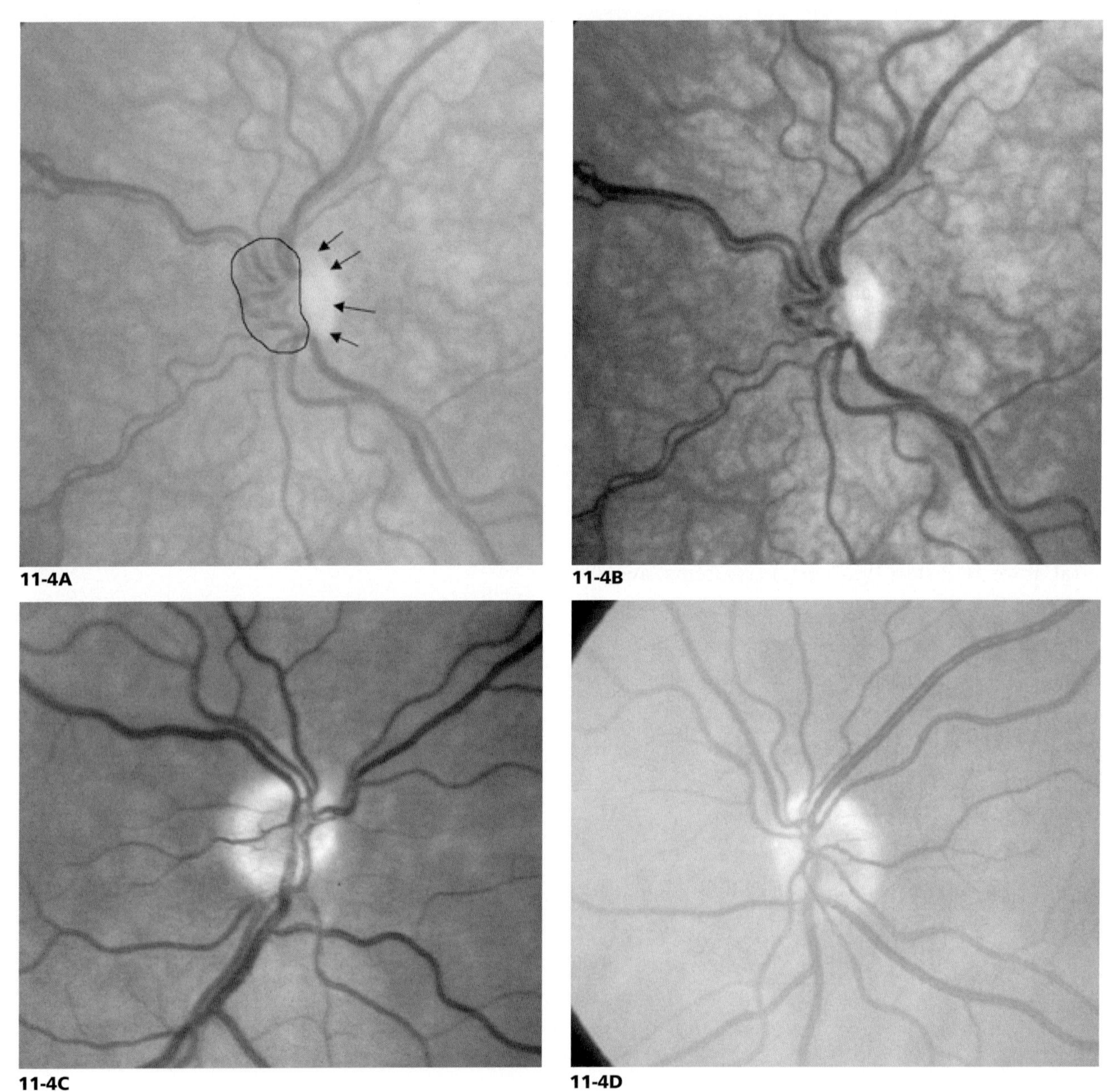

Figure 11-5. A,B. This young girl was referred for anomalous discs. The arrowheads in A mark the optic disc. There is a thinning of the nerve fiber layer, and one might suspect optic atrophy.[10] The color of the disc is variable from gray to white and may be normal; therefore, look at its size, not the color, for the diagnosis of this condition. Fortunately, she had relatively good vision (20/30) and no other endocrinologic or neurologic problems.

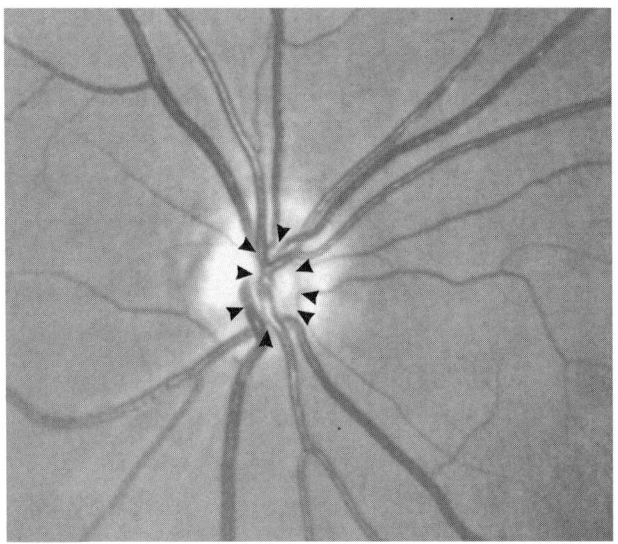

11-5A

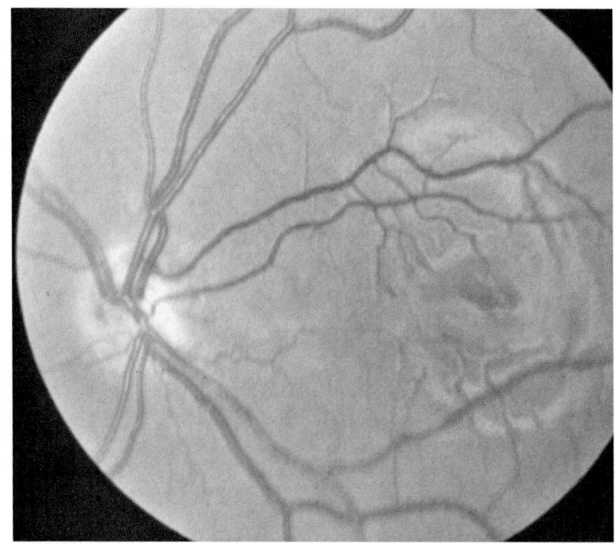

11-5B

The most serious central nervous system defects associated with optic disc hypoplasia are abnormal midline structures within the brain. Septo-optic dysplasia (de Morsier's syndrome) is the association of optic disc hypoplasia with an absent septum pellucidum and agenesis or thinning of the corpus callosum. Dr. Georges de Morsier, a Swiss neuropathologist writing in the 1940s, called attention to the absent septum pellucidum and small visual pathways. Later, pituitary dwarfism was described in conjunction with the optic nerve anomaly.[11] These patients may also have other pituitary hormonal deficiencies such as diabetes insipidus, growth hormone deficiency, hypothyroidism, and hypocorticoidism. Magnetic resonance (MR) imaging in such cases shows the absence of the pituitary infundibulum.[12]

Figure 11-6. (opposite page) A. **The sagittal view shows thinning of the corpus callosum (*black arrow*). The chiasm is markedly thinned (*white arrow*).** B. **The axial view demonstrates thinned optic nerves.** C. **The coronal view shows the absent septum pellucidum, thinned optic chiasm, and almost absent pituitary gland.** D. **The T2-weighted axial MR shows also the absent septum pellucidum. (Photographs courtesy of Judith Warner, M.D.)**

Van Dalen found that in his examination of 25 patients with bilateral optic nerve hypoplasia, only five had a completely normal neurologic history and examination. Mental retardation was the most common neurologic abnormality found, and few had epilepsy.[6] Other central nervous system abnormalities like hypopituitarism, agenesis of the septum pellucidum, and cerebral palsy have been reported; reported endocrinologic abnormalities include hypothyroidism, panhypopituitarism, diabetes insipidus, and hyperprolactinemia.[12]

The MR shows cerebral hemispheric abnormalities in children with neurologic abnormalities or developmental delay.

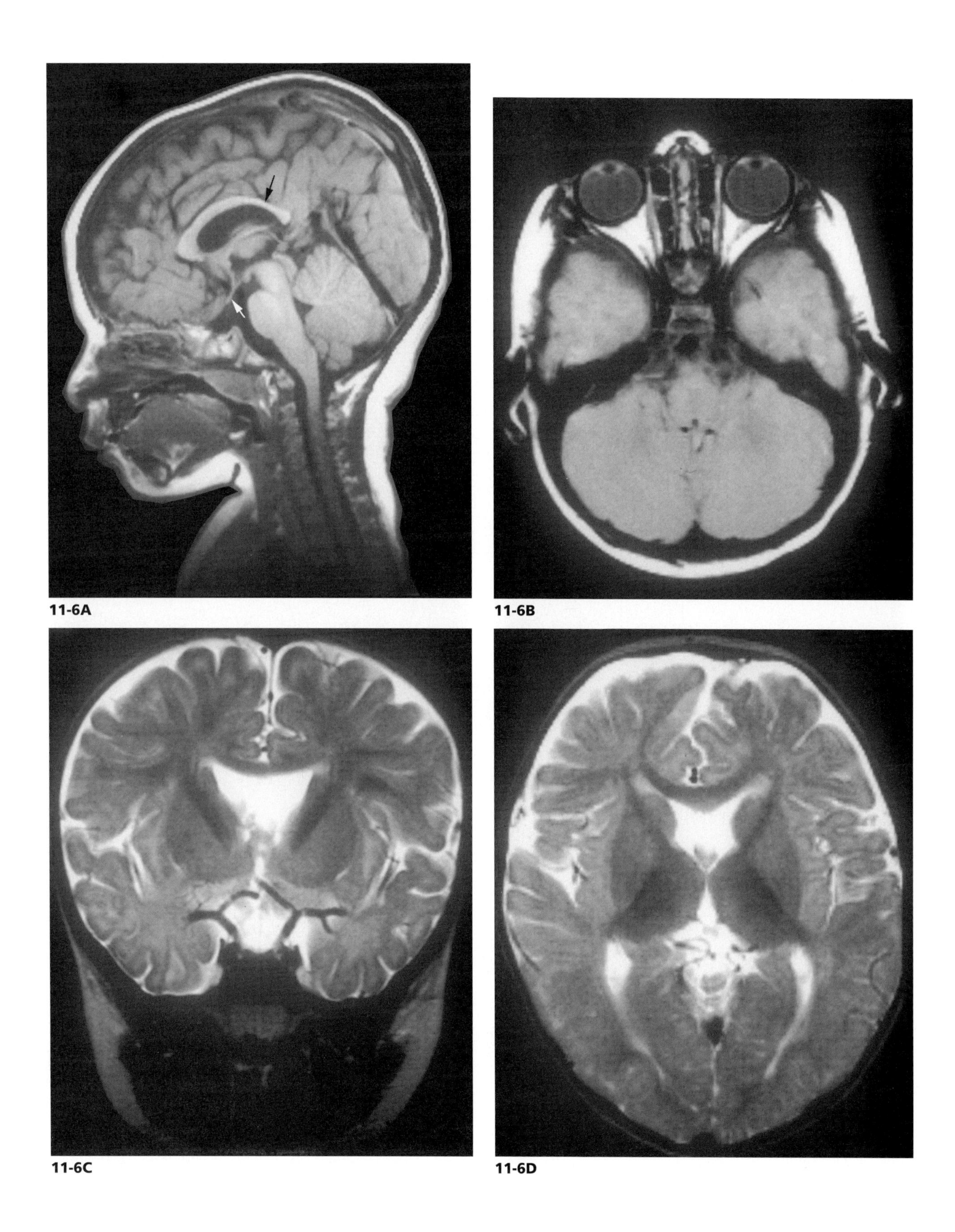
11-6A
11-6B
11-6C
11-6D

Figure 11-7. A–D. **In each of these examples, try to identify and outline where the actual disc tissue is.**

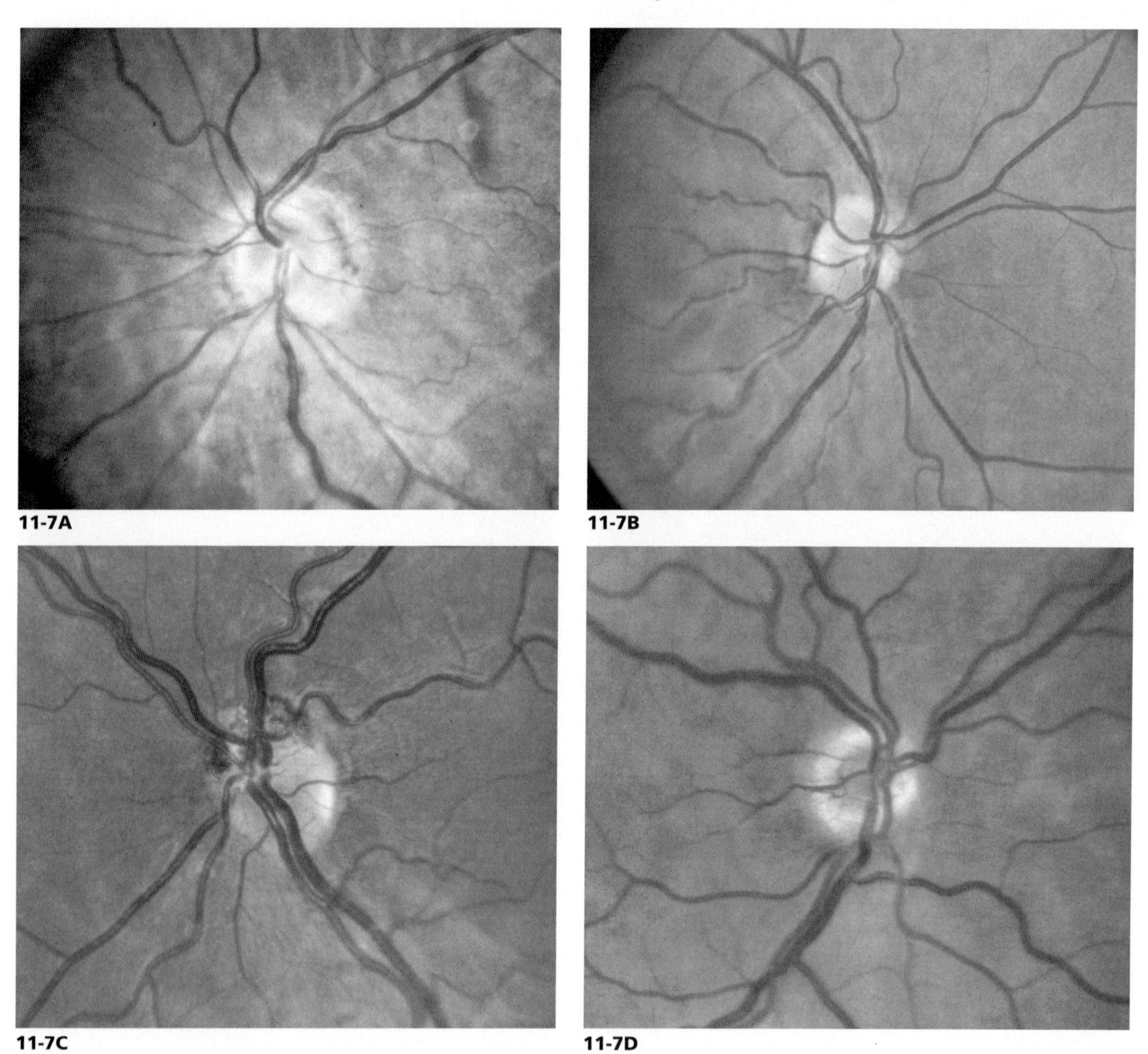

Table 11-7. Systemic Associations of Optic Nerve Hypoplasia

Central nervous system	Short stature
Anencephaly	Arched palate
Microcephaly	Congenital heart disease (ventricular septal defect)
Hydrencephaly	Trisomy 18
Oxycephaly	Chromosome 13q
Hydrocephalus	Trisomy 21 (Down syndrome)
Septo-optic dysplasia	Trisomy D
Encephalocele—basal	Skin abnormalities
Hypopituitarism	Albinism
Anterior (dwarfism)	Fetal alcohol syndrome
Posterior (diabetes insipidus)	Eye deformities
Panhypopituitarism	Albinism
Agenesis of the septum pellucidum	Aniridia
Cerebral palsy	Microphthalmos
Psychomotor retardation	Strabismus
Epilepsy/seizures	Ptosis
Porencephaly	Duane's syndrome
Developmental delay	Blepharophimosis
Precocious puberty	Aicardi's syndrome
Facial and head abnormalities	Apert's syndrome
Facial hemiatrophy	Others
Mandibulofacial dysostosis	Klippel-Trenaunay-Weber syndrome
Oxycephaly	Goldenhar's syndrome
Palatoschisis	Linear sebaceous nevus syndrome
Deafness	Meckel syndrome
Glucose-6 phosphatase deficiency	Osteogenesis imperfecta
Chondrodysplasia punctata	Potter syndrome
Medial facial cleft syndrome	Dandy-Walker syndrome
Saddle-nose deformity	Delleman syndrome
Hypertelorism	
Frontal bossing	
Short neck	

Source: Adapted in part from references 3,12–16.

Optic disc aplasia is extremely rare. In this condition there is total absence of the optic nerve, retinal vessels, and ganglion cell layer. Optic disc aplasia is associated with micro-ophthalmus, cataracts, and colobomas.[14]

Table 11-8. Imaging Findings with Optic Disc Hypoplasia

Magnetic resonance finding	Frequency of finding	Clinical neurologic correlation	Other associations
Thinning of optic nerve/chiasm	Common	Variable acuity	—
Posterior pituitary ectopia	Approximately 15%	Growth delay; neurodevelopmental deficits	Abnormal anterior pituitary hormone deficiency—growth hormone, thyroid, corticotropin deficiency, antidiuretic hormone deficiency
Absent septum pellucidum	Common	Usually nothing specific; may see ventricular enlargement	Usually no pituitary dysfunction
Thinning or absence of the corpus callosum	Common	Neurodevelopmental problems when associated with cerebral hemisphere abnormalities	—
Hemispheric migration abnormalities (e.g., schizencephaly, cortical heterotopia)	Present in 20%	Seizures; mental retardation possible	—
Encephalomalacia—after intrauterine or perinatal hemispheric injury	Seen in 25%	Developmental delay; spastic diplegia, hemiplegia, seizures	—

Source: Adapted from reference 12.

The association of optic nerve hypoplasia with maternal diabetes has been recognized for more than 20 years.[15] Other central nervous system and ocular anomalies in children of diabetic mothers are common (3–9 times the normal rate of anomalies),[15] including holoprosencephaly, neural tube defects, microcephaly, and deafness.

Table 11-9. Causes of Optic Nerve Hypoplasia

Causes
Familial
Diabetic mothers
Young mothers
Maternal use of
Alcohol
Phenytoin
Quinine
LSD
PCP
Maternal infections
Cytomegalovirus
Syphilis
Rubella
Toxemia of pregnancy
Polyhydramnios

SEGMENTAL HYPOPLASIA

Occasionally, the optic disc hypoplasia is only segmental. *Superior segmental optic nerve hypoplasia* has an associated inferior visual field defect; this can be seen in maternal diabetes mellitus, but usually there are no other associated systemic abnormalities.[5] Kim et al. reported four characteristic findings with superior segmental optic hypoplasia termed *topless discs*, including the relative superior entrance of the central retinal artery, superior peripapillary scleral halo, pallor of the superior optic disc, and thinning of the superior nerve fiber layer.[17] In these patients, the visual acuity is usually normal, and the patient does not recognize the inferior visual field defect. If not looked for carefully, these subtle findings may be missed. More recently, there have been reports of segmental hypoplasia—topless discs—in children of mothers who were not diabetic.[18]

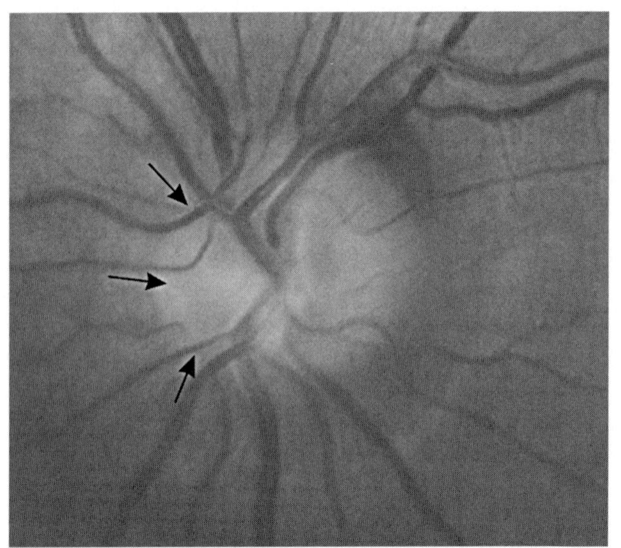

11-8A

Figure 11-8. A. This disc is only segmentally hypoplastic—in other words, part of it looks almost normal (*arrows*). B,C. This woman presented with normal visual acuity. You can see that there is very little tissue superiorly; hence the term *topless disc*. D. The same patient had irregular inferior visual field defects, however.

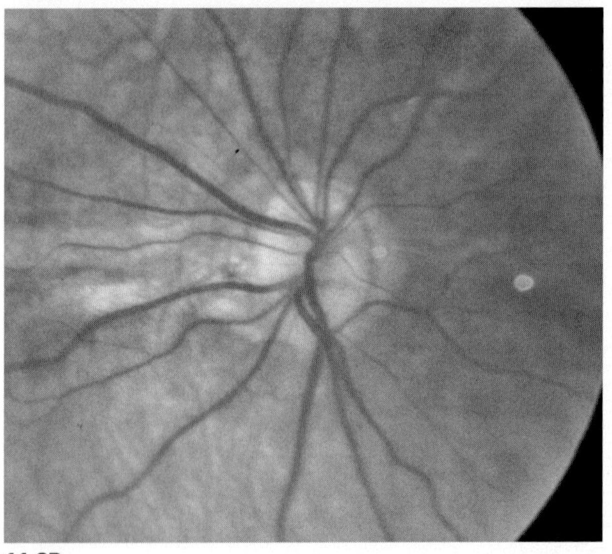

11-8B

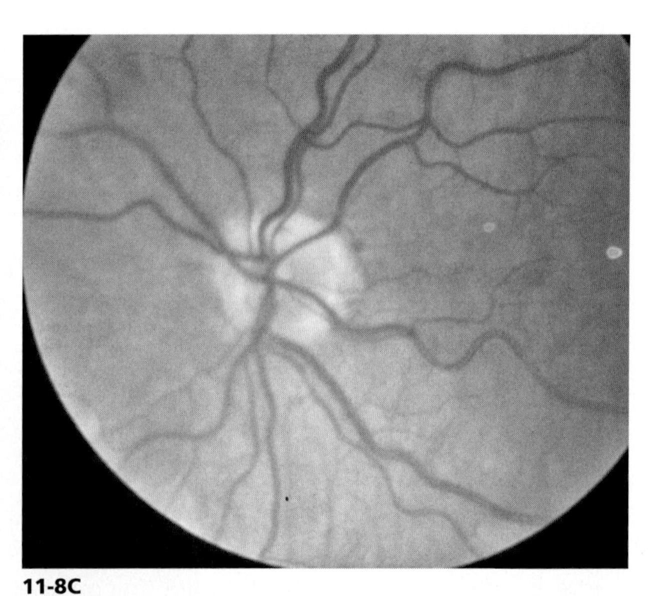

11-8C

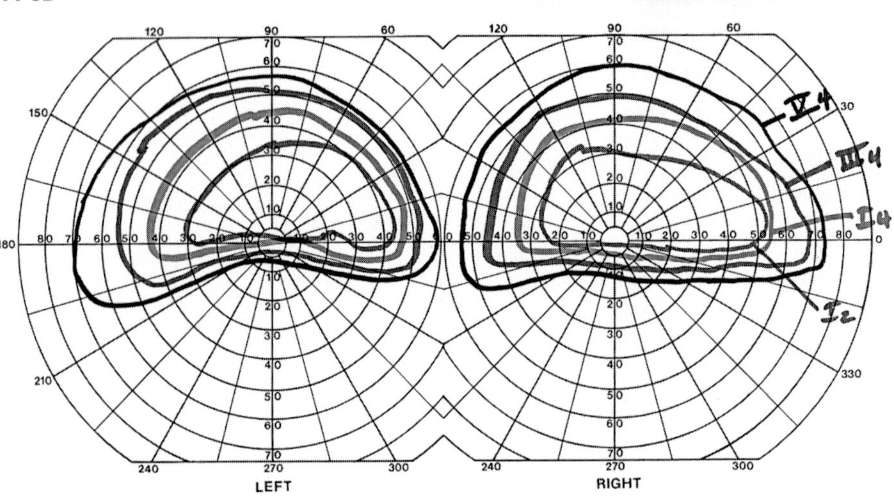

11-8D

Congenital cerebral hemispheric lesions can produce asymmetrical segmental hypoplasia from transsynaptic degeneration. Hoyt et al. termed this *homonymous hemioptic hypoplasia.*[19] Not only does the child have a homonymous hemianopia, but the disc has a distinct appearance of a normal disc ipsilateral to the degeneration and a "bow-tie" appearance contralaterally (see also hemioptic hypoplasia in Chapter 4, Figure 4-43). In children with a congenital insult, look for this defect.

Figure 11-9. A. **This diagram illustrates the formation of hemioptic hypoplasia. In the diagram, A represents the normal hemiretina. B represents the contralateral hypoplastic retina that has no ganglion cells but does have nerve fibers transversing the area. These would have been the crossed fibers. C represents the hypoplastic fundus of both eyes that has no ganglion cells and no nerve fiber layers. (Reprinted with permission from reference 19.)** ***Continued***

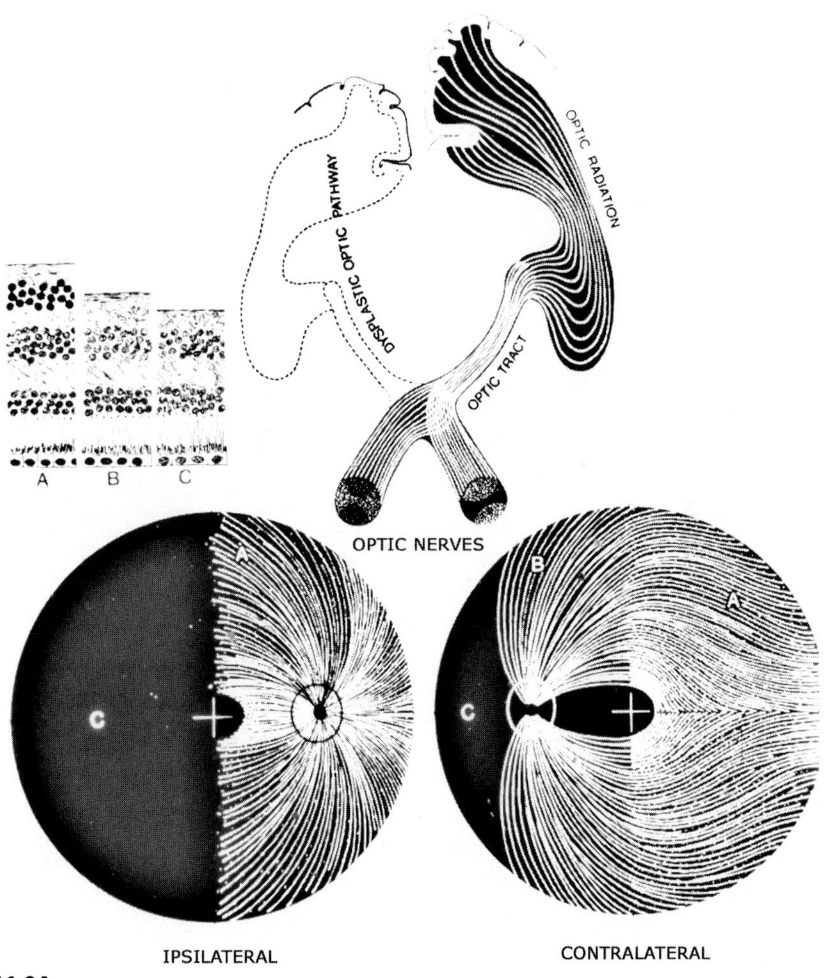

11-9A

Figure 11-9. ***Continued.*** **The right (B) and left discs (C) of a child with bilateral optic disc hypoplasia and abnormal formation of the occipital lobes. The sagittal (D) and axial (E) MR shows congenital malformation of the occipital lobes.**

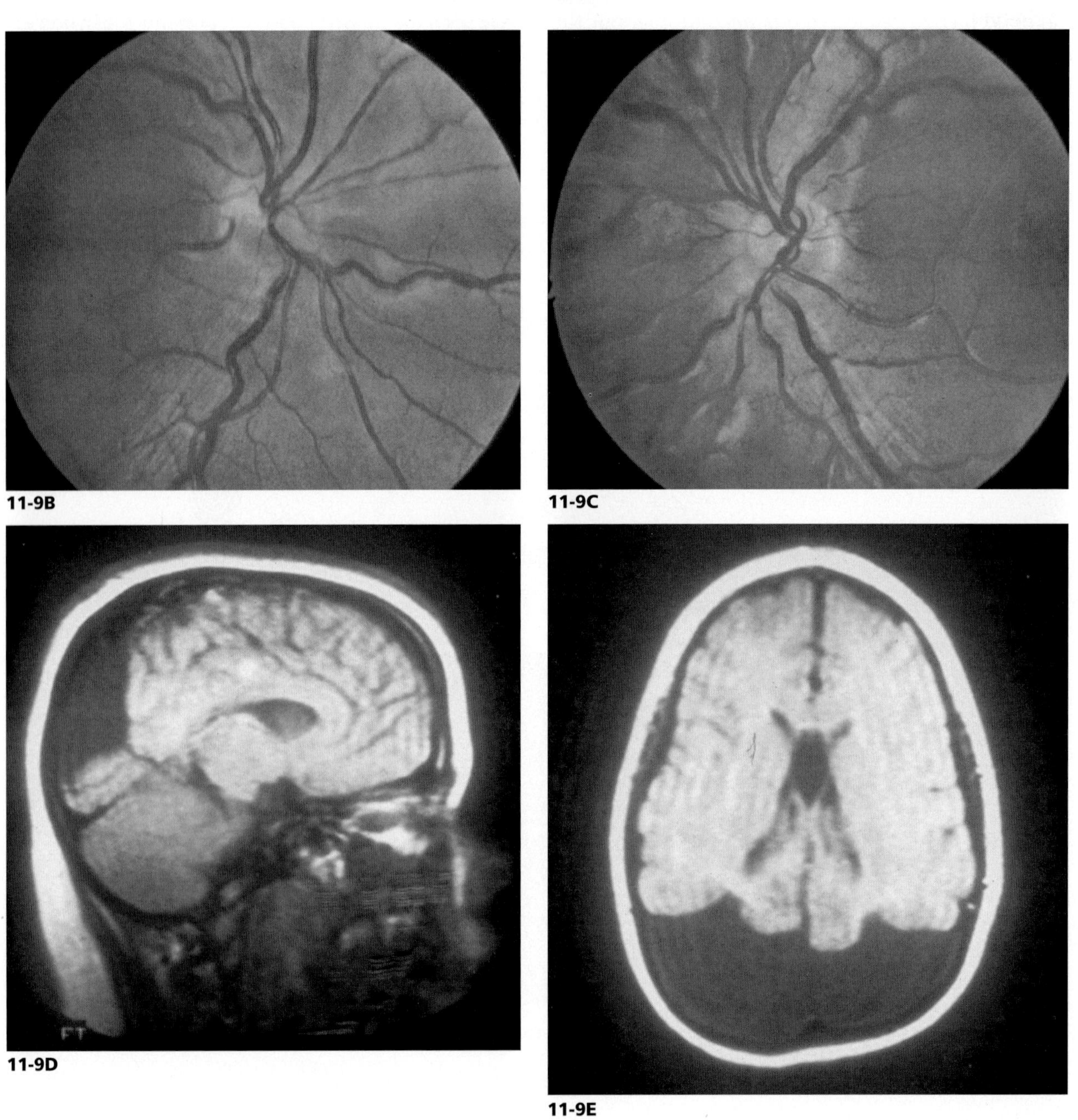

11-9B

11-9C

11-9D

11-9E

Another anomaly of the optic disc to be aware of is the optic disc associated with periventricular leukomalacia (PVL). PVL is periventricular white matter disease especially around the lateral horns of the ventricles caused by ischemia or hypoxia in the fetus between 29 and 34 weeks' gestation. One investigator found that children who were born preterm and had normal MR showed only abnormal patterns of vascularity on the disc. However, children born preterm and with periventricular (PVL) white matter changes displayed normal disc size with enlarged cups.[20] Approximately one-third of all premature infants can have PVL. PVL is associated with decreased visual acuity, visual field constriction (especially inferiorly), various visual-cognitive disorders (e.g., trouble reading), and spasticity. Optic nerve hypoplasia is a known accompaniment; however, normal-sized discs with abnormally large optic cups accompanied by a neuroretinal rim have also been reported. The disc looks like glaucomatous cupping. There is no associated endocrine deficit, unlike optic nerve hypoplasia. The mechanism is thought to be that the scleral canal develops normally; however, because of the periventricular damage around the lateral posterior horns of the ventricles, there is injury to the optic radiations that results in transsynaptic degenerations of the retinogeniculate axons and, hence, cupping of the optic disc. Although this type of disc can be confused with glaucoma, the disproportionate amount of inferior visual field loss to neuroretinal rim changes helps to solidify the diagnosis.[21] When seeing a child with enlarged cup-to-disc ratios with normal intraocular pressure, remember to ask about prematurity. Look for problems with reading comprehension and abnormal spastic gait. See Brodsky's article for an example of the discs, visual field, and MR findings.[22]

Is the Disc Too Large?

Again, use the small aperture of the ophthalmoscope to tell whether the disc is much larger than the aperture. What if it is too big?

MYOPIA

Even a normal disc may look large with a direct ophthalmoscope if the refractive error of myopia is not corrected, because myopia magnifies the disc. Myopia alone, however, may be associated with changes in the disc. We have seen in Chapter 2 (Figure 2-6) that there can be some changes in the disc with simple myopia, including temporal crescent, with or without a pigmented rim.

MEGALOPAPILLA

Megalopapilla is a term for a large disc (greater than 2.1 mm in diameter) that appears otherwise normal in its configuration.[23] The cup is usually enlarged but, as opposed to glaucomatous cups, there are no notches. Megalopapillae are usually bilateral. Most of the time there is no underlying neurologic disorder, except for occasional midfacial abnormalities or altered optic nerve function. Because the disc and cup are large and the nerve fibers are spread out over a larger area, the disc color can mimic optic disc pallor. Cilioretinal arteries are more prevalent in these discs. The only abnormality reported with megalopapilla is progressive enlargement of the disc associated with an orbital optic glioma.[24]

Figure 11-10. A,B. **This girl has a unilateral megalopapilla—notice the size difference between her normal right disc** (A) **and the large left one** (B). **The magnification is the same.** C. **Another child with normal vision and unilateral megalopapilla. The disc is enlarged, and so is the cup. Compare picture** C **with her normal left disc, shown here** (D).

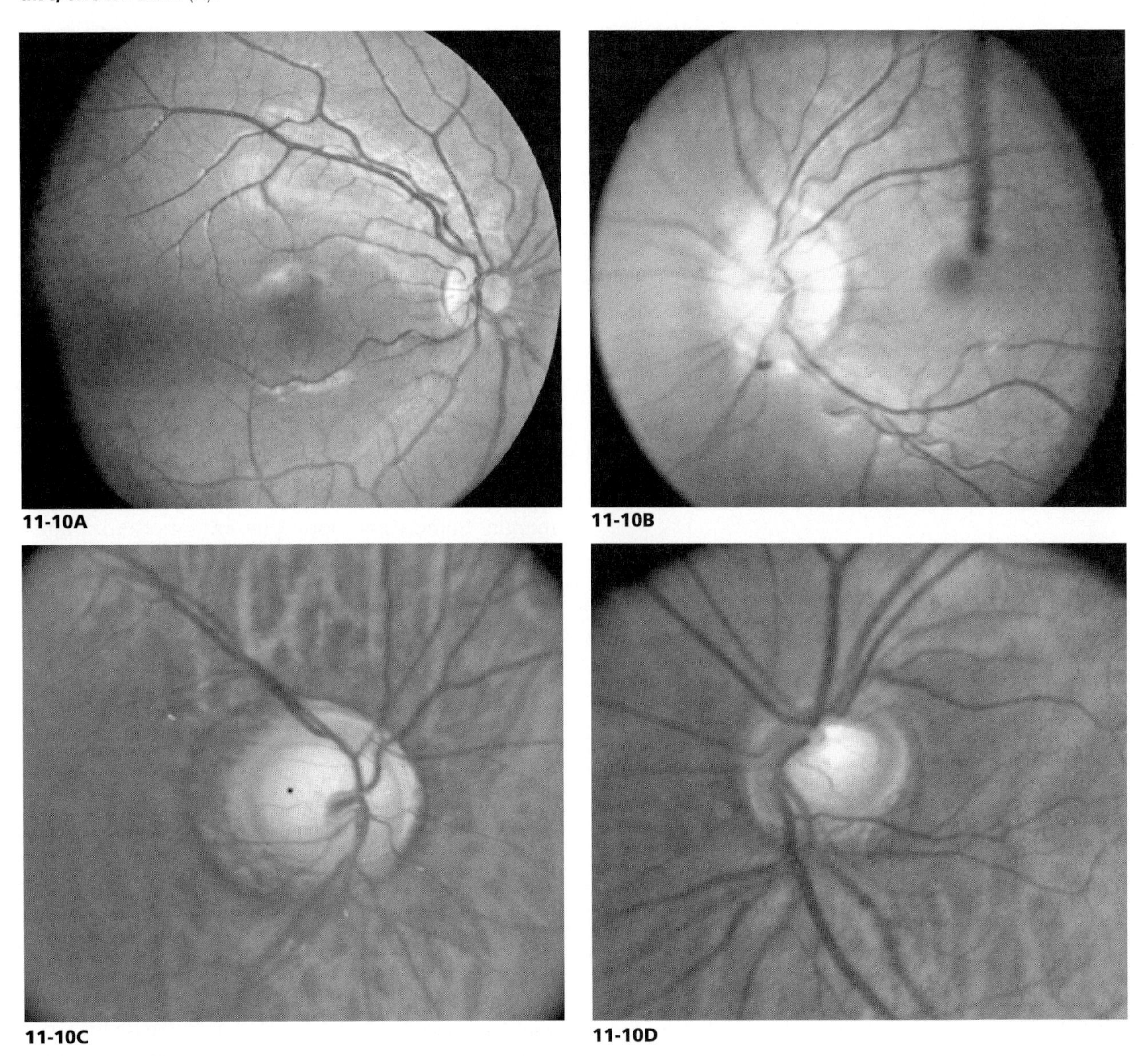

FUNDUS ECTASIA

Tilted discs with nasal fundus ectasia and other tilted disc variants are related to an oblique insertion of the optic nerve to the globe, thought to be owing to

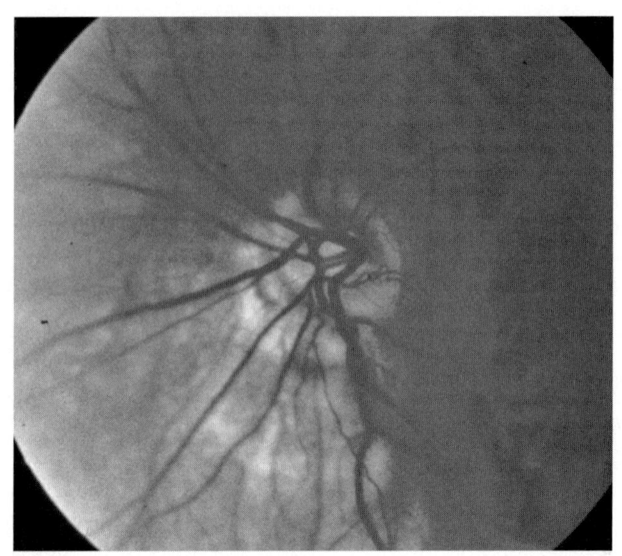

11-11

a defect in the closure of the embryonic fissure. See the discussion of these otherwise functionally normal ectatic variants in Chapter 2, Figures 2-13–2-16.

Figure 11-11. **An inferiorly tilted disc. Note the inferior scleral crescent; the vessels leave the disc nasally at first—situs inversus. There is also some inferior thinning of the retina.**

CONGENITAL PIT

A *congenital pit* is a developmental abnormality in the fetus that occurs when the epithelial papilla differentiates into neural and pigment epithelial cells. Pits were first described in 1882 by Wiethe (reviewed by Chang).[25] Pits are uncommon, occurring in approximately 1/11,000 people.[14] Most pits are unilateral, although bilateral pits are seen in approximately 15% of reported cases. An optic pit appears to be a small (one-eighth to one-half of disc diameter) hole that can be seen on the lateral disc margin. Some think optic pits are inherited.[26] Some have thought them to be closely allied with a coloboma.[27] Because it is associated with pigmented cells, the pit may often appear pigmented. The color of a pit is variously gray, white, yellow, or black. It is most frequent in the temporal disc region and is close to the disc margin at 8 o'clock in the right eye and 5 o'clock in the left eye, but it may be central.

Figure 11-12. (opposite page) A–F. **A pit is a round or oval depression in the temporal portion of the disc. The size is variable—from small to large. There is usually only one pit per nerve. The color is most often gray or olive, but yellow, white, or even black can occur. The margin of the disc is preserved, and the physiologic cup is still present.** A. **A grayish-appearing pit on the temporal aspect of the disc at approximately 8 o'clock (*arrow*).** B. **This grayish pit occurs temporally in the left eye (*arrow*).** C. **A large pit is present at approximately 9 o'clock. The arrows mark the nasal margin of the pit.** D. **An optic pit with a serous retinal detachment (*arrows*). The arrowheads mark the sides of the pit.** E. **In this darkly pigmented fundus, you can appreciate another serous retinal detachment (*arrows*).** F. **There is a large yellow pit in this disc. Notice the three cilioretinal arteries that come out of the margin of the disc (*arrows*). (Photographs in** D–F **courtesy of Madison Slusher, M.D.)**

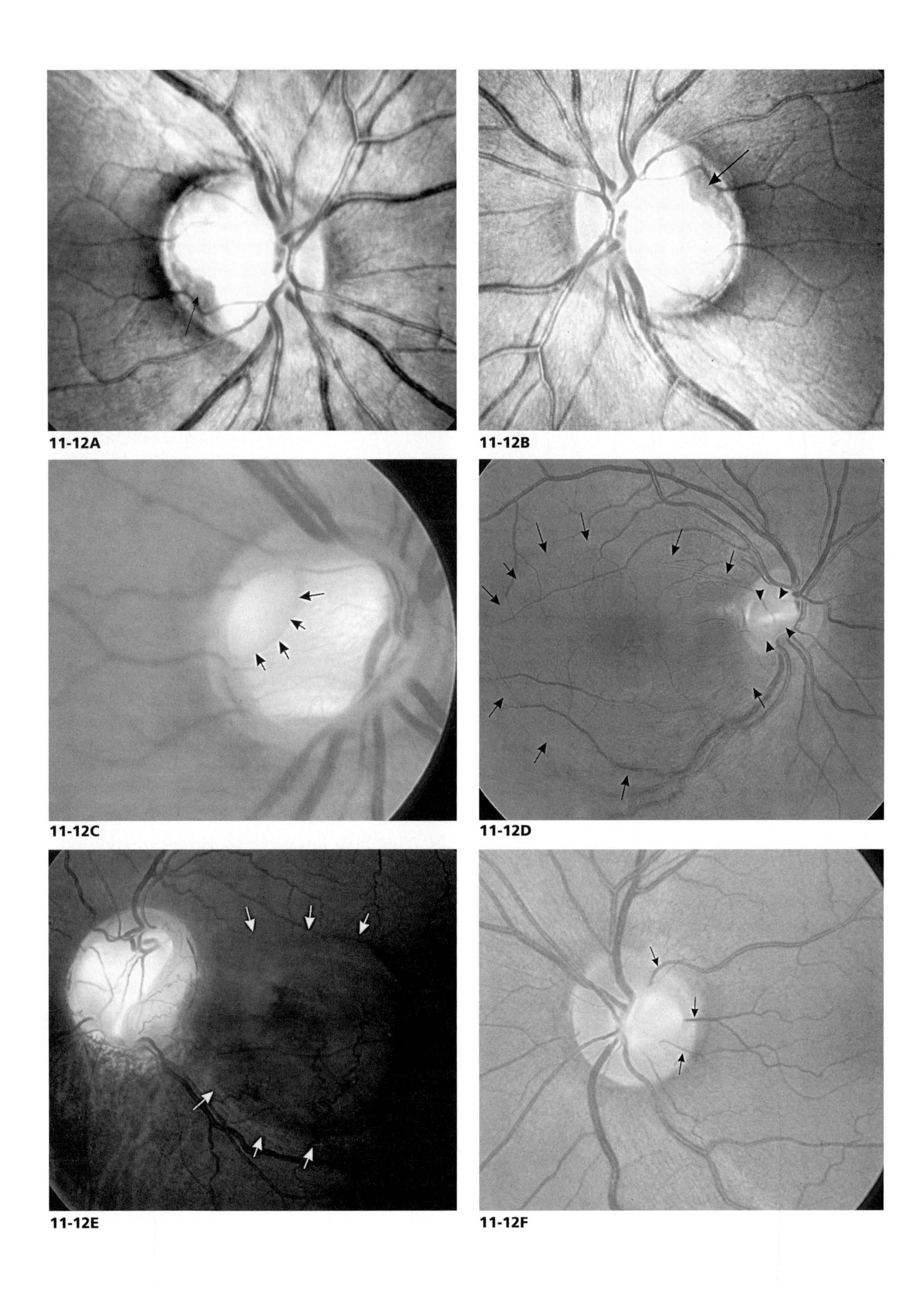
11-12A
11-12B
11-12C
11-12D
11-12E
11-12F

There are no visual or associated systemic symptoms unless a serous retinal detachment occurs, which is fairly common, seen in 25–75% of eyes with a pit.[3,28]

Figure 11-13. A,B. **The major complication of an optic pit is a serous retinal detachment. Look for a serous retinal detachment that looks like shiny plastic wrap stretched from the pit toward the macula (*arrows*). The arrowheads mark the sides of the pit.**

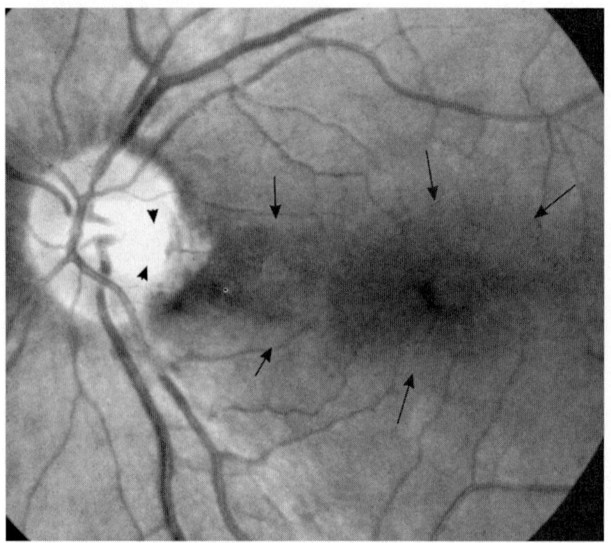

11-13A

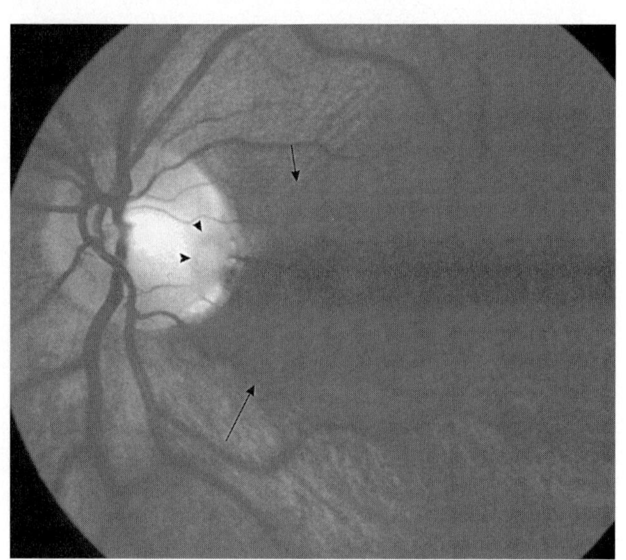

11-13B

Although the detachment may occur at any time, it is most frequent in adulthood—specifically, the 40s. This may be owing to vitreal traction on the disc due to posterior vitreous detachment. The vitreous tends to liquefy as we age, and it may pull away from the disc and retina. The symptom of a detachment is blurred vision. An ophthalmologist should be asked to see a patient with a known optic pit who has visual blurring; however, most serous detachments caused by optic pits do not require surgical intervention.

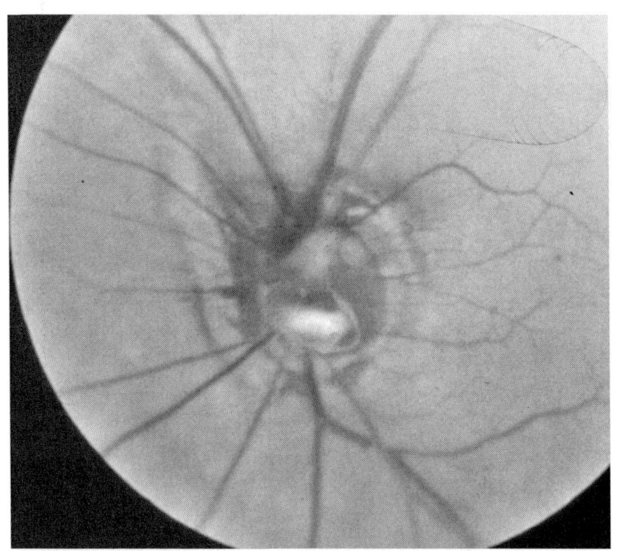

11-14A

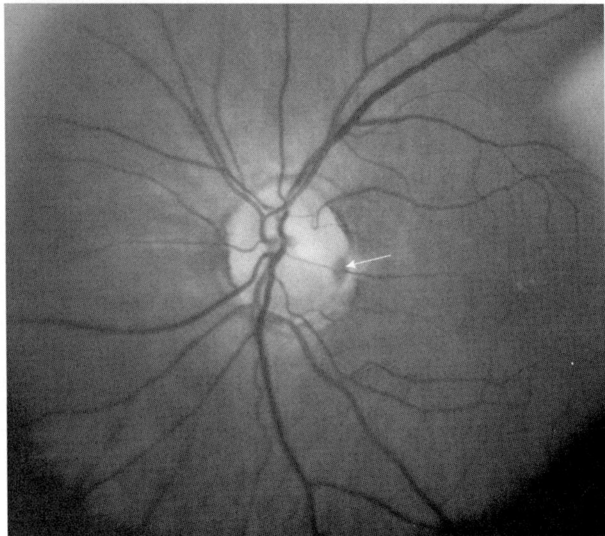

11-14B

Figure 11-14. A. **This pit is black, thus it is no wonder that the differential diagnosis is sometimes a melanocytoma (see Figure 8-8 A,B).** B. **The pit is black (*arrow*).**

The differential diagnosis of an optic pit includes tumors of the disc including a melanocytoma, astrocytic hamartoma, glaucoma, optic neuritis, central serous retinopathy, and optic disc colobomas.[29]

Fluorescein angiography may confirm a pit. There will be no leakage of dye, but hyperfluorescence of the pit occurs and fades late. In addition, if present, a serous detachment may be demonstrated.

COLOBOMA

Coloboma in Greek means a "gap," and can be used to describe any fissure, hole, or gap in the eye. The general term refers to any congenital gap in the disc, retina, choroid, and the iris or eyelid; the embryologic usage of the term is restricted to a congenital defect in one part of the eye (i.e., pupil, disc, retina, choroid).

Colobomas occur because the embryonic fissure fails to fuse. The optic fissure closure begins in what becomes the inferior retina and continues up to the iris and pupil region including the optic nerve; thus, colobomas are usually inferior to the disc. Colobomas can involve the optic nerve or retina-choroid complex. When they are of the optic nerve, colobomas can mimic optic atrophy. If the coloboma extends to the pupil, iris colobomas can also be present.

Figure 11-15. A,B. **These "cat's eye" pupils are elongated owing to pupillary colobomas—inferior gaps of the pupil. (Photographs courtesy of William T. Shults, M.D.)**

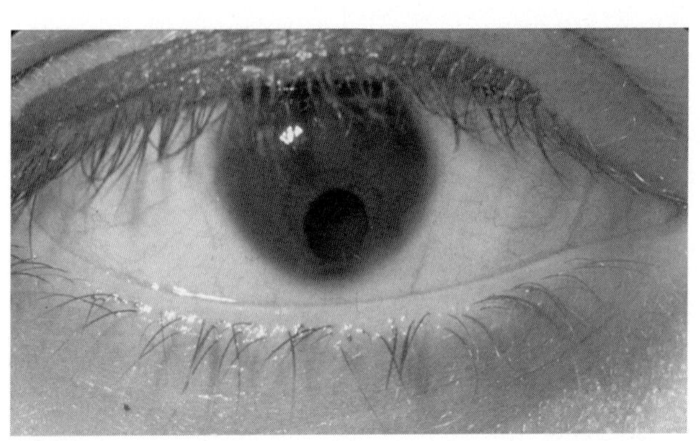

11-15A

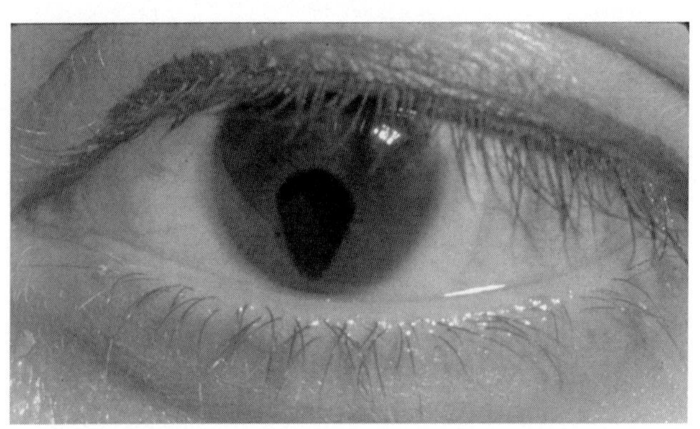

11-15B

Optic nerve colobomas are associated with enlargement of the peripapillary area and variably severe excavation of the inferior portion of the optic nerve; the color of the disc can be shades of white to gray, and blood vessels exit and enter from the edge of the defect. Because what you see within the gap is the sclera, the defect usually appears white. Colobomas are usually oval and make the disc appear enlarged. The retinal vessels also appear abnormal. Importantly, optic disc colobomas can be recognized by their inferior placement, with the neuroretinal rim being absent inferiorly and largely intact superiorly.

Optic nerve colobomas may be autosomal dominantly inherited.[30] Unilateral and bilateral colobomas occur with about equal frequency.[5]

The importance of recognizing a coloboma is threefold: First, vision may be affected and amblyopia can be present. Second, colobomas indicate the need to look for multisystem diseases or syndromes.[31] The acronym *CHARGE* has been suggested to summarize the systemic associations[31] seen in 85% of patients with *bilateral* colobomas:

*C*oloboma
*H*eart defects
*A*tresia choanae
*R*etarded growth and development
*G*enital hypoplasia
*E*ar anomalies

Figure 11-16. A. The superior aspect of the disc is usually spared from the defect. B. This inferior coloboma almost has the appearance of an inferior optic disc tilt. C. Around the disc, hyperpigmentation and hypopigmentation can be seen, but the peripapillary area is frequently normal. This disc appears large. D. The disc appears enlarged and has pigmentary changes around it. The vessels may exit the center of the nerve and branch on the disc, or they may enter and exit from the border of the disc, as in this case.

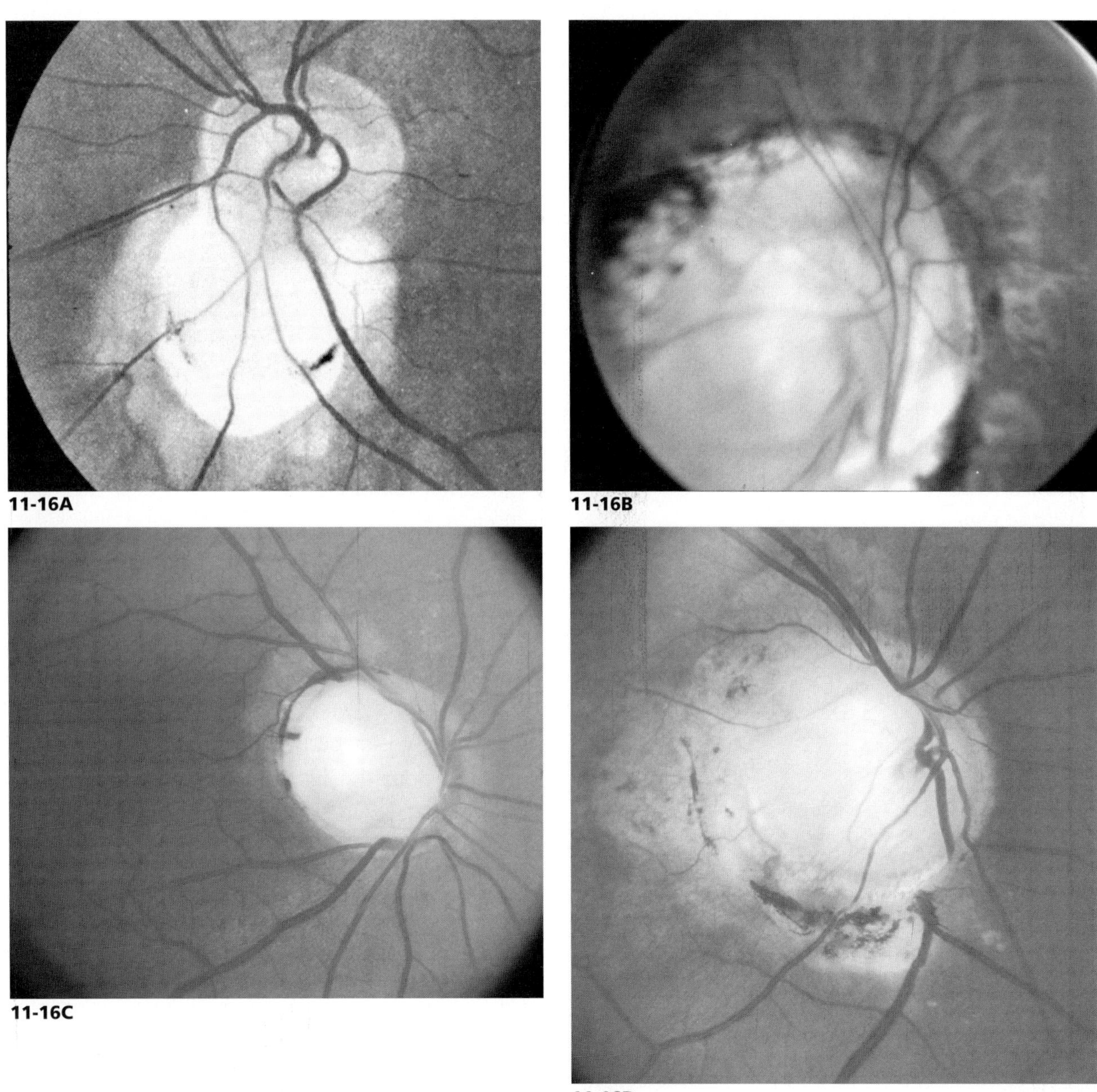

11-16A

11-16B

11-16C

11-16D

Table 11-10. Associations with Optic Disc and Retinal Colobomas

Genetic disorders
Lenz syndrome
Goltz syndrome
Basal cell nevus syndrome
CHARGE (*c*oloboma, *h*eart defects, *a*tresia choanae, *r*etarded growth and development, *g*enital hypoplasia, *e*ar anomalies)
Meckel syndrome
Walker-Warburg syndrome
Aicardi's syndrome
Rubinstein-Taybi syndrome
Linear sebaceous nevus syndrome
Goldenhar's syndrome
Chromosomal abnormalities
Trisomy 13
Triploidy
Cat's eye syndrome

Source: Adapted from references 5,30.

Thirdly, and very rarely, a transsphenoidal encephalocele—a bony defect in the roof of the sphenoid sinus through which brain and meninges variably prolapse—has rarely been reported.[27,32]

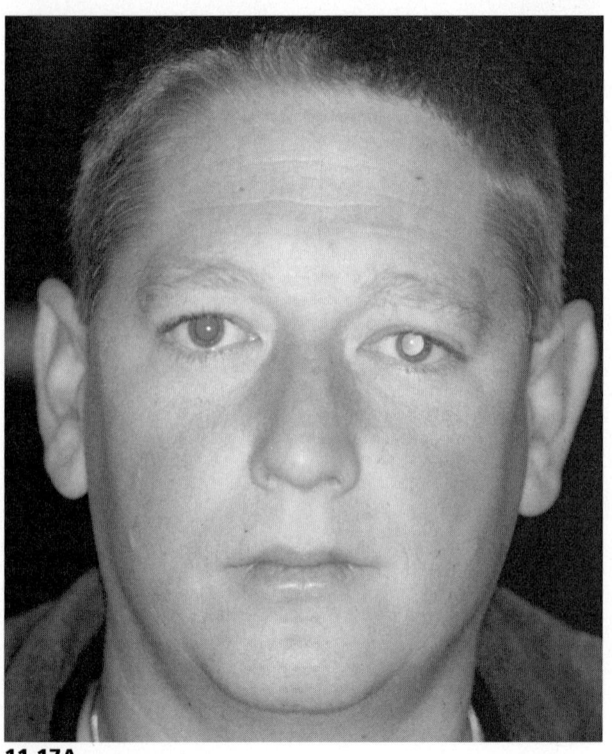

11-17A

Figure 11-17. (A, left; B–E, opposite page) A. **This man presented with fluctuating vision. The red reflex shows an ever-so-slight change, which might tip you off that the left disc is anomalous.** B. **The normal right eye and the colobomatous left optic nerve** (C) **are shown taken at the same magnification as the fellow normal eye. His colobomatous disc looks large.** D. **An MR sagittal view demonstrates the transsphenoidal encephalocele (*arrow*). The arrowhead points to the lamina terminalis. Notice also the pituitary stalk.** E. **Coronal T1-weighted MR showing the encephalocele and dipping of the chiasm toward the encephalocele (the *arrow* points to the chiasm).**

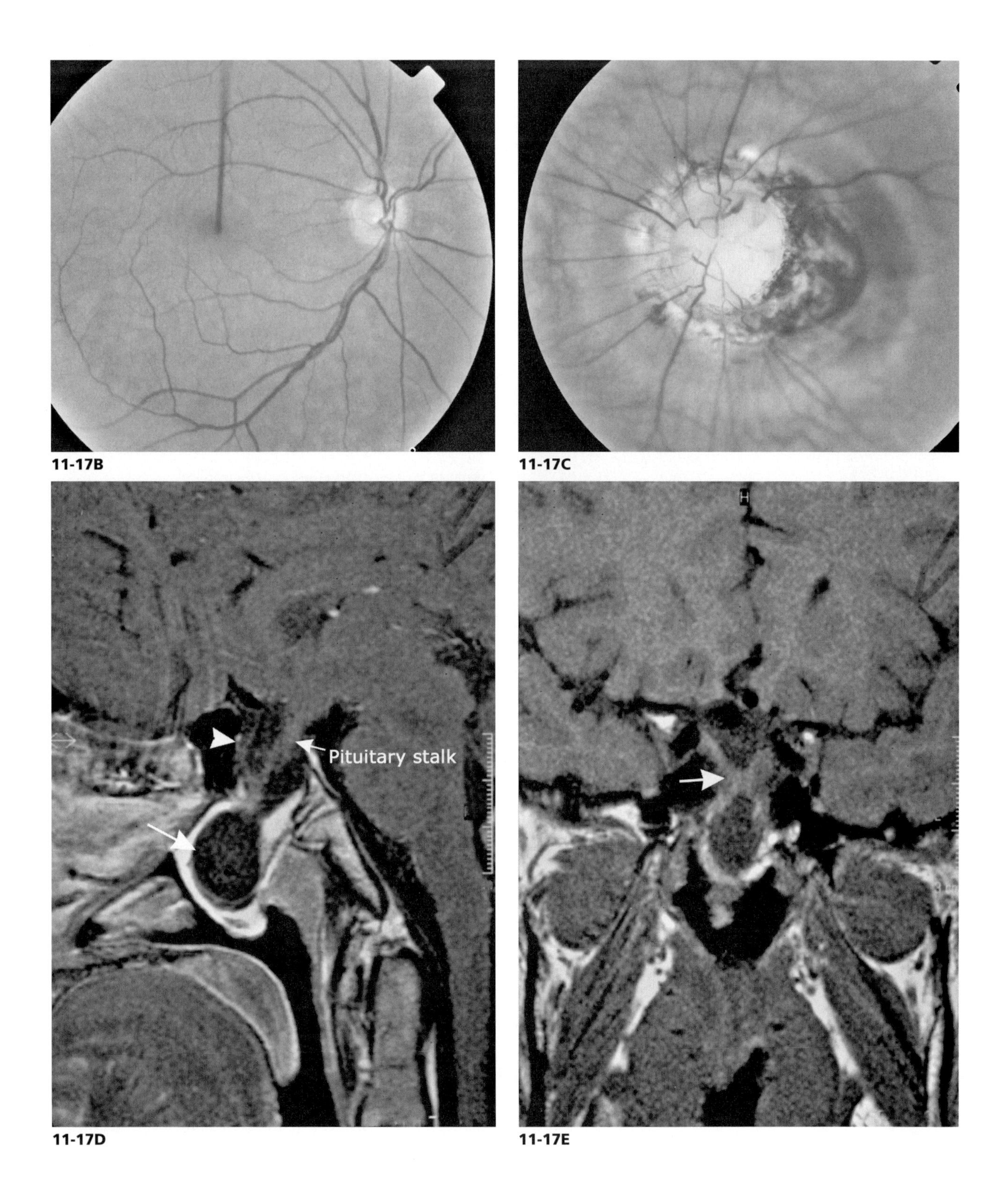

11-17B

11-17C

11-17D

11-17E

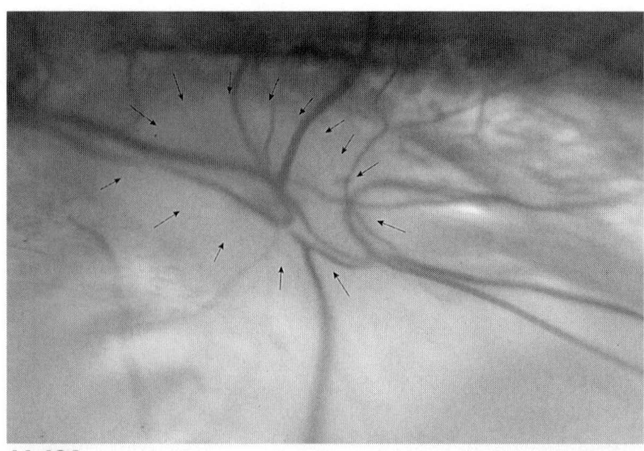

11-18A

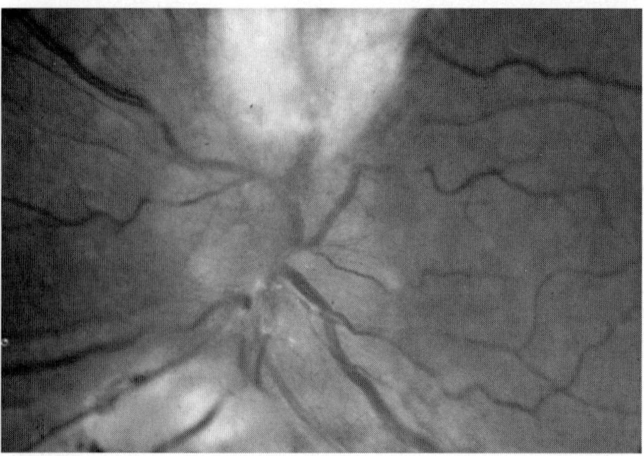

11-18B

Thus, when you identify a coloboma look at ears, fingers, and radiographically visualize the kidneys, brain, and genitourinary system. Do not worry so much about encephaloceles or other midline facial defects.

Retinal/choroidal colobomas can be autosomal dominantly inherited because the closure of the optic cleft is under gene control.[30,31] Retinochoroidal colobomas are associated with retinal detachments that may need repair. The disc may be normal and outside of the coloboma, but more frequently the disc and the fundus are both colobomatous.[33] Furthermore, retinal/choroidal colobomas are more likely to have associated iris colobomas (versus pure optic disc coloboma).[33]

Figure 11-18. A. **The disc here is almost normal (outlined by *arrows*), but inferiorly there is a dramatic gap of the retina and choroid typical of a retinal coloboma. If you were to view this with a direct ophthalmoscope, you might be confused as to what is disc and what is retina.** B. **To complicate matters, the woman, who is also pictured in Figure 11-15 with the colobomatous irides, developed a brain tumor that presented with transient visual obscuration. The left disc showed papilledema. In addition, she had myelinated nerve fibers seen superiorly. Remember that individuals with anomalous discs are not immune to other conditions. If the history suggests other conditions, further evaluation is indicated. (Photographs courtesy of William T. Shults, M.D.)**

The major ocular complication of disc colobomas is serous macular detachment, and retinochoroidal colobomas can be associated with rhegmatogenous detachments (detachment of the retina caused by a tear or rent), which can be hard to repair and often recur.

MORNING GLORY DISC

Morning glory disc is a unique developmental anomaly. Although some have called it a true optic disc coloboma,[6] others[3,5] maintain that there are important distinguishing characteristics that should separate the two. Still others place the morning glory disc in a spectrum of disc anomalies from elevated posterior persistent hyperplastic primary vitreous to staphyloma.[34] Although Handmann described the disc in 1928, Kindler named this disc in 1970.[35]

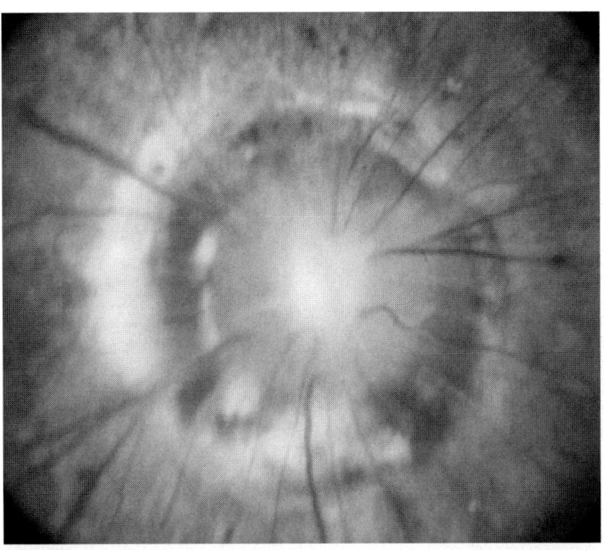

11-19A

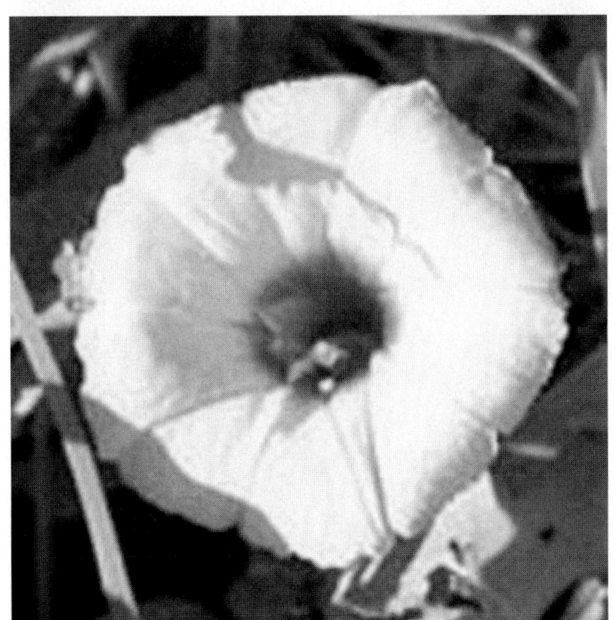

11-19B

Figure 11-19. A. **The morning glory disc looks funnel-shaped, with a white center surrounded by chorioretinal pigmentary changes.** B. **The name comes from the appearance of the blood vessels exiting the disc in a radial fashion—much like the morning glory flower (*Convolvulus arvensis*).**

In this anomaly, the vessels are markedly abnormal. Frequently, there are more vessels on the nerve than is normal, but the central retinal artery branches early, which is to say "deep in the disc tissue," and overlying gliotic tissue obscures the origin of the vessels. Thus, the vessels also appear to arise from the periphery of the optic disc, whereas the disc actually lies within the excavation. The lamina cribrosa appears to be "prolapsed" posteriorly through a large scleral canal.

The morning glory disc is most often unilateral and more often seen in women (ratio, 2:1). It is a rarer defect than a coloboma.[3]

Figure 11-20. A–F. **The ophthalmoscopic appearance of a morning glory disc is as follows:** A. **White central tissue.** B. **Large, excavated optic nerve.** C. **The vessels exit in a radial fashion, with branching of the arteries having taken place posterior to the visualized disc. There is no central retinal vasculature. Veins and arteries are hard to differentiate.** D. **There is frequently a chorioretinal ring around the disc; there may be white glial tissue on top of the disc.** ***Continued***

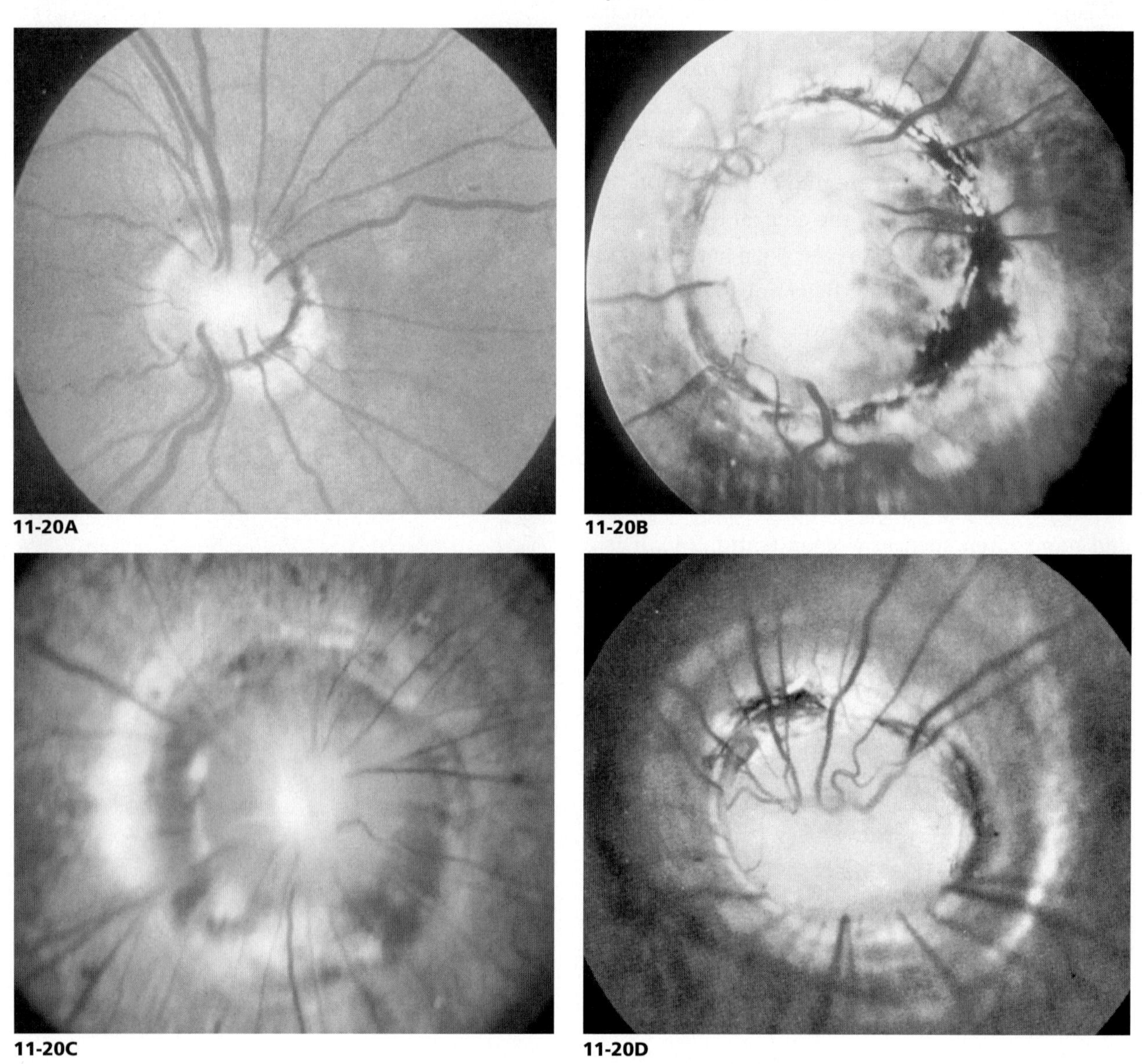

11-20A **11-20B** **11-20C** **11-20D**

Figure 11-20. ***Continued.*** E. **There is often a halo of light and variably pigmented tissue around the disc. The vessels can be sheathed.** F. **The color may be orange to pink; white glial tissue may be on the top. (See the corresponding color figure on the accompanying CD-Rom.) (Photographs in** E,F **courtesy of William T. Shults, M.D.)**

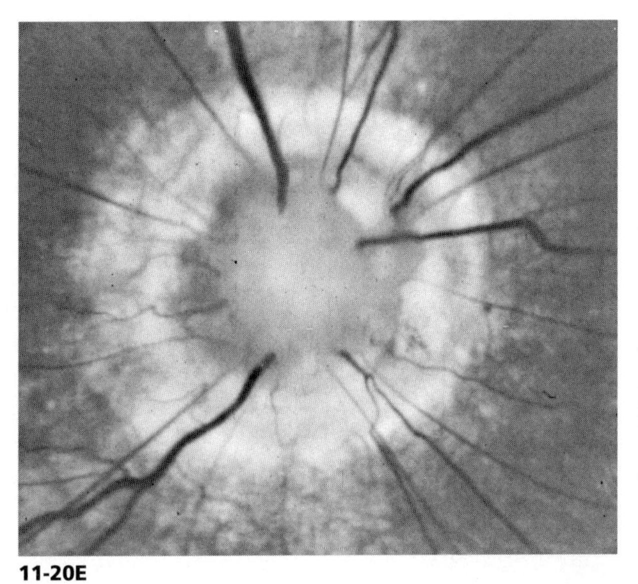

11-20E

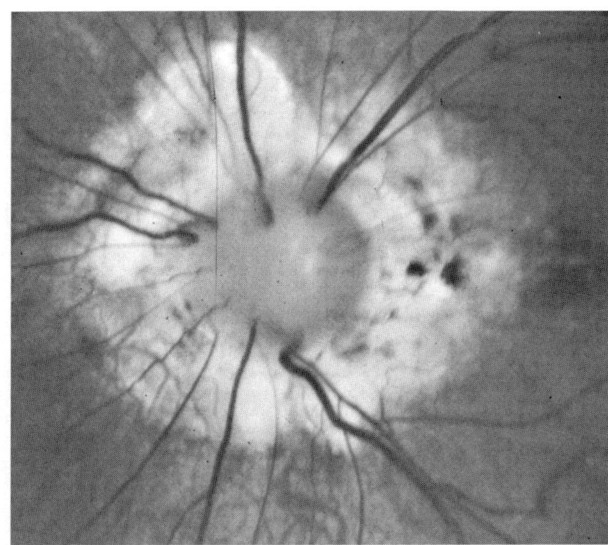

11-20F

Interestingly, contractile movements occasionally have been reported in the morning glory optic disc. These movements may be owing to fluctuation of fluid[36] or secondary to a periodic contraction of a ring of smooth muscle around the disc.

The importance of recognizing a morning glory disc is that although a child may have normal visual acuity or correctable amblyopia, a transsphenoidal basal encephalocele is commonly associated with this anomaly, and furthermore, hypopituitarism is common when an encephalocele is present. Look at the facial features if you see someone with a morning glory disc—is there widening of the nasal bridge? Recently, cases of pituitary dwarfism owing to pituitary hormone deficiencies have been reported, especially growth hormone deficiency.[37]

Another reason to recognize a morning glory disc is that some of these anomalies are associated with ipsilateral hypoplasia or agenesis of the carotid and cerebral arteries, suggesting that a regional vascular dysgenesis (e.g., moya moya syndrome) may underlie the anomaly.[38] MR and MR angiography have been used successfully in looking for intracranial vascular anomalies.

Figure 11-21.

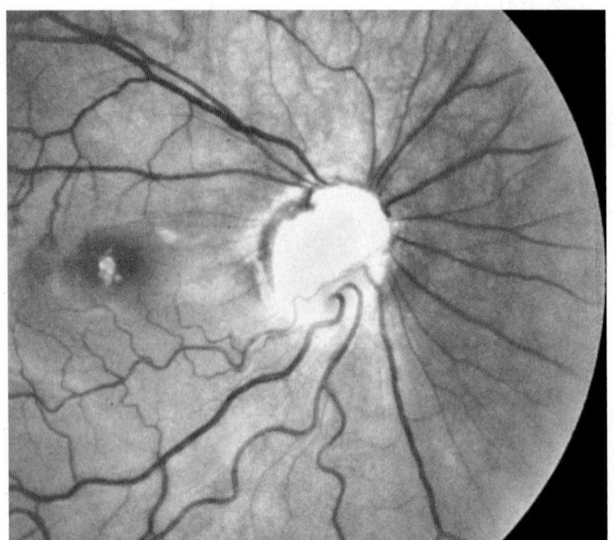

11-21A

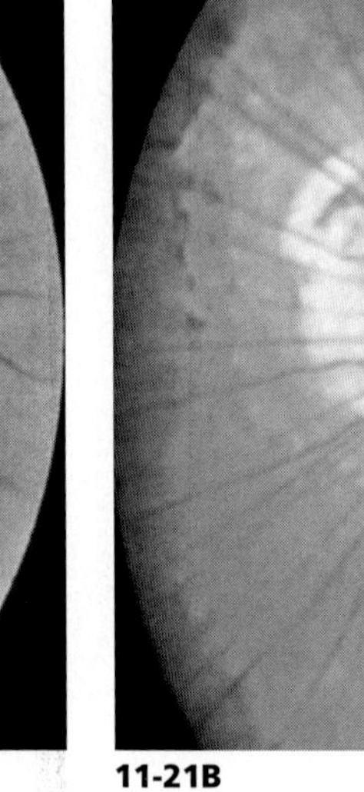

11-21B

Table 11-11. Differentiating Excavation Defects

Colobomas (Figure 11-21A)	Morning glory anomaly (Figure 11-21B)
Excavation lies within the disc	Disc lies within the scleral excavation
Disc defect is very asymmetrical, usually inferior	Disc defect is symmetrical
Minimal peripapillary pigment disturbance	Prominent pigment disturbance inferiorly
Color variable, more white	Color may be orange–pink
Retinal vasculature normal	Retinal vasculature anomalous, exiting in a radial fashion
No sex predilection	Women > men, 2:1
Familial	Not usually familial
Bilateral	Unilateral
Associated with multisystem genetic disorders (CHARGE)	Rare associations with genetic disorders; may see moya moya syndrome
Basal encephalocele rare	Basal encephalocele common

CHARGE = coloboma, *h*eart defects, *a*tresia choanae, *r*etarded growth and development, *g*enital hypoplasia, *e*ar anomalies.
Source: Adapted in part from references 3,5,38.

PAPILLORENAL SYNDROME

Papillorenal syndrome is another rare developmental disorder in which the disc looks excavated like a coloboma or morning glory disc but is actually devoid of central retinal arterial vessels—there are only cilioretinal vessels providing blood for the inner retina. Fluorescein angiography shows only filling of the cilioretinal vessels at the same time as the choroid (confirming that they are indeed cilioretinal vessels). The typical visual field defect is superior nasal field loss. The disc defect is a genetic trait because it has been found in families. The importance of knowing about this syndrome is that these discs are associated with renal hypoplasia.[39]

PERIPAPILLARY STAPHYLOMA

Peripapillary staphyloma is a rare peripapillary excavation in which a normal disc appears telescoped backward into a round peripapillary excavation. This anomaly occurs when there is a defect in the sclera at embryogenesis and the disc prolapses through the defect.[3,5] What you see is an almost normal–looking disc (there may be some pallor) at the bottom of a scleral excavation. The excavation has a rim of choroid/retinal pigment surrounding the staphyloma. The retinal vasculature is normal; there is no glial tuft. The staphyloma can contract.[40] The patient is usually myopic. There is usually no systemic or central nervous system abnormality; however, an occasional encephalocele has been reported.[41] Seybold and Rosen reported transient visual obscuration associated with a peripapillary staphyloma.[42]

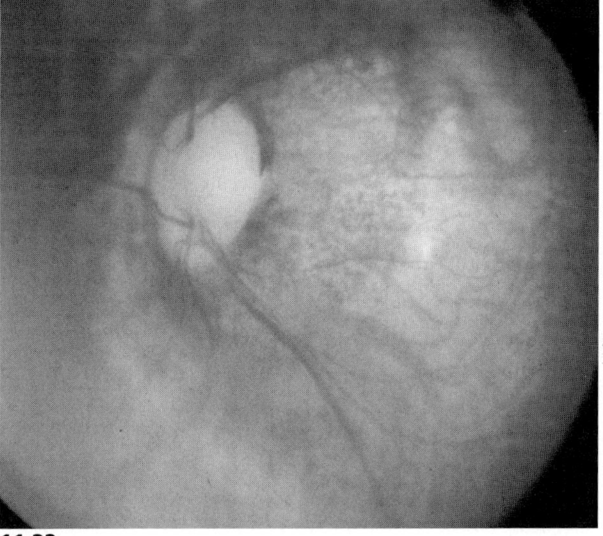

11-22

Figure 11-22. This is a myopic disc with staphyloma. The patient had a linear nevus syndrome. (Photograph courtesy of Michael Brodsky, M.D.)

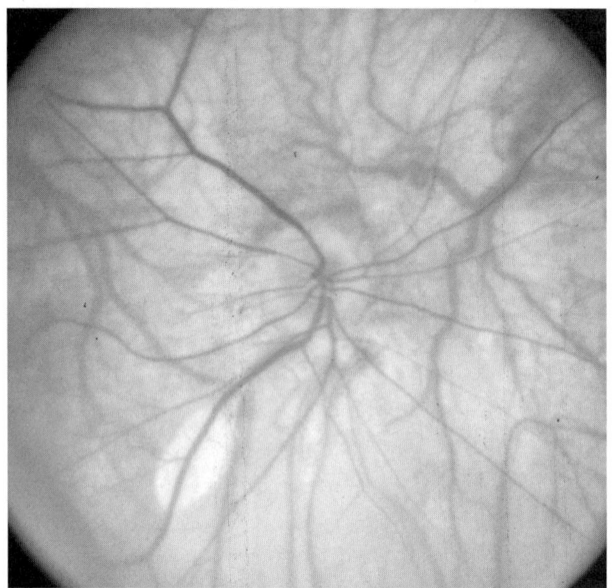

11-23A

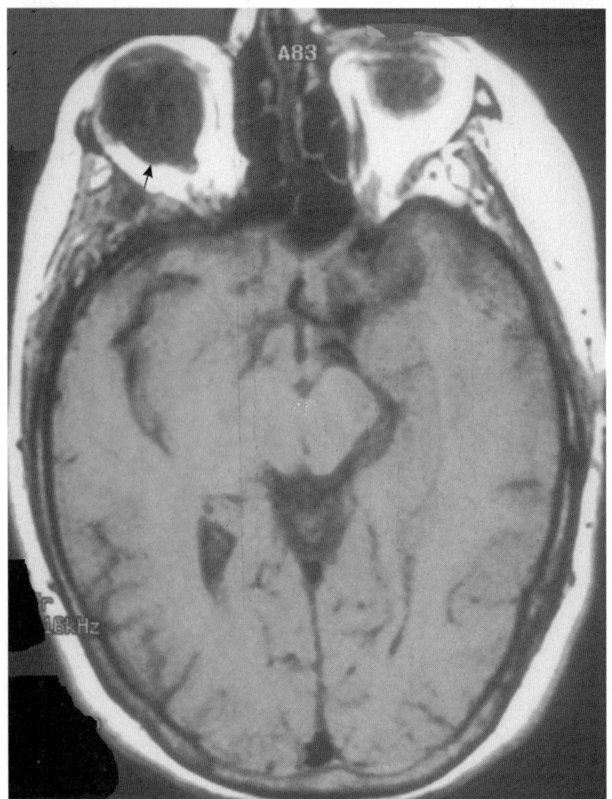

11-23B

Figure 11-23. A. **This woman has high myopia with a staphyloma just inferior to the disc.** B. **Notice the outpouching on the MRI (*arrow*).**

MYOPIA

Myopia is a common cause of vision loss that can be corrected with spectacles. Simple myopia (usually slight in degree, less than 5 diopters) is a static process and no further change in the eye occurs. Pathologic myopia can occur when the refraction is –5.0 to –7.5 diopters and the globe is congenitally long. If myopia becomes progressive (malignant myopia) there are also profound changes in the disc and peripapillary retina. Women are more prone to development of malignant myopia and the subsequent degenerative changes.

Malignant myopia causes vision loss that is not correctable with glasses and is associated with progressive elongation of the globe. This progressive elongation may cause degenerative changes within the fundus. Not only is there a myopic crescent around the disc, but there can also be advancing retinal degeneration around the disc, macular degeneration, and, finally, degeneration of the peripheral retina. Macular degeneration can occur after a macular hemorrhage or macular edema, which accumulates as the globe elongates. The degenerative changes in the retina can be progressive as well; these can be associated with the vitreous detaching from the retina (i.e., vitreal detachment). Symptoms of vitreous detachment include an increase in the number of floaters and occasionally flashing lights. If the retina is adherent to the vitreous, a small hole may form and cause a retinal detachment. High myopes are prone to retinal detachments, and myopic patients with sudden flashes and floaters should be examined by an ophthalmologist for a retinal detachment. Finally, choroidal atrophy can also occur in myopic degeneration. Choroidal atrophy looks like punched-out white spots with variable pigment around them. These white spots can occur around the disc or in the retina.

Table 11-12. Findings in Pathologic Myopia

Myopic appearance to the disc—large cup, temporal crescent
Staphyloma in one-third
Vitreous detachment in one-third
Cobblestone degeneration 14%
Retinal detachment 10%
Retinal pits, holes, or tears 8%
Lattice degeneration 5%

Source: Adapted from reference 43.

The appearance of myopia forms a spectrum—from a simple temporal crescent to degeneration of the choroid and retina around the disc. A crescent usually exhibits a white, sharply defined border, because sclera is showing through; this is because the choroid and retina do not reach the disc. Eighty percent of crescents are temporal in myopia. When a patient has greater than 6 diopters of myopia, crescents are almost always seen.

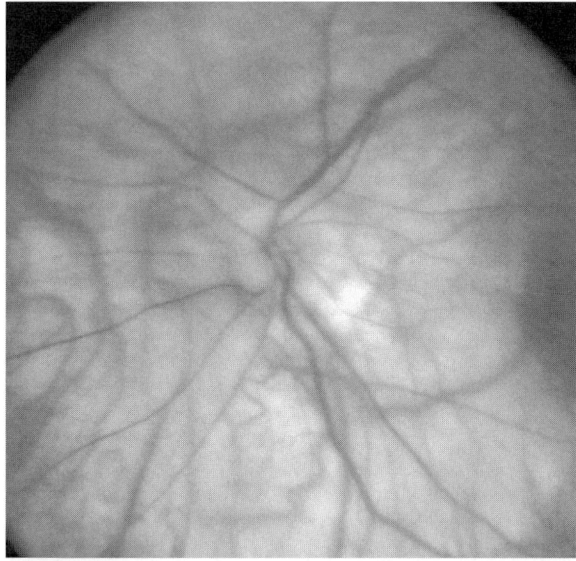

11-24A

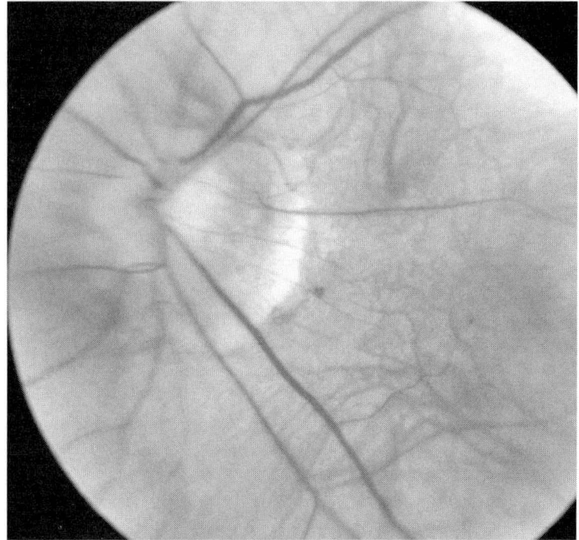

11-24B

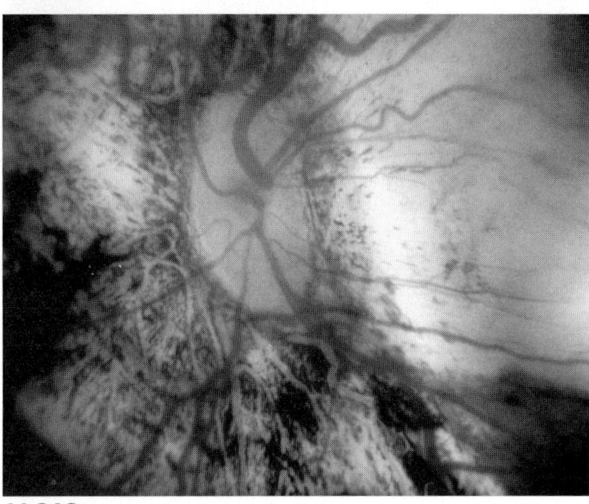

11-24C

Figure 11-24. A. **Myopic-appearing discs frequently have a temporal crescent. You may have trouble focusing on the disc because of the power required to view the disc. This example is in a very blonde fundus.** B. **Here you can appreciate the temporal crescent and the slightly tilted disc.** C. **Patients with high myopia like this are at risk for retinal detachments. Myopic patients with sudden flashes and floaters should be referred emergently for examination by an ophthalmologist to look for retinal detachments.**

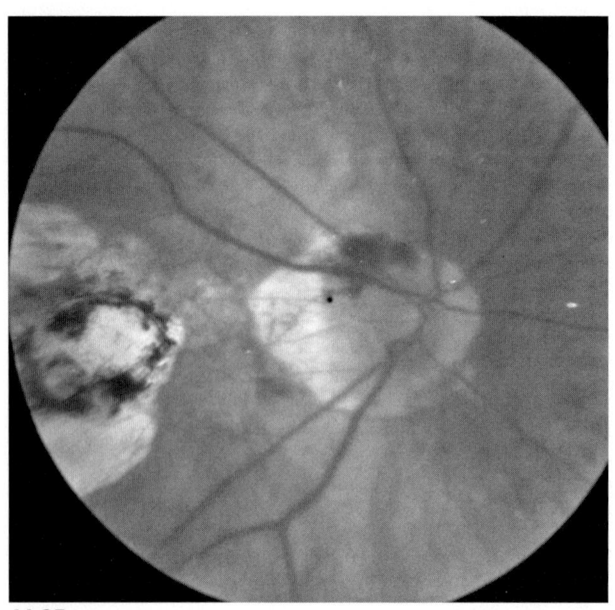

11-25

Figure 11-25. The disc not only has a temporal crescent with pigmentary changes around the disc, but there is pigmentary change in the macula as well. These are characteristics of "malignant" myopia.

PERSISTENT HYPERPLASTIC PRIMARY VITREOUS OR PERSISTENT FETAL VASCULATURE

A remnant of the Bergmeister papilla can also cause the disc to appear anomalous (see the discussion in Chapter 2, Figures 2-18 and 2-19). These discs are related to disturbance in the regression of the Bergmeister papillae. The appearance may even resemble morning glory disc. Sometimes these remnants have fibrous proliferation from the disc to the lens that can cause traction on the retina and even retinal detachment; this proliferation has been named *persistent hyperplastic primary vitreous*. Recently, Dr. Goldberg suggested categorizing it with a broader term, *persistent fetal vasculature*,[44] because the term is more accurate and clinically useful. Persistent hyperplastic primary vitreous be detected at birth with a change in the red reflex, and there may also be pronounced changes in the lens and the ciliary processes.[14] Furthermore, visual acuity may be affected.[45] In addition, the eye may also be smaller than normal. Persistent hyperplastic primary vitreous is the most frequent cause of a white pupil[29] and the most frequent process mistaken for retinoblastoma.

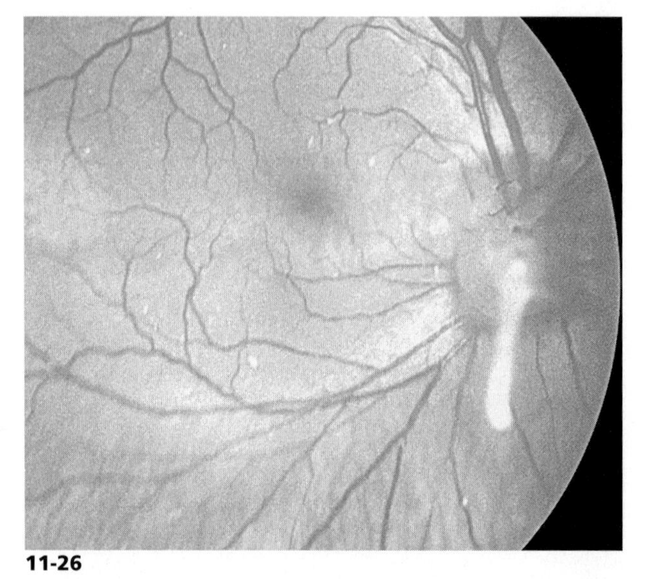

11-26

Figure 11-26. This woman has a persistent hyperplastic primary vitreous. The disc appears small, and hypertrophic tissue is pulled into the vitreous. Her vision is light perception in this eye. (Photograph courtesy of Paula Morris, CRA.)

Other Disc Anomalies

IS THE COLOR OF THE DISC ABNORMAL?

See Chapter 8, on pigmentary changes of the disc and retina.

Gray optic discs can be a normal finding in infants who have a delay in visual maturation. The gray tint disappears as the baby grows; this type of pigmentation is not thought to be melanin, but rather an "optical effect."[46] This type of gray disc has also been seen in children with disorders of proteolipid protein metabolism (formerly, Pelizaeus Merzbacher) and true albinism. Truly gray discs are caused by melanin deposition into the lamina cribrosa. These discs may be associated with congenital defects such as optic nerve hypoplasia and a deletion on chromosome 17.[46] Simultaneous optic disc anomalies (e.g., hypoplasia, pseudopapilledema) are often detected when congenital optic disc pigmentation associated with visual impairment is seen.

See Figure 8-7 for a view of a gray disc in infants.

IS THE OPTIC DISC DOUBLED?

When the optic disc is doubled, check to be sure that your direct ophthalmoscopic lens is correctly adjusted, that you are not between two lenses on your ophthalmoscope, and that you are not viewing through the edge of your bifocals, all of which may produce a double disc.

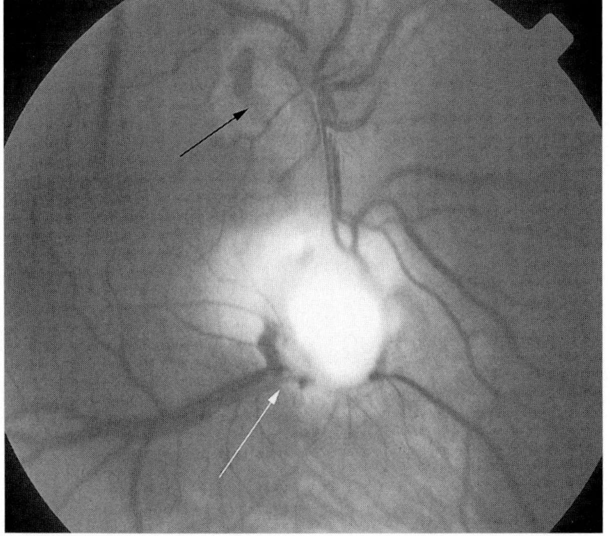

11-27

Figure 11-27. This disc appears to be doubled, but if you look closely, it is simply a colobomatous defect that resembles another optic disc in size, color, and configuration. The colobomatous defect also appears to have its own blood supply. The real disc above (*black arrow*) is not as prominent as the colobomatous defect below (*white arrow*).

True doubling of the optic disc is a rare developmental anomaly that has been documented in lower animals, but never in humans. Most purported cases are actually colobomatous defects associated with decreased vision.[14]

DOES THE DISC LOOK TOO BIG AND TOO WHITE?

If the disc looks big and white, consider the following—could there be myelinated nerve fibers? Myelination of the optic nerve is not really an anomaly, but, rather, a continuation of a normal process. See the examples of myelinated nerve fibers in Chapter 2, Figure 2-17.

Evaluation of Acquired Optic Nerve Disorders in Children

SWOLLEN DISC

Review the chapter on the swollen disc (Chapter 3), because many of the principles pertain to children, as well as adults. There are also several caveats that are special to children.

First, is it true swelling? Anomalous discs can fool you. Check the parents, because many of them also have elevated discs; this is particularly true when a child has no complaints of headache or vision loss. If you are in doubt, refer the child for ophthalmologic evaluation. Papilledema is too important to miss. If the discs are judged anomalous, they should be photographed and the photos made part of the permanent medical records.

If the discs are swollen bilaterally and vision is normal or nearly so, it could be papilledema. Review the disc appearance of papilledema in Chapter 3. The etiologies in children are similar to those in adults, but consider the causes of papilledema in children shown in Table 11-13.

Table 11-13. Causes of Papilledema in Children

Causes
Increased intracranial pressure owing to neurologic disease
Brain tumor (posterior fossa); gliomatosis cerebri
Hydrocephalus
Vascular malformations: arteriovenous, dural venous fistulas
Venous thrombosis (dural or deep)
Meningitis
Spinal cord tumors with high protein in cerebrospinal fluid
Premature closure of the sutures
Increased intracranial pressure owing to trauma
Shaken baby syndrome
Subdural hematoma
Increased intracranial pressure owing to systemic disease
Malnutrition (feeding after)
Autoimmune disease (systemic lupus; angiitis)
Endocrinologic disease: Addison's disease, hypothyroidism (especially after treatment)
Hematologic disease (anemia)
Renal disease (hypertension)
Increased intracranial pressure owing to medications
Tetracycline/minocycline
Vitamin A (exogenous or skin preparations)
Quinolones, including nalidixic acid, ciprofloxacin
Thyroid replacement in hypothyroidism
Primary idiopathic intracranial pressure

Source: Adapted in part from reference 3 and S Lessell. Pediatric pseudotumor cerebri (idiopathic intracranial hypertension). Surv Ophthalmol 1992;37:155–166.

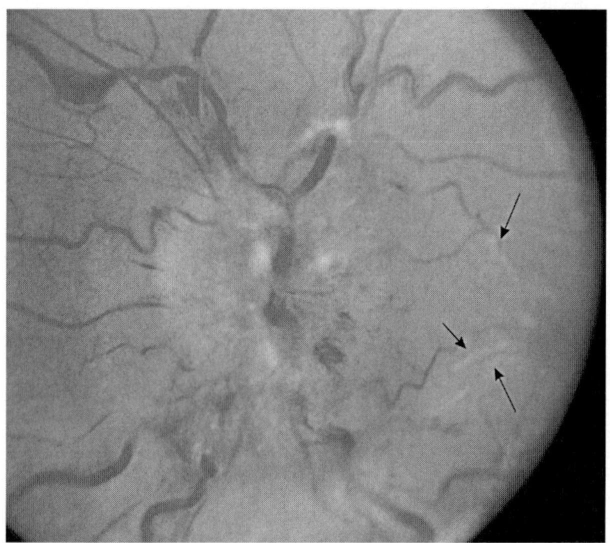

11-28A

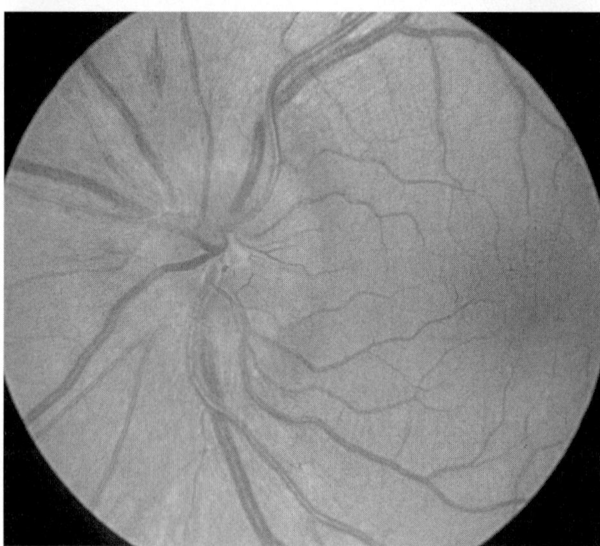

11-28B

Figure 11-28. A. **This 14-year-old girl had severe papilledema owing to use of tetracycline. The tetracycline was stopped, and the papilledema improved. Notice a hint of a "macular star" temporal to the disc (*arrows*). Although there are millions of teens placed on tetracycline for acne, few develop increased intracranial pressure.** B. **This 15-year-old boy presented with new-onset headache and papilledema. Spinal fluid showed a pleocytosis owing to a meningeal process.**

The evaluation of papilledema in children should proceed as with the adult, including imaging of the brain and venous sinuses, usually with MR. Look carefully for a mass in the posterior fossa. A spinal fluid examination to check the intracranial pressure and fluid constituents should be performed only after an MR or computed tomography, unless there is strong suspicion of meningitis. The visual function of children can be affected insidiously by papilledema and children can lose vision; therefore, attention to confrontation, formal visual fields (Goldmann and kinetic perimetry or Humphrey static perimetry, if the child can perform), and color vision is important.

Swollen discs can occur in children owing to other disorders as well. In many of these cases, the patient may complain of decreased vision or have other constitutional and neurologic symptoms (e.g., fever, lethargy, and coma).

Table 11-14. Other Causes of Disc Swelling in Children

Optic neuritis
Ocular disc edema with macular star, often related to infections
Leber's optic neuropathy
Diabetic papillopathy
Sarcoidosis
Leukemia

OPTIC NEURITIS

The most common cause of disc swelling that is not papilledema is bilateral optic neuritis, related to a flulike respiratory illness or gastroenteritis. In many of these cases, severe vision loss may ensue. Evaluation should include MR and cerebrospinal fluid examination.[47]

Some think optic neuritis in children under the age of puberty is a *forme fruste* of acute demyelinating encephalomyelitis, whereas optic neuritis after puberty may be a clue to multiple sclerosis. Multiple sclerosis is a less common sequel to optic neuritis in children than in adults. Brodsky et al. reported, in a review of the natural history of optic neuritis in children, that only 7–50% of children with a mean follow-up of 4–7 years developed multiple sclerosis (versus 50–70% of adults).[3]

In children, check the history of bee stings, tick bites, cat scratches, and immunizations. The examination should include a thorough look for lymphadenopathy (e.g., cat-scratch disease, sarcoid, virus), skin rash, and hepatosplenomegaly (e.g., leukemia).

Figure 11-29. A,B. **This boy had a flulike illness and within 1 week complained of decreased vision. His examination showed no light perception vision in the left eye and count fingers vision in the right eye. Intracranial pressure was normal on cerebrospinal fluid examination. He recovered vision. No organism was found. Note the elevated optic nerves, widening, and tortuosity of the retinal veins (**A, **right eye;** B, **left eye).** C. **His visual fields revealed complete loss in the left eye initially.** D. **At follow-up, his visual fields were normal.**

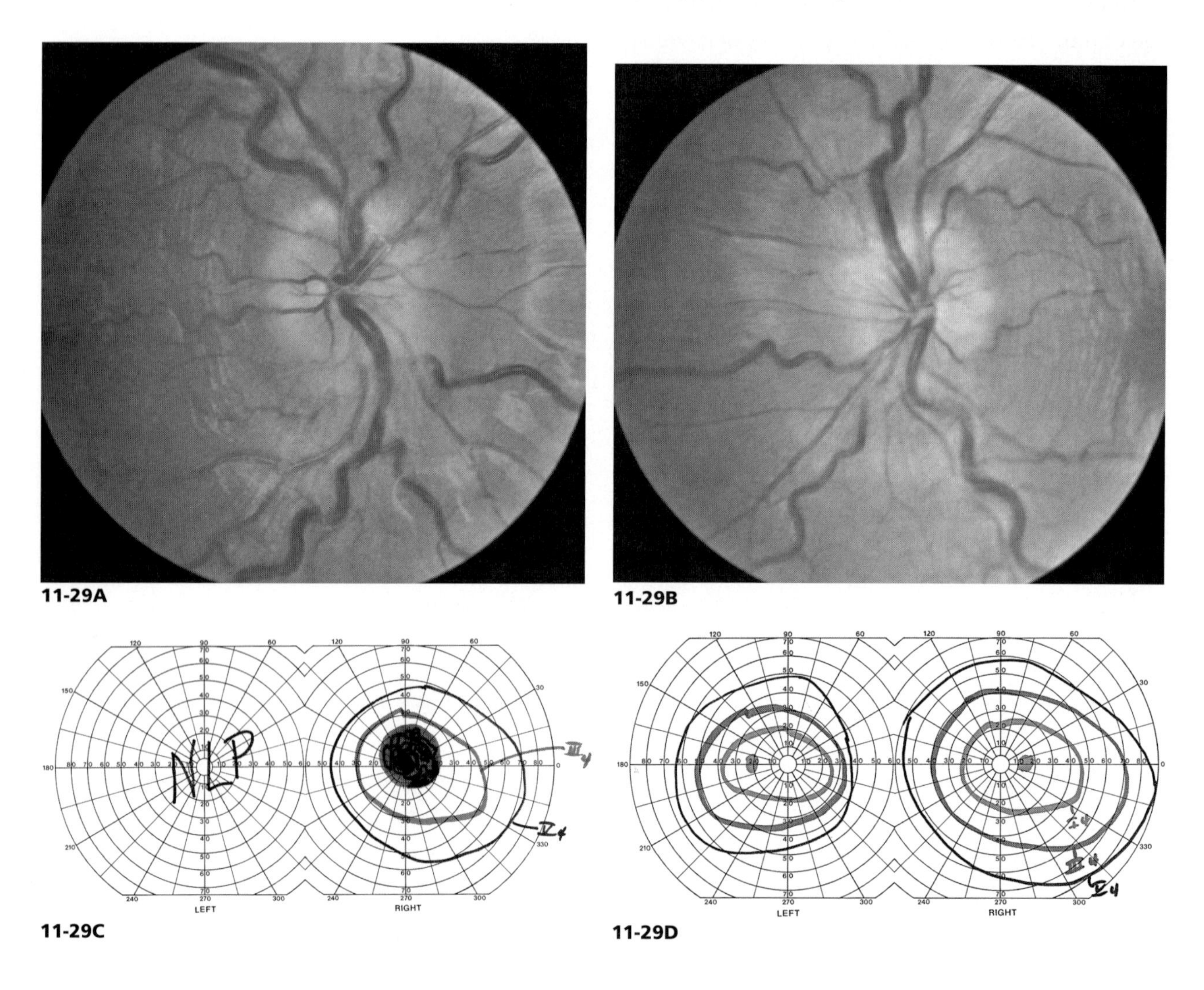

Table 11-15. Causes of Childhood Optic Neuritis

Infections/Postinfections
Measles (rubeola)
Mumps (paramyxovirus)
Chicken pox
Whooping cough (pertussis)
Lyme disease (*Borrelia burgdorferi*)
Mononucleosis (Epstein-Barr)
Cat-scratch fever (*Bartonella henselae*)
Toxocara canis
Toxoplasmosis
Rickettsial diseases
Coxiella burnetii
Brucellosis
Tuberculosis
Vaccinations
Bee venom
Other
Vasculitis
Sarcoid
Idiopathic

Source: Reprinted with permission from reference 3.

Treatment of bilateral optic neuritis in childhood is controversial. Intravenous steroids are sometimes helpful for 3–5 days, followed by a variable taper of oral steroids.

Thus, there are three important differences in optic neuritis between children and adults. In children, optic neuritis is usually bilateral, is usually papillitis, and usually follows or is part of a viral (infectious) condition.

PALE DISC

The *pale disc*, either unilateral or bilateral, deserves attention. Review Chapter 4, on disc pallor. Remember that the color of the nerve can be misleading. Does the accompanying vision loss go along with the pale disc?

The history is key to the diagnosis, and imaging studies are usually indicated to evaluate for treatable conditions. Optic nerve and chiasmal tumors may cause painless optic atrophy. Besides looking for tumors, look also for hydrocephalus, another common cause of bilateral optic atrophy in children and young adults (see Figures 4-41 and 4-51).

In children, congenital and hereditary causes of optic atrophy should be explored. Furthermore, metabolic disorders of childhood should be considered (see Tables 11-16 and 11-17). Although the main cause of optic atrophy remains acquired neurologic disorders, the main congenital causes include dominant optic atrophy and Leber's optic atrophy.

Table 11-16. Congenital Optic Neuropathies

Leber's optic atrophy
Dominant optic atrophy
Recessive optic atrophy
Behr's hereditary optic atrophy
Retinitis pigmentosa
Charcot-Marie-Tooth disease
Metachromatic leukodystrophy
Subacute sclerosing panencephalitis
Cerebral birth injuries
Craniosynostosis
Metabolic disorders
Osteopetrosis
Morquio's disease
Tay-Sachs disease
Niemann-Pick disease

Adapted in part from reference 3.

For a complete list of optic atrophies with genetic disorders see references 3 and 49.

Table 11-17. Hereditary Causes of Optic Atrophy

Genetic syndrome	Genetic disorder	Characteristics of syndrome	Age and gender	Ophthalmic characteristics	Optic nerve characteristics	Diagnosis
Leber's hereditary optic neuropathy	Mitochondrial defect; maternal transmission; mutations 11778, 3460, 14482, 15257, 4160	Primarily an optic atrophy	Usually male (9:1 in United States); onset age 20–30 yrs	20/20 to no light perception; usually almost simultaneous onset (within days to months); central scotoma	Initially edema of disc, blood vessels show tortuosity and sometimes extra vessels; no leakage on fluorescein angiogram	Send blood for studies; electrocardiogram
Dominant optic atrophy (Kjer's optic atrophy)[49]	Autosomal dominant; chromosome 3 and 18[50]; most common inherited optic neuropathy (1:50,000)[51]	Usually decreased vision on routine screening in school; insidious loss	Onset age 4–8 yrs; onset frequently after age 10 yrs	Visual acuity 20/25–20/400; see tritan color defect (blue-yellow); central/cecocentral scotoma	Classically: discrete temporal pallor with loss of papillomacular bundle on examination of nerve fiber layer	Visual evoked potential reduced amplitude and delayed latency; in the future, chromosomal studies
Simple recessive optic atrophy	Very rare	Optic atrophy primary sign	Age variable; young	More pronounced vision loss than dominant; diagnosis in first years of life; associated nystagmus	Severe diffuse atrophy and deep cupping; arteriolar attenuation	Need electroretinogram to differentiate from congenital retinal syndromes; in this disorder, electroretinogram OK
Behr's optic atrophy	Recessive	Vision loss with ataxia, hypertonia, mental retardation, pes cavus	Early childhood	Optic atrophy, nystagmus	Severe optic atrophy	Test for 3-methylglutaryl-conic acid

Continued

Table 11-17. *Continued*

Genetic syndrome	Genetic disorder	Characteristics of syndrome	Age and gender	Ophthalmic characteristics	Optic nerve characteristics	Diagnosis
DIDMOAD syndrome (Wolfram syndrome)	Sporadic, autosomal recessive, possibly mitochondrial	*D*iabetes *i*nsipidus, *d*iabetes *m*ellitus; optic *a*trophy, *d*eafness, nystagmus, ptosis, seizure, anosmia, ataxia	<15 years of age	Vision 20/200; pigmentary retinopathy in some; usually plateaus around 20/200	Disc diffuse atrophy	MR may show signal in posterior pituitary; atrophic brain
Optic atrophy and deafness syndromes (see reference 3)	Autosomal dominant, recessive, and x-linked	Variable findings: spasticity, peripheral neuropathy, posterior column, mental retardation, myopathy	Variable	Moderate to severe vision loss; some with ophthalmoplegia	Diffuse atrophy	May need electroretinogram to separate from retinal dystrophies
Cone dysfunction—leads to optic atrophy	Autosomal dominant, recessive and x-linked	Often no other finding	Young to age 50–60 yrs	See subtle changes in the macula to bull's eye in macula	Temporal optic nerve pallor; central scotoma	Electroretinogram is diagnostic; color vision is proportionately diminished

Source: Data adapted from references 3,48.

Figure 11-30. This mother (A, B) and son (C, D) have an autosomal dominant optic atrophy. Leber's mutation was not found. Notice the profound wedge-shaped temporal pallor characteristic of the dominant optic atrophies. The son's case fulfills the diagnostic criteria of (1) an established autosomal dominant link (his mother), (2) insidious onset before age 10 years, (3) bilateral neuropathy, (4) mild drop in acuity, (5) central or cecocentral scotomas with normal periphery on visual fields, (6) decreased color vision, and (7) temporal disc excavation (look especially at his mother's discs).[49] Often there is no family history of optic atrophy because there is an increased spontaneous mutation rate in this disorder. Also, ask about hearing loss, because a small subgroup does experience it.

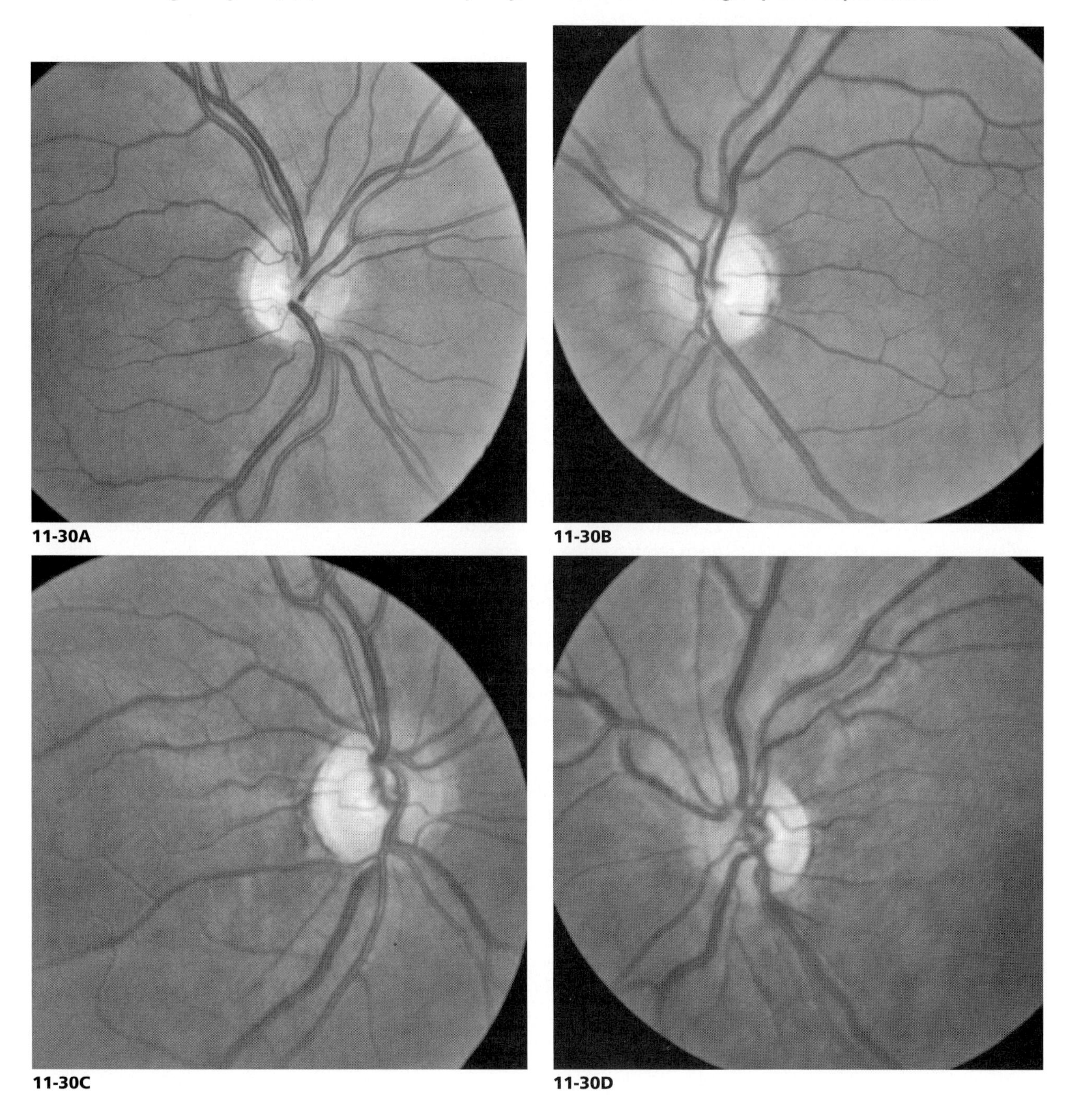

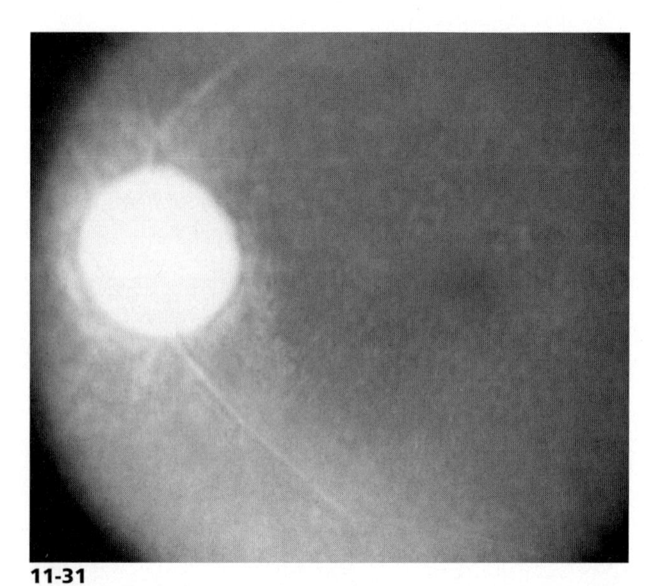
11-31

Neurologic diseases that produce optic atrophy generally affect white matter, whereas those that affect the gray matter cause seizures without much optic atrophy.

Figure 11-31. This child had complete blindness and mental deterioration Batten's disease (neuronal ceroid lipofuscinosis). Notice the extreme whiteness to the disc and threadlike narrowing of the retinal vessels. There is a roughened appearance of the macula as well. Batten's disease is associated with seizures, ataxia, and dementia. The diagnosis can be made with a skin biopsy.

Table 11-18. Neurodegenerative Conditions Associated with Optic Atrophy

Condition	Major features	Other eye findings	Optic nerve features
Hereditary ataxias			
Friedreich's ataxia	Autosomal recessive; before age 25 yrs; ataxia, dysarthria, loss of deep tendon reflexes, extensor plantars, pes cavus; cardiac disease, diabetes, infection	Mild vision loss	Optic atrophy in some
Spinocerebellar ataxias—(olivocerebellar ataxia)	Autosomal dominant, CAG repeat disease; progressive ataxia; SCA-3 has optic atrophy; SCA-7 has a maculopathy	Vision loss mild–moderate; ophthalmoplegia and nystagmus in some	Optic atrophy in some
Hereditary polyneuropathies			
Charcot-Marie-Tooth disease	Autosomal dominant; childhood onset; progressive demyelinating neuropathy	Vision loss variable; presents in teenage years or later; visual evoked potential may be abnormal in asymptomatic individuals	May see mild optic atrophy
Riley-Day syndrome	Dysautonomia; peripheral neuropathy	Vision loss variable; severe in some with progression; lack of tears; decreased corneal reflex	Optic atrophy

Continued

Condition	Major features	Other eye findings	Optic nerve features
White matter degenerative conditions			
Krabbe's disease	Autosomal recessive; normal at birth, then at 4 months progressive spasticity, seizure, deafness and blindness; galactocerebroside deficiency; some late onset forms	Facial weakness; deafness; opisthotonos	Optic atrophy
Canavan's disease	Autosomal recessive; aspartoacylase deficiency; infantile: hypotonia; large head	Deafness; macrocephaly; seizures	Optic atrophy
Leigh's disease	Autosomal recessive; mitochondrial; presents infant, child, adult; spasticity; see increased lactate and pyruvate; MR characteristic—demyelination of thalamus and pons	Deafness	Optic atrophy
Abnormalities in proteolipid metabolism (Pelizaeus Merzbacher)	X-linked; poor head control; chorea; MR demyelination	Nystagmus; head shaking	Atrophy
Adrenoleukodystrophy	Autosomal recessive and X-linked; seizure, dementia, polyneuropathy; infant, child, and young adult; long chain fatty acid accumulation abnormal	Pigmentary retinopathy; other causes of vision loss—cortical blindness or visual field cuts	Optic atrophy
Metachromatic leukodystrophy	Autosomal recessive; peripheral neuropathy; spasticity and gait disorder; speech slow; arylsulfatase deficiency	Cortical vision loss	Optic atrophy
Infantile neuronal axonal dystrophy	Autosomal recessive; motor delay, arrested mental development, seizures; see eosinophilic spheroids in the nervous system	Blindness	Optic atrophy
Gray matter degenerations			
Hallervorden-Spatz syndrome (neuroaxonal dystrophy)	Autosomal recessive; chorea and gait disorder; MR shows iron in globus pallidus and substantia nigra	Retinopathy; occasional cherry-red spot	Optic atrophy
Batten's disease (neuronal ceroid lipofuscinosis)	Autosomal recessive; seizure, ataxia, dementia; skin biopsy shows storage material	Pigment in retina	Optic atrophy

Continued

Table 11-18. *Continued*

Condition	Major features	Other eye findings	Optic nerve features
Mucopolysaccharidosis			
MPS IH-Hurler (absence of α-L-iduronidase; storage material is dermatan and heparan sulfate); MPS IS-Scheie (dermatan sulfate); MPS HIS (Hurler-Scheie) (α-L-iduronidase deficiency; dermatan sulfate); MPS II (Hunter—iduronosulfate sulfatase), MPS III (Sanfilippo syndrome) (α-glucosaminidase; *N*-acetylglucosamine; heparan sulfate); MPS IV (Morquio syndrome) (deficiency of *N*-acetylgalactosamine-6-sulfatase or β-galactosidase; keratan sulfate); and MPS VI (Maroteaux-Lamy) (deficiency of *N*-acetylgalactosamine-4-sulfatase or arylsulfatase B—accumulate dermatan sulfate)	Autosomal recessive; see hepatomegaly; characteristic facies; hydrocephalus, poor cerebrospinal fluid absorption	Lens changes; corneal clouding; glaucoma	Optic atrophy; papillodema may precede optic atrophy in some patients
Lipidosis			
Neuronal ceroid lipofuscinoses (juvenile form: Batten's disease)	Onset childhood–adulthood; seizures, ataxia, blindness; electronic microscopy of lymphocytes may show fingerprint inclusions; lipofuscin in neurons, conjunctiva, liver, rectum	Pigmentary changes in retina; attenuated arterioles; electroretinogram extinguished	Optic atrophy—sometimes from the retinal disorder

Source: Adapted from references 3,48,52.

Importantly, the appearance of the disc does not reflect the cause of the condition. You have to judge neurologic and metabolic disorders of optic atrophy by the company they keep—hearing loss, organomegaly, ataxia.

Retinal degenerations and retinitis pigmentosa can cause vision loss in children. See Chapter 8,

Table 8-4 (on pigmentation in the retina) and Chapter 9, Table 9-11 for further descriptions.

CHERRY-RED MACULA

What if there is a *cherry-red macula*? Although cherry-red spots are associated with central retinal artery occlusion in the adult, in children there are specific inherited conditions that present with a cherry-red macula. The red spot is formed because the ganglion cells are filled with abnormal metabolic products, which opacify the perifoveolar retina. The normal color of the macula exists because in this region there are no engorged ganglion cells overlying the retina. As the child loses vision and the nerve becomes atrophic, the cherry-red spot disappears.

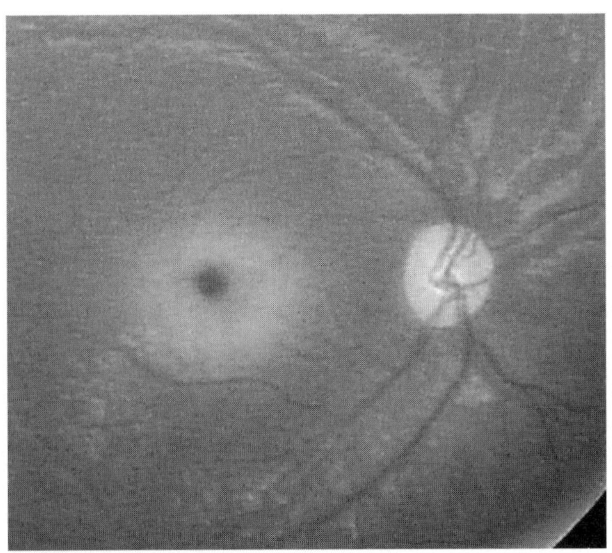

11-32

Figure 11-32. This cherry-red spot is caused by Tay-Sachs disease. The macula appears cherry red because the ganglion cells, filled with abnormal metabolic products, opacify the retina. Because the fovea has no ganglion cells, the normal red color of the macula is seen. When the child loses vision, the nerve becomes atrophic, and the cherry-red spot disappears. (Photograph courtesy of Robert Hoffman, M.D.)

Table 11-19. Causes of a Cherry-Red Spot

Condition	Enzyme defect	Major features	Other
Vascular			
Central retinal artery defect	None	Loss of vision; usually owing to embolic disease	
Other			
Quinine toxicity		History of quinine use	
Retinal edema after trauma		History of trauma	
Subacute sclerosing panencephalitis	Measles	History of measles encephalitis; neurologic and white matter disease	Cortical blindness, nystagmus, supranuclear gaze palsies
Storage diseases			
GM-2 gangliosidosis type 1: Tay-Sachs disease	Hexosaminidase A	Jewish or French ancestry; gait and speech abnormal; age 3–7 yrs; psychomotor retardation	Limited up-gaze
GM-2 gangliosidosis; type 2: Sandhoff's disease	Hexosaminidase A and B	Hepatosplenomegaly, renal and heart disease; macrocephaly, macroglossia	Serum and leukocyte assays
Generalized gangliosidosis, type 1	β-Galactosidase	Spasticity and seizures	Fibroblasts show enzyme defect
Niemann-Pick type C disease	Sphingomyelinase	Organomegaly, myoclonic jerks, xanthoma; psychomotor deterioration	Loss of down-gaze and vertical saccades
Sialidoses: Cherry-red spot myoelonus	Neuraminidase	Myoclonus; seizures; normal IQ; ascites, cataract	Conjunctival biopsy shows vacuoles in cytoplasm
Nephrosialidosis	Neuraminidase	Ascites	Bone marrow shows foam cells
Goldberg's syndrome—type II sialidosis	Neuraminidase	Dementia, ataxia; hearing loss; blindness; corneal clouding	Conjunctival biopsy shows fibrillogranular inclusions
Late-onset cerebellar ataxia	Hexosaminidase B	Rare	
Farber's disease (lipogranulomatosis)	Ceramidase	Arthropathy, hoarseness, and subcutaneous nodules	Ceramidase activity in fibroblasts, leukocytes
Metachromatic leukodystrophy	Arylsulfatase A	Most common white matter degeneration in children; peripheral neuropathy	Optic atrophy; strabismus
Gaucher's disease—type II	Glucocerebrosidase	Seizures and spasticity	Horizontal gaze abnormal
Krabbe's disease	Glucosylceramidase	Protruding ears; fevers (episodic)	Measure enzyme in leukocytes or fibroblasts
Hallervorden-Spatz syndrome	Elevated cystine and cysteine owing to reduced cysteine dioxygenase	Progressive spasticity	Iron on MR

Source: Adapted from references 3,52–55.

Hemorrhages in an Infant or Child—Be Aware of Shaken Baby Syndrome

Shaken baby syndrome is a constellation of clinical findings characteristic of child abuse in which there is evidence of intraocular and intracranial trauma without any external signs of direct head trauma.

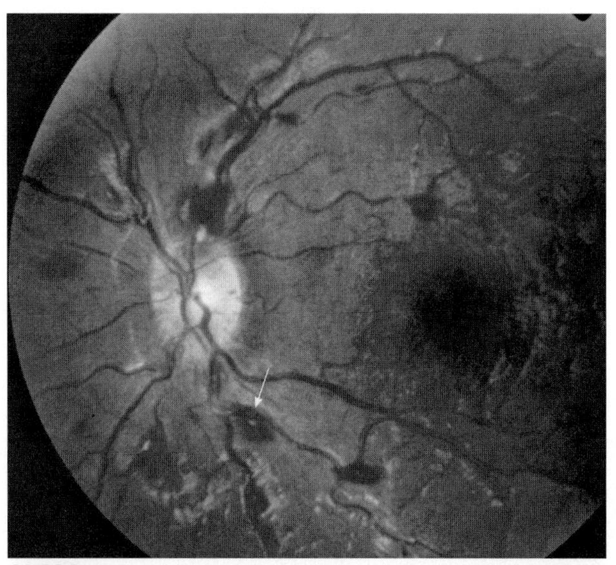

11-33A

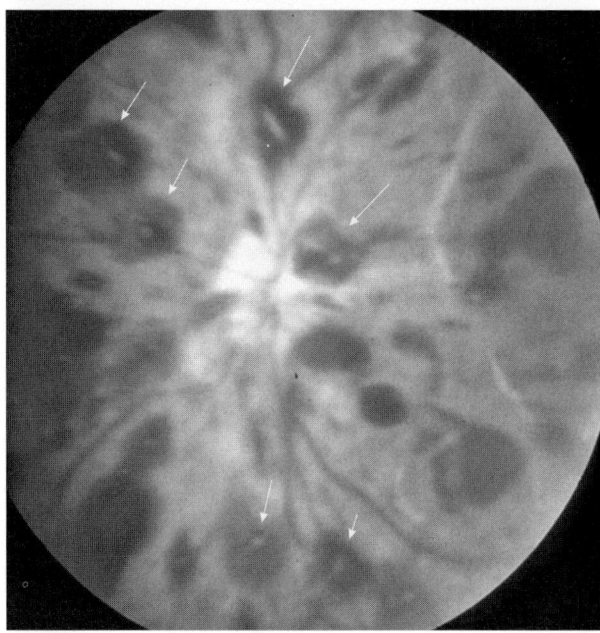

11-33B

Figure 11-33. A. **In shaken baby syndrome, bilateral retinal hemorrhages (*arrow*) are the most common ocular finding, although unilateral hemorrhages have been reported. These hemorrhages are found at all ocular and retinal levels, including vitreal, preretinal, nerve fiber layer, and deep retinal or subretinal. Hemorrhages are usually seen in the posterior pole.** B. **Roth's spots may also be present (*arrows*). There may be papilledema if there is severely increased intracranial pressure.**

The eye is involved in shaken baby syndrome approximately 5–10% of the time, and it is usually detected by a non-ophthalmologist who is examining the baby. The child is usually younger than 12 months of age but always younger than 3 years of age. The typical story is that the child became sleepy and unarousable, or that allegedly minor trauma occurred, such as falling off of a bed.

A dilated fundus examination using direct and indirect techniques should be performed by an experienced ophthalmologist in cases of suspected shaken baby syndrome. Neurologic examination is critical. Systemic examination may show nothing, but one should look for bruising, namely, imprints of the perpetrator on the body. Often, fresh or healed fractures, or both, are found. Skeletal x-rays should be performed. A computed tomographic scan without contrast should be performed looking for evidence of subarachnoid hemorrhage, subdural hematomas, or signs of contusions. The etiology of shaken baby syndrome is a whiplash injury to the brain with rapid increase of intracranial pressure. Other mechanisms include thorax compression and, therefore, decrease in venous return from the eyes and head, and sudden deceleration from the baby being put down suddenly. Treatment of the hemorrhages is usually not necessary, although, if extensive, vitrectomy may be required. Close follow-up watching for amblyopia is wise. By law in most states, physicians are obliged to report cases of suspected child abuse to authorities. Complications of shaken baby syndrome include mental retardation, cortical blindness, and macular injury causing vision loss.

The absence of papilledema is an important sign because this indicates that only the shaking during increased venous pressure could produce the finding. Papilledema may be present later if there is intracranial hemorrhage or increased intracranial pressure from brain swelling; in this case, the papilledema ensues many days later.

Differential diagnosis of hemorrhages in infants is extensive, and one should always rule out leukemia, ROP, sickle cell retinopathy, meningitis, intracranial bleeding from a venous malformation, and severe hypertension. One study was performed in which accidental traumatic head injury in 79 children younger than 3 years old found no evidence of retinal hemorrhages; they concluded that finding retinal hemorrhages in a child after a head injury suggested nonaccidental cause.[56] Even after cardiopulmonary arrest, only one child out of 45 had retinal hemorrhages[57]; however, bilateral retinal hemorrhages have been reported in an infant with ROP and cardiopulmonary resuscitation.[58]

Table 11-20. Differential Diagnosis of Hemorrhages in Infants and Children

Condition	Distinguishing features	Other characteristics	Outcome
Neonatal hemorrhage	Occurs within hours of birth	Splinter, dot and blot	Normal
Shaken baby; abuse	Frequently have nonaccidental trauma (65–89%)	All retinal layers; vitreous; look for other signs of trauma—bruise, fracture, brain injury	Can cause permanent damage; close follow-up for amblyopia
Subarachnoid hemorrhage (rare in children)	Occurs after intracerebral hemorrhage from aneurysm, arteriovenous malformation; frequency approximately 20%	Preretinal	Usually good; may require vitrectomy
Leukemia and blood dyscrasias (e.g., anemia, pancytopenia, coagulopathy)	Very frequent	All layers	Good outcome if there is a remission
Hyperviscosity (e.g., cryoglobulinemia, paraproteinemia, macroglobulinemia; cystic fibrosis)	Occasional	All layers; all types; seen with cystic fibrosis	Good
Persistent hyperplastic primary vitreous (developmental anomaly)	Occasional	Vitreal and intraretinal; see other anomalies like cataract, micro-ophthalmus	Poor visual outcome
Retinopathy of prematurity	Frequent finding; premature infant	Vitreal and intraretinal hemorrhage near junction of the vascularized and nonvascularized premature retina; watch for neovascularization	Fair visual outcome; prematurity itself causes other problems
Retinopathy owing to infection (e.g., cytomegalovirus, herpes, rickettsia, ocular toxoplasmosis, bacterial endocarditis)	Frequent with cytomegalovirus, immune deficiency syndrome	See cotton-wool spots and retinal necrosis	Variable—depends on severity
Hypertension	Frequent with papilledema; look for renal disease	Flame-shaped, peripapillary, exudates	Good if blood pressure controlled
Coats' disease (rare retinal telangiectasia sometimes seen in facial scapulohumeral dystrophy)	Frequent with intraretinal and vitreal hemorrhage	Also see neovascularization	Poor outcome
Retinal dysplasia	Frequent in site of dysplastic retina	Look for glaucoma; Norrie's disease	Poor

Source: Adapted in part from reference 59.

Retinopathy of Prematurity

Since the 1950s, great advances have been made in premature fetal outcome, allowing ever younger infants to survive. *Retrolental fibroplasia*, the former name for ROP, was initially thought to be a disorder of the hyaloid system (like persistent hyperplastic primary vitreous). However, ROP now is known to be a specific retinopathy of premature infants who have been exposed to higher than normal levels of oxygen and the bright lights of a neonatal intensive care unit.[60] ROP occurs in approximately 38% of infants that weigh less than 1,200 g, and it increases to 52% of infants between 501 and 1,250 g. The risk factors include apnea, parenteral nutrition, hypoxia, hyperoxia, hypercarbia, ventilator hours, respiratory distress, low birth weight, gestational age, blood transfusions, maternal bleeding, and exposure to light. ROP is caused by immaturity of the premature infant's retinal and retinal vascular development—the retinal circulation does not start until approximately 4 months' gestation. Immature infants are unable to cope with the stresses of life outside of the uterus at such a young age. Ophthalmologic examination should be performed before discharge of a preterm baby from the nursery and again at approximately 7–9 weeks of age. Involution of disease seemed to occur at approximately 38 weeks postmenstrual age, with more than 90% involution of retinopathy by 44 weeks postmenstrual age.[61]

Appearance of the disc depends on the stage of disease. The International Classification of Retinopathy of Prematurity (reviewed in reference 61) is based on the following:

1. Location of disease (zones I, II, III are zones concentrically centered around the optic disc, with zone I around the disc and macula and zone III the far periphery)
2. Extent of disease (described by hours of a clock around the disc)
3. Stage of disease

Table 11-21. Staging in Retinopathy of Prematurity

Stage	Finding
1. Demarcation line	Seeing a line separating the avascular retina from the posterior vascular retina
2. Ridge	Vessels enter the ridge
3. Ridge with fibrovascular proliferation	Can be mild, moderate, or severe depending on how much fibrovascular proliferation
4. Partial retinal detachment	Occurs owing to effusions
5. Total retinal detachment	Funnel-shaped retinal detachment
6. "Plus" disease	Tortuous and dilated retinal vessels, pupil is immobile, vitreous is hazy

Source: Adapted from reference 60.

In one study, non-ophthalmologists were successful in identifying stage 3 or worse disease with a direct ophthalmoscope. However, we suggest that all of these infants be referred for full evaluation by an experienced ophthalmologist, because treatment has centered on cryotherapy and photocoagulation.[62]

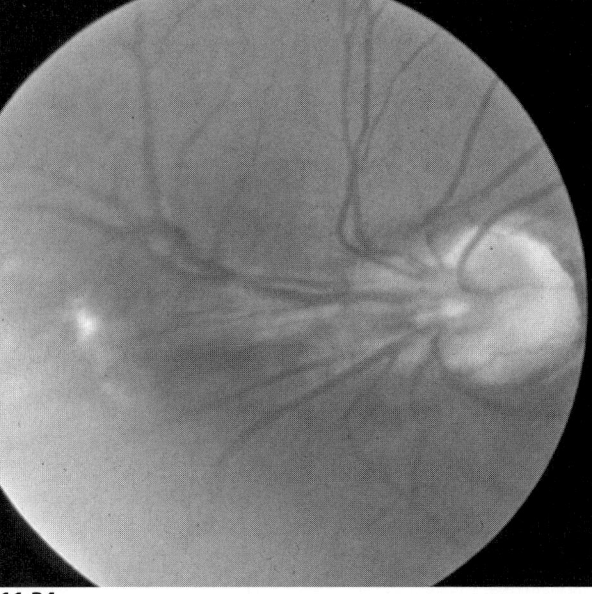

11-34

Figure 11-34. This disc is the typical dragged disc of a child with a history of ROP. After ROP there can be longstanding findings. The child has other features of the history of ROP, including myopia, astigmatism, and pigmentation of the retina.

Table 11-22. Findings on Eye Examination in Parents after Retinopathy of Prematurity

Myopia
Refractive errors like astigmatism
Early cataract
Glaucoma
Disc
Dragging of retina on disc
Vessel tortuosity
Retina: pigmentary changes
Macula: dragging or distortion
Vasculature: tortuosity
Optic atrophy owing to neovascular hemorrhage

Source: Adapted from reference 63.

Practical Essentials to Viewing in Children

1. Examine the anomalous nerve with the presenting problem (if any) in mind—is it an incidental finding, or is it affecting vision?
2. When an anomaly is present, look for an associated systemic or neurologic abnormality.
3. Look for evidence of amblyopia.
4. If there is no overt retinal abnormality or myopia, usually poor vision is secondary to a perinatal insult (e.g., intraventricular leukomalacia). Amblyopic vision loss could also be present.
5. If the disc is hypoplastic, look for endocrinologic abnormalities. Is the mother diabetic?
6. If the disc is a coloboma, look for an associated heart defect.
7. If the disc is a morning glory disc, look for basal encephalocele or abnormalities in cranial circulation (moya moya syndrome).
8. If there is a swollen disc, look for brain tumor, increased intracranial pressure, and optic neuritis.
9. If the disc is pale, examine the parents.
10. If there are hemorrhages in the retina of an infant, look for signs of shaken baby syndrome.
11. Premature infants should be examined by an ophthalmologist.

References

1. Gowers W. A Manual and Atlas of Medical Ophthalmoscopy. London: J & A Churchill, 1879.
2. Olitsky SE, Nelson LB. Common ophthalmologic concerns in infants and children. Pediatr Clin North Am 1998;45:993–1102.
3. Brodsky MC, Baker RS, Hamed LM. Pediatric Neuro-ophthalmology. New York: Springer, 1996;42–75.
4. Hellström A, Hård AL, Chen Y, et al. Ocular fundus morphology in preterm children. Invest Ophthalmol Vis Sci 1997;38:1184–1192.
5. Brodsky MC. Congenital optic disk anomalies. Surv Ophthalmol 1994;39:89–112.
6. Van Dalen JT, Delleman JW. Congenital Anomalies of the Eye. Amersfoort: Holland Ophthalmic Publishing Center, 1983.
7. Skarf B, Hoyt CS. Optic nerve hypoplasia in children. Association with anomalies of the endocrine and CNS. Arch Ophthalmol 1984;102:62–67.
8. Deiner MS, Kennedy TE, Fazell A, et al. Netrin-1 and DCC mediate axon guidance locally at the optic disc: loss of function leads to optic nerve hypoplasia. Neuron 1997;19:575–589.
9. Hellström A, Wiklund LM, Svensson E, et al. Optic nerve hypoplasia with isolated tortuosity of the retinal veins. Arch Ophthalmol 1999;117:880–884.
10. Hoyt CS, Good WV. Do we really understand the difference between optic nerve hypoplasia and atrophy? Eye 1992;6:201–204.
11. Roessmann U. Septo-optic dysplasia (SOD) or DeMorsier syndrome. J Clin Neuroophthalmol 1989; 9:156–159.
12. Brodsky MC, Glasier CM. Optic nerve hypoplasia. Arch Ophthalmol 1993;111:66–74.
13. Brodsky MC. Septo-optic dysplasia: a reappraisal. Semin Ophthalmol 1991;6:227–232.
14. Brown G, Tasman W. Congenital Anomalies of the Optic Disc. New York: Grune & Stratton, 1983.
15. Nelson M, Lessell S, Sadun AS. Optic nerve hypoplasia and maternal diabetes mellitus. Arch Neurol 1986;43:20–25.
16. Zeki SM, Dutton GN. Optic nerve hypoplasia in children. Br J Ophthalmol 1990;74:300–304.
17. Kim RY, Hoyt WF, Lessell S, Narahara MH. Superior segmental optic hypoplasia. A sign of maternal diabetes. Arch Ophthalmol 1989;107:1312–1315.
18. Hashimoto M, Ohtsuka K, Nakagawa T, Hoyt WF. Topless optic disk syndrome without maternal diabetes mellitus. Am J Ophthalmol 1999;128:111–112.
19. Hoyt WF, Rios-Montenegro EN, Behrens MM, Eckelhoff RJ. Homonymous hemioptic hypoplasia. Br J Ophthalmol 1972;56:537–545.
20. Hellström A. Optic nerve morphology may reveal adverse events during prenatal and perinatal life-digital image analysis. Surv Ophthalmol 1999;44 (Suppl 1):S63–S73.
21. Jacobson L, Hellström A, Flodmark O. Large cups in normal-sized optic discs. A variant of optic nerve hypoplasia in children with periventricular leukomalacia. Arch Ophthalmol 1997;115:1263–1269.
22. Brodsky MC. Periventricular leukomalacia: an intracranial cause of pseudoglaucomatous cupping. Arch Ophthalmol 2001;119:626–627.
23. Franceschetti A, Bock RH. Megalopapilla: a new congenital anomaly. Am J Ophthalmol 1950;33:227–235.
24. Grimson BS, Perry DD. Enlargement of the optic disk in childhood optic nerve tumors. Am J Ophthalmol 1984;97:627–631.
25. Chang M. Pits and crater-like holes of the optic disc. Ophthalmic Semin 1976;1:21–61.
26. Stefko ST, Campochiaro P, Wang P, et al. Dominant inheritance of optic pits. Am J Ophthalmol 1997;124:112–113.
27. Corbett JJ, Savino PJ, Schatz NJ, Orr LS. Cavitary developmental defects of the optic disc. Arch Neurol 1980;37:210–213.
28. Postel EA, Pulido JS, McNamara JA, Johnson MW. The etiology and treatment of macular detachment associated with optic nerve pits and related anomalies. Trans Am Ophthalmol Soc 1998;96:73–93.
29. Apple DJ, Rabb MF, Walsh PM. Congenital anomalies of the optic disc. Surv Ophthalmol 1982;27:3–41.
30. Pagon RA. Ocular coloboma. Surv Ophthalmol 1981;25:223–236.
31. Pagon RA, Graham JM, Zonana J, Yong SL. Coloboma, congenital heart disease, and choana atresia with multiple anomalies: CHARGE association. J Pediatr 1981;99:223–227.
32. Brodsky MC, Hoyt WF, Hoyt CS, et al. Atypical retinochoroidal coloboma in patients with dysplastic optic discs and transsphenoidal encephalocele. Arch Ophthalmol 1995;113:624–628.

33. Gopal L, Badrinath SS, Kumar KS, et al. Optic disc in fundus coloboma. Ophthalmology 1996;103:2120–2127.
34. Beyer WB, Quencer RM, Osher RH. Morning glory syndrome. Ophthalmology 1982;89:1362–1367.
35. Kindler P. Morning glory syndrome: unusual congenital optic disk anomaly. Am J Ophthalmol 1970;69:376–384.
36. Pollack S. The morning glory disc anomaly: contractile movement, classification, and embryogenesis. Doc Ophthalmol 1987;65:439–460.
37. Eustis HS, Sanders MR, Zimmerman T. Morning glory syndrome in children. Arch Ophthalmol 1994;112:204–207.
38. Massaro M, Thorarensen O, Liu GT, et al. Morning glory disc anomaly and moyamoya vessels. Arch Ophthalmol 1998;116:253–254.
39. Parsa CF, Silva ED, Sundin OH, et al. Redefining papillorenal syndrome: an underdiagnosed cause of ocular and renal morbidity. Ophthalmology 2001;108:738–749.
40. Kral K, Svarc D. Contractile peripapillary staphyloma. Am J Ophthalmol 1971;71:1090–1092.
41. Hodgkins P, Lees M, Lawson J, et al. Optic disc anomalies and frontonasal dysplasia. Br J Ophthalmol 1998;82:290–293.
42. Seybold ME, Rosen PN. Peripapillary staphyloma and amaurosis fugax. Ann Ophthalmol 1977;9:1139–1141.
43. Grossniklaus HE, Green WR. Pathologic findings in pathologic myopia. Retina 1992;12:127–133.
44. Goldberg MF. Persistent fetal vasculature (PFV): An integrated interpretation of signs and symptoms associated with persistent hyperplastic primary vitreous (PHPV). LIV Edward Jackson Memorial Lecture. Am J Ophthalmol 1997;124:587–626.
45. Joseph N, Ivry M, Oliver M. Persistent hyperplastic primary vitreous at the optic nerve head. Am J Ophthalmol 1972;73:580–583.
46. Brodsky MC, Buckley EG, McConkie-Rosell A. The case of the gray optic disc! Surv Ophthalmol 1989;33:367–372.
47. Farris BK, Pickard DJ. Bilateral post-infectious optic neuritis and intravenous steroid therapy in children. Ophthalmology 1990;97:339–345.
48. Newman NJ. Hereditary optic neuropathies. In NR Miller, NJ Newman (eds), Walsh and Hoyt's Clinical Neuro-ophthalmology. Baltimore: Williams & Wilkins, 1998;741–773.
49. Kline LB, Glaser JS. Dominant optic atrophy. Arch Ophthalmol 1979;97:1680–1686.
50. Kerrison JB, Arnould VJ, Sallum F, et al. Genetic heterogeneity of dominant optic atrophy, Kjer type. Arch Ophthalmol 1999;117:805–810.
51. Johnston RL, Seller MJ, Behnam JT, et al. Dominant optic atrophy. Ophthalmology 1999;106:123–128.
52. Rosenberg RN, Prusiner SB, DiMauro S, Barchi RL. Clinical Companion to the Molecular and Genetic Basis of Neurologic Disease. Boston: Butterworth, 1998.
53. Rizzo JF. Neuroophthalmologic Disease of the Retina. In DM Albert, FA Jakobiec (eds), Principles and Practice of Ophthalmology. Philadelphia: Saunders, 1994;2507–2529.
54. Kivlin JD, Sanborn GE, Myers GG. The cherry red spot in Tay-Sachs and other storage diseases. Ann Neurol 1985;17:356–360.
55. Kelly J, Maumenee IH. Hereditary macular diseases. Int Ophthalmol Clin 1999;39(4):83–115.
56. Buys YM, Levin AV, Enzenauer RW, et al. Retinal findings after head trauma in infants and young children. Ophthalmology 1992;99:1718–1723.
57. Kanter RK. Retinal hemorrhage after cardiopulmonary resuscitation or child abuse. J Pediatr 1986;108:430–432.
58. Polita A, Au Eong KG, Repka MX, Pieramici DJ. Bilateral retinal hemorrhages in a preterm infant with retinopathy of prematurity immediately following cardiopulmonary resuscitation. Arch Ophthalmol 2001;119:913–914.
59. Kaur B, Taylor D. Fundus hemorrhages in infancy. Surv Ophthalmol 1992;37:1–17.
60. Ben Sira I, Nissenkorn I, Kremer I. Retinopathy of prematurity. Surv Ophthalmol 1988;33:1–16.
61. Repka MX, Palmer EA, Tung B. Involution of retinopathy of prematurity. Arch Ophthalmol 2000;118:645–649.
62. Saunders RA, Bluesten EC, Berland JE, et al. Can non-ophthalmologists screen for retinopathy of prematurity? J Pediatr Ophthalmol Strabismus 1995;32:302–304.
63. Palmer EA, Patz A, Phelps DL, Spencer R. Retinopathy of prematurity. In SJ Ryan, AP Schachat, RP Murphy (eds), Retina. St. Louis: Mosby, 1994;1473–1498.

12 What to Look for in Aging

Primary care physicians often ask themselves, "When do I need a consultation?" My answer is simple: whenever it "niggles" you; whenever you feel something isn't just right.

Eugene Guazzo[1]

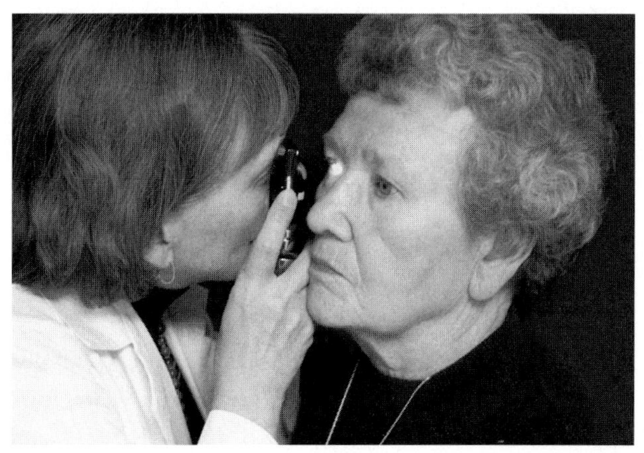

12-1

Figure 12-1. Viewing the optic disc and fundus in older people is important in the prevention of unnecessary vision loss. Look for evidence of cataract, glaucoma, diabetic retinopathy, and macular degeneration.

Approximately 13% of the U.S. population is older than 65 years. Furthermore, this statistic will increase to almost 20% by the year 2020. Vision and other senses fail as we age. A recent study showed that visual acuity was worse than 20/40 in 4% of the people from ages 65–74 years and 16% in ages 80–84 years. More than one-third of these individuals required refraction to improve acuity; the other two-thirds had cataract, glaucoma, and diabetic retinopathy.[2] Therefore, it is important that we recognize observable visual changes in the elderly that can be ameliorated to preserve or improve quality of life. How do you view the optic disc and fundus in the elderly?

The eye has many changes that occur as we age. The lens becomes more rigid and loses accommodation (i.e., we need glasses to read the paper).

There are no known changes to the disc incident to aging, but there are four ocular disease processes that the primary care physician should be able to recognize using the ophthalmoscope in the elderly: cataract, open-angle glaucoma, diabetic retinopathy, and macular degeneration.[1] In addition, the elderly are more susceptible to vascular disease that affects the eye. Many of these can be diagnosed using an ophthalmoscope.

Table 12-1. Vision and Aging

Part of the eye	Aging change	Effect on vision	What to look for
Cornea	Thickens; dryness	Can scatter light; blur	Opacification; a fluorescein strip to stain the cornea can be viewed with the blue light of the ophthalmoscope
Lens	Thickens, yellows; loses accommodation; when diseased can produce cataract	Needs glasses for near in presbyopia; with cataract may become more myopic and be able to read without glasses; scatters light	Through a dilated pupil, examine the lens with the red reflex—has dark, irregular center if cataract is present
Retina	Gradual loss of cells; depigmentation in the periphery; more prominent choroidal vasculature (tigroid fundus) becomes more common[4]	Usually not noticed; may complain that night vision is affected	With the ophthalmoscope, view the retina
Macula	Gradual loss of cells; loss of the prominent light reflex; when diseased produces macular degeneration	When diseased affects central vision	Use the ophthalmoscope to look for macular degeneration
Retinal vessels	Age as the blood vessels in the body age	No obvious symptoms	With the ophthalmoscope, look for vascular attenuation
Disc	Usually no changes; increased risk of anterior ischemic optic neuropathy and glaucoma	No symptoms; may report visual field narrowing	With the ophthalmoscope, look for enlarged cup-to-disc ratio; pallor of the disc

Source: Adapted and revised from references 1,3.

Because the pupil becomes smaller with age, it is essential to dilate the pupil to view any of the aforementioned conditions (see Chapter 1). Dilation aids the examiner in viewing the lens, the vitreous, the fundus, and the disc.

Figure 12-2. The tigroid fundus accentuates the outline of the choroidal vessels and changes in choroidal melanin that occur with aging.[4] A. There is also loss of the macular reflex with aging. B. The optic disc does not usually change, although older individuals are at risk for the development of glaucoma. C. The tigroid fundus is prominent here.

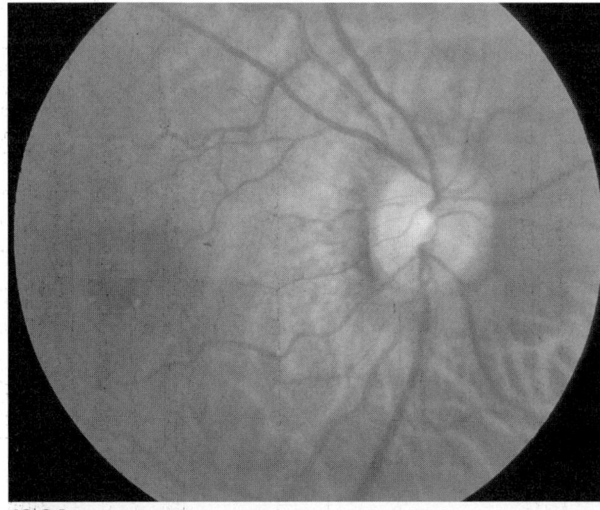

12-2A

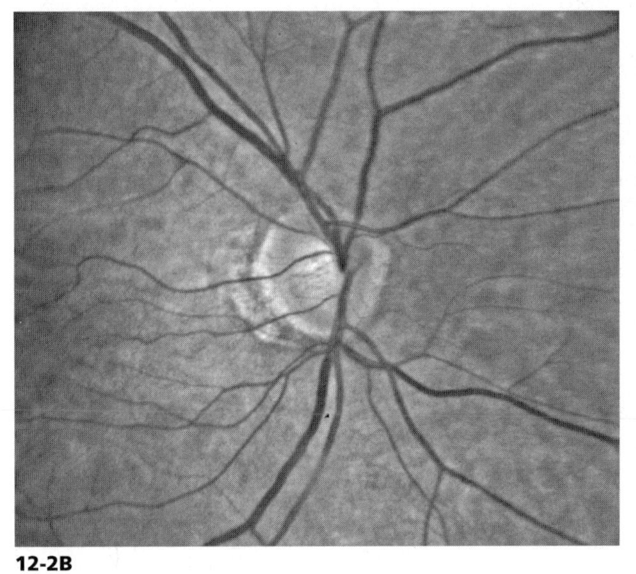

12-2B

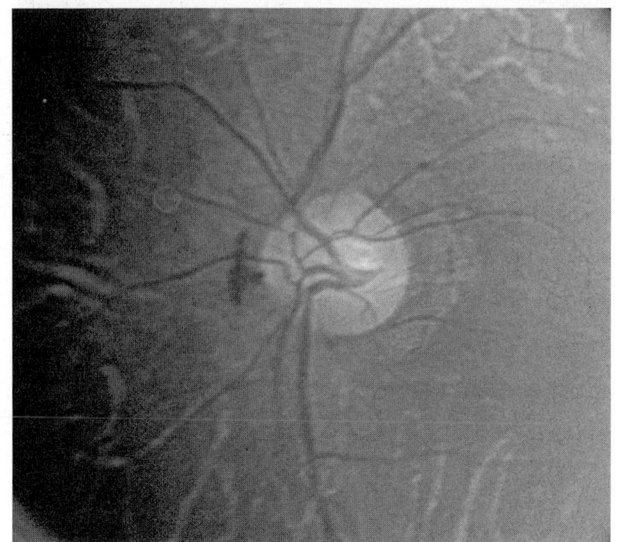

12-2C

What questions should you ask your older patients about their vision? First, "have you noticed any sudden changes in your vision?"[1] (Most changes with aging are slow and gradual, and a sudden change should be evaluated.) Next, "can you read the newspaper?" (Check visual acuity.) "Can you drive at night?" (If not, the patient may have cataract.) "Have you had an eye examination in the last 2 years?" (Most recommend an eye examination by an eye care professional every 2 years.)

The examination should evaluate visual acuity (near card; Snellen chart). The most common cause of visual impairment with age is an uncorrected refractive error—13% of those older than 80 years have uncorrected refractive error.[5] Look for a relative afferent pupillary defect. Look at the angle of the eye. Test the visual field to confrontation. Measure the intraocular pressure if you have a Tono-Pen or Shiötz tonometer. Observe the disc through a dilated pupil; 0.5% tropicamide (Mydriacil) is recommended.[1] Although some physicians are reluctant to dilate because of the potential to precipitate glaucoma, Butler et al. believe that you are doing the patient a favor, because you will refer this patient immediately to an ophthalmologist (within 24 hours).[1] Topical mydriatics, which cause the most problems in the elderly, include cyclopentolate (Cyclogyl). Adrenergic agents such as phenylephrine may cause tachycardia and hypertension.[6] If the patient is aphakic (i.e., they have had cataract surgery and no longer have their lens), the absorption of dilating drops may be affected.

With aging, there are four major diseases that affect vision. First, cataract is a change in the lens that is easily remediable with surgery. In patients younger than 70 years, Weih did not find a significant vision-threatening prevalence of cataract; however, the prevalence tripled by decade.[5] By age 90 years, 12% had vision-threatening cataract. The risk factors for cataracts include sun exposure, diet (diets low in green vegetables), and smoking. Recognize cataract by its symptoms—blurring of vision and scattering of light at night. View the lens by dilating the patient and using the red reflex with the ophthalmoscope to look for cataract.

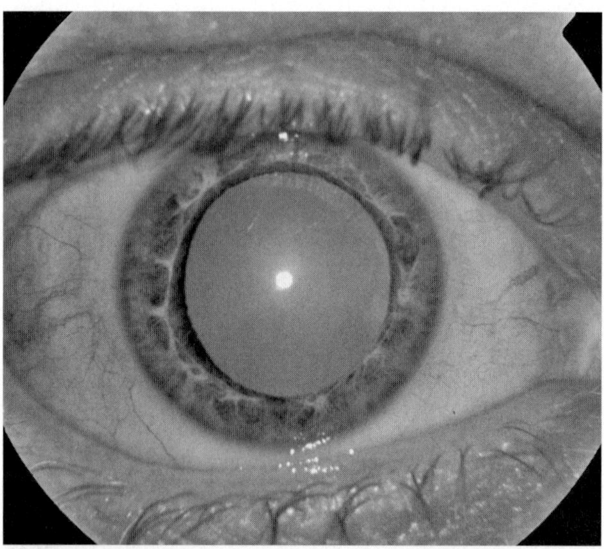

12-3A

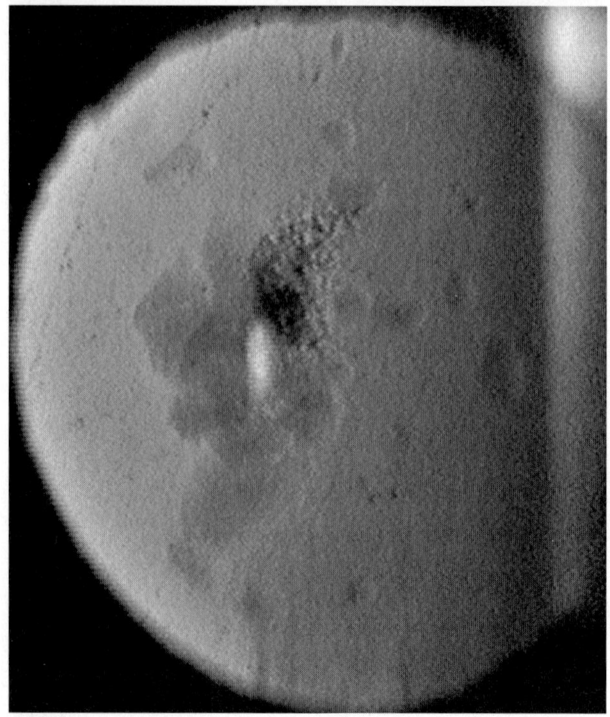

12-3B

Figure 12-3. A. **First view the red reflex with your ophthalmoscope.** B. **Look for lens opacities typical of cataract.**

The incidence of ocular hypertension increases with age, and with it the chance of open-angle glaucoma. The prevalence of glaucoma in those younger than 79 years was less than 1% at Weih's screening.[5] However, after age 80 years the prevalence jumped to 1.4% and the severity definitely increased with age. Although pressure plays an important role in glaucoma, some people may have elevated pressures that are asymptomatic; others can have profound glaucomatous changes in the optic nerve with only slight pressure elevations. Symptoms of glaucoma, as discussed in Chapter 4, are not dramatic. Some complain of halos around lights and blurring of vision, but most have no complaints. Besides age alone, another risk factor that the elderly experience is the use of medications—drops like steroid eye drops increase intraocular pressure in many older individuals. Furthermore, other systemic medications with parasympathomimetic properties used in the treatment of depression (tricyclic antidepressants) may further increase the possibility of increased intraocular pressure.[7]

There are three things to look for in glaucoma. First, check the angle as described in Chapter 1, Figure 1-20. Second, measure the intraocular pressure of the eye—this can be done with a simple pen tonometer in an office. Third, look at the disc—is there asymmetrical cupping? Are there notches in the neuroretinal rim? Is there peripapillary atrophy? Whether or not one is *sure*, referral to an ophthalmologist is important (see Chapter 4, Figures 4-27–4-36).

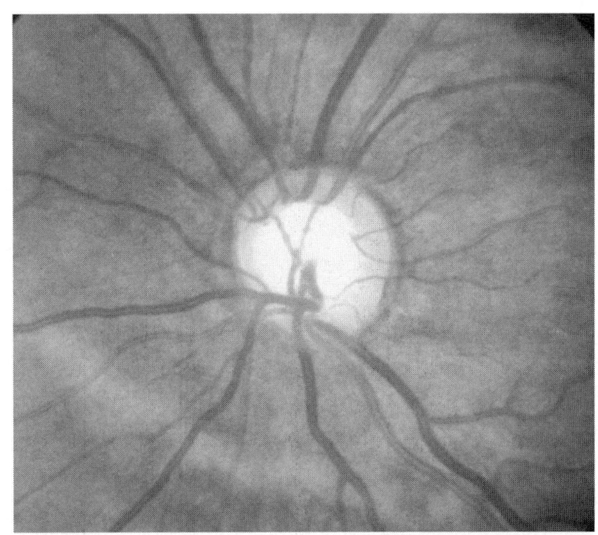

12-4A

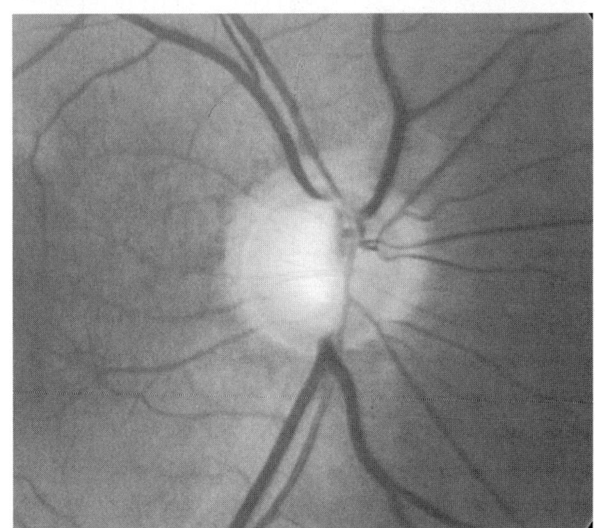

12-4B

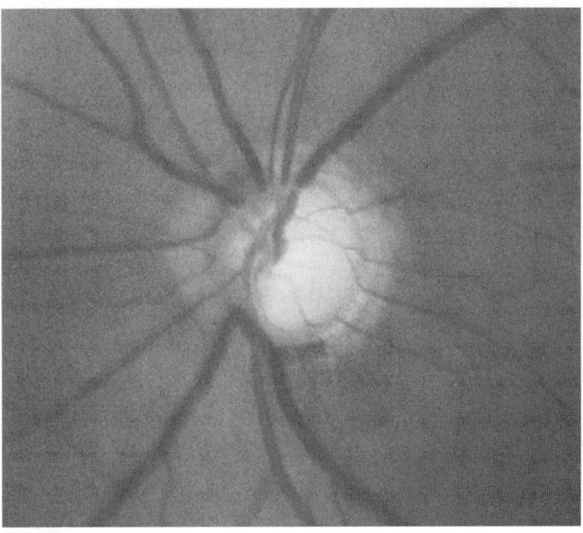

12-4C

Figure 12-4. A. **Glaucoma occurs more frequently as patients age. Remember to check the cup-to-disc ratio in older individuals. Notice the tigroid fundus changes as well as the enlarged cup-to-disc ratio. This older individual has glaucoma and should be referred to an ophthalmologist. The right** (B) **and left** (C) **disc of an older individual with glaucoma.**

The incidence of diabetes increases as people age. Remember that even younger individuals may have diabetes. If your patient is diabetic, carefully

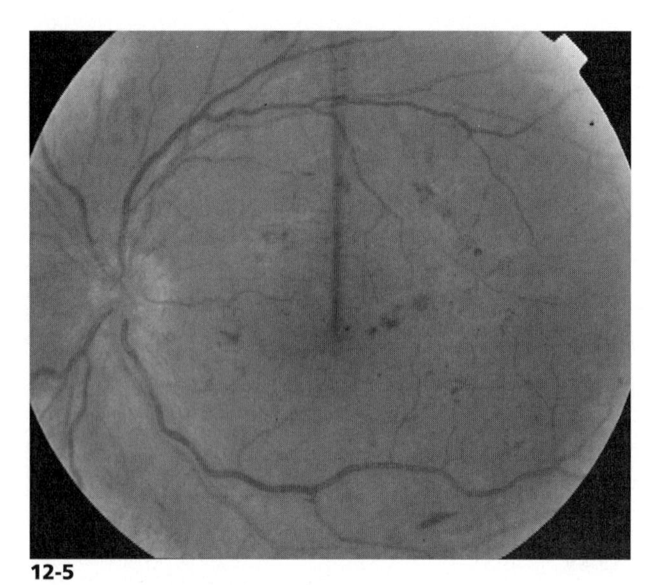

12-5

assess the retina for hemorrhages or cotton-wool spots. Review Chapters 6, 7, and 9 for how to look for these. All patients with a new diagnosis of diabetes should see an ophthalmologist. If retinopathy is present, the patient should be screened every 6 months.

Figure 12-5. Diabetes becomes more prevalent as individuals age. View the optic fundus in all of your diabetic patients. Here you see features that suggest early proliferative diabetic retinopathy.

Finally, macular degeneration occurs in the elderly and has a profound effect on the quality of life of an individual. Weih found that those individuals younger than 70 years were not likely to have visual impairment with age-related macular degeneration; however, the prevalence tripled by decade (1% in ages 70–79 but 16% in their 90s). This is certainly a disease of aging.[5] Because macular degeneration destroys central vision, everyday tasks like reading and driving are affected.

The most common symptom is blurring of the central vision, leading to difficulty with reading and seeing fine detail.

Ways to test for macular degeneration include first checking visual acuity. An Amsler's grid is also helpful.

Figure 12-6. A. The Amsler's grid is helpful in screening for macular degeneration in your office. See the use of the Amsler's grid in Chapter 10, Figure 10-5. Ask the patient to stare at the center dot to see if any of the lines are missing, absent, or distorted. In particular, macular degeneration affects the central area of the grid. B. Macular degeneration is one of the leading causes of blindness in the elderly. This individual was diagnosed with macular degeneration. Early on, the visual acuity was not severely affected. C. Three years later, however, this same individual had progressive macular changes with a fall in central visual acuity.

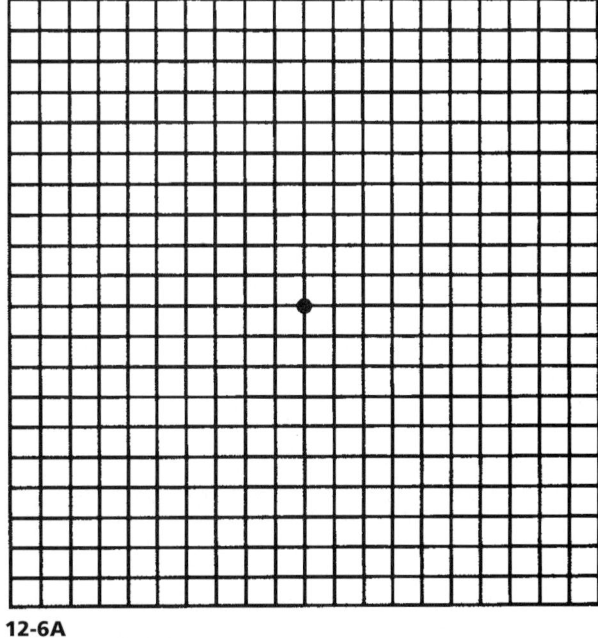

12-6A

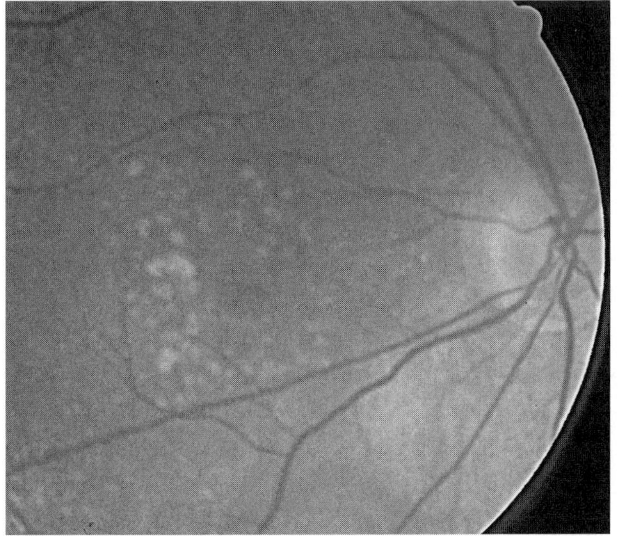

12-6B

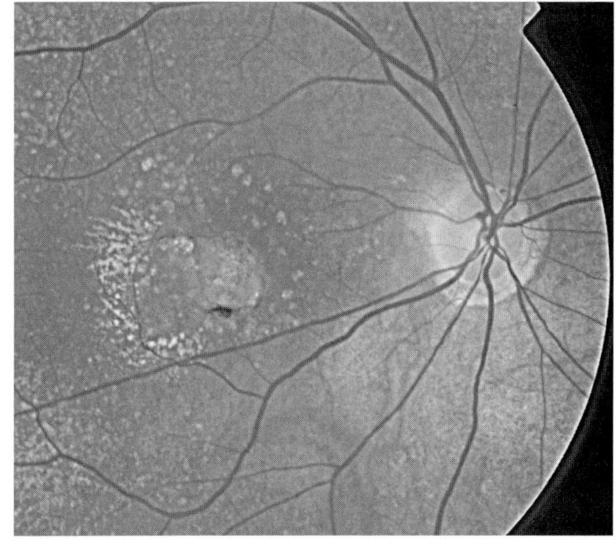

12-6C

Finally, be sure to dilate the pupil. The changes of the macula are visible only in a dilated state. Observe the macula as discussed in Chapter 10. Normal changes with aging include changes in the color of the retina and the presence of drusen. Interestingly, there may be extensive changes in the macula and little effect on the visual acuity. Look for drusen and any hemorrhages. Patients in whom you suspect macular pathology should be sent to an ophthalmologist for examination.

Other diseases of the macula can occur as a person ages, including myopic macular degeneration (see Figure 11-24) and macular hole. See Chapter 10, Figure 10-14.

Conditions of the Disc That Occur More Commonly with Aging

Although there are not age-specific causes of diseases of the disc, there are disc disorders that are more common with aging; these should be reviewed and refreshed by anyone who takes care of an older person.

Anterior ischemic optic neuropathy (AION) can occur in the young, but it is much more common in the older patient. Older individuals with hypertension and vascular disease are more likely to acquire this disc disorder. Aside from hypertension and diabetes, individuals with small cup-to-disc ratios are at risk for AION. In particular, the arteritic form is *specific* to the elderly, with few if any cases diagnosed in individuals younger than 65 years. Review the sections on AION—nonarteritic and arteritic (see Table 5-6)—for presentation and appearance.

Figure 12-7. A. Nonarteritic AION becomes more prevalent as individuals age. The patient typically presents with loss of visual acuity, a relative afferent pupillary defect, and a change in visual field. The disc is swollen. B. Arteritic AION is exclusively a disease of the older patient. Always suspect the arteritic form in patients older than 65 years. Westergren sedimentation rate, C-reactive protein, or both are important tests to order. A temporal artery biopsy should be performed if you suspect the arteritic form. C. A normal right disc with a large (0.6) cup-to-disc ratio. D. The chalky-white swollen disc obliterates the cup. The view is indistinct owing to cataract. This disc is typical of arteritic AION.

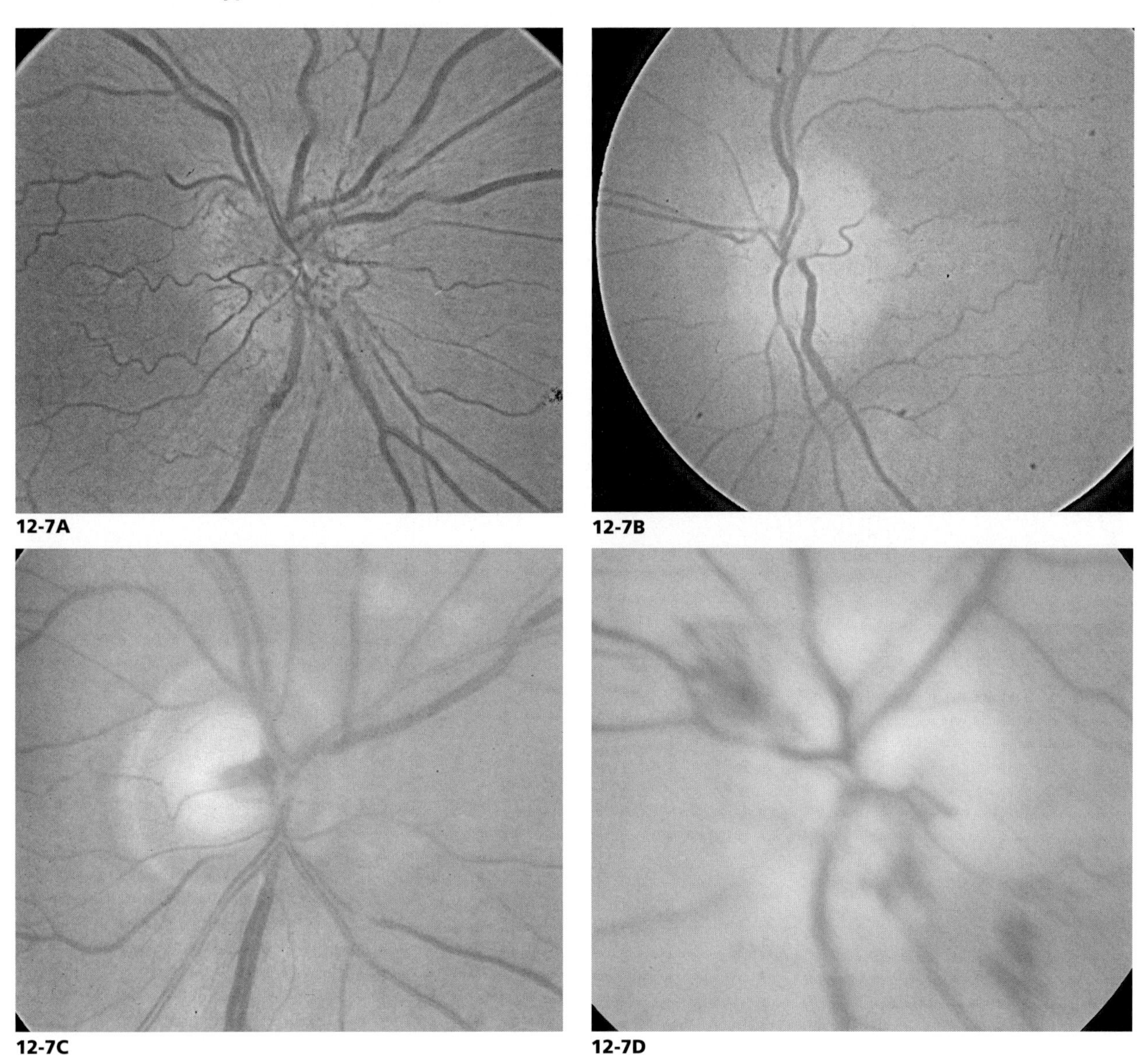

Central and branch retinal artery occlusions are more common in the elderly, and although less common than vein occlusion, are important to recognize as signs of significant systemic vascular disease that requires treatment.

Central retinal vein occlusion is common in older individuals. Look for accompanying glaucoma. See Chapter 5, Figure 5-27.

Finally, an eye specialist should evaluate the aging patient with visual complaints, because there are many treatable conditions causing vision loss.

Practical Viewing Essentials

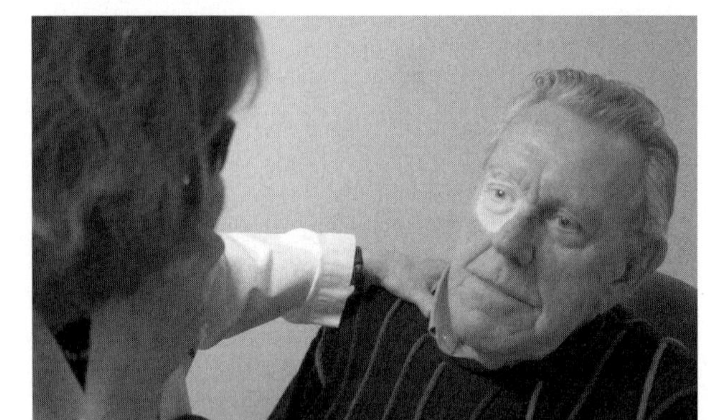

12-8

Figure 12-8. Use your ophthalmoscope to view the fundus in all of your older patients.

1. An eye specialist should see all aging patients with vision loss for diagnosis of treatable conditions from whatever cause, from acuity change to macular degeneration.
2. The common eye problems to recognize in aging patients are refractive error, cataract, macular degeneration, glaucoma, and diabetic retinopathy.
3. Vascular changes are important to recognize, including retinal artery and vein occlusion and ischemic optic neuropathy.
4. Arteritic AION is a disease that occurs only in patients older than 50 years.

References

1. Butler RN, Faye EE, Guazzo E, Kupfer C. Keeping an eye on vision. Primary care of age-related ocular disease. Geriatrics 1997;52:30–41.
2. Munoz B, West SK, Rubin GS, et al. Causes of blindness and visual impairment in a population of older Americans: The Salisbury Eye Evaluation Study. Arch Ophthalmol 2000;118(6):819–825.
3. Caird FI, Williamson J. The Eye and its Disorders in the Elderly. Bristol, UK: Wright, 1986.
4. Yoo SH, Adamis AP. Retinal manifestations of aging. Int Ophthalmol Clin 1998;38:95–101.
5. Weih LM, Van Newkirk MR, McCarty CA, Taylor HR. Age-specific causes of bilateral visual impairment. Arch Ophthalmol 2000;118:264–269.
6. Brodie SE. Aging and disorders of the eye. In JC Brocklehurst, RC Tallis, HM Fillit (eds), Textbook of Geriatric Medicine and Gerontology. Edinburgh, UK: Churchill Livingstone, 1992;472–479.
7. Millichamp NJ. Toxicity in specific ocular tissues. In GCY Chiou (ed), Ophthalmic Toxicology. Philadelphia: Taylor and Francis, 1999;43–87.

13 Viewing the Disc in Pregnancy

Of puerperal eclampsia Gowers said, "Moreover, even when other signs of uremia are absent, albuminuric retinitis often testifies to the intensity of the influence on the system exerted by renal disease."

William Gowers[1]

Figure 13-1.

Pregnancy causes a multitude of physiologic changes—hormonal, cardiovascular, immunologic, and metabolic—that can affect the possibility of visual disorders in pregnancy. Vascular disorders and neurologic disorders in pregnancy become more frequent because of this fact. Because the disc and the retina are key in the diagnosis of vascular events and changes, an ophthalmoscopic examination should be performed on all women who are pregnant.

Pregnancy itself does not change the disc, retina, or blood vessels in the eye. In fact, vision for the most part is unaffected in pregnancy except for some refractive changes owing to fluid shifts in the cornea and a decrease in intraocular pressure.

As far as we know, there are no neuro-ophthalmic changes in a normal pregnancy.

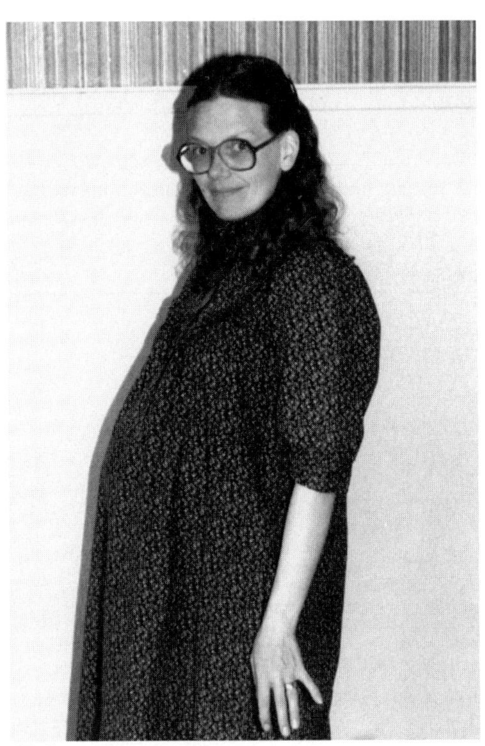

13-1

Table 13-1. Physiologic Changes of Pregnancy

Change	Effect	Possible pathology
Cardiovascular	Cardiac output increases 30–50%	Hyperdynamic system—underlying cardiac or vascular disease may worsen
	Blood volume increases 30–50%	
	Blood pressure decreases in pregnancy	
Pulmonary	Increased respiratory rate	
Renal	Increased renal blood flow	
Gastrointestinal	Decreased motility	
Hematologic	Decreased hematocrit; decreased platelets	Anemia
Coagulation factors	Increased plasminogen, fibrinogen, factors VII, VIII, IX, X	Tendency toward hypercoagulability
Hormonal changes	High estrogen	

Source: Adapted in part from reference 3.

Table 13-2. Physiologic Changes of the Eye in Pregnancy

Change	Complaint	Etiology
Alterations in cornea	Unable to wear contacts; blurred vision	Changes in corneal thickness and sensitivity
Intraocular pressure	Reduced intraocular pressure	Improvement of outflow aqueous
Accommodation	Can't read well at near	Changes in accommodation related to pregnancy and lactation

Source: Adapted in part from JS Sunness. The pregnant woman's eye. Surv Ophthalmol 1988;32:219–238.

Physiologic Changes during Labor

During labor, an extra 500 cc of blood is infused to the maternal circulation with each contraction. Furthermore, in approximately one-third of women who "push" in the second stage of labor, intracranial pressure rises.[2]

Postpartum Physiologic Changes

After delivery, there is a profound diuresis within 2 weeks. Furthermore, there is a decrease in fibrinolysis and a slight increase in clotting factors, making this portion of parturition particularly prone to thrombosis.

What Should You Notice in Every Pregnant Woman's Eye?

On the first visit, check visual acuity and look at the optic disc. Note the shape and size of the disc, if there is a cup, and if the disc is normal in color. Are there venous pulsations? Note that there is no sign of disc swelling. Note the size and caliber of the retinal vessels.

Knowing the systemic changes and changes in the eye, what conditions are more frequent in pregnancy because of these systemic changes? What clues can we get from viewing the fundus of the eyes?

Table 13-3. Ophthalmoscopic Findings to Be on the Lookout for in Pregnant Women

Finding	What to look for	Why are you looking?
Normal fundus	Look for a normal fundus on the first day's visit. Document the normal findings: shape and color of the disc; retinal vessels; venous pulsations.	If there is a change, you will know about it.
Optic disc swelling	Hyperemia that develops, elevation, swelling of the nerve fiber layer, hemorrhages, exudates.	Early signs of intracranial pathology such as brain tumor, idiopathic intracranial hypertension, venous thrombosis.
Optic nerve pallor	Loss of nerve fiber layer, new pallor of the disc.	Optic neuritis.
Optic disc hemorrhage	Hemorrhage on the disc.	Early glaucoma.
Retinal vessels	Narrowing; spasm of vessels.	Early signs of severe pre-eclampsia.
Retina	In diabetics, look for hemorrhages or exudates.	Refer regularly to ophthalmologist for full evaluation.

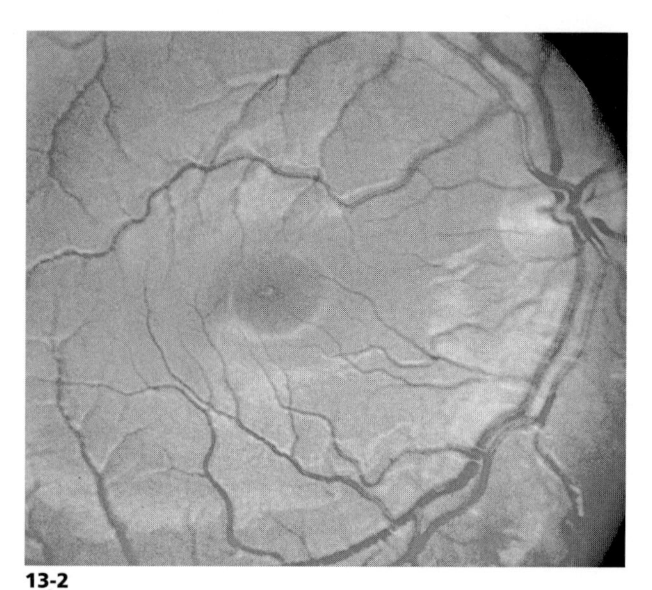

13-2

Figure 13-2. Although obstetricians often have remarked on "retinal sheen" in evaluating pregnant women who are believed to have eclampsia, retinal sheen is normal in healthy-appearing young adult retinas. Retinal sheen is the reflection off of the internal limiting membrane. This photograph is from a 12-year-old boy and shows retinal sheen. By itself, it is not pathologic.

Review the chapters on optic disc swelling (Chapter 3), optic pallor (Chapter 4), vascular abnormalities (Chapter 5), and retinal changes (Chapter 9).

Because pregnancy is a somewhat hypercoagulable, hyperdynamic vascular state, neurovascular events can occur.

Table 13-4. Vascular Conditions with Increased Frequency in Pregnancy

Condition	Symptoms	What to look for	Diagnosis
Stroke: Branch retinal artery occlusion; central retinal artery occlusion	Sudden onset of a spot in the vision that does not go away	Follow the central retinal artery through the branches; visual field	Fluorescein angiogram; blood tests for hypercoagulability—proteins C and S, Factor V Leiden, homocysteine
Stroke: Apoplexy	Sudden vision loss and headache	Visual field abnormalities—discs may be normal initially	MR shows hemorrhage in the pituitary gland
Venous sinus thrombosis	Headache, obscuration of vision; seizure	Papilledema	MR and MR venography shows venous sinus occlusion
Subarachnoid hemorrhage	Sudden onset of "worst headache"	Vitreal hemorrhage	Computed tomography looking for blood; MR angiography or angiogram to look for aneurysm
AVM leakage	Sudden headache; seizure; hemiparesis	Vitreal hemorrhage	MR or computed tomography of brain

AVM = arterioventricular malfunction.
Source: Adapted from reference 3.

Table 13-5. Causes of Acute Vascular Events in Pregnancy

- Arterial occlusive disease
  - Thrombotic cause
    - Atherosclerotic
    - Fibromuscular dysplasia
  - Embolic source
    - Cardiac
      - Peripartum cardiomyopathy
      - Mitral valve prolapse
      - Rheumatic heart disease
      - Endocarditis (bacterial and nonbacterial)
      - Paradoxical embolus (Patent foramen ovale)
    - Amniotic/air embolism
- Venous occlusive disease
  - Hypercoagulable state
  - Infection
- Drug abuse—cocaine, sympathomimetics
- Hypotensive disorders
- Watershed infarction
- Sheehan's pituitary necrosis
- Hematologic disorders
  - Lupus anticoagulant
  - Thrombocytopenic purpura
  - Sickle cell disease
  - Protein C, antithrombin III, protein S deficiencies; homocysteine elevation
  - Factor V Leiden mutation
- Arteritis
  - Systemic lupus erythematosus
  - Infectious arteritis (syphilis, tuberculosis, meningococcal)
  - Cerebral angiitis
  - Takayasu's arteritis
- Intracerebral hemorrhage
  - Eclampsia and hypertensive disorders
  - Venous thrombosis
  - Choriocarcinoma
  - Arteriovenous malformation
  - Vasculitis
- Subarachnoid hemorrhage
  - Aneurysm (saccular, mycotic)
  - Arteriovenous malformation (cerebral, spinal cord)
  - Eclampsia
  - Vasculitis
  - Choriocarcinoma
  - Venous thrombosis
- Other
  - Carotid cavernous fistula
  - Dural vascular malformation

Source: Adapted in part from reference 3.

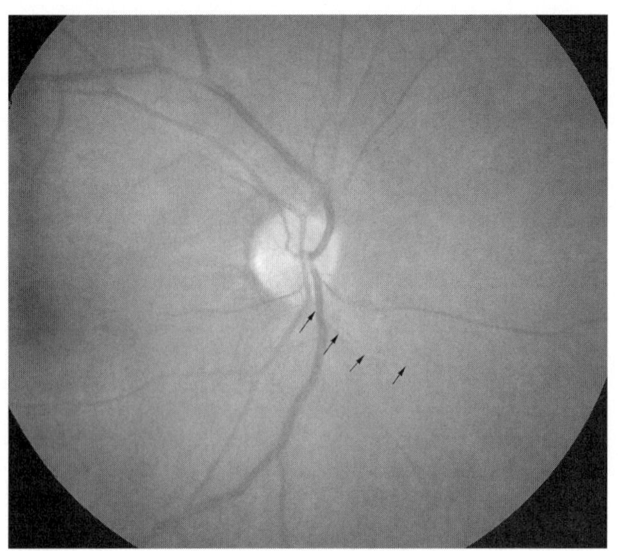

13-3A

Figure 13-3. A,B. **This 28-year-old gravida 1, para 0 woman had a sudden spot in her vision that did not go away. Her fundus examination** (A) **showed a branch retinal artery occlusion (*arrows*). The visual field showed a large corresponding defect in the right eye.** B. **An extensive evaluation for an embolic source, including carotid ultrasonography and esophageal echocardiogram, were normal. Blood work for hypercoagulable state (e.g., proteins C, S; antithrombin III; antiphospholipid antibodies; homocysteine, factor V Leiden; platelets and fibrinogen) was unrevealing. The visual field persisted. She did well on aspirin without any further event.**

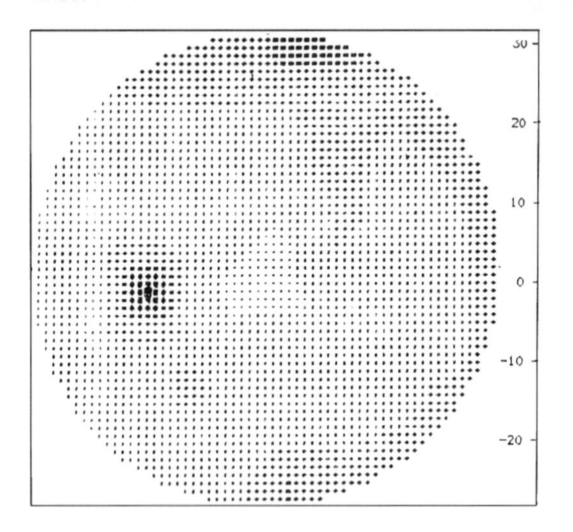

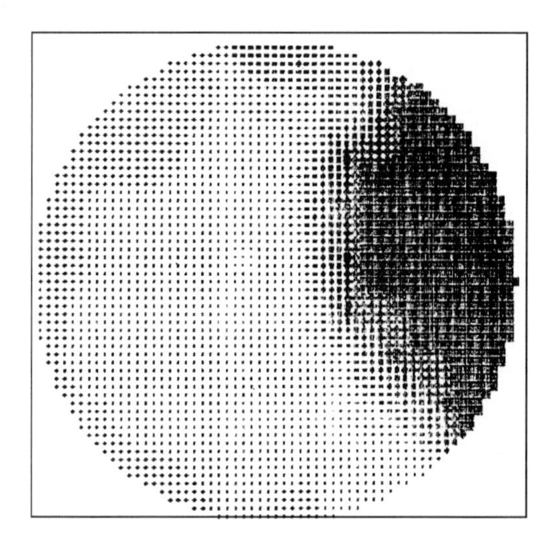

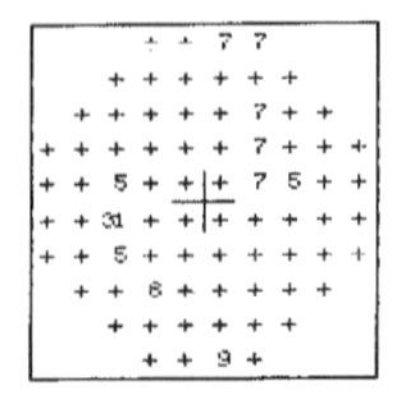

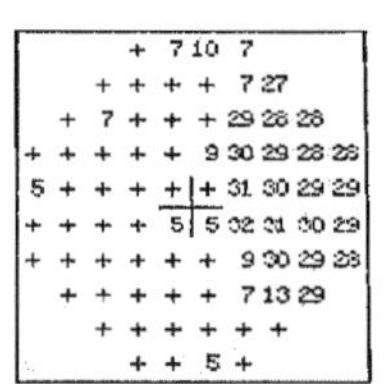

13-3B

Figure 13-4. This woman also had a sudden spot in her vision. A. **A small embolus was found near the macula (*arrow*).** B. **A small visual field defect was detected centrally. An equally extensive evaluation showed a patent foramen ovale. She was placed on aspirin and did well without further events.**

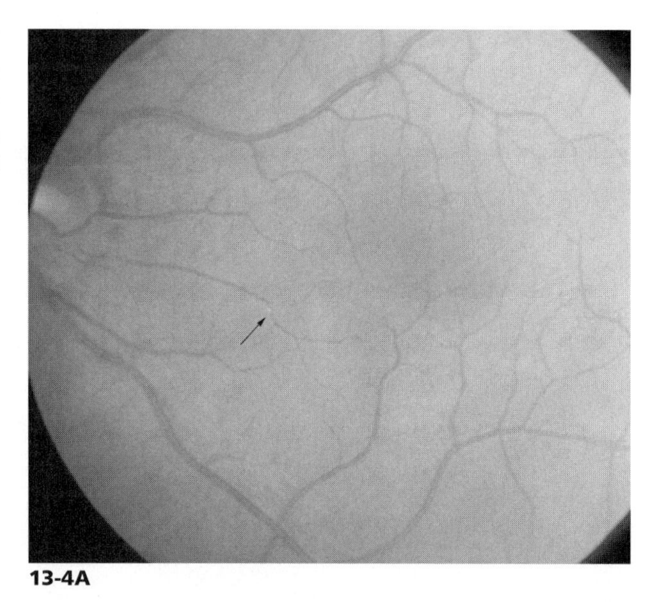

13-4A

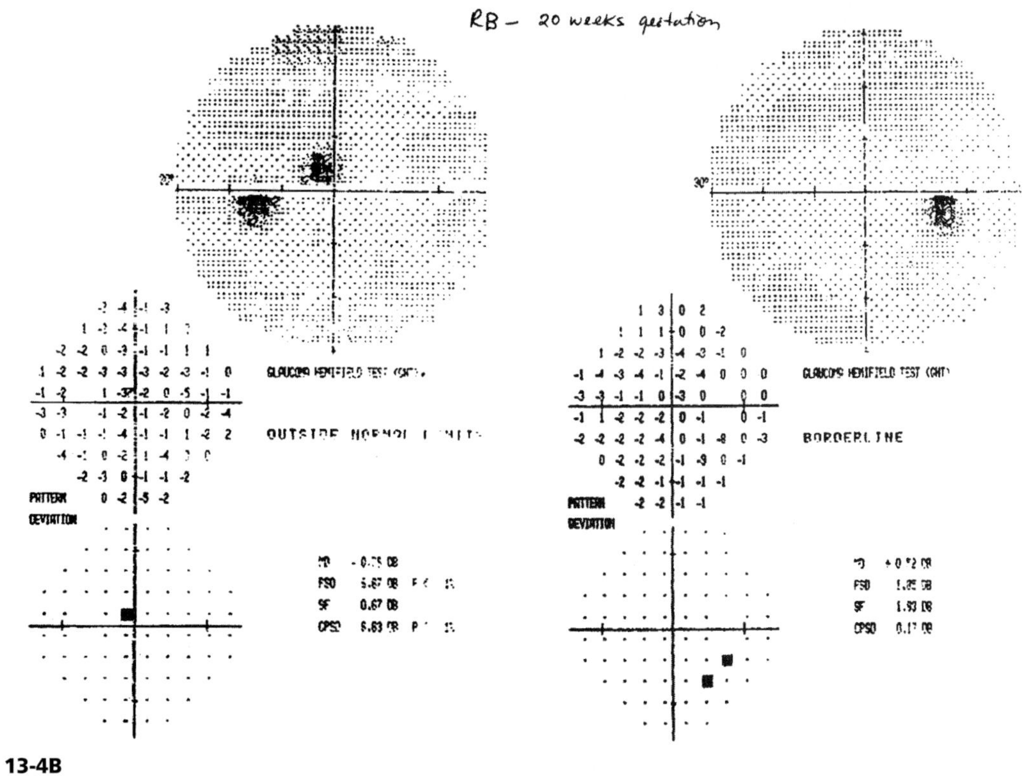

13-4B

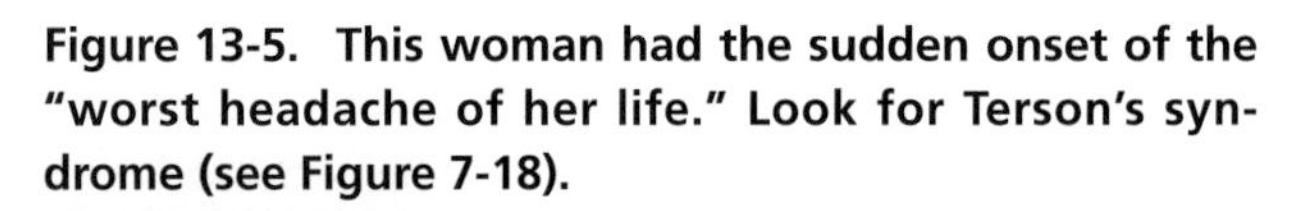

Figure 13-5. This woman had the sudden onset of the "worst headache of her life." Look for Terson's syndrome (see Figure 7-18).

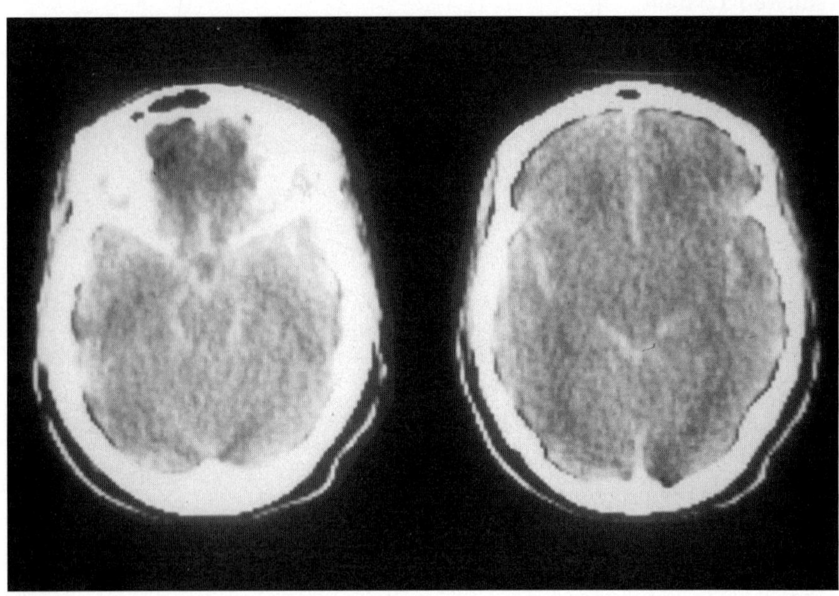

13-5

Venous sinus occlusion in pregnancy and postpartum is not rare. Although traditionally thought to be more frequent in the postpartum time, venous sinus occlusion can occur at any time during pregnancy. Dural sinus thrombosis and deep cerebral vein thrombosis have both been reported in pregnancy.

Table 13-6. Comparing Dural and Cerebral Venous Sinus Thrombosis

	Dural venous sinus thrombosis	Deep cerebral venous thrombosis
Occurs in pregnancy	++	+
Symptoms	Seizure, headache, visual blurring	Seizure, headache, coma
Signs	Focal deficits	Focal deficits; coma
Funduscopic findings	Papilledema or normal	May be normal initially
Findings on magnetic resonance	Look for venous abnormality in dural sinuses	Look at the thalamus and deep brain structures
Outcome	Good if recognized and treated	Often fatal because not diagnosed quickly

+ = can occur, less common; ++ = more common.
Source: Adapted from reference 4.

Figure 13-6. This 24-year-old woman who was at 30 weeks' gestation complained of headaches to her obstetrician. She then developed transient monocular/ binocular blindness. Only after an ophthalmoscopic examination weeks later was papilledema discovered (A, right eye; B, left eye). A thorough evaluation, including MR venography, showed that she had venous thrombosis of her sagittal (C) and transverse venous sinuses (D) (*arrows*). Compare the normal sinus on the right (*arrow*) with the absent sinus on the left (*arrow*). She was treated with subcutaneous heparin for the duration of her pregnancy. A protein C deficiency was eventually detected.

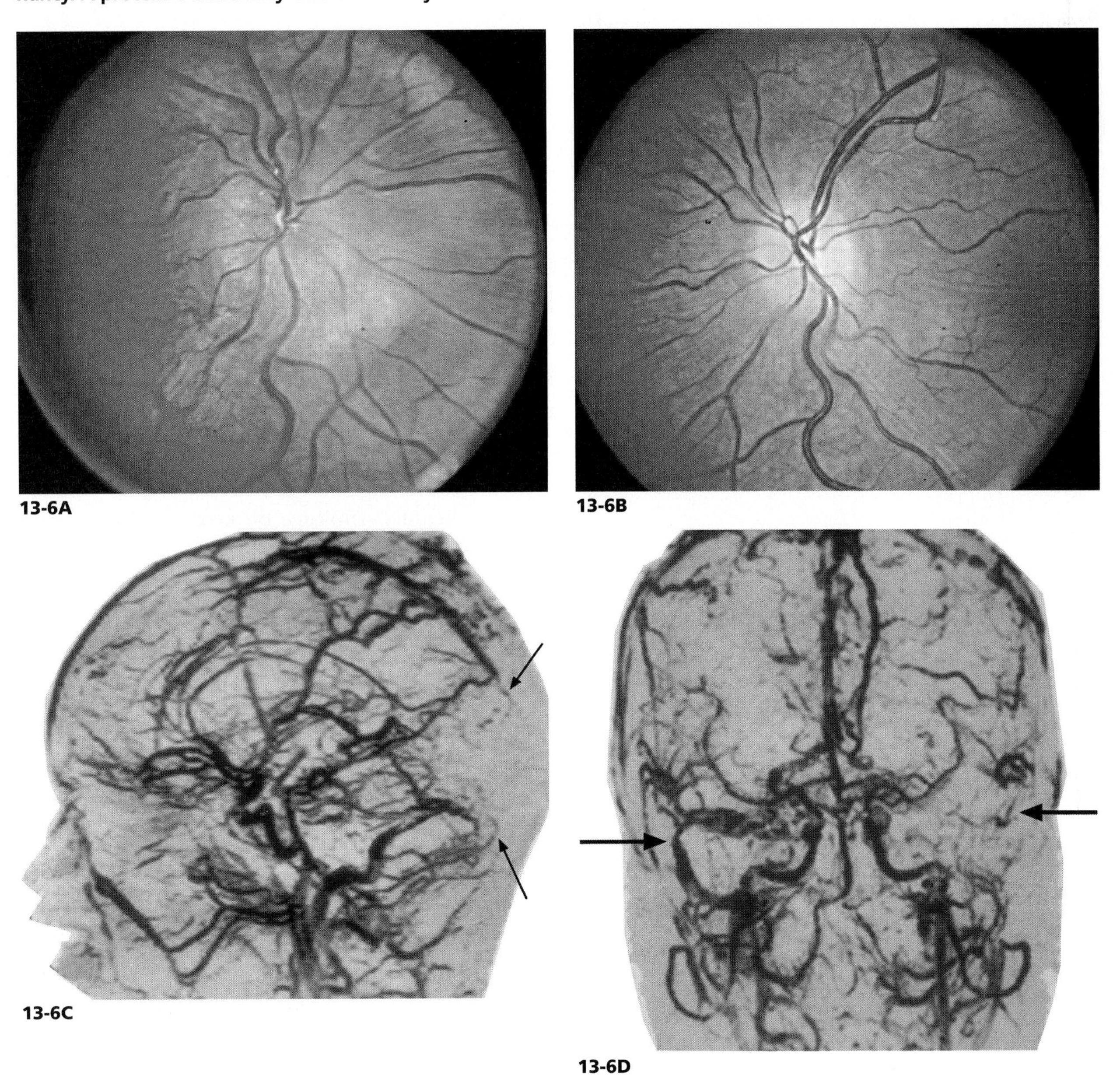

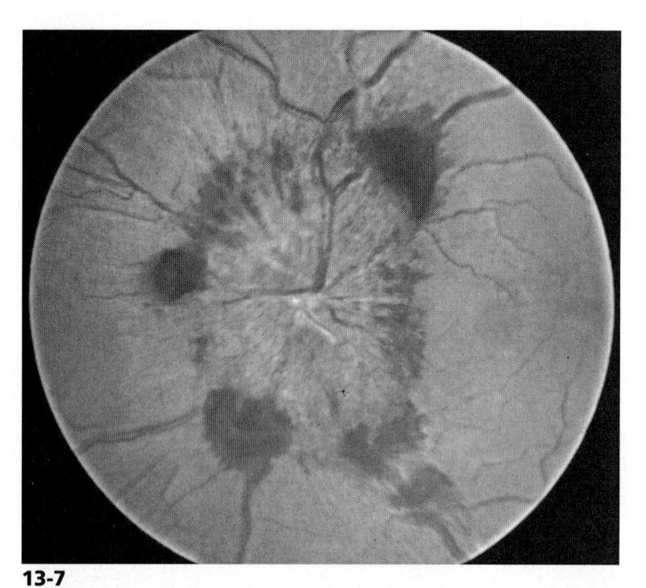

13-7

Figure 13-7. This 26-year-old woman was 3 weeks postpartum when she began having headaches. Her obstetrician recognized papilledema, and after appropriate evaluation, venous thrombosis was found. She was treated with warfarin without further consequence. She had significant papilledema, which resolved after treatment with anticoagulants.

Conditions in Pregnancy That May Affect the Fundus

Headache is probably the most common neurologic complaint in pregnancy. Most of the time, the headache is a benign, primary headache disorder such as migraine or tension headache, and does not signify significant pathology. Be alert to characteristics of the history and examination of the eye, which give you a clue to the diagnosis (see Table 13-7).

Special conditions in pregnancy include *diabetes.* Patients who have retinopathy at the time of pregnancy have a high likelihood of worsening retinopathy during pregnancy. This must be taken into consideration in following pregnant diabetic women.

Retinopathy is found in approximately one-fourth of pregnant women who are diabetic. If nonproliferative retinopathy is present in the beginning of pregnancy, progression occurs in approximately 10%.[5] If the pregnant woman has proliferative retinopathy, however, progression is seen in approximately one-fourth.[5,6]

Table 13-7. Differential Diagnosis of Headache in Pregnancy

Headache source	Headache characteristic	History	Examination	Fundus examination	Evaluation
Migraine with or without aura	Throbbing with photo/phonophobia; nausea ± vomiting; aura precedes the headache	Family history; previous migraine; car sickness	Normal eye and neurologic examination	Normal disc; look for venous pulsations	None
Tension	Tight, bandlike pain	May have family history of migraine; worse as the day goes on	Normal eye and neurologic examination	Normal—venous pulsations	None
Increased intracranial pressure (idiopathic intracranial hypertension, venous thrombosis, tumor)	Daily headache; may be frontal or occipital; may have "whooshing noises" in head; awaken at night; worse with cough	Other neurologic complaints: seizure, focal weakness	May see focal neurologic deficits	Papilledema; loss of venous pulsations	Magnetic resonance scan of brain; if normal, lumbar puncture to assess opening pressure
Subarachnoid hemorrhage; intracranial hemorrhage	Sudden onset of "worst headache"	Lethargy; coma	May see focal deficit; check visual fields	Look for vitreal hemorrhage (Terson's syndrome)	Computed tomography scan
Severe preeclampsia/eclampsia	Spots in the vision; headache and spots concurrent	Swelling, headache	Hyperreflexia; abnormalities on Amsler's grid	Arterial narrowing; focal narrowing of vessels	Magnetic resonance scan shows characteristic curvilinear abnormalities at the gray-white junction of the parietal/occipital lobe

Multiple sclerosis and *optic neuritis* can occur during pregnancy because both occur in women of childbearing age. The evaluation should proceed as in the nonpregnant state.

PITUITARY TUMORS IN PREGNANCY

The pituitary increases in size during pregnancy. If there is an undiagnosed pituitary adenoma, the adenoma can be come symptomatic in pregnancy. Macroadenomas are more likely to be symptomatic in pregnancy (approximately 35% of the time), versus microadenomas (only 5%).[7] The disc may show band atrophy or pallor.

OTHER TUMORS IN PREGNANCY

Meningiomas and gliomas may become symptomatic in pregnancy. The woman may present with focal neurologic deficits or headache and papilledema.

A tumor specific to pregnancy is choriocarcinoma, which is rare, but presents as brain metastases with increased intracranial pressure (possible papilledema), as a subarachnoid hemorrhage, and as possible Terson's syndrome.[7]

IDIOPATHIC INTRACRANIAL HYPERTENSION IN PREGNANCY

Idiopathic intracranial hypertension is a condition of obese women in their childbearing years. The diagnosis is established by symptoms (e.g., headache, diplopia) and signs (e.g., papilledema, sixth nerve palsy) of intracranial hypertension without other localizing findings (hemiparesis). Imaging studies (magnetic resonance [MR], including a normal MR venography to rule out venous thrombosis) are totally normal. A lumbar puncture is essential to not only establish elevated cerebrospinal fluid pressure (>250 mm CSF), but to be sure that protein, glucose, and cells are normal. Although pregnancy has been thought to be a provoking factor for the condition, studies have shown that the prevalence parallels the age of the women with the condition.[8] Evaluation of papilledema should be as in the nonpregnancy state. Weight gain should be limited. If vision loss ensues, an optic nerve sheath fenestration is the preferred treatment when medical treatment fails.[9]

Figure 13-8. This woman had idiopathic intracranial hypertension during pregnancy. Her optic discs remained swollen throughout the pregnancy. She delivered without problems. Later when she lost weight, her discs returned to normal. A, **right eye;** B, **left eye.**

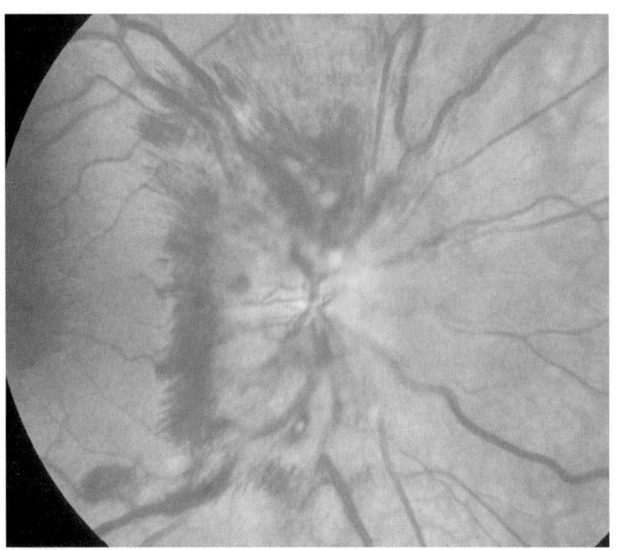

13-8A

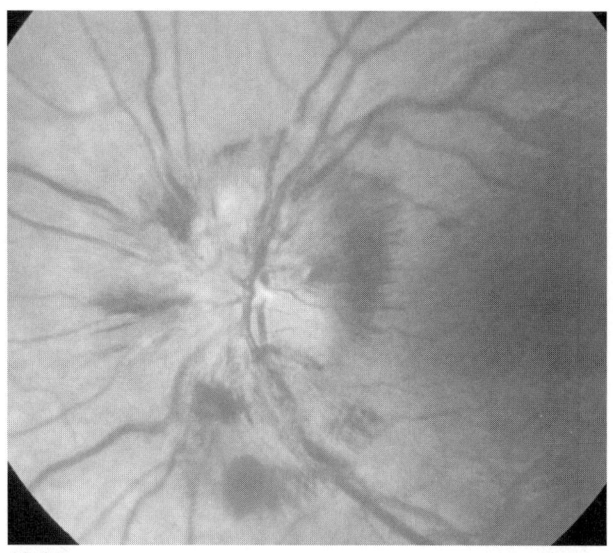

13-8B

Pregnancy-Specific Conditions Having an Effect on the Optic Nerve and Fundus—Severe Pre-Eclampsia and Eclampsia

Severe pre-eclampsia and eclampsia are pregnancy-specific conditions characterized clinically by elevated blood pressure, peripheral swelling, altered liver function tests, and proteinuria. Severe pre-eclampsia has the aforementioned features, and eclampsia has the same features plus a seizure or coma. Visual complaints are very frequent. In fact, *eclampsia* comes from the Greek word meaning "to

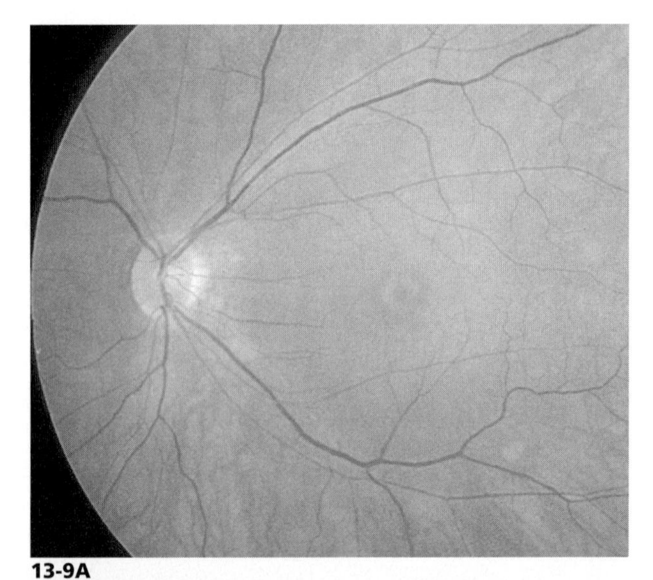

13-9A

shine forth," referring to the visual phenomenon reported frequently with this condition.

Severe pre-eclampsia and eclampsia are more common in patients with underlying hypertension. Look for retinal signs of hypertension in all women with pregnancies.[10]

Figure 13-9. A. **This 38-year-old gravida 2, para 1 woman had systemic hypertension throughout her pregnancy. Notice the diffuse arterial narrowing.** B. **Others may show A-V nicking (*arrow*).** C. **Even nerve fiber layer hemorrhages and cotton-wool spots (*arrows*) may be seen in women with superimposed hypertension in pregnancy (review Chapter 9, Figure 9-23).**

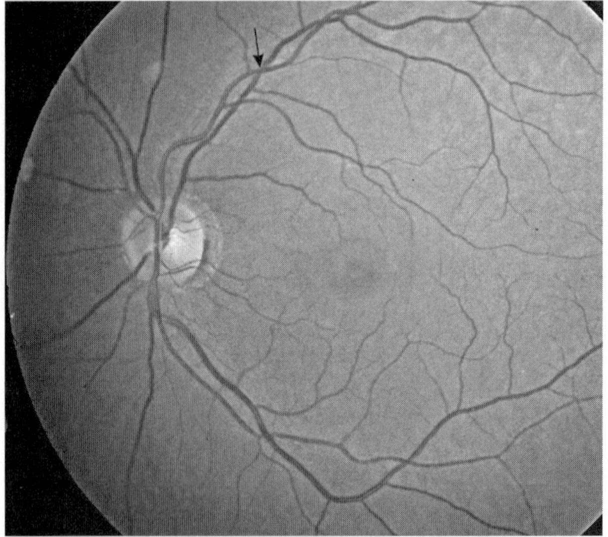

13-9B

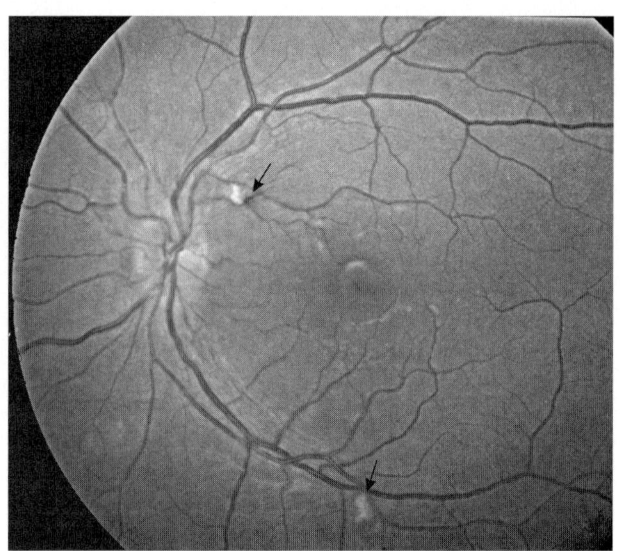

13-9C

There are multiple sites in the visual system that can be affected in severe pre-eclampsia or eclampsia.

Vision loss in severe pre-eclampsia and eclampsia may be from any of the previously mentioned sites. The most common findings on ophthalmoscopic examination are abnormalities of the retina, the retinal vasculature, and the optic disc. The retinal findings of severe pre-eclampsia and eclampsia are owing to acute hypertension. First, there is vascular narrowing or focal vascular narrowing. Peripapillary hemorrhages may be present.

Table 13-8. Causes of Vision Loss in Severe Pre-Eclampsia and Eclampsia

Source	Symptom	Ophthalmoscopic finding	Evaluation	Diagnosis
Retina	Blurred vision	Nerve fiber hemorrhage; cotton-wool spots; arterial narrowing; hypertensive retinopathy; serous retinal detachment	Amsler's grid abnormalities	Fluorescein angiogram showing leakage; dilated ophthalmoscopic evaluation by ophthalmologist/retinal specialist
Choroid	Blurred vision; spots	May see little; changes in color vision; Elschnig's spot	Amsler's grid may be abnormal	Fluorescein angiogram
Optic nerve—Papilledema	Transient visual obscuration	Papilledema	MR imaging, light perception for opening pressure and cells	MR, MR venography; lumbar puncture
Ischemic optic neuropathy	Loss of vision—one eye	Swollen disc—unilateral	Visual field	
Central retinal artery spasm	Loss of vision—one eye	Vasoconstriction of the arteries	Amsler's grid, visual field	Clinical; possible fluorescein angiogram
Brain—Migraine-like symptoms	Spots in front of the eyes	Normal	Normal examination	Clinical; possible MR if focal findings
Brain—Cortical blindness	Blindness; achromatopsia, prosopagnosia, Balint's syndrome	Normal	Visual field abnormalities	Brain MR shows characteristic changes

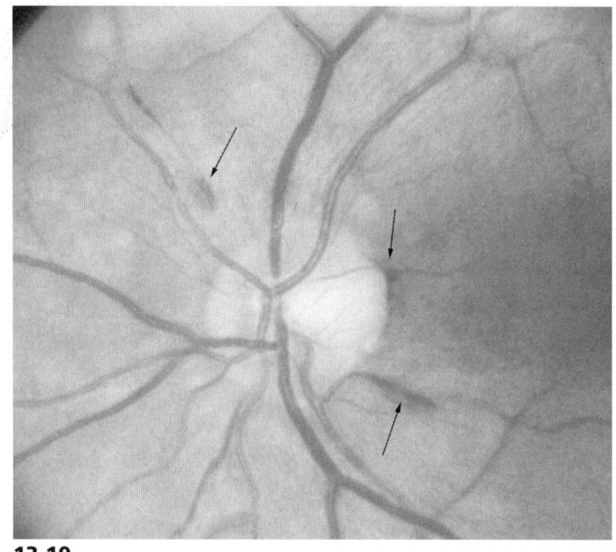

13-10

Figure 13-10. This previously normotensive woman developed severe pre-eclampsia and blurred vision. Ophthalmoscopic examination showed nerve fiber layer hemorrhages around her disc (*arrows*). After delivery, her symptoms resolved. Her disc and peripapillary retina returned to normal.

If the hypertension is severe enough, choroidal changes—in the form of infarction—from microvascular disease may cause a yellow spot from the choroid (an Elschnig's spot). These lesions are hard to see, and frequently fluorescein angiography is required to view them. Anton Elschnig first described these spots (see also Chapters 5 and 9).

Figure 13-11. A,B. **This 28-year-old prima gravida had severe pre-eclampsia and visual blurring. Dilated examination revealed subtle changes in the choroid, sometimes referred to as *Elschnig's spots*. Note that they are hard to see (the *arrows* in** A **point to a few of them).** C,D. **Fluorescein angiogram shows the defect well in the choroid. The arrows in** C **point to a few of the defects. This examination revealed choroidal infarction and staining. Elschnig's spots are really infarctions in the choroid.**

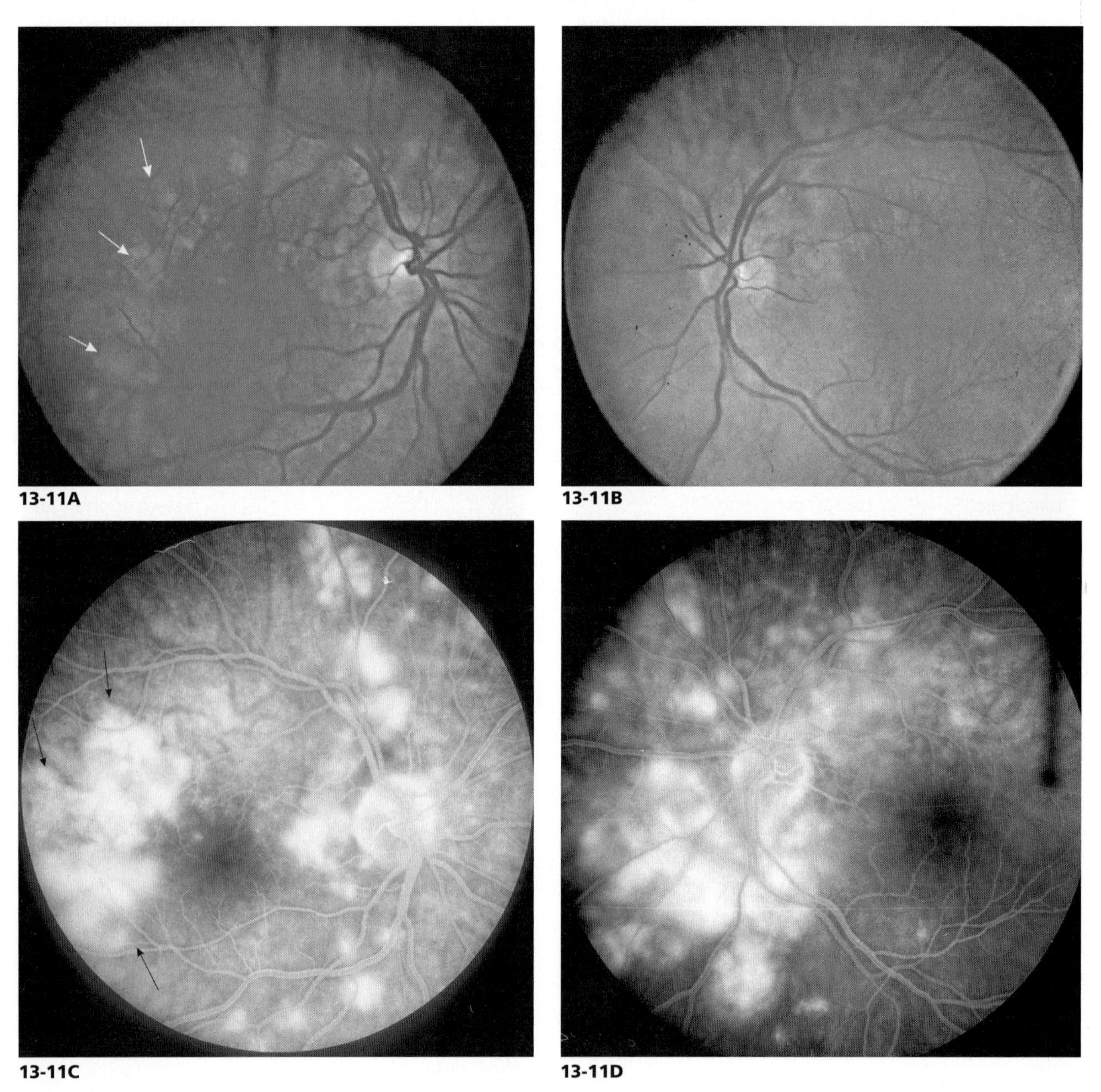

13-11A **13-11B**

13-11C **13-11D**

If the choroid infarcts, fluid escapes under the retina, forming serous retinal detachments. These look like a "blister" or a sheet of plastic food wrap bubbled around the peripapillary area. The Amsler's grid is abnormal and you may see the serous detachment by viewing the peripapillary area with the ophthalmoscope. Fluorescein angiography is helpful in viewing the choroidal changes.

Figure 13-12. A. **This woman developed severe preeclampsia and complained of blurred vision. She had changes in her Amsler's grid. Ophthalmoscopy showed a serous retinal detachment (*arrows*).** B. **The fluorescein confirmed leakage of fluid around the disc and leakage of dye from choroidal infarctions. Arrows demarcate the edge of the serous detachment. (Photographs from reference 11, with permission.)**

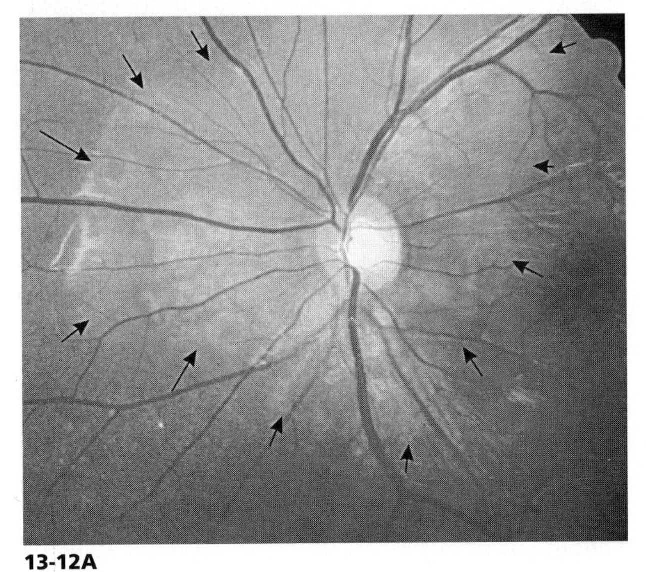

13-12A

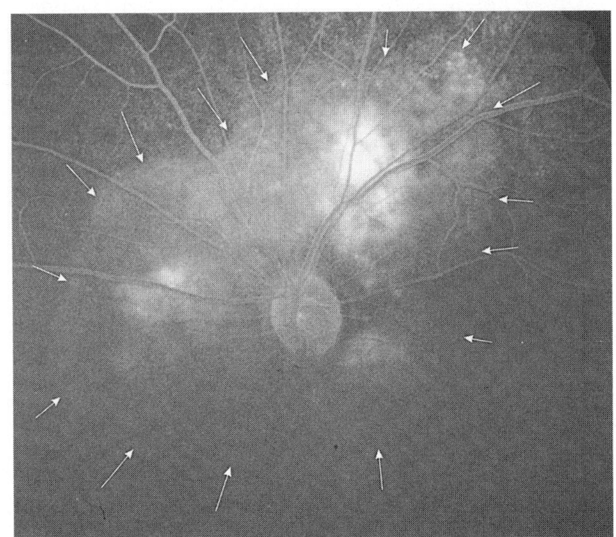

13-12B

Vascular narrowing and focal arterial stenosis can be seen on the arterial vessels as they leave the disc.

Figure 13-13. A,B. **This woman had severe pre-eclampsia and blurred vision. Acutely before delivery, her inferior retinal artery shows vasospastic changes (*arrows,* A) photographed with a hand-held Kowa fundus camera that resolved after delivery** (B)**. Similar changes were seen in the contralateral eye.**

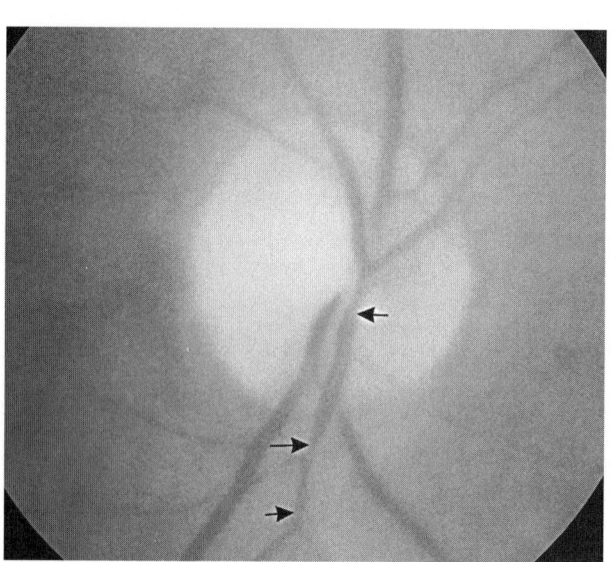

13-13A

13-13B

On occasion in severe pre-eclampsia and eclampsia, the optic disc may be swollen—either from ischemic optic neuropathy or owing to increased intracranial pressure. Be sure to review other causes of papilledema, however, including venous thrombosis.

Imaging in severe pre-eclampsia and eclampsia is helpful because there are frequently characteristic curvilinear signals on the MR–spin echo and T2-weighted images in the parietal-occipital junction. Interestingly, a patient with Amsler's grid findings (and changes on the funduscopic examination) predicted abnormalities on MR.[11]

Figure 13-14. A. **This woman suffered a generalized tonic-clonic seizure after reporting difficulty seeing. The typical MR findings in eclampsia include T2 curvilinear signals at the gray-white junction in the parietal-occipital lobes. In addition, there are signals in the basal ganglia. All of these changes resolved after delivery when the patient became normotensive.** B. **The typical features of MR in severe pre-eclampsia are summarized in this diagram.** C. **The MR findings correlate nicely with what is known to occur pathologically within the brain. This diagram represents the reported pathologic changes. (Reprinted with permission from reference 12.)**

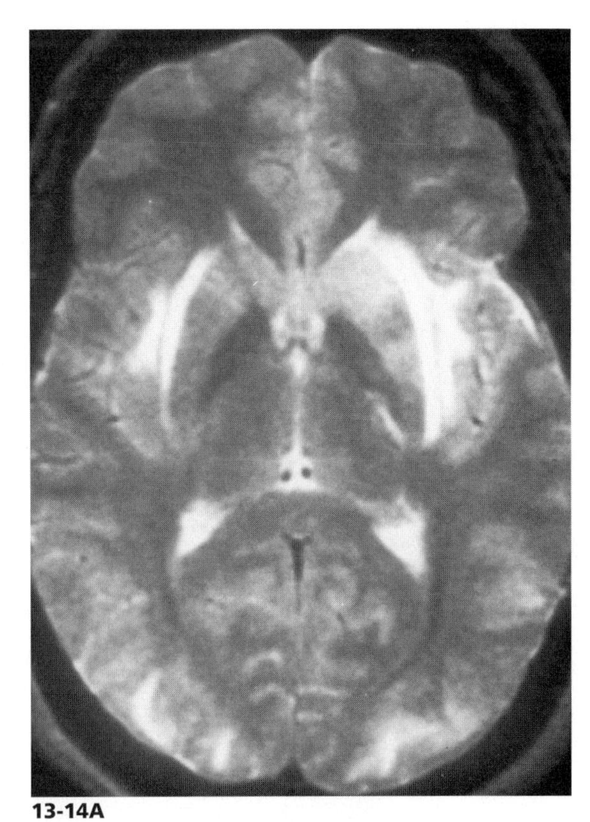

13-14A

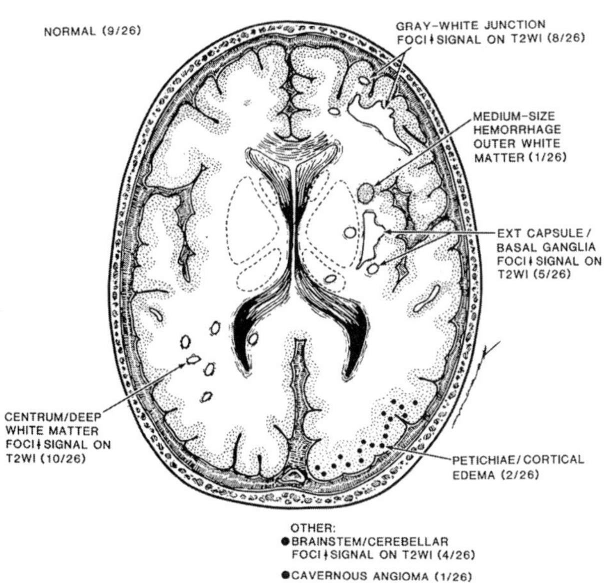

13-14B

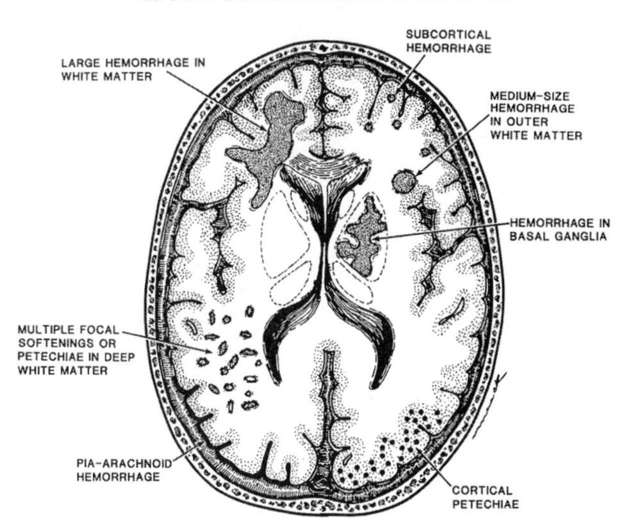

13-14C

Practical Viewing Essentials

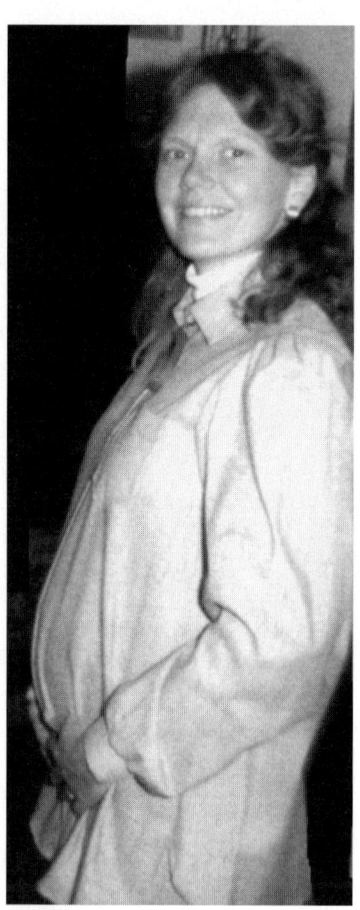
13-15

Figure 13-15.

1. Practice looking at the pregnant woman's eye because the eyes may be a clue to an underlying condition.
2. Verify a normal optic nerve, fundus, and vascular examination on the first visit.
3. Watch for signs of papilledema, vascular narrowing, and optic disc pallor.
4. In a diabetic, be aware of progression of diabetes.
5. Look for specific retinal findings in all pregnant women with pre-eclampsia.
6. Take complaints of visual changes seriously in women who are pregnant. Refer for further evaluation if there is any doubt in your examination.

References

1. Gowers WR. A Manual of Diseases of the Nervous System (2nd ed). Darien, CT: Hafner, 1970.
2. McCausland AM, Holmes F. Spinal fluid pressure during labor. West J Surg Obstet Gynecol 1957;65: 220–233.
3. Digre KB, Varner MW. Diagnosis and Treatment of Cerebrovascular Disorders in Pregnancy. In HP Adams (ed), Handbook of Cerebrovascular Diseases. New York: Marcel Dekker, 1993;258.
4. Crawford S, Digre KB, Palmer CA, et al. Thrombosis of the deep venous drainage of the brain in adults. Arch Neurol 1995;52:1101–1108.
5. Rodman HM, Singerman U, Aiello LM, Merkatz IR. Diabetic Retinopathy and Its Relationship to Pregnancy. In IR Merkatz, PA Adam (eds), The Diabetic Pregnancy: A Perinatal Perspective. New York: Grune & Stratton, 1979;73–91.
6. Klein BE, Moss SE, Klein R. Effects of pregnancy on progression of diabetic retinopathy. Diabetes Care 1990;132:34–40.
7. Donaldson JO. Neurology of Pregnancy. London: Saunders, 1989.
8. Digre KB, Varner M, Corbett JJ. Pseudotumor cerebri in pregnancy. Neurology 1984;34(6):721–729.
9. Digre KB, Corbett JJ. Idiopathic intracranial hypertension: a reappraisal. The Neurologist, 2001.
10. Jaffe G, Schatz H. Ocular manifestations of preeclampsia. Am J Ophthalmol 1987;103:309–315.
11. Digre KB, Varner MW. Pregnancy. In Gold DH, Weingeist TA (eds), The Eye in Systemic Disease. Philadelphia: J.B. Lippincott, 1990.
12. Digre KB, Varner MW, Osborne AO, Crawford S. Cranial magnetic resonance imaging in severe preeclampsia vs eclampsia. Arch Neurol 1993;50:399–406.

14 Practical Viewing of the Optic Disc and Retina in the Emergency Department

Injuries to the head, blows, falls, &c, frequently cause ocular symptoms and often very marked ophthalmoscopic signs.

William Gowers[1]

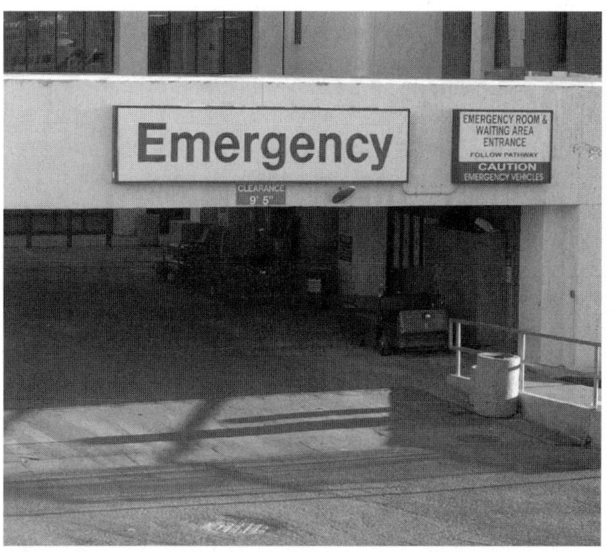

14-1

Figure 14-1. The Emergency Room provides many opportunities to view the optic disc.

Visual complaints make up 3% of all visits to the emergency room.[2] Although most of these complaints are related to external disease, such as corneal disease, foreign body, and so forth, the emergency department physician has many more patients in whom a quick and accurate look at the optic disc aids the diagnosis. From looking for papilledema in someone with headache to viewing the retinal arteries for signs of long-standing hypertension, the physician in the emergency department (ED) makes a more accurate diagnosis using the ophthalmoscope.

The history is important in determining how the vision loss occurred using the principles of history outlined in Chapter 2.

The examination in the ED of a patient with any visual complaint should include corrected near visual acuity (or distance acuity with pinhole), pupillary light reaction with the swinging flashlight test to look for an afferent pupillary defect, ocular motility, confrontation visual field testing, and direct ophthalmoscopy. Slit-lamp examination is also preferred when there is a suspicion of a corneal or foreign body problem.

Complaints that should prompt a look at the optic disc include sudden vision loss (present at the time of the visit or in the past), headache, and trauma to the eye.

Table 14-1. Complaints That Patients Have and What to Look for

Complaint	Examination tips	What to check on the disc	What to do
Sudden vision loss	Visual acuity; look for an APD; check visual field to confrontation	Look for a central retinal artery occlusion, hemorrhage (see below)	Refer to ophthalmology
Headache	Take a careful history	Papilledema? Spontaneous venous pulsations	Treat as directed by history and examination
Trauma	Visual acuity; look for an APD; full eye examination; intraocular pressure	Optic nerve avulsion; hemorrhages around the disc; retinal changes—hemorrhages	If there is any concern for globe perforation or injury, ophthalmology consult; if afferent pupillary defect present, ophthalmology consult to look for canal fracture
Pain in the eye	Visual acuity; APD; fluorescein drops to look for corneal abrasion	Disc swelling; cupping asymmetry	Refer to ophthalmology
Any infant—consider abuse	Complete examination	Hemorrhages around the disc	Contact child protective services

APD = afferent pupillary defect.

Reasons for Not Dilating a Patient

Most of the time, there is no contraindication to dilating the patient. The concern for glaucoma after dilating drops is mostly theoretical; besides, if the patient has pain and blurred vision after dilation, a visit with the ophthalmologist to treat the unsuspected glaucoma is in the patient's best interest.

Patients, however, often arrive at the ED in coma or with multiple severe traumas. In these cases of altered consciousness, in which the neurologic examination may be important to follow for progression, pupillary dilation is relatively contraindicated.

In cases in which there is no obvious abnormality of the eyes or optic nerve but the patient still cannot see, think of the following: optic neuritis, apoplexy of the pituitary gland (is there a headache or confusional state?), cortical vision loss (the pupils will work, but the patient cannot see), and functional disorders. You need to use your judgment, because magnetic resonance (or computed tomography) scanning is appropriate with some of these disorders.

Table 14-2. Emergency Conditions

Condition	What to look for	Causes	Treatment
Vitreal hemorrhage	Red reflex may show hemorrhage; view of disc obscured	Trauma, diabetic retinopathy, subarachnoid hemorrhage	Ophthalmologic examination and follow-up
Central retinal artery occlusion	Cherry-red spot; boxcar segments of arteries and veins	Embolism; atherosclerosis	Massage the globe; possible anterior chamber tap by ophthalmology; IV acetazolamide to lower intraocular pressure; consider TPA; call ophthalmology
Retinal detachment	Gray or opaque retina	Trauma; spontaneous	Refer to ophthalmology at once
Central retinal vein occlusion	Diffuse retinal hemorrhages and venous dilation	Hypertension, diabetes, glaucoma	Refer to ophthalmology
Ischemic optic neuropathy*	Swelling of the optic disc; usually unilateral	Hypertension, diabetes	Check erythrocyte sedimentation rate; refer to ophthalmology for temporal artery biopsy or possible treatment
Glaucoma	Pain in the eye; red eye with high pressure; may see asymmetrical cupping	Family history	IV acetazolamide; pressure-lowering drops; refer to ophthalmology for treatment
Papilledema	Usually not symptomatic; transient vision loss; usually has headache	Brain tumor, cerebral venous thrombosis, idiopathic intracranial hypertension	Magnetic resonance scan; possible lumbar puncture; neurologic evaluation; ophthalmologic evaluation of vision
Neuroretinitis	Unilateral disc swelling with edema and exudates into the macula	Infectious process usually	Refer to ophthalmology/neurology
Optic neuritis	See an afferent pupillary defect but no abnormality of the disc	Multiple sclerosis	Magnetic resonance scan; refer to ophthalmologist or neurologist

*The arteritic form is a true emergency.
Source: Information adapted from reference 3.

Trauma: What Should We Look for?

Trauma to the head, face, or body can result in changes in the eye and vision. The first obvious job in the emergency room is to be sure that the patient has cardiovascular and pulmonary stability. The next job is to be sure that the globe itself is not perforated or injured. A complete examination should be performed by an ophthalmologist if there is any concern for the eye itself. Once you are sure about these conditions, what else is there to do? Vision can be reduced by injury to the rest of the visual apparatus.

Traumatic optic neuropathy occurs when there is an injury to the optic nerve anywhere along its course. The single best test to detect an optic nerve disorder is the swinging flashlight test, which looks for an afferent pupillary defect. If present, this should signal further evaluation, including a possible computed tomography scan of the bony orbit looking for a canal fracture. The optic disc may not show any changes acutely. In fact, disc swelling is *not* a response to acute closed head injury within the first 5 days. Bilateral or unilateral disc swelling seen in an acute setting is almost invariably the result of a pre-existing condition. In traumatic optic neuropathy, the appearance of the optic nerve after acute trauma most usually is normal.

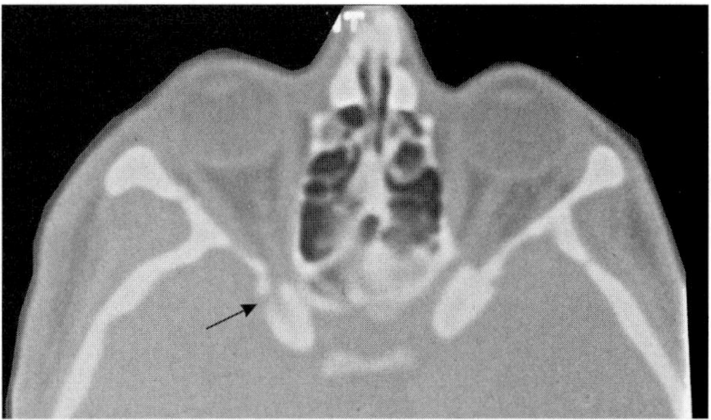

14-2A

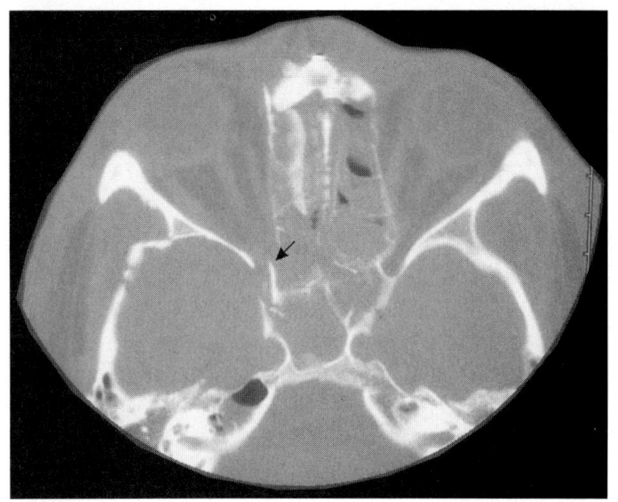

14-2B

Figure 14-2. A. **After a motor vehicle accident, this individual complained of absent vision in the right eye. You can see the displacement of the optic canal (*arrow*).** B. **Another case where there is a fracture through the ethmoid air cells displacing bony fragments into the right optic canal (*arrow*), as seen in this bone window computed tomography scan.**

A dramatic appearance of optic nerve trauma is optic nerve avulsion, in which the optic nerve is literally torn from the back of the eye. Avulsion of the disc is a rare occurrence. This can be diagnosed with the direct ophthalmoscope.

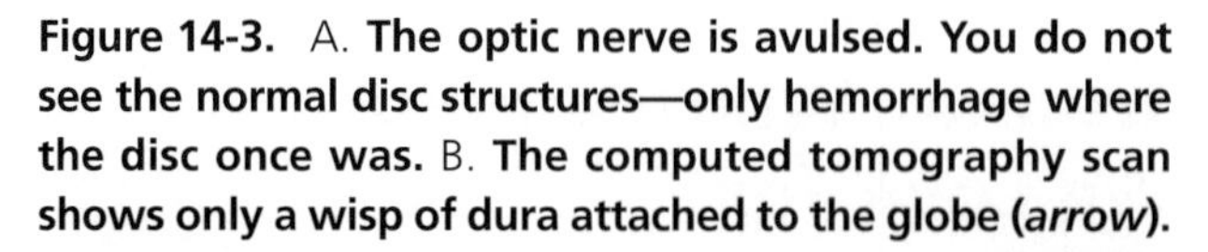

Figure 14-3. A. **The optic nerve is avulsed. You do not see the normal disc structures—only hemorrhage where the disc once was.** B. **The computed tomography scan shows only a wisp of dura attached to the globe (*arrow*).**

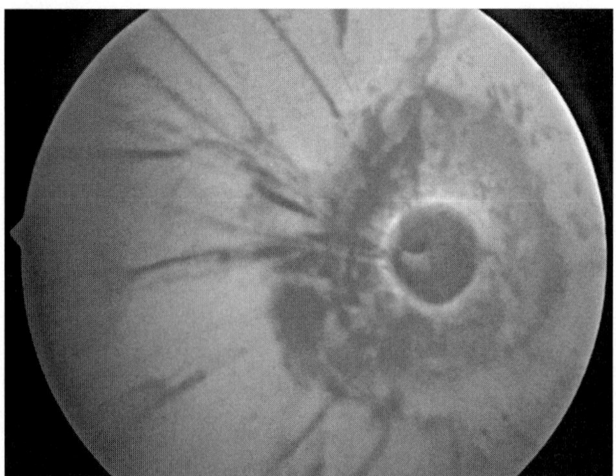

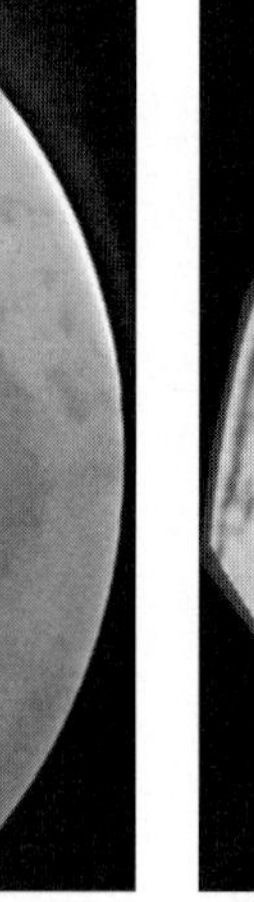

14-3A

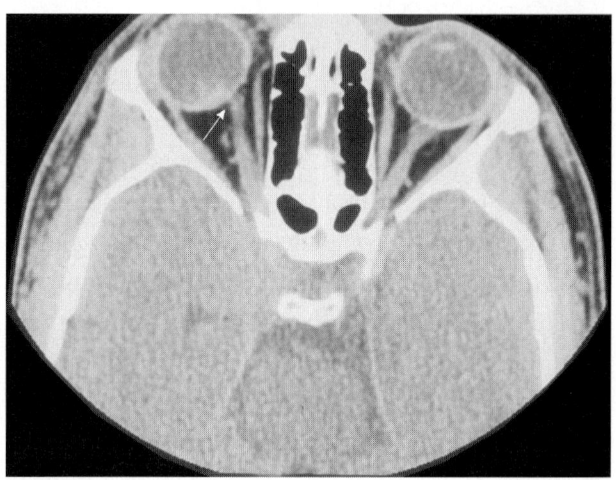

14-3B

There are two forms of optic nerve trauma: direct trauma (e.g., stabbing, gunshot wound, and intrusion of bone fragments into the nerve), which accounts for approximately 20% of optic nerve trauma, and indirect trauma caused by a blow to the head, most commonly to the brow above the orbit, causing damage to the optic nerve, especially in the bony intracanalicular portion of the optic nerve.[4] Anterior indirect injury can result in optic nerve avulsion and is rare. However, the more common traumatic optic nerve injury is posterior. Furthermore, the optic nerve may swell days later owing to increased intracranial pressure related to the head trauma.

Figure 14-4. A,B. **This individual not only suffered optic nerve trauma, but also developed papilledema related to increased intracranial pressure from brain trauma. The swelling did not appear until several days after trauma.** C. **Later, optic atrophy ensued.**

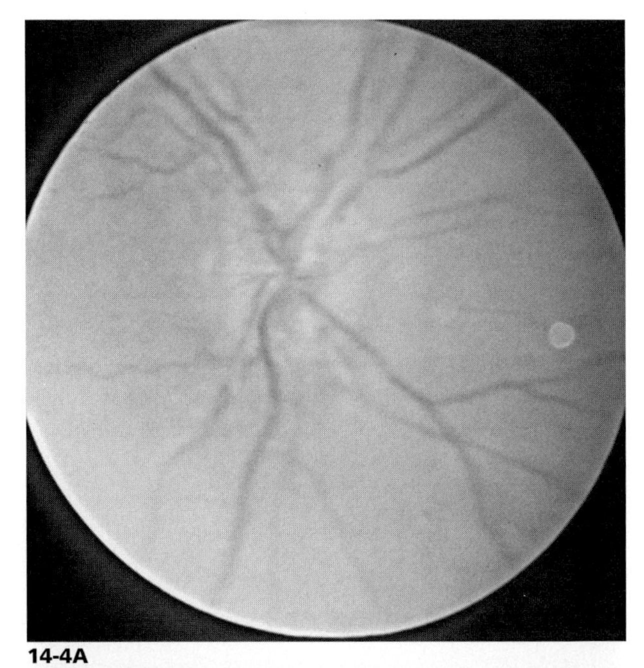

14-4A

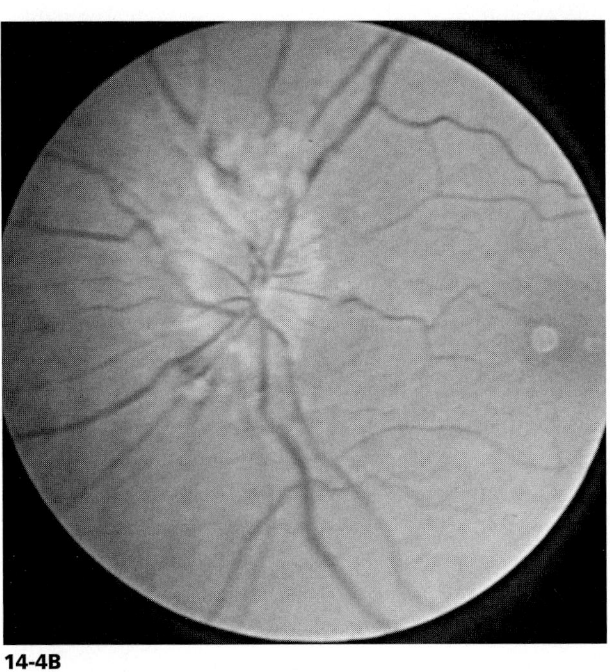

14-4B

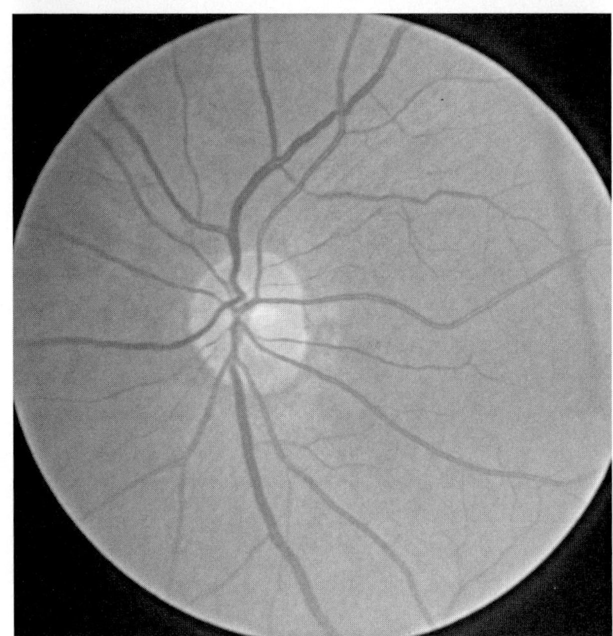

14-4C

Sometimes the discs do not simply develop pallor, but become cupped in the absence of glaucoma, as a result of axonal loss and loss of tissue bulk.

Injury to the rest of the visual pathway, including chiasm and occipital lobe, should be considered in anyone with vision loss and no afferent pupillary defect. Again, imaging is essential.[5]

Figure 14-5. A,B. **Acutely, chiasmal injury may show no changes in the optic nerve. However, weeks after chiasmal trauma, the disc may show bow-tie atrophy. The arrows point to a section of atrophy.** C. **Computed tomography shows a hemorrhage (*arrow*) around the chiasm.** D. **A plain-film radiograph shows the fracture through the sella (*arrow*).**

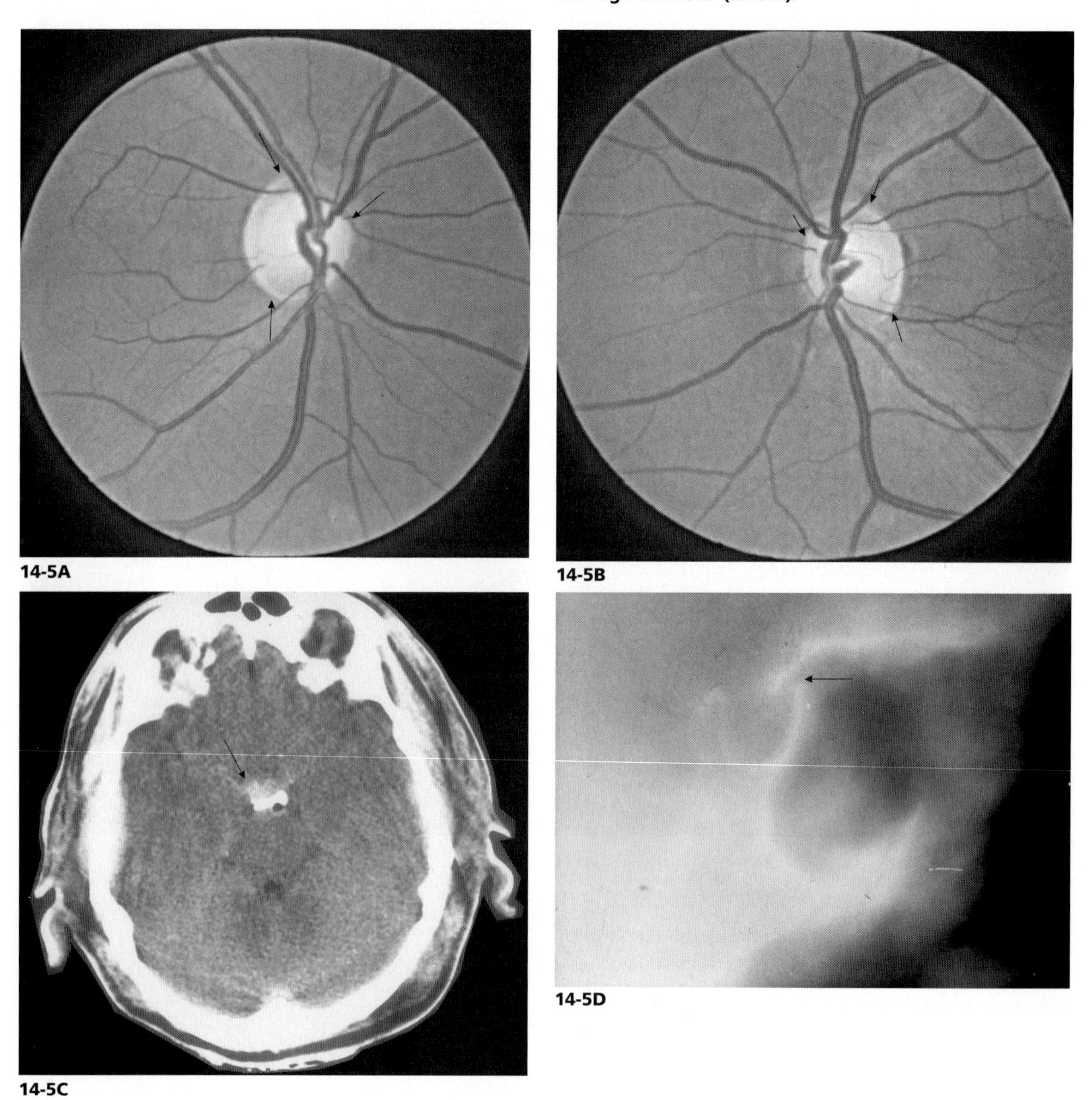

14-5A **14-5B** **14-5C** **14-5D**

Other traumatic conditions include the following conditions: Trauma to the retina directly from injury is called *commotio retinae*. This type of injury is owing to direct injury to the eye. It is caused by a sheer injury to the rods and cones. Retinal edema that forms looks like gray-white opacification, and on occasion hemorrhages can be seen; it is sometimes called *Berlin's edema* (named for Rudolf Berlin, who wrote about commotio retinae in 1873).[6] Although the retina and vision may normalize, sometimes there is enough damage to the retinal pigment epithelium that pigmentary changes can occur in the periphery that mimic retinitis pigmentosa.

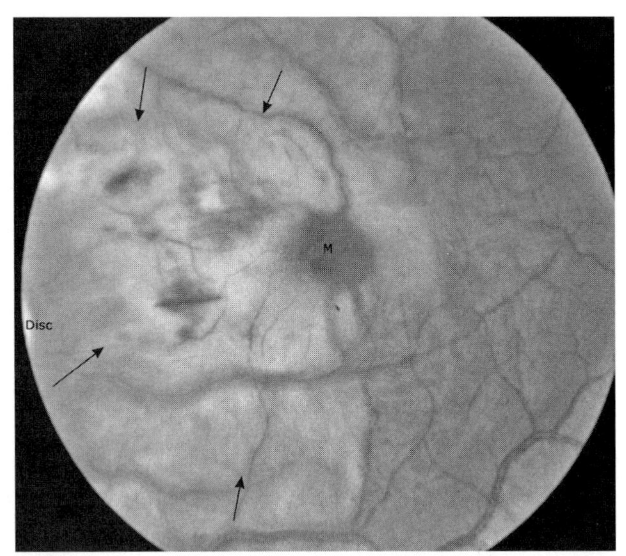

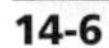
14-6

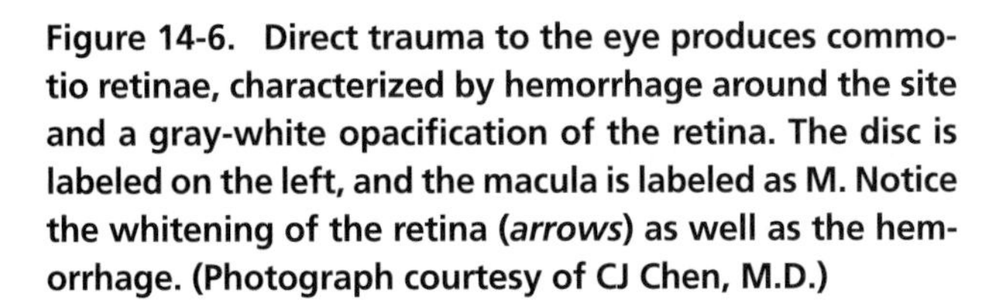
Figure 14-6. Direct trauma to the eye produces commotio retinae, characterized by hemorrhage around the site and a gray-white opacification of the retina. The disc is labeled on the left, and the macula is labeled as M. Notice the whitening of the retina (*arrows*) as well as the hemorrhage. (Photograph courtesy of CJ Chen, M.D.)

Do not forget to look at the fundus of a lethargic infant for signs of shaken baby syndrome, discussed in Chapter 11.

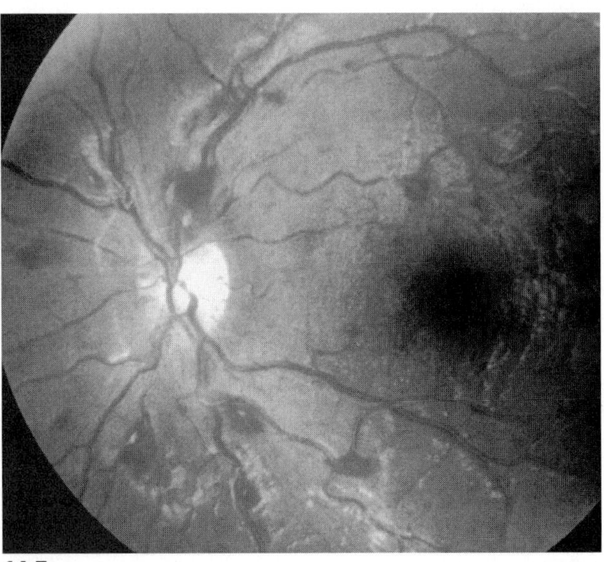
14-7

Figure 14-7. Hemorrhages seen on the ophthalmoscopic examination of any baby in the emergency department should alert the physician to the possibility of shaken baby syndrome. (Photograph courtesy of Marie Acierno, M.D.)

Purtscher's retinopathy is named for Othmar Purtscher, a German, who reported in 1910 on a traumatic retinopathy characterized by hemorrhages and white spots in a man who fell out of a tree.[7] Since this report, numerous other cases have been reported owing to injuries in which there is sudden elevation of intravascular pressure in the upper part of the body, especially the chest. The changes have been called *traumatic retinal angiopathy* or *Purtscher's disease*.[8] The retinopathy is seen usually within 2 days of the injury and is characterized by "cumulus clouds" (cotton-wool spots) and retinal and preretinal hemorrhages. The retinoscopic findings may last for months. Although there is usually decreased vision, vision tends to return to normal. There may be optic atrophy. See Table 14-3 for other causes of Purtscher's retinopathy.

Table 14-3. Causes of Purtscher's Retinopathy

Chest compression from a rapid injury
Valsalva maneuver (severe) (e.g., severe vomiting; pushing during labor)
Fat emboli
Anoxia
Extreme deceleration force in pilots traveling at speed of sound
A retinopathy similar to Purtscher's has been seen in:
Acute pancreatitis
Lupus
Dermatomyositis
Central retinal artery occlusion
Amniotic fluid embolism
Retrobulbar injections[10]
Thrombotic thrombocytopenic purpura/hemolytic uremic syndrome[11]

Source: Adapted in part from references 7,9.

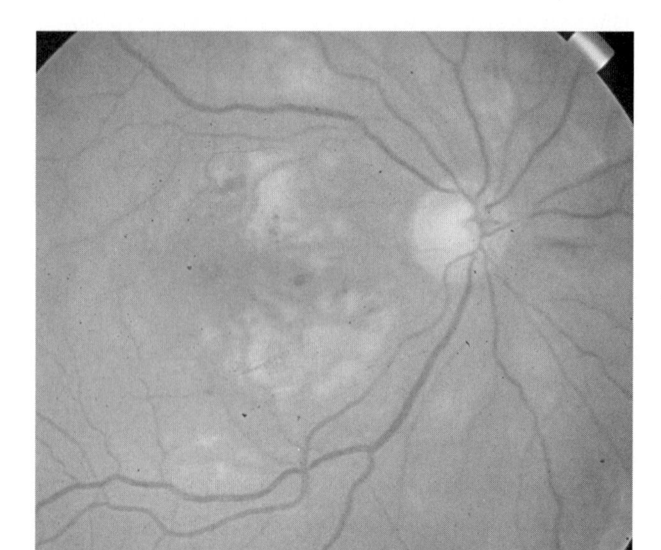

14-8A

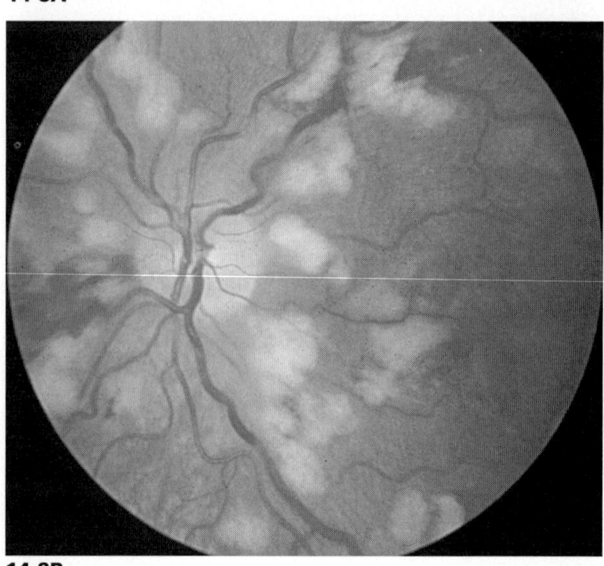

14-8B

Figure 14-8. A. **Cotton-wool spots, along with hemorrhages—both retinal and preretinal—characterize Purtscher's retinopathy. (Photograph courtesy of CJ Chen, M.D.)** B. **In this case, the Purtscher's retinopathy has many cotton-wool spots.**

Air embolism can occur owing to injury to the chest, rib fractures, wounds to the jugular veins, or pneumothorax. This type of injury is rarely observed, because most of the time it is transient. However, visual acuity may be affected for days.

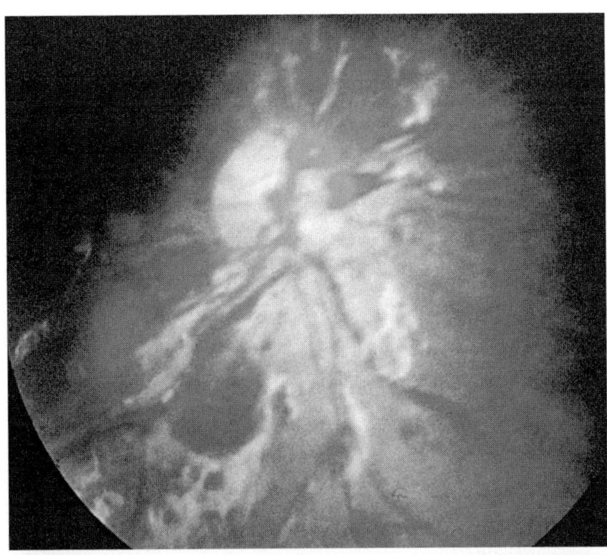
14-9A

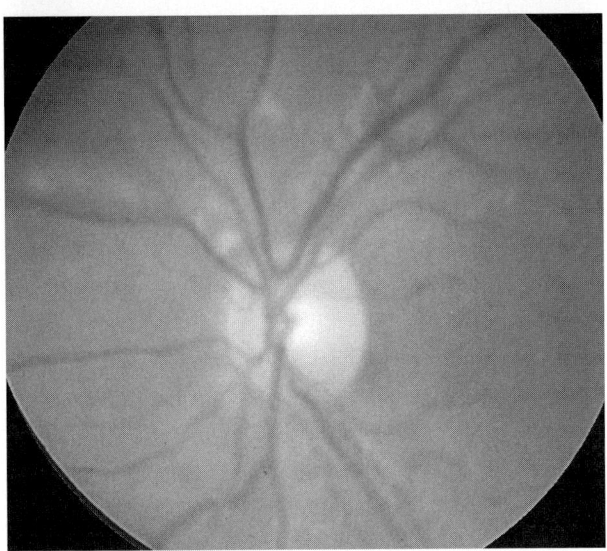
14-9B

Figure 14-9. A. **Air embolism often causes only a hemorrhage or cotton-wool spots, as are seen here.** B. **After long bone trauma, fat emboli may be seen. Cotton-wool spots and hemorrhages centered in the posterior pole, and, rarely, fat globules have been noted.**

Fat embolism can occur after trauma to a long bone and with pancreatitis. In fact, it is seen in approximately 4% of long bone fractures.[12] In the study of 100 consecutive long bone fractures, only one person was visually symptomatic, whereas four patients had evidence of cotton-wool spots and hemorrhages.[12] Cotton-wool spots and hemorrhages are centered in the posterior pole. Rarely, fat globules have been noted.

Choroidal rupture occurs after blunt trauma to the globe. There may only be a choroidal hemorrhage. Choroidal ruptures are seen around the disc and have a crescent shape. Later, white and pigmented lines around the disc may be present. If the fovea is involved, visual acuity falls.[13]

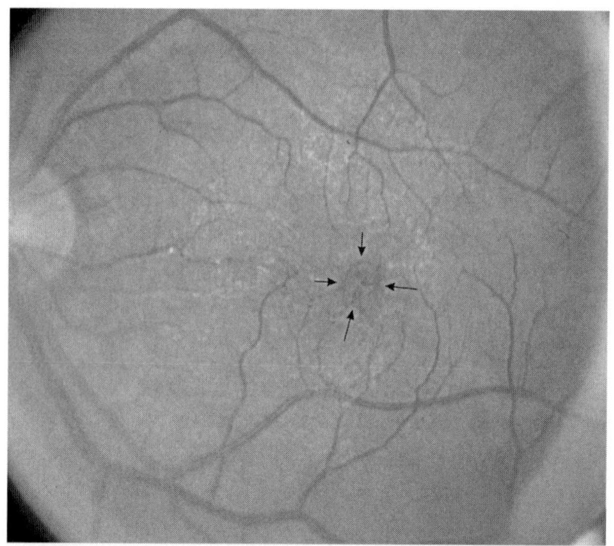

14-10A

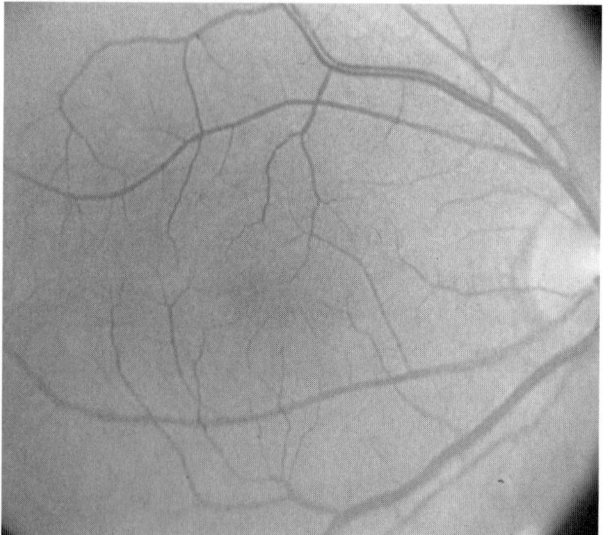

14-10B

Figure 14-10. A. **This man was involved in work-related trauma. He complained of persistent decreased acuity in the left eye. A dilated examination revealed macular trauma and a choroidal rupture (*arrows*).** B. **Compare with his normal right macula.**

Traumatic maculopathy may occur with blunt trauma to the globe and also by whiplash.

Barometric decompression (e.g., during scuba diving) can affect vision. Very little direct visualization of the retina has been reported. Some hypothesize the injury to be similar to air embolism.[7]

Hyperbaric oxygen has recently received favor for the treatment of radiation retinopathy. However, the treatment itself has been associated with vascular constriction and cotton-wool spots.[7]

Altitude changes (i.e., lowered barometric pressure and hypoxia) are usually seen at over 12,000 feet. Aside from decreased visual acuity and decreased color perception, there is constriction of the visual field and changes in the brain. According to Walsh and Hoyt, retinal and cortical functions are affected simultaneously.[7] Ophthalmoscopic changes include widening of the retinal veins and vasodilation. Hemorrhages can occur when there is some pre-existing disease, such as hypertension.

Table 14-4. Traumatic Retinopathy

Characteristics	Commotio retinae	Purtscher's retinopathy	Fat embolism
Type of injury	Blunt, to the eye	Compression of chest	Long bone fracture; pancreatitis
Systemic findings	None	May see upper body discoloration	Multiple petechiae hemorrhages; cerebral symptoms/signs
Vision	Variable: 20/200	Variable	Normal or reduced
Fundus examination	Retinal edema; hemorrhage	Hemorrhage and exudates	See hemorrhage, exudate and edema
Time to findings	Within hours	Within 1–2 days	After 1–2 days
Recovery	Usually good	Good	Good

Source: Adapted in part from reference 7.

Neurologic Conditions in Which Viewing the Disc Is Helpful

Headache is the most common single symptom for which patients are seen in the emergency department. Most of the time, headache represents a benign recurrent primary disorder such as migraine, but occasionally headache may be the clue to a serious underlying condition.

Table 14-5. Headache—What to Look for

Headache disorder	Features	Disc/fundus finding	What to do
Primary headache (migraine)	Throbbing, nausea, photo/phonophobia; worse with movement; recurrent; family history	Normal disc with venous pulsation	Treat primary headache
Secondary headaches			
Subarachnoid hemorrhage	Sudden onset of the "worst headache of patient's life"	See preretinal hemorrhage around disc; Terson's syndrome	Computed tomographic scan without contrast; lumbar puncture
Venous thrombosis	Headache, seizure, coma	Disc swelling—papilledema	MR/MR venography
Tumor	New headache; may have focal neurologic deficits	Disc swelling—papilledema	MR scan
Idiopathic intracranial hypertension	Headache; pulsatile tinnitus; obesity	Papilledema	MR/MR venography; cerebrospinal fluid with opening pressure
Meningitis	New headache; possible nuchal rigidity; altered consciousness	Possibly normal	MR; cerebrospinal fluid evaluation
Carotid dissection	Headache; Horner's syndrome	Look for central or branch retinal artery occlusion	MR and MR angiography

Other acute neurologic symptoms such as sudden weakness, coma, and seizure all deserve a look at the optic disc, because a clue may emerge as to the cause.

What About General Medical Disorders—Should I View the Disc?

As we have pointed out all along, viewing the optic disc may give you a clue to an underlying condition that you didn't suspect. *View* the disc—look for hemorrhages and exudates that could be due to diabetes, or disc swelling caused by increased cerebrospinal fluid pressure.

Practical Viewing Essentials

1. Always view the optic disc in a patient in the emergency department.
2. If there is a visual complaint, an eye examination is especially important.
3. Check for an afferent pupillary defect if you suspect an optic nerve injury.
4. Look for papilledema in all patients with headache.
5. A fundus examination should be done in any child brought to the emergency room with injuries of suspicious origin.
6. If there is any question about the fundus in the emergency department, dilate the pupils of the patient for a better look.

References

1. Gowers W. A Manual and Atlas of Medical Ophthalmoscopy. London: J & A Churchill, 1879.
2. Handler JA, Ghezzi KT. General ophthalmologic examination. Emerg Med Clin North Am 1995;13: 521–538.
3. LaVene D, Halpern J, Jagoda A. Loss of vision. Emerg Med Clin North Am 1995;13(3):539–560
4. Anderson RL, Panje WR, Gross CF. Optic nerve blindness following blunt forehead trauma. Ophthalmol 1982;89:445–455.
5. Lessell S. Traumatic optic neuropathy and visual system injury. In BJ Shingleton, PS Hersh, KR Kenyon (eds), Eye Trauma. St. Louis: Mosby, 1991;371–379.
6. Williams DF, Mieler WF, Williams GA. Posterior segment manifestations of ocular trauma. Retina 1990;10(Suppl 1):S35–S44.
7. Walsh FB, Hoyt WF. Clinical Neuro-ophthalmology. Baltimore: Williams & Wilkins, 1969;2445–2446.
8. Marr WG, Marr EG. Some observations on Purtscher's disease: Traumatic retinal angiopathy. Am J Ophthalmol 1962;54:692–702.
9. Cogan DG. Neurology of the Visual System. Springfield, IL: Charles C Thomas, 1967.
10. Chaudhry NA, Flynn HW, Mieler WF. Ocular trauma. In RK Parrish II (ed), Atlas of Ophthalmology. Boston: Butterworth–Heinemann, 2000;313–324.
11. Patel MR, Bains A, O'Hara JP, et al. Purscher retinopathy as the initial sign of thrombotic thrombocytopenic purpura/hemolytic uremic syndrome. Arch Ophthalmol 2001;119:1388–1389.
12. Chuang EL, Miller FS, Kalina RE. Retinal lesions following long bone fractures. Ophthalmology 1985;92: 370–374.
13. Dugel PU, Opber RR. Posterior segment manifestations of closed-globe contusion injury. In JJ Ryan, CP Wilkerson (eds), Retina. St. Louis: Mosby, 2001;2381.

Index

Note: Page numbers followed by *f* refer to figures; page numbers followed by *t* refer to tables.